Cytokines and Cell Homeostasis in the Gastrointestinal Tract

FALK SYMPOSIUM 113

Cytokines and Cell Homeostasis in the Gastrointestinal Tract

EDITED BY

**T. Andus, G. Rogler,
K. Schlottmann, E. Frick**

*University of Regensburg, University Hospital
Department for Internal Medicine I
Regensburg, Germany*

G. Adler

*University of Ulm
University Hospital
Department for Internal Medicine
Ulm, Germany*

M. Zeitz

*University of the Saarland
University Hospital
Department for Internal Medicine II
Homburg, Germany*

W. Schmiegel

*University of Bochum
Department for Internal Medicine
Knappschaftskrankenhaus
Bochum, Germany*

J. Schölmerich

*University of Regensburg
University Hospital
Department for Internal Medicine I
Regensburg, Germany*

*Proceedings of the Falk Symposium 113 held in Regensburg, Germany,
16–18 September, 1999*

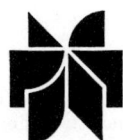

KLUWER ACADEMIC PUBLISHERS
DORDRECHT / BOSTON / LONDON

Library of Congress Cataloging-in-Publication Data is available.

ISBN 0-7923-8758-9

Published by Kluwer Academic Publishers, BV
P.O. Box 17, 3300 AA Dordrecht, The Netherlands.

Sold and distributed in North, Central and South America
by Kluwer Academic Publishers,
101 Philip Drive, Norwell, MA 02061, USA.

In all other countries, sold and distributed
by Kluwer Academic Publishers, Distribution Center,
P.O. Box 322, 3300 AH Dordrecht, The Netherlands

Printed on acid-free paper

Printed and bound in Great Britain by MPG Books, Bodmin, Cornwall.

Contents

CONTENTS

SECTION II: LIVER

CONTENTS

CONTENTS

List of Principal Authors

G. Adler
Innere Medizin I
Medizinische Klinik und Poliklinik
Klinikum der Universität Ulm
Robert-Koch-Str. 8
D-89081 Ulm
Germany

K. E. Barrett
Department of Medicine
UCSD Medical Center, 8414
200 W. Arbor Dr.
San Diego
CA 92103
USA

U. Böcker
Department of Medicine IV
  (Gastroenterology)
University Hospital of Heidelberg at
  Mannheim
Theodor-Kutzer-Ufer
68167 Mannheim
Germany

D. Brenner
University of North Carolina at
  Chapel Hill
CB# 7038,156 Glaxo Building
Chapel Hill
NC 27599-7038
USA

P. Brissot
Clinique des Maladies du Foie
Hôpital Pontchaillou
Centre Hospitalier Régional
rue Henri Le Guilloux
F-35033 Rennes Cedex
France

A. M. Diehl
Gastroenterology Division
Johns Hopkins University
918 Ross Research Building
720 Rutland Street
Baltimore
MD 21205-21090
USA

G. S. Evans
The University of Sheffield
Division of Child Health
The Sheffield Children's Hospital
West Bank
Sheffield
S10 2TH
UK

G. Feldmann
INSERM U327
Faculté de Médecine Xavier Bichat
16 rue Henri Huchard
F-75018 Paris
France

J.-N. Freund
INSERM Unité 381
Ontogenese et Pathologie du
  Système Digestif
3 avenue Molière
F-67200 Strasbourg
France

P. R. Galle
I Medizinische Klinik und Poliklinik
Klinikum der Universität
Langenbeckstr. 1
D-55131 Mainz
Germany

J. Gauldie
Department of Pathology & Molecular
  Medicine
McMaster University
1200 Main Street West
Hamilton
Ontario
L8N 3Z5
Canada

M. N. Göke
Department of Gastroenterology &
  Hepatology
Medical School of Hannover
Carl-Neuberg-Straße 1
30625 Hannover
Germany

G. J. Gores
Department of Medicine
Mayo Clinic
200 First Street SW
Rochester
MN 55905-0001
USA

A. M. Gressner
Institut für Klinische Chemie und
  Pathobiochemie
Zentrallaboratorium
RWTH Universitätsklinikum
Pauwelsstr. 30
D-52074 Aachen
Germany

S. Grüne
Klinik und Poliklinik für Innere
  Medizin I
Klinikum der Universität Regensburg
D-93042 Regensburg
Germany

M. Hebrok
Diabetes Research Center
Department of Medicine
University of California
San Francisco
513 Parnassus Ave., HSW 1112
San Francisco, CA 94143-0573
USA

P. C. Heinrich
Institut für Biochemie Neuklinikum
Universitätsklinikum der RWTH
  Aachen
Pauwelsstraße 30
D-52057 Aachen
Germany

C. Jobin
Division of Digestive Diseases and
  Nutrition
University of North Carolina at
  Chapel Hill
CB #7038 Rm, 146 Glaxo Building
Chapel Hill
NC 27599-7080
USA

S. C. Lu
University of California
Division of Gastrointestinal & Liver
  Diseases
HMR Building 415
Dept. of Medicine, USC School of
  Medicine
2011 Zonal Ave
Los Angeles
CA 90033
USA

A. Mallat
INSERM U99
Hôpital Henri Mondor
F-94000 Créteil
France

D. Moradpour
Abteilung Innere Medizin II
Medizinische Universitätsklinik
Hugstetter Str. 55
D-79106 Freiburg
Germany

M. F. Neurath
I Medizinische Klinik
Klinikum der Universität
Langenbeckstr. 1
D-55131 Mainz
Germany

C. S. Potten
Department of Epithelial Cell Biology
Paterson Institute for Cancer
  Research
Christie Hospital NHS Trust
Wilmslow Road
Manchester
M20 9BX
UK

H. A. Reber
Section of Gastrointestinal Surgery,
  72-256 CHS
UCLA School of Medicine
10833 Le Conte Avenue
Los Angeles
CA 90095
USA

G. Rogler
Klinik und Poliklinik für Innere
  Medizin I
Klinikum der Universität Regensburg
  Franz-Josef-Strauße-Allee II
D-93042 Regensburg
Germany

K. Schlottmann
Klinik und Poliklinik für Innere
  Medizin I
Klinikum der Universität Regensburg
Franz-Josef-Strauße-Allee 11
D-93042 Regensburg
Germany

R. M. Schmid
Abteilung Innere Medizin I
Medizinische Klinik und Poliklinik
Klinikum der Universität Ulm
Robert-Koch-Str. 8
D-89081 Ulm
Germany

C. J. Steer
Department of Medicine
Mayo Mail Code 36
University of Minnesota Medical
  School
420 Delaware Street, SE
Minneapolis
MN 55455
USA

M. L. Steer
Department of Surgery
Beth Israel Deaconess Medical
  Center & Harvard Medical School
330 Brookline Avenue
Boston
MA 02215-5491
USA

J. Sträter
Institut für Pathologie
Universität Ulm
Albert-Einstein-Allee 11
D-89081 Ulm
Germany

W. Strober
Mucosal Immunity Section
National Institute of Allergy and
  Infectious Diseases
10 Center Drive MSC 1890
Bethesda
MD 20892-1890
USA

R. G. Thurnan
Laboratory of Hepatobiology and
  Toxicology
Department of Pharmacology
University of North Carolina at
  Chapel Hill
CB# 7365, Mary Ellen Jones Building
Chapel Hill
NC 27599-7365

C. Trautwein
Abteilung für Gastroenterologie und
  Hepatologie
Medizinische Hochschule Hannover
Carl-Neuberg-Str. 1
D-30625 Hannover
Germany

J. L. Wallace
Department of Pharmacology and
  Therapeutics
University of Calgary
3330 Hospital Drive NW
Calgary
Alberta
T2N 4N1
Canada

S. Werner
Institute of Cell Biology
Swiss Federal Institute of Technology
ETH-Hönggerberg
CH-8093 Zürich
Switzerland

G. D. Wu
600 Clinical Research Building
415 Curie Boulevard
Philadelphia
PA 19104-6144
USA

Preface

The gastrointestinal tract has a number of unique features. Its extensive surface is formed by a single layer of rapidly renewing cells, the intestinal epithelial cells. These cells are in contact with a number of other cell populations, including the largest part of the immune system, and with an excessive luminal antigen load, including vast numbers of bacteria. Furthermore two more organs, namely liver and pancreas, are part of the system. The rapid renewal of the epithelial layer, the interactions of different cell types, the balance between cell proliferation and death in the gut as well as in the liver and to some extent in the pancreas have been fascinating subjects of studies during the last years. Much has been learned, and cytokines have emerged as important mediators for many of these interactions and the homeostasis of the system.

The symposium on "Cytokines and cell homeostasis in the gastrointestinal tract" provided a forum for basic scientists and interested clinicians to exchange ideas, to discuss concepts and to plan further studies. This book contains most of the presentations at this symposium. The first section deals with the intestine and is divided into 15 chapters including mechanisms of mucosal inflammation, repair and wound healing, and apoptosis. The second section is devoted to the liver and includes 16 chapters devoted again to inflammation, fibrosis, transport, and apoptosis induced by different mechanisms. The third section comprises the pancreas and includes 5 chapters ranging from acute inflammation to pancreatic cancer.

The editors of this book want to thank all the contributors, others involved in the running of this symposium, in particular the moderators, and the members of the Department of Internal Medicine I of the University of Regensburg, as well as Miss Rombach from the congress division of the Falk Foundation. Particular thanks go to Dr. Herbert Falk who provided the opportunity to hold this exciting meeting and to produce its contents in book form.

T. Andus, G. Rogler, K. Schlottmann, E. Frick, G. Adler, W. Schmiegel, M. Zeitz, J. Schölmerich

Section I
Intestine

1
Counter-regulation in the mucosal immune system and the mechanism of mucosal inflammation

W. STROBER, I. FUSS and A. KITANI

INTRODUCTION

In recent years a large number of murine models of mucosal inflammation have appeared which, in aggregate, are adding immeasurably to our understanding of how immune responses are regulated in the mucosal immune system in normal animals and how dysregulation of such responses leads to human inflammatory bowel disease (IBD). In general, the mucosal inflammation occurring in these models is due to exaggerated or excessive Th1 T cell responses or, less commonly, to exaggerated or excessive Th2 T cell responses; alternatively, they are due to insufficient counter-regulatory responses that ordinarily control (suppress) Th1 and Th2 T cell responses in the mucosal immune system (Fig. 1 and Table 1)[1–22]. A clear example of an experimental inflammation caused by an exaggerated response is provided by mice who bear a transgene for STAT-4, the intracellular signalling molecule that transduces IL-12 signals and thus is necessary for Th1 T cell responses (Fig. 2)[1]. In these transgenic mice the STAT-4 transgene is under the control of a CMV promoter; thus when it is activated by systemic administration of DNP-KLH (an antigen capable of inducing cross-reactive responses to gut antigens) unregulated STAT-4 signalling occurs which leads to a colitis characterized by excessive production of IFN-γ and TNF-α. In addition, if spleen and colonic T cells from mice bearing this STAT-4 transgene are activated *in vitro* by intestinal microflora and then are adoptively transferred to SCID mice they induce colitis in the latter. These results, taken together, indicate that the intestinal microflora can conceivably be a driving force of an excessive Th1 T cell response leading to colonic inflammation.

A similar situation is thought to underlie TNBS colitis, i.e. the colitis induced in SJL/J mice administered the contactant TNBS by an intrarectal route[3]. In this case the TNBS induces a massive Th1 T cell response, perhaps due to a geneti-

3

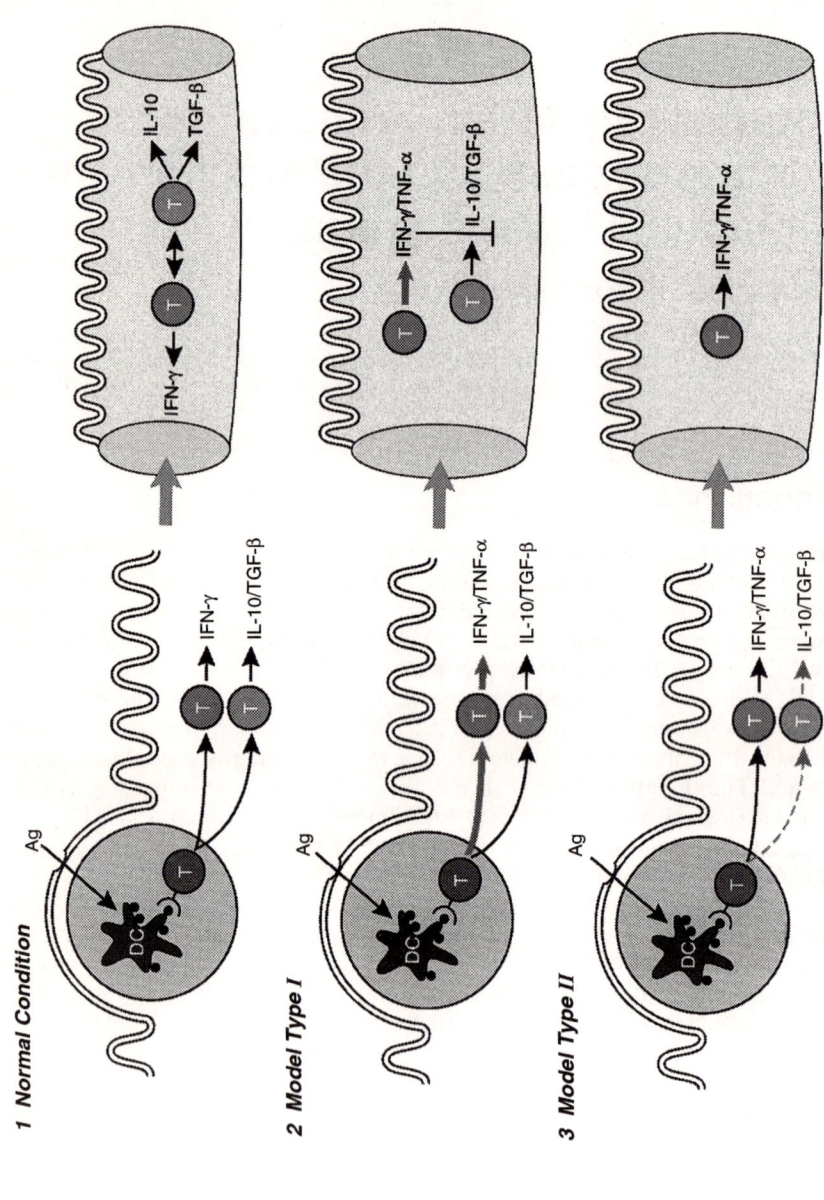

Figure 1 Major types of experimental mucosal inflammation

4

Table 1

	Comments
Type 1 model	
STAT-4 Tg	Increased intracellular IL-12 signalling leading to the overexpression of inflammatory cytokines IFN-γ and TNF-α.
TNBS	Dysregulated IL-12/IFN-α response in certain animal strains (SJL/J).
Gi2α	Increased production of IL-12 and subsequently IFN-γ from activated T cells secondary to absence of G-protein.
TNF-$^\Delta$ARE	Absence of the TNF AU-rich elements (ARE) responsible for TNF mRNA destabilization and translational repression leads to overexpression of TNF-α.
BM$\rightarrow$Tgϵ26	Expression of inflammatory cytokines IFN-γ/TNF-α from TCR $\alpha\beta$ and TCR $\gamma\delta$+ T cells. IL-12 can influence the nature of the response in that reconstitution with BM from STAT-4 deficient mice or treatment with anti-IL-12 can ameliorate disease.
Type 2 model	
CD45 RB^{hl}$\rightarrow$SCID	Transfer of CD45RB^{lo} regulatory T cells which produce IL-10 and/or TGF-β can ameliorate disease.
IL-10$^{-/-}$	Chronic enterocolitis mediated by CD4+ Th1 cells producing IFN-γ secondary to deficient IL-10 response and overproduction of IL-12.
IL-2$^{-/-}$	Lack of Th2 (IL-4) and TGF-β response leads to increased IL-12-mediated IFN-γ T cell response.
TCR $\alpha^{-/-}$	Overexpression of IL-4 from TCR β^{dim} T cells. Transfer of TCR$^{-/-}$ T cells to Ig mu$^{-/-}$ mice leads to more severe disease. Suppressive role of B cells (?).

cally determined hyper-responsiveness to concomitant stimulation of the mucosal immune system by substances in the mucosal environment, such as bacterial LPS, which necessarily accompanies TNBS exposure. The Th1 response thus initiated quickly overcomes any possible counter-regulatory response and the mouse develops colitis.

There are also several models in which mucosal inflammation is attributed to weak counter-regulation (Table 1)[10–22]. Most notably, this mechanism of colitis is seen in the 'SCID-transfer' model wherein SCID mice are adoptively transferred with either CD45Rb^{hi} T cells (naive T cells) in which case they develop colitis, or with both CD45Rb^{hi} and CD45Rb^{lo} (mature T cells) in which case they do not develop colitis (Fig. 2)[10–12]. The CD45Rb^{lo} T cell population can thus be assumed to contain a subpopulation of counter-regulatory or suppressor T cells (see further discussion below). Another, less known, murine colitis model in which the development of colitis is dependent on the failure of counter-regulatory mechanisms, is the colitis developing in IL-2 knockout

Model Type 1

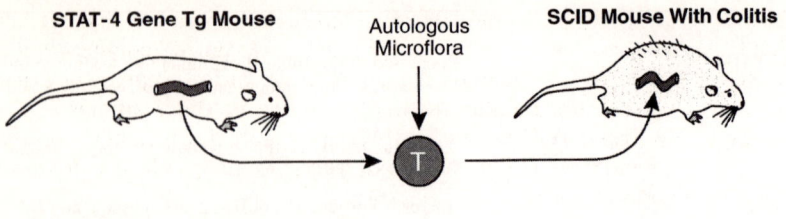

STAT-4 Gene Tg Mouse   Autologous Microflora   **SCID Mouse With Colitis**

Model Type 2

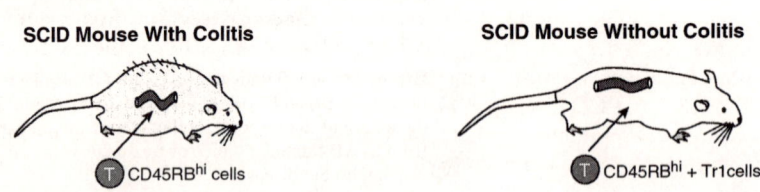

SCID Mouse With Colitis   **SCID Mouse Without Colitis**

CD45RB^{hi} cells   CD45RB^{hi} + Tr1cells

Figure 2   Representative models of mucosal inflammation

mice[13,14]. In this case colitis can be induced by parenteral administration of a normally harmless antigen TNP-KLH, presumably because, as already mentioned, this antigen induces cells which cross-react with mucosal antigens. Paradoxically, however, induction of colitis is prevented if TNP-KLH administration is accompanied by anti-CD3 antibody administration, i.e. administration of a polyclonal stimulant of T cells. Analysis of the mechanism of such colitis induction (or lack thereof in the case of anti-CD3 administration) shows that TNP-KLH administration alone elicits a strong Th1 T cell response in the colon which is the cause of the inflammation, whereas TNP-KLH plus anti-CD3 administration does not elicit a Th1 response; on the contrary, TNP-KLH plus anti-CD3 administration elicits an IL-4 response associated with the production of the suppressor cytokine, TGF-β[14,23]. Thus, while the reason why anti-CD3 induces a counter-regulatory response remains unclear, the fact that it does so explains its ability to inhibit induction of colitis. Parenthetically, the cause of this kind of response pattern in IL-2 deficiency is only now becoming clear: IL-2 is necessary for the T cell proliferation that allows the maturation of IL-4-producing T cells and it is the latter that normally hold Th1 responses in check.

A third model of mucosal inflammation in which the inflammation induced is due to decreased regulatory control is the spontaneous colitis occurring in IL-10 knockout mice[15-18]. Here again a Th1 T cell-mediated inflammation develops which may in this case be due to the well-established fact that IL-10 suppresses IL-12 production and thus one may presume that endogenous stimulation of mucosal T cells in the IL-10 knockout leads inevitably to an excessive IL-12 response and a Th1 T cell-mediated colitis.

MECHANISMS OF COUNTER-REGULATION IN MODELS OF MUCOSAL INFLAMMATION

Current studies of mouse models of mucosal inflammation that are due to inadequate counter-regulation quite obviously turn on the counter-regulatory mechanisms involved, particularly the nature of the various suppressor cytokines mediating the counter-regulation. In the course of these studies two such cytokines, IL-10 and TGF-β, have so far been identified, which alone or in combination appear to have major counter-regulatory activity. These cytokines will thus be the focus of our further discussion.

The data supporting a role for IL-10 as a counter-regulatory cytokine in mucosal interaction comes mainly from the aforementioned IL-10 knockout mouse. Thus, in the relevant studies it has recently been shown that transfer of CD45RB^{lo} cells from an IL-10 knockout mouse does not provide the normal counter-regulatory effect of wild-type CD45RB^{lo} cells in the SCID transfer model and, perhaps more importantly, treatment of SCID mice transferred with CD45RB^{hi} and CD45RB^{lo} cells which normally do not develop colitis, do so if they are concomitantly administered anti-IL-10R antibody[24]. Finally, it has also recently been shown that antigen-specific T cell clones induced *in vitro* in cultures containing IL-10 develop into 'Tr1 T cells' which produce IL-10 and which prevent development of colitis when administered to SCID mice previously treated with CD45RB^{hi} T cells only, which would otherwise lead to colitis (Fig. 2)[25,26]. Taken together these data provide a compelling case for the concept that IL-10 is a major counter-regulatory cytokine that is involved in the prevention of mucosal inflammation.

The second cytokine implicated as a counter-regulatory factor involved in the regulation of mucosal inflammation, TGF-β, has previously been identified as

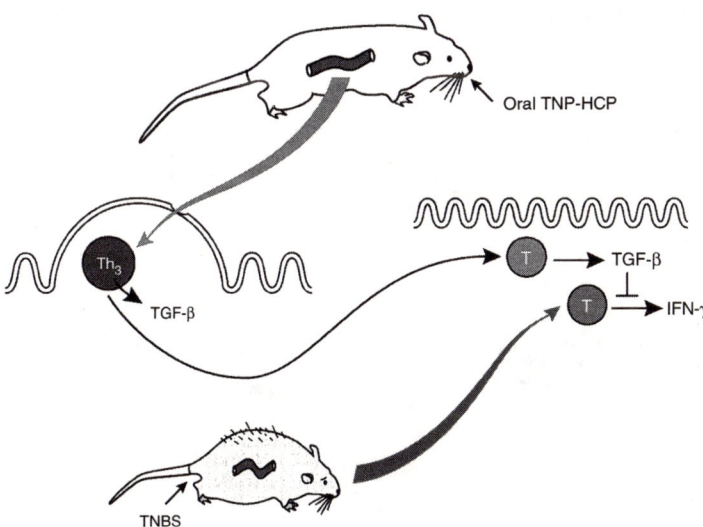

Figure 3   Counter-regulation in TNBS colitis

the cytokine that mediates oral tolerance. In particular, it has been shown that one important mechanism of oral tolerance is the induction of suppressor T cells producing TGF-β, so-called Th3 T cells. This fact links the control of mucosal inflammation with the control of mucosal responses in general[27,28].

There are data supporting the role of TGF-β as a counter-regulatory cytokine in murine models of colitis. First, in the SCID transfer model, it has been shown that administration of anti-TGF-β to SCID mice adoptively transferred CD45RB[hi] T cells and CD45RB[lo] T cells (and which thus do not ordinarily develop colitis) leads to the development of colitis[29]; this, of course, implies that the counter-regulatory CD45RB[lo] T cells preventing colitis do so by secreting TGF-β. Similarly, in the IL-2 knockout model of colitis, the aforementioned prevention of colitis that follows co-administration of anti-CD3 antibody is associated with increased production of TGF-β by mucosal cells and co-administration of both anti-CD3 and anti-TGF-β is again associated with the development of colitis[23]. Finally, in the model of TNBS colitis occurring in SJL/J mice, TGF-β also plays a role. This is seen in experiments in which it is shown that feeding mice TNP-substituted colonic protein prior to TNBS administration per rectum elicits a TGF-β/IL-10 response in the mucosa which blocks the subsequent induction of colitis (Fig. 3)[30,31]; moreover, administration of anti-TGF-β blocks the protective effect of feeding. These studies thus suggest that TNBS colitis produced by intrarectal TNBS administration is accompanied by a Th1 T cell response that shuts off a nascent TGF-β-mediated counter-regulatory response; however, if the latter is induced first by feeding antigen, it can prevent TNBS colitis.

Somewhat paradoxically, the above data indicate that at least two cytokines can counter-regulate experimental mucosal inflammation, IL-10 and TGF-β, in a more or less complete manner. This is seen best in studies of the SCID-transfer model of colitis already mentioned, wherein it was shown that, on the one hand, CD45RB[lo] cells from IL-10 knockout mice do not protect against the develop-

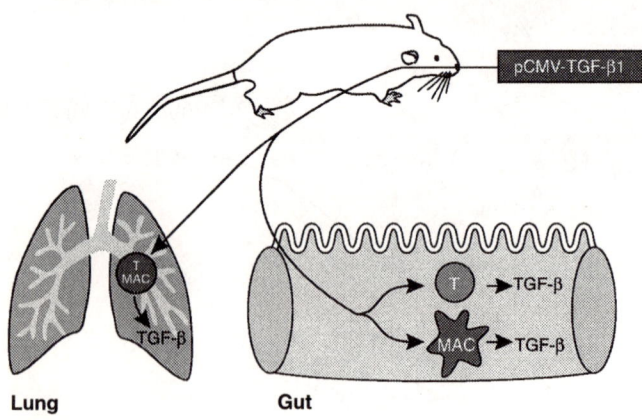

Figure 4 Intrarectal TGF-β-encoding plasmid (pCMV-TGF-β_1) induces TGF-β-producing cells in the lung and gastrointestinal tract

ment of colitis and, on the other, anti-TGF-β administration along with CD45RB^{lo} T cells abrogates protection[11,24,29]. This ability of both IL-10 and TGF-β to provide more or less complete counter-regulation strongly suggests that these suppressor cytokines do not act independently, but rather are essential to each other's activity.

Studies of the regulation of mucosal inflammation by a plasmid expressing TGF-β_1

To further our understanding of the relation of TGF-β secretion to experimental mucosal inflammation, we have recently conducted studies in which we evaluate the effects of TGF-β secretion utilizing a plasmid vector TGF-β under the control of a CMV promoter. This plasmid allowed us to, in effect, create cells producing TGF-β during induced mucosal inflammation. It should be noted that the TGF-β_1 DNA in the plasmid encodes 'activated' TGF-β_1, i.e. TGF-β_1 that is not associated with an encapsulating 'latency' protein that ordinarily inhibits TGF-β_1 activity until the latency protein is cleaved.

In initial experiments the TGF-β_1 plasmid was administered intranasally to SJL/J mice undergoing induction of TNBS colitis via intrarectal instillation of TNBS (Kitani *et al.*, manuscript in preparation, also cf. ref. 32). These experiments showed first that plasmid administration leads to the production of TGF-β in mice undergoing initiation of colitis, but only modest amounts of TGF-β in mice lacking inflammation; thus, inflammation was necessary to activate the CMV promoter and thus induce TGF-β secretion. Second, they showed that TGF-β was produced by both macrophages and T cells present in lung, spleen, and gastrointestinal tract, indicating that intranasal administration of plasmid is an efficient way of inducing the formation of cells capable of TGF-β_1 production (Fig. 4). Third, and finally, they showed that administration of plasmid completely prevented development of colitis and that such treated mice, in contrast to untreated mice, produced little or no IFN-γ. Thus, administration of a TGF-β_1-producing plasmid is a powerful means of preventing experimental colitis, and may therefore be applicable to the treatment of human IBD.

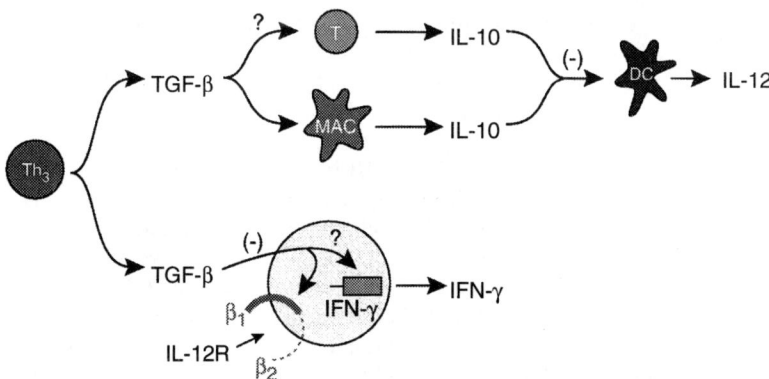

Figure 5 Mechanisms of TGF-β_1-mediated counter-regulation of mucosal responses

9

Additional studies were directed towards understanding the mechanism of the above TGF-β effect. For this purpose, mice were administered the TGF-β_1-producing plasmid with and without anti-IL-10 to probe the relation of IL-10 counter-regulatory activity to that of TGF-β. In these studies it was found that intranasal TGF-β_1 plasmid administration profoundly inhibited IL-12 production in the lamina propria of mice undergoing induction of TNBS colitis by intrarectal administration of TNBS. However, this effect of the plasmid could be shown to be mediated mainly, if not exclusively, by IL-10 since: (1) plasmid administration induced cells producing large amounts of IL-10; and (2) mice administered plasmid along with anti-IL-10 led to levels of IL-12 production seen in mice undergoing TNBS colitis in the absence of plasmid administration, i.e. high levels of IL-12 production (Fig. 5). From these studies one can infer first that the mechanism of TGF-β_1 counter-regulation is due in part to the suppression of IL-12 secretion via IL-10, and second, that TGF-β is sufficient unto itself, as a suppressor factor, at least in relation to the prevention of TNBS colitis, i.e. it does not require the presence of IL-10 in this circumstance.

A further and perhaps more interesting observation in relation to the co-administration of anti-IL-10 is that TGF-β plasmid administration was able to prevent the induction of TNBS colitis even in the presence of anti-IL-10 and indeed it greatly inhibited IFN-γ production even though anti-IL-10 administration led to normal or increased IL-12 levels (Fig. 5). Thus, it was apparent that the protective effect of the plasmid does not only depend on IL-10 (and suppression of IL-12 secretion). Since, as mentioned, TGF-β plasmid administration inhibits IFN-γ but not IL-12 production in the presence of anti-IL-10, one can infer that TGF-β_1 also prevents development of TNBS colitis by interfering with IFN-γ production. However, whether such interference is in the IL-12 signalling pathway, or on the transcription at the IFN-γ gene, will require further studies.

SUMMARY

Taken together, these studies offer several important insights into the relation between TGF-β and IL-10 in the counter-regulation of experimental mucosal inflammation. First, they illustrate that while IL-10 is a key component of one mechanism of TGF-β-induced suppression (suppression of IL-12 production) it plays no role in a second mechanism (interference with IL-12 signalling or IFN-γ transcription); thus, TGF-β is at least partly independent of IL-10. It should be noted, however, that IL-10 may be necessary for endogenous TGF-β secretion, i.e. secretion by normal T cells not containing a TGF-β1 plasmid. Second, they illustrate that since the IL-10 induced by TGF-β in these studies led to the down-regulation of IL-12 production, and the latter is normally inhibitory of TGF-β production, it is possible that IL-10 normally acts as a facilitator of TGF-β secretion rather than as a direct suppressor cytokine. This possibility is not ruled out by the studies described above in which IL-10 knockout mice were the source of CD45R6^{lo} T cells in the SCID transfer model, since these studies can also be explained by the fact that IL-10 functions to facilitate TGF-β secretion. Overall, therefore, while it is clear that both IL-10 and TGF-β are both counter-regulatory cytokines, the data for the TGF-β plasmid studies are most compatible with an interactive role between IL-10 and TGF-β in suppression, in which the IL-10 effect is indirect and the TGF-β effect is direct.

How do these findings impact on our knowledge and understanding of human IBD? On the surface of things, one would postulate from the studies reviewed here that some forms of IBD are in fact due to sub-optimal TGF-β production. Unfortunately, however, the data supporting this idea are marginal at best, primarily because it is difficult to accurately measure immunoregulatory TGF-β levels in tissues. In particular, while a great deal of TGF-β can be identified in both normal and inflamed mucosal sites[33], it is not yet possible to determine the component of TGF-β present that is actually involved in immunoregulation. Until techniques for quantitating TGF-β associated with particular cells become available, key questions about the role of TGF-β in human IBD will remain unanswered.

These difficulties with our current knowledge of the pathogenesis of IBD notwithstanding, the studies discussed suggest for the first time that it may be possible to treat human IBD (both Crohn's disease and ulcerative colitis) with an easily administered suppressor cytokine. The fact that the plasmid that generates the latter acts quickly and completely in prevention of experimental mucosal inflammation (and in studies not described in the cure of established colitis) suggests that TGF-β can be administered in a way that does not lead to one of the side-effects of TGF-β, the induction of fibrosis. Further work, however, will be necessary to verify this point.

References

1. Wirtz S, Finotto S, Kanzler S *et al*. Chronic intestinal inflammation in STAT-4 transgenic mice: characterization of disease and adoptive transfer by TNF-plus IFN-γ producing CD4+ T cells that respond to bacterial antigens. J Immunol. 1999;162:1884–8.
2. Simpson SJ, Shah S, Comiskey M *et al*. T cell-mediated pathology in two models of experimental colitis depends predominantly on the interleukin 12/Signal transducer and activator of transcription STAT-4 pathway, but is not conditional on interferon gamma expression by T cells. J Exp Med. 1998;187:1225–34.
3. Neurath MF, Fuss I, Kelsall BL, Strober W. Antibodies to interleukin 12 abrogate established experimental colitis in mice. J Exp Med. 1995;182:1281–90.
4. Rudolph U, Finegold MJ, Rich SS *et al*. Gi2 alpha protein deficiency: a model of inflammatory bowel disease. J Clin Immunol. 1995;15(Suppl.):101–5S.
5. Hornquist CE, Lu X, Rogers-Fani PM *et al*. G(alpha)i2-deficient mice with colitis exhibit a local increase in memory CD4+ T cells and proinflammatory Th1-type cytokines. J Immunol. 1997;158:1068–77.
6. Spiegel AM, Elson CO, Sartor RB, Tennyson GS, Riddell RH. G protein gene knockout hits the gut. Experimental models of inflammatory bowel disease. Nat Med. 1995;1:522–4.
7. Kontoyiannis D, Pusparakis M, Pizarro TT, Cominelli F, Kollias G. Impaired on/off regulation of TNF biosynthesis in mice lacking TNF AU-rich elements; implications for joint and gut-associated immunopathologies. Immunity. 1999;10:387–98.
8. Hollander GA, Simpson SJ, Mizoguchi E *et al*. Severe colitis in mice with aberrant thymic selection. Immunity. 1995;3:27–38.
9. Simpson SJ, Hollander GA, Mizoguchi E *et al*. Expression of pro-inflammatory cytokines by TCR alpha beta+ and TCR gamma delta+ T cells in an experimental model of colitis. Eur J Immunol. 1997;27:17–25.
10. Powrie F, Mason D. OX-22 high CD4+ T cells induce wasting disease with multiple organ pathology: prevention by the OX-22low subset. J Exp Med. 1991;172:1701–8.

11. Powrie F, Leach MW, Mauze S, Menon S, Caddle LB, Coffman RL. Inhibition of Th1 responses prevents inflammatory bowel diseases in SCID mice reconstituted with CD45RBhi CD4+ T cells. Immunity. 1994;1:553–62.
12. Leach MW, Bean AG, Mauze S, Coffman RL, Powrie F. Inflammatory bowel disease in C.B.-17 SCID mice reconstituted with the CD45Rbhigh subset of CD4+ T cells. Am J Pathol. 1996;148:1503-515.
13. Sadlack B, Merz H, Schorle H, Schimpl A, Feller AC, Horak I. Ulcerative colitis-like disease in mice with a disrupted interleukin-2 gene. Cell. 1993;75:253–61.
14. Ehrhardt RO, Ludviksson BR, Gray B, Neurath M, Strober W. Induction and prevention of colonic inflammation in IL-2-deficient mice. J Immunol. 1997;158:566–73.
15. Kühn R, Löhler J, Rennick D, Rajewsky K, Müller W. Interleukin-10-deficient mice develop chronic enterocolitis. Cell. 1993;75:263–74.
16. Berg DJ, Davidson N, Kühn R et al. Enterocolitis and colon cancer in interleukin-10-deficient mice are associated with aberrant cytokine production and CD4+ Th1-like responses. J Clin Invest. 1996;98:1010–20.
17. Fort MM, Leach MW, Rennick DM. A role for NK cells as regulators of CD4+ T cells in a transfer model of colitis. J Immunol. 1998;161:3256–61.
18. Davidson NJ, Hudak SA, Lesley RE, Menon S, Leach MW, Rennick DM. IL-12, but not IFN-gamma, plays a major role in sustaining the chronic phase of colitis in IL-10 deficient mice. J Immunol. 1998;161:3143–9.
19. Mombaerts P, Mizoguchi E, Grusby MJ, Glimcher LH, Bhan AK, Tonegawa S. Spontaneous development of inflammatory bowel disease in T cell receptor mutant mice. Cell. 1993;75:275–82.
20. Mizoguchi A, Mizoguchi E, Chiba C et al. Cytokine imbalance and autoantibody production in T cell receptor-α mutant mice with inflammatory bowel disease. J Exp Med. 1996;183:847–56.
21. Takahashi I, Kiyono H, Hamada S. CD4+ T-cell population mediates development of inflammatory bowel disease in T-cell receptor α chain-deficient mice. Gastroenterology. 1997;112:1876–86.
22. Mizoguchi A, Mizoguchi E, Smith RN, Preffer FI, Bhan AK. Suppressive role of B cells in chronic colitis of T cell receptor alpha mutant mice. J Exp Med. 1997;186:1749–56.
23. Ludviksson BR, Ehrhardt RO, Strober W. TGF-beta production regulates the development of the 2,4,6-trinitrophenol-conjugated keyhole limpet hemocyanin-induced colonic inflammation in IL-2-deficient mice. J Immunol. 1997;159:3622–8.
24. Asseman C, Mauze S, Leach MW, Coffman RL, Powrie F. An essential role for interleukin 10 in the function of regulatory T cells that inhibit intestinal inflammation. J Exp Med. 1999;190:995–1004.
25. Groux H, O'Garra A, Bigler M, Antonenko S, de Vries JE, Roncarolo MG. A CD4+ T-cell subset inhibits antigen-specific T cell responses and prevents colitis. Nature. 1997;389:737–42.
26. Asseman C, Powrie F. Interleukin 10 is a growth factor for a population of regulatory T cells. Gut. 1998;42:157–8.
27. Strober W, Kelsall B, Marth T. Oral tolerance. J Clin Immunol. 1998;18:1–30.
28. Weiner HL. Oral tolerance. Proc Natl Acad Sci USA. 1994;91:10764–5.
29. Powrie F, Carlino J, Leach MW, Mauze S, Coffman RL. A critical role for transforming growth factor-beta but not interleukin 4 in the suppression of T helper type 1-mediated colitis by CD45RB(low) CD4+ T cells. J Exp Med. 1996;183:2669–74.
30. Neurath MF, Fuss I, Kelsall BL, Presky DH, Waegell W, Strober W. Experimental granulomatous colitis in mice is abrogated by induction of TGF-beta-mediated oral tolerance. J Exp Med. 1996;183:2605–16.
31. Elson CO, Beagley KW, Sharmanov AT et al. Hapten-induced model of murine inflammatory bowel disease: mucosa immune response and protection by tolerance. J Immunol. 1996;157:2174–85.
32. Fuss IJ, Kitani A, Nakamura K, Chua K, Strober W. Successful treatment of experimental (TNBS) colitis by intranasal transfer of DNA encoding active TGF-β. Gastroenterology. 1999;116:63130 (abstract).
33. Babyatsky MW, Rossiter G, Podolsky DK. Expression of transforming growth factors alpha and beta in colonic mucosa in inflammatory bowel disease. Gastroenterology. 1996;110:975–84.
34. McKaig BC, Hawkey JC, Mahida YR. Differential expression of transforming growth factor β (TGF-β) isoforms by normal, ulcerative colitis and Crohn's disease intestinal myofibroblasts. Gastroenterology. 1999,116:G33330 (abstract).

2
A novel therapy for colitis utilizing PPARγ ligands to inhibit the epithelial inflammatory response

C. G. SU, X. WENG, S. T. BAILEY, W. JIANG, S. M. RANGWALA, S. A. KEILBAUGH, A. FLANIGAN, S. MURTHY, M. A. LAZAR and G. D. WU

INTRODUCTION

Delicately balanced mechanisms maintain the intestinal mucosa in a quiescent state of inflammation. In humans, loss of this balance leads to inflammatory bowel disease (IBD). The intestinal inflammatory phenotype observed in many immune receptor and cytokine knockout mice models lends support to the notion that cytokines help to regulate and maintain this quiescent state[1]. More recently it has become apparent that the intestinal epithelium, which is the interface between the highly antigenic luminal environment and the mucosal immune system, itself plays an active role in the immune responsiveness of the intestinal mucosa. Intestinal epithelial cells not only express various immune receptors traditionally believed to be expressed primarily by myeloid cell lineages[2], but can also produce a wide array of immune modulatory substances such as cytokines and complement factors[3,4]. Indeed, specific perturbation of the intestinal epithelium can lead to intestinal inflammation[5,6].

Many immune response genes are regulated by homo- and heterodimeric complexes of the NF-κB/Rel family of transcription factors. We have previously shown that binding of proteins to the NF-κB element in the IL-8 promoter is critical for IL-1β-mediated activation of this promoter in intestinal cell lines[7]. In most cells NF-κB/Rel factors are maintained in an inactive state in the cytoplasm bound to members of the IκB family of inhibitory proteins[8]. Upon cell stimulation by a variety of immunomodulatory substances such as IL-1, TNF-α, PMA, or oxygen radicals, these IκB proteins are rapidly phosphorylated and degraded via the ubiquitin–proteosome pathway[9]. This allows NF-κB/Rel proteins to translocate from the cytoplasm into the nucleus and activate gene transcription. Inhibitors of NF-κB activation, such as glucocorticoids, have been shown to be very potent anti-inflammatory agents[10].

Peroxisome proliferator-activated receptor γ (PPARγ) is a member of the nuclear hormone receptor superfamily whose ligands include several prostanoids, including 15-deoxy-$\Delta^{12,14}$ prostaglandin J$_2$ (15d-PGJ$_2$), polyunsaturated fatty acids, a variety of nonsteroidal anti-inflammatory drugs (NSAIDS), and a new class of oral antidiabetic agents, the thiazolidinediones (TZDs)[11–13]. PPARγ ligands are best characterized as regulators of adipocyte differentiation and glucose homeostasis[14,15]. However, PPARγ ligands have been shown to inhibit the expression of various cytokines in monocytes and macrophages, principally by preventing the activation of NF-κB/Rel by an unknown mechanism[16,17].

PPARγ is also expressed at high levels in both the colonic epithelium and in colon cancer cell lines[18–22]. The function of PPARγ in the colonic epithelium is currently unknown. This is reinforced by recent studies which report that PPARγ ligands can either increase or decrease colonocyte proliferation depending on the model system studied[20–23]. Here we show that the role of PPARγ in the colon may not be solely or even primarily to regulate growth and differentiation, but rather to regulate immune responsiveness. PPARγ ligands dramatically interfere with the activation of NF-κB and the ability of colonocytes to express immune modulating cytokines. Moreover, PPARγ ligands interfere with the colonic inflammatory process *in vivo*, and thus have promise as preventive and therapeutic agents against IBD.

METHODS

Cell culture

Caco-2 and HT-29 cells (from ATCC) were maintained in Dulbecco's modified Eagle's medium (DMEM) containing 10% fetal bovine serum and penicillin/streptomycin.

RNA analysis

Caco-2 and HT-29 cells were treated with various concentrations of either 15d-PGJ$_2$, BRA 49653, or ethyl acetate for 24 h. After RNA isolation and blotting, the Northern blots were hybridized with cDNA probes for IL-8, MCP-1, and ribosomal 7S[38].

Protein analysis

Proteins were isolated from cells in culture by suspension in RIPA buffer (1 $\times$ PBS, 1% nonidet P-40, 0.5% sodium deoxycholate, 0.1% SDS) containing 100 μg/ml PMSF, 60 μg/ml aprotinin, and 1 mM sodium orthovanadate. Cell lysates were centrifuged and the supernatants were collected and subjected to Western analysis using a 1:200 dilution of an affinity-purified IκB-α antibody (#sc-203, Santa Cruz). Following washing in 1 $\times$ TTBS containing 0.1% Tween and a 1 h incubation at room temperature with a horseradish peroxidase conjugated anti-rabbit Ab (1:5000 dilution, BMB), the proteins were visualized by ECL (Amersham).

Electrophoretic mobility shift assays were performed using Caco-2 cells, treated with either methylacetate (solvent) or 15d-PGJ$_2$ (30 μM) for 24 h, which were stimulated with complete medium containing IL-1β (5 ng/ml) for various periods of time as indicated. Nuclear proteins were isolated from both unstimulated and IL-1β-stimulated Caco-2 cells. Double-stranded oligonucleotides spanning the NF-κB element of the IL-8 promoter[7] were labelled with ^{32}P. Binding reactions, each containing 10 μg of nuclear proteins, were performed as previously described[39] and subsequently separated on a 4% polyacrylamide gel.

Transient cell transfections

Caco-2 cells were transiently co-transfected with the IL-8 promoter luciferase reporter plasmid (wt)LUC[7] and pCMV-β-Gal (transfection control) using the calcium phosphate precipitation method[40]. At 48 h after transfection the cells were treated with either methylacetate (solvent control) or 15d-PGJ$_2$ (30 μM) for 24 h. Designated cells were stimulated with IL-1β (5 ng/ml) for 6 h followed by assays for luciferase and β-galactosidase activity as described previously[41].

Animal treatments

Female, 8-week-old Swiss Webster mice, weighing 25–30 g, were fed standard mice chow pellets and had access to tap water. Acute colitis was induced by feeding the mice 4% dextran sodium sulphate (DSS, 30–40 kDa mol. wt dissolved in drinking water) for 7 days. Two treatment studies were performed, one with troglitazone (RezulinT^M) and one with BRL 49653. The two studies contained eight animals in each treatment group. In the first protocol, troglitazone was suspended in 0.75% methylcellulose solution. Then 0, 10, 30, and 100 mg/kg per day of troglitazone (0.1 ml/mouse) was administered by gavage on the day DSS feeding was initiated. After induction of colitis, DSS was discontinued on day 7. Therapy with troglitazone was continued until the mice were sacrificed on day 15. In the second protocol, colitis was initiated with DSS for 7 days followed by therapy with BRL 49653 (suspended in 0.75% methylcellulose at 0 or 20 mg/kg per day gavaged p.o.) for an additional 8 days, at which time the animals were sacrificed for histological analysis. A disease activity index (DAI) was determined on a daily basis for each animal and consists of a calculated score based upon change in body weight, stool consistency, and intestinal bleeding as described previously[27]. Parameters for the DAI were measured by an investigator (A.F.) blinded to the protocol. A significant decrease in the DAI is considered an endpoint of successful therapy.

Histology and immunohistochemistry

Mouse colonic tissues embedded in OCT were cut into 5 μm sections, dried, and fixed in 4% paraformaldehyde. Following a rinse in 1 $\times$ PBS, they were treated with 1.5% H$_2$O$_2$ in methanol for 20 min at room temperature. The sections were then microwaved for 12 min in 10 mM citrate acetate, pH 6.0. Blocking was performed with 1 $\times$ PBS containing 5% normal goat serum for 10 min and incubated with an affinity-purified polyclonal antibody for PPARγ[42] at 1:500 dilution for 30 min. After washing with 1 $\times$ PBS the slides were incubated with a biotinylated goat anti-rabbit secondary antibody (Vector Laboratories) at a dilution of 1:200 for 30 min. Staining was detected by using the horseradish peroxidase Vectastain Elite ABC kit (Vector Laboratories) and DAB

(3,3′-diaminobenzidine, Sigma). The slides were counterstained in haematoxylin, dehydrated in ethanol and xylene, and mounted with mounting media.

RESULTS

Treatment of the Caco-2 intestinal cell line, previously shown to express PPARγ, with 15d-PGJ$_2$ strongly inhibited IL-1β-induced expression of both the neutrophil chemoattractant interleukin 8 (IL-8) as well as the monocyte chemoattractant, MCP-1 (Fig. 1A). The 15d-PGJ$_2$ also inhibited the induction of IL-8 expression in a second intestinal cell line, HT-29, in response to stimulation with either IL-1β or TNF-α (Fig. 1B). A different TZD ligand for PPARγ, BRL 49653, also inhibited IL-8 gene expression (Fig. 1B). This effect of PPARγ ligands was dose-dependent with ED$_{50}$ of 15–30 μM and 50–100 μM for 15d-PGJ$_2$ and BRL49653, respectively. The increased potency of 15d-PGJ$_2$ relative to BRL 49653 contrasts with the direct binding affinities of these compounds but is consistent with their relative potencies as anti-inflammatory agents[16]. Interestingly, although the PPARα isoform has been shown to be expressed in colon cancer cell lines[24], treatment of either Caco-2 or HT-29 cells with the PPARα specific ligand, WY 14643, did not inhibit the expression of IL-8 (data not shown). This finding is in direct contrast to those observed in vascular smooth muscle cells, in which ligands for PPARα but not PPARγ inhibit the inflammatory response[25]. Therefore, although both PPARα and γ heterodimerize with RXR and bind to similar *cis*-acting elements, their effects on immune responsiveness appear to be tissue-specific.

We next investigated the mechanism by which PPARγ ligands inhibit IL-8 gene expression in colon cancer cells. Consistent with its effect on IL-8 gene expression, 15d-PGJ$_2$ inhibited the ability of IL-1β to activate a reporter gene regulated by the IL-8 promoter (Fig. 2A). The NF-κB element plays the most critical role in the activation of this promoter[7]. Electrophoretic mobility shift assays (EMSAs) show that the treatment of Caco-2 cells with 15d-PGJ$_2$ dramatically reduced nuclear protein binding to the NF-κB element of the IL-8 promoter (Fig. 2B).

In response to immune stimulation, degradation of the IκB family of proteins plays a critical role in the activation of NF-κB[8]. The rapid and transient expression of IL-8 mRNA in Caco-2 cells in response to IL-1β stimulation is consistent with regulation by IκB-α expression. An immunoblot of IκB-α in Caco-2 cells showed that IκB-α protein was rapidly degraded within 10 min after stimulation with IL-1β followed by reappearance of the protein at 80 min due to autoregulatory induction of this gene by NF-κB[26] (Fig. 2C). In contrast, IκB-α was resistant to degradation in IL-1β-stimulated Caco-2 cells treated with 15d-PGJ$_2$ (Fig. 2C) consistent with the absence of NF-κB binding noted on EMSA (Fig. 2B).

In order to determine if ligands for PPARγ can attenuate intestinal inflammation *in vivo*, we studied the effect of two different TZD PPARγ ligands on a well-established murine model of colonic inflammation which is commonly used to screen pharmacological agents[1]. Animals fed 4% dextran sodium sulphate (DSS) develop colonic inflammation within 7 days; upon termination of

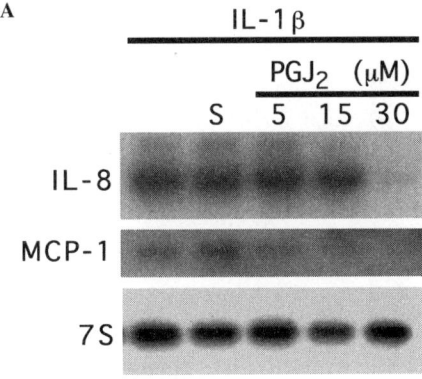

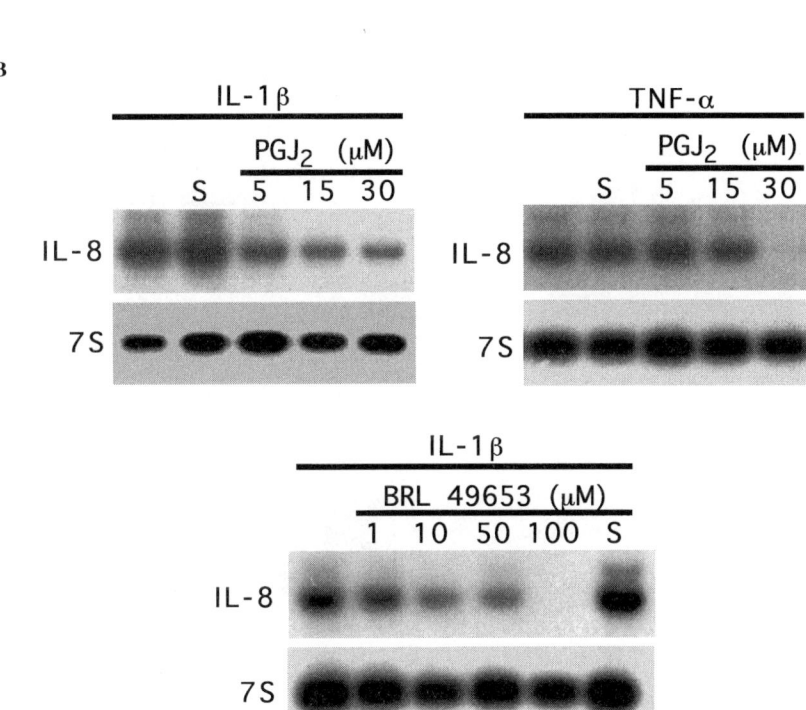

Figure 1 PPARγ ligands inhibit cytokine gene expression in colon cancer cell lines. **A**: The Caco-2 colon cancer cell line was treated with various concentrations of 15d-PGJ$_2$ or ethylacetate (solvent control-S) for 24 h prior to immune stimulation with IL-1β for 90 min. **B**: HT-29 cells were treated for 24 h with either 15d-PGJ$_2$, BRL 49653, ethyl acetate or DMSO (solvent controls – S) followed by stimulation with either IL-1β or TNF-α for 90 min

A

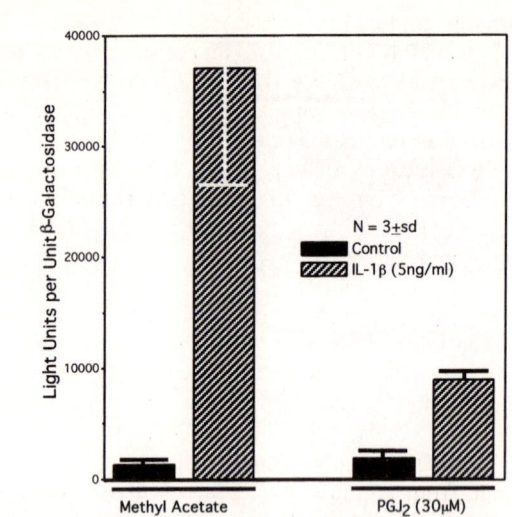

B

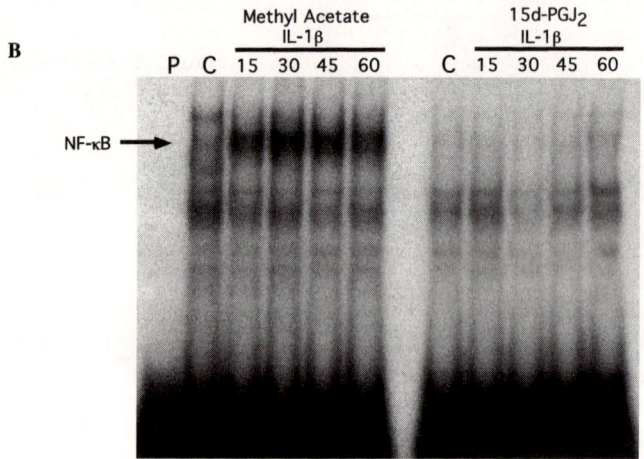

C

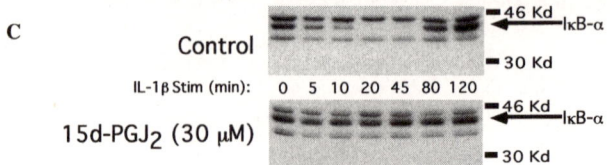

DSS administration, colonic inflammation slowly resolves[27]. The DAI provides a well-characterized method of quantitating disease severity in this model, which correlates well with histological healing[27]. Two treatment studies were performed, one with troglitazone and one with BRL 49653. In the first study the mice were treated throughout the entire protocol with various concentrations of troglitazone. The DAI for each study group demonstrated that 7 and 8 days after DSS was discontinued, troglitazone (100 mg/kg per day) led to a 47% and 70% decrease in the DAI, respectively, compared to the placebo-treated group (Fig. 3A). Also noted was a trend towards a decrease in the DAI observed in mice treated with an intermediate dose of troglitazone (30 mg/kg per day) suggestive of a dose-dependent response. Therapeutic efficacy was also determined for BRL 49653 in the same model. BRL 49653 was administered once colitis was established after 7 days of DSS. This eliminated the possibility that the compound altered water consumption while the disease was being initiated with DSS during the first 7 days. Figure 3B shows that BRL dramatically decreased the DAI by 67% and 70% on days 7 and 8, respectively.

Colonic tissue from animals which received vehicle alone showed intense mucosal inflammation with a chronic inflammatory infiltrate, oedema, and marked thickening of the bowel wall (Fig. 3C). In contrast, histological sections from the colon of animals treated with 8 days of BRL 49653 showed a remarkable decrease in inflammation with only a mild inflammatory infiltrate, no oedema, and normal bowel wall thickness. Immunostaining of these tissue sections demonstrated that PPARγ is expressed primarily in the colonic epithelium even in the presence of intense inflammation (Fig. 3C). The inflammatory cells expressed comparatively little PPARγ, consistent with the colonic epithelium itself being the target of PPARγ ligands.

DISCUSSION

There is significant interest in the biological consequences of PPARγ activation in the colon. Due to the differentiating and antiproliferative effects of PPARγ in adipose and breast tissue[14,15,28,29], it has been proposed that ligands for this receptor may have therapeutic potential in chemoprevention or the treatment of colorectal neoplasia[20,23]. Recent studies, however, suggest that these same ligands actually enhance colon polyp and tumour formation in the *min* mouse model of familial adenomatous polyposis coli[21,22]. Here we show that PPARγ ligands have another major effect on colon epithelial cells; namely to regulate the inflammatory response. Several historical observations are consistent with

◀ **Figure 2** 15d-PGJ$_2$ inhibits the transcriptional activation of the IL-8 promoter by preventing the activation of NF-κB via an IκB-α dependent pathway. **A:** Caco-2 cells co-transfected with an IL-8 promoter luciferase reporter gene and CMV-β galactosidase (transfection control) were treated with either 15d-PGJ$_2$ (30 μM) or methyl acetate for 24 h. Designated cells were stimulated with IL-1β (5 ng/ml). **B:** EMSAs of nuclear extracts isolated from Caco-2 cell treated with either 15d-PGJ$_2$ or methyl acetate for 24 h followed by IL-1β stimulation (5 ng/ml) for the times indicated. A double-stranded oligonucleotide spanning the NF-κB element in the IL-8 promoter was used as a probe. **C:** IκB-α Western blot of proteins isolated from Caco-2 cells treated with 15d-PGJ$_2$ or methyl acetate for 24 h followed by IL-1β stimulation (5 ng/ml) for the times indicated

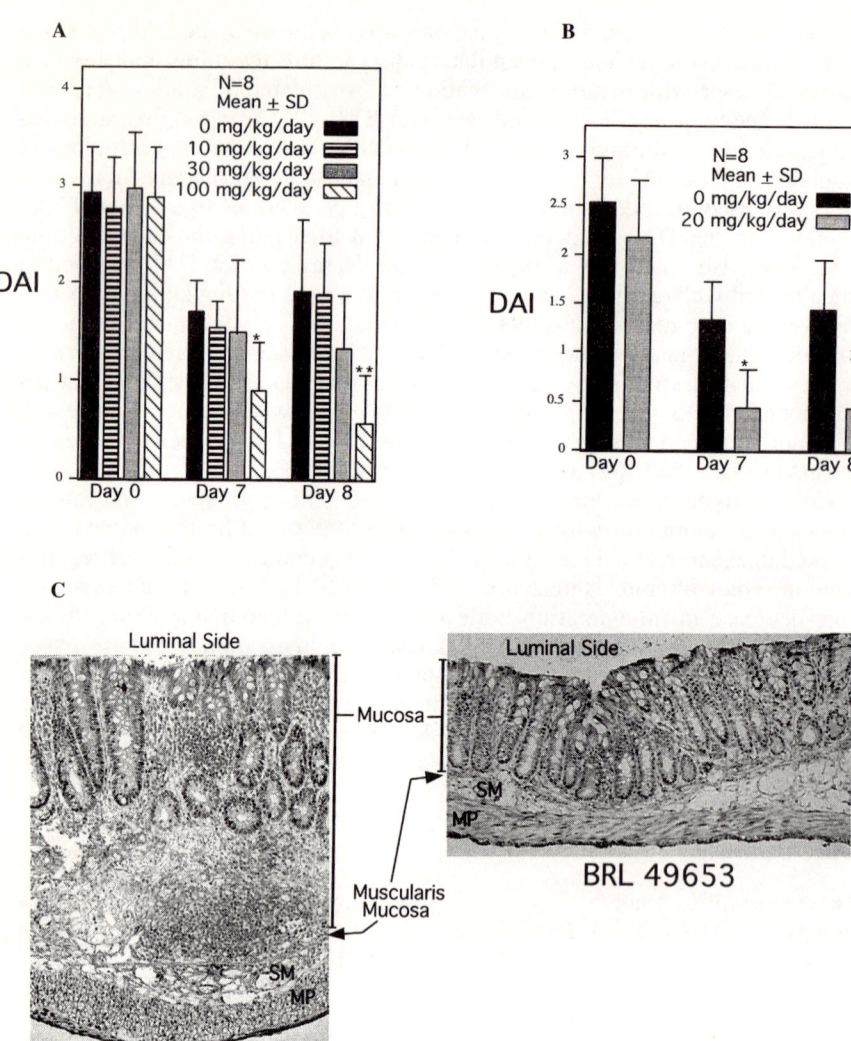

Figure 3 PPARγ ligands inhibit inflammation and reduce disease severity in the DSS model of murine colitis. **A**: Colitis was established after 7 days of 4% DSS. Day 0 refers to the day that DSS treatment ended. Throughout the entire course of the study the mice were treated with the various amounts of troglitazone indicated. A disease activity index (DAI) was determined daily for each animal in the study. $*p = 0.009$, $**p = 0.003$ by unpaired t-test. **B**: Colitis was established after 7 days of 4% DSS. Day 0 refers to the day that DSS treatment ended and BRL 49653 administration was begun. $*p = 0.001$, $**p = 0.008$. **C**: Immunohistochemistry for PPARγ was performed on frozen sections of colonic tissue obtained from mice in the BRL 49653 study, vehicle alone or BRL 49653 (20 mg/kg per day), sacrificed on day 8. Original magnification × 100; MP = muscularis propria, SM = submucosa

the possible utility of PPARγ activation in the treatment of colonic inflammation. First, polyunsaturated fatty acids, such as provided in fish oil, have been shown to be potent activators of PPARγ and have efficacy in the treatment of IBD[30,31]. Second, there is evidence that thiazolidinediones may decrease insulin resistance by decreasing the production of TNF-α by adipose tissue and/or by inhibiting TNF-α-mediated signal transduction[32]. Inhibition of TNF-α activity by the use of anti-TNF antibodies has been shown to be an effective treatment modality for refractory Crohn's disease[33].

We show that two different classes of ligands for PPARγ potently inhibit cytokine expression in two different PPARγ-expressing colon cell lines[20,23]. PPARγ ligands inhibit activation of NF-κB via an IκB-α dependent pathway by inhibiting the immune response-induced degradation of IκB-α. Although further investigation will be required to elucidate the upstream mechanisms by which PPARγ inhibits the degradation of IκB-α, inhibition of both IL-1β and TNF-α-induced IL-8 gene expression suggests that activation of PPARγ alters functional elements common to both these pathways. The use of an antisense oligonucleotide to inhibit the expression of p65 has established the utility of targeting NF-κB as therapeutic approach to treat intestinal inflammation[34].

Although previous studies have shown that activation of PPARγ inhibits the inflammatory response in monocytes and macrophages, immunolocalization of PPARγ primarily to colonocytes, even in the presence of inflammation, strongly suggests that these epithelial cells are the target of PPARγ ligands in IBD. This provides evidence that immune modulation of the intestinal epithelium alone may be efficacious in the treatment of intestinal inflammatory states. The role that PPARγ ligands play in neoplasia need not be necessarily viewed as a disparate effect. Indeed, it is well known that chronic intestinal inflammation not only alters patterns of cellular proliferation and differentiation in the intestinal epithelium but is also a significant factor in the development of colorectal neoplasia[35,36]. Further investigation into the effect of PPARγ ligands on neoplastic transformation in the setting of IBD may provide important insights into the biology of the colonic epithelium.

In addition, PPARγ ligands represent a novel approach to the treatment of IBD. The DAI used to quantitate disease activity in our study are comprehensive functional measures that are analogues to the subjective clinical symptoms observed in humans with ulcerative colitis. In this model the results with either troglitazone or BRL 49653 show a greater level of therapeutic efficacy than that observed with Olsalazine (150 mg/kg per day), a drug that has been commonly used in the treatment of IBD[37]. Troglitazone is currently in widespread use as a treatment for type 2 diabetes, and the doses of troglitazone administered in this study were within the concentrations that have been shown to be well tolerated by mice[20]. The demonstration that TZD ligands have potent anti-inflammatory effects *in vivo* represents a new concept in the therapeutic approach to IBD, a chronic debilitating disease which affects millions of people worldwide.

Acknowledgements

This work was supported by NIH grants DK47709 (G.W.), AI39368 (G.W.), Center Grant P30 DK50306, DK49780 (M.A.L.) and DK49210 (M.A.L.).

References

1. Elson CO, Sartor RB, Tennyson GS, Riddell RH. Experimental models of inflammatory bowel disease. Gastroenterology. 1995;109:1344–67.
2. Reinecker HC, Podolsky DK. Human intestinal epithelial cells express functional cytokine receptors sharing the common γc chain of the interleukin 2 receptor. Proc Natl Acad Sci USA. 1995;92:8353–7.
3. Jung HC, Eckmann L, Yang SK et al. A distinct array of proinflammatory cytokines is expressed in human colon epithelial cells in response to bacterial invasion. J Clin Invest. 1995;95:55–65.
4. Andoh A, Fujiyama Y, Bamba T, Hosoda S. Differential cytokine regulation of complement C3, C4, and factor B synthesis in human intestinal epithelial cell line, Caco-2. J Immunol. 1993;151:4239–47.
5. Hermiston ML, Gordon JI. Inflammatory bowel disease and adenomas in mice expressing a dominant negative N-cadherin. Science. 1995;270:1203–7.
6. Baribault H, Penner J, Iozzo RV, Wilson-Heiner M. Colorectal hyperplasia and inflammation in keratin 8-deficient FVB/N mice. Genes Dev. 1994;8:2964–73.
7. Wu GD, Lai EJ, Huang N, Wen X. Oct-1 and C/EBP bind to overlapping elements within the IL-8 promoter: the role of Oct-1 as a transcriptional repressor. J Biol Chem. 1997;272:2396–403.
8. Verma IM, Stevenson JK, Schwarz EM, Antwerp DV, Miyamoto S. Rel/NF-κB/IκB family: intimate tales of association and dissociation. Genes Dev. 1995;9:2723–35.
9. Brown K, Gerstberger S, Carlson L, Franzoso G, Siebenlist U. Control of IκB-α proteolysis by site-specific, signal-induced phosphorylation. Science. 1995;267:1485–8.
10. Auphan N, DiDonate JA, Rosette C, Helmberg A, Karin M. Immunosuppression by glucocorticoids: inhibition of NF-κB activity through induction of IκB synthesis. Science. 1995;270:286–90.
11. Yu K, Bayona W, Kallen CB et al. Differential activation of peroxisome proliferator-activated receptors by eicosanoids. J Biol Chem. 1995;270:23975–83.
12. Kliewer SA, Lenhard JM, Willson TM, Patel I, Morris DC, Lehmann JM. A prostaglandin J2 metabolite binds peroxisome proliferator-activated receptorγ and promotes adipocyte differentiation. Cell. 1995;83:813–19.
13. Forman BM, Tontonoz P, Chen J, Brun RP, Spiegelman BM, Evans RM. 15-Deoxy delta 12,14-prostaglandin J2 is a ligand for the adipocyte determination factor PPARγ. Cell. 1995;83:803–12.
14. Tontonoz P, Hu E, Spiegelman BM. Stimulation of adipogenesis in fibroblasts by PPARγ2, a lipid-activated transcription factor. Cell. 1994;79:1147–56.
15. Chawla A, Schwarz EJ, Dimaculangan DD, Lazar MA. Peroxisome proliferator-activated receptor γ (PPARγ): adipose predominant expression and induction early in adipocyte differentiation. Endocrinology. 1994;135:798–800.
16. Ricote M, Li AC, Willson TM, Kelly CJ, Glass CK. The peroxisome proliferator-activated receptor-γ is a negative regulator of macrophage activation. Nature. 1998;391:79–82.
17. Jiang C, Ting AT, Seed B. PPAR-γ agonists inhibit production of monocyte inflammatory cytokines. Nature. 1998;391:82–6.
18. Fajas L, Auboerf D, Raspe E et al. The organization, promoter analysis, and expression of the human PPARγ gene. J Biol Chem. 1997;272:18779–89.
19. Dubois RN, Gupta R, Brockman J, Reddy BS, Kradow SL, Lazar MA. The nuclear eicosanoid receptor, PPARγ, is aberrantly expressed in colonic cancers. Carcinogenesis. 1998;19:49–53.
20. Sarraf P, Mueller E, Jones D et al. Differentiation and reversal of malignant changes in colon cancer through PPARγ. Nature Med. 1998;4:1046–52.
21. Saez E, Tontonoz P, Nelson MC et al. Activators of the nuclear receptor PPARγ enhance colon polyp formation. Nature. Med. 1998;4:1058–61.
22. Lefebvre AM, Chen I, Desreumaux P et al. Activation of the peroxisome proliferator-activated receptorγ promotes the development of colon tumors in C57BL/6J-APC^{Min}/+ mice. Nature Med. 1998;4:1053–7.
23. Brockman JA, Gupta RA, Dubois RN. Activation of PPARγ leads to inhibition of anchorage independent growth of human colorectal cancer cells. Gastroenterology. 1998;115:1049–55.
24. Suzuki R, Suruga K, Goda T, Takase S. Peroxisome proliferator enhances gene expression of cellular retinol-binding protein, type II in Caco-2 cells. Life Sci. 1998;62:861–71.
25. Staels B, Koenig W, Habib A et al. Activation of human aortic smooth-muscle cells is inhibited by PPARα but not by PPARγ activators. Nature. 1998;393:790–3.

26. Sun SC, Ganchi PA, Ballard DW, Greene WC. NF-κB controls expression of inhibitor IκBα: evidence for an inducible autoregulatory pathway. Science. 1993;259:1912–15.

27. Cooper HS, Murthy SNS, Shah RS, Sedergran D. Clinicopathologic study of dextran sulfate sodium experimental murine colitis. Lab Invest. 1993;69:238–49k.

28. Tontonoz P, Hu E, Graves RA, Budavari AI, Spiegelman BM. mPPARγ2: tissue-specific regulator of an adipocyte enhancer. Genes Dev. 1994;8:1224–34.

29. Mueller E, Sarraf P, Tontonoz P et al. Terminal differentiation of human breast cancer through PPARγ. Mol Cell. 1998;1:465–70.

30. Kliewer SA, Sundseth SS, Jones SA et al. Fatty acids and eicosanoids regulate gene expression through direct interactions with peroxisome proliferator-activated receptors α and γ. Proc Natl Acad Sci USA. 1997;94:4318–23.

31. Belluzzi A, Brignola C, Campieri M, Pera A, Boschi S, Miglioli M. Effect of enteric-coated fish-oil preparation on relapses in Crohn's disease. N Engl J Med. 1996;334:1557–60.

32. Peraldi P, Xu M, Spiegelman BM. Thiazolidinediones block tumor necrosis factor-α-induced inhibition of insulin signaling. J Clin Invest. 1997;100:1863–9.

33. Targan SR, Hanauer SB, van Deventer SJH et al. A short-term study of chimeric monoclonal antibody CA2 to tumor necrosis factor (alpha) for Crohn's disease. N Engl J Med. 1997;337:1029–35.

34. Neurath MF, Pettersson S, Büschenfelde KHM, Strober W. Local administration of antisense phosphorothioate oligonucleotides to the p65 subunit of NF-κB abrogates established experimental colitis in mice. Nature Med. 1996;2:998–1004.

35. Serafini EP, Kirk AP, Chambers TJ. Rate and pattern of epithelial cell proliferation in ulcerative colitis. Gut. 1981;22:648–52.

36. Bachwich DR, Lichtenstein GR, Traber PG. Cancer in inflammatory bowel disease. Med Clin N Am. 1994;78:1399–412.

37. Murthy S, Murthy NS, Coppola D, Wood DL. The efficacy of BAY γ 1015 in dextran sulfate model of mouse colitis. Inflamm Res. 1997;46:224–33.

38. Huang N, Katz JP, Martin DR, Wu GD. Inhibition of IL-8 gene expression in Caco-2 cells by compounds which induce histone hyperacetylation. Cytokine. 1997;9:27–36.

39. Traber PG, Wu GD, Wang W. Novel DNA-binding proteins regulate intestine-specific transcription of the sucrase-isomaltase gene. Mol Cell Biol. 1992;12:3614–27.

40. Chen C, Okayama H. High-efficiency transformation of mammalian cells by plasmid DNA. Mol Cell Biol. 1987;7:2031–4.

41. Wu GD, Wang W, Traber PG. Isolation and characterization of the human sucrase-isomaltase gene and demonstration of intestine-specific transcriptional elements. J Biol Chem. 1992;267:7863–70.

42. Xue JC, Schwartz EJ, Chawla A, Lazar MA. Distinct stages in adipogenesis revealed by retinoid inhibition of differentiation after induction of PPARγ. Mol Cell Biol. 1996;16:1567–75.

3
Prostaglandins and nitric oxide: down-regulators of intestinal inflammation

M. N. AJUEBOR and J. L. WALLACE

INTRODUCTION

From a drug development standpoint, much attention has been devoted to identifying pro-inflammatory mediators that play a crucial role in diseases such as inflammatory bowel disease (IBD). If a key mediator could be identified, it should be possible to develop drugs that block the synthesis or action of that mediator, and therefore reduce the severity of the disease. However, one of the problems with this approach is that there is tremendous redundancy in terms of the actions of pro-inflammatory mediators. Inhibiting the production of one chemotactic factor, for example, may have little effect on the magnitude of an inflammatory response if numerous other chemotactic factors are still being produced in the tissue. On the other hand, one could focus on the mediators that are produced in the context of inflammation that exerts anti-inflammatory effects. For example, the cytokines IL-10 and IL-4 are known to exhibit a number of anti-inflammatory and immunoregulatory actions. The importance of IL-10 in this regard is underscored by the observation that mice lacking the gene for this cytokine spontaneously develop colitis[1].

Two groups of mediators that have been the focus of a great deal of research pertaining to IBD, both of which have the capacity to act in both pro- and anti-inflammatory capacities, are nitric oxide and the prostaglandins. Interestingly, both of these mediators were initially thought to be important in the pathogenesis of IBD, but more recent data suggest that their primary role in the inflamed intestine is to down-regulate inflammatory responses. In this chapter, we review the evidence in support of this hypothesis, and highlight the potential for nitric oxide- and prostaglandin-based anti-inflammatory drugs.

PROSTAGLANDINS

Prostaglandins belong to a family of 20-carbon polyunsaturated fatty acids known as eicosanoids. Other members of this family include thromboxane and leukotrienes. Eicosanoids are derived from arachidonic acid found within cell membrane phospholipids. Arachidonic acid is liberated from these phospholipids via the action of phospholipases. Arachidonic acid can then be metabolized by the enzyme cyclooxygenase, which exists in at least two isoforms (COX-1 and COX-2), to form prostaglandin H_2. PGH_2 is rapidly transformed, enzymatically or non-enzymatically, to one of several prostaglandins (PGE_2, PGD_2, $PGF_2\alpha$, PGI_2) or to thromboxane (TXA_2). Which particular prostanoid is formed largely depends on the presence within the cell of specific prostanoid synthase enzymes (e.g. PGI_2 synthase, TXA_2 synthase, etc.).

A number of prostaglandin receptors have now been identified[2]. The receptor for PGD_2 is termed the DP receptor, whilst the receptors for PGE_2, $PGF_2\alpha$, and PGI_2 are termed EP, FP and IP, respectively. There are at least four subclasses of the EP receptor.

As mentioned above, two isoforms of COX have been identified[3]. COX-1 is constitutively expressed in many tissues, including the gastrointestinal tract[4-6]. In contrast, COX-2 is expressed at low levels in normal intestine but is strongly expressed at sites of intestinal inflammation[5,6].

A role for prostaglandins in the pathogenesis of IBD was first suggested more than two decades ago. Rectal biopsies from patients with active ulcerative colitis were found to produce very high levels of prostaglandins[7-11], and it was proposed that they contributed to the infiltration of inflammatory cells, tissue injury and diarrhoea that characterized IBD. However, suppression of prostaglandin synthesis with nonsteroidal anti-inflammatory drugs (NSAIDs) was found to exacerbate, rather than abrogate, the symptoms of IBD[12,13]. Studies using a model of colitis in the rat confirmed the ability of NSAIDs to exacerbate tissue injury and inflammation[14]. Additional evidence that prostaglandins played a beneficial role in the context of intestinal inflammation came from animal studies in which administration of PGE_2 or PGE_2 analogues was found to significantly reduce the severity of colitis[15-17].

How would prostaglandins down-regulate inflammation in the intestine? Prostaglandins are capable of inhibiting a number of events in the inflammatory cascade. For example, PGE_2 and PGI_2 are potent inhibitors of neutrophil adherence to the vascular endothelium and can suppress the production of reactive oxygen metabolites by neutrophils[18-20]. There is good evidence from animal models of colitis that neutrophils are a primary effector cell in terms of the production of tissue injury[21,22], and that the damage produced by neutrophils is largely mediated via the release from these cells of reactive oxygen metabolites[23]. Prostaglandins can also inhibit the release of leukotriene B_4 and interleukin-8 from neutrophils[24-26]. Leukotriene B_4 and IL-8 are potent chemotaxins that play roles both in the recruitment of neutrophils and in stimulating the release from these cells of other mediators and proteases. Thus, the release of these mediators from infiltrating neutrophils is a positive feedback signal to amplify an inflammatory response. Prostaglandins can also suppress the release of a number of other inflammatory mediators. For example, Hogaboam et al.[27]

demonstrated that prostaglandin E_2 analogues could inhibit the release of platelet-activating factor from mucosal or peritoneal mast cells at concentrations in the picomolar to nanomolar range. Kunkel and colleagues[28,29] have demonstrated that prostaglandins play an important role in regulating the release of interleukin-1β and tumour necrosis factor-α from macrophages.

A number of recent studies have attempted to determine which isoform of COX was responsible for prostaglandin synthesis in the inflamed colon. Reuter et al.[5] demonstrated that most of the prostaglandins produced by the inflamed rat colon are derived from COX-2. COX-2 mRNA and protein expression were found to be markedly up-regulated within hours of induction of colitis, and remained elevated for at least 2 weeks thereafter. Suppression of COX-2 activity, using agents such as L-745,337 (a selective COX-2 inhibitor), resulted in significant exacerbation of colonic injury. Moreover, with continued administration of COX-2 inhibitors over the course of a week, perforation of the colon was observed, leading to death[5]. The importance of COX-2 as the primary source of anti-inflammatory prostaglandin production was further demonstrated by studies utilizing mice in which the gene for COX-2 was disrupted. COX-2-deficient mice exhibited markedly more severe colitis, induced by dextran sodium sulphate, than wild-type controls or COX-1-deficient mice[30,31].

The concept that prostaglandins derived from COX-2 exert important anti-inflammatory effects is supported by two recent studies of peripheral inflammation. First, carrageenan-induced paw edema in COX-2-deficient mice was found to persist for more than 7 days, while in wild-type control mice the inflammatory response to carrageenan injection was resolved within 24 h[32]. This suggests that COX-2-derived prostaglandins normally play a role in 'turning off' the inflammatory response. Second, Gilroy et al.[33] recently reported that COX-2 was markedly up-regulated in experimental pleurisy during the period of resolution of the inflammation. They demonstrated that PGD2 derived from COX-2 suppressed the infiltration of leucocytes into the inflamed pleural cavity. Selective inhibition of COX-2 resulted in a propagation of the inflammatory response.

In summary, prostaglandins appear to play a very important role in down-regulating inflammatory responses in the intestine, and probably elsewhere. COX-2 appears to be the primary source of prostaglandin synthesis in the inflamed intestine, and inhibition of its activity leads to exacerbation of the inflammatory response. It may be possible to design anti-inflammatory therapies that act through specific prostaglandin receptors that mediate the down-regulation of inflammation produced by this group of mediators.

NITRIC OXIDE

Nitric oxide is a free radical produced as a secondary product in the conversion of L-arginine to L-citrulline. It has an extremely short half-life, but is an important mediator of a number of physiological processes (e.g. regulation of blood pressure, neurotransmission). NO is also believed to be an important mediator of inflammatory responses and, like the prostaglandins, has both pro- and anti-inflammatory actions. There is tremendous controversy surrounding the role of NO in intestinal inflammation. Several studies have suggested that NO, either directly or through a reaction with superoxide anion to form peroxynitrite[34], is a major contributor to the tissue injury that characterizes IBD. Other studies suggest that NO does not play an important role in this process, and may even be more important as a protective factor in the mucosa.

The evidence supporting the role of NO as a mediator of inflammation and injury in IBD includes the demonstration that production of this mediator is markedly elevated in human IBD and in several models of enterocolitis, and that there is increased activity and expression of inducible nitric oxide synthase (NOS)[34–38]. Increased formation of peroxynitrite has also been detected in the inflamed intestine, via staining for nitrotyrosine residues[37,38]. One problem with these latter data is that it is now clear that nitrotyrosine residues can be formed independently of peroxynitrite formation[39]. Further support for a role of NO in the pathogenesis of IBD was provided by studies of inhibitors of NOS in experimental models of enterocolitis. Inhibition of NO synthesis, with agents now regarded as non-selective (i.e. not discriminating very well between constitutive NOS and inducible NOS), were able to reduce the severity of intestinal injury and inflammation[37,40–42].

In recent years the role of NO in IBD has become less clear, as a number of studies have emerged which reported data contradicting the earlier studies. First, inhibition of NOS with more selective inhibitors of the inducible isoform of NOS failed to consistently produce beneficial effects in experimental colitis[43,44]. Second, mice that lacked the gene for iNOS were found to have increased, rather than decreased, susceptibility to chemically induced colitis[45]. Finally, McCafferty et al.[46] recently demonstrated that the production of NO increased in a parallel manner with the development of enterocolitis in IL-10-deficient mice. However, when they crossed the IL-10-deficient mice with mice lacking the gene for inducible NOS, they found that the NO production reduced to the levels of control mice, but enterocolitis developed to the same extent as in the IL-10-deficient mice[46].

As mentioned above, NO is capable of exerting several anti-inflammatory activities, including inhibition of neutrophil adherence to the vascular endothelium[47], inhibition of the release of several inflammatory mediators from mast cells[48,49] and suppression of platelet aggregation and secretion[50]. Moreover, NO has been reported to contribute to the healing of tissue injury, including that in the gastrointestinal tract. For example, NO donors can accelerate the healing of experimental gastric ulcers[51] and have been used clinically to accelerate the healing of anal fissures in Crohn's disease[52]. Recently, we tested the hypothesis that, because of the anti-inflammatory and ulcer healing properties of NO, a NO donor would have beneficial effects in experimental colitis. We have previously found that injury to the stomach and small intestine induced by NSAIDs could be almost completely abolished by agents that slowly release NO[53]. Thus, we used the same approach to test the hypothesis stated above. A NO-releasing group was coupled to 5-aminosalicylic acid (5-ASA) through an ester linkage. 5-ASA is among the most commonly used drugs for the treatment of IBD, but is only modestly effective. When given intracolonically to rats with colitis, the NO-releasing 5-ASA derivative (NCX-456) markedly reduced the severity of colonic damage and the infiltration of granulocytes into the colonic tissue[54]. The effects of NCX-456 were statistically superior to those of 5-ASA. One of the

27

mechanisms responsible for the enhanced anti-inflammatory activity of NCX-456 over the parent drug is likely to be the ability of the former to suppress leucocyte adherence to the vascular endothelium. We found that NCX-456, but not 5-ASA, prevented chemotaxin-induced leucocyte adherence within post-capillary mesenteric venules[54]. NCX-456 was also found to suppress the release of IL-1β and interferon-γ from lymphocytes, which could further contribute to its beneficial actions in colitis.

SUMMARY

A number of recent studies have provided compelling evidence that prostaglandins produced by the inflamed gut play a critical role in down-regulating the inflammatory response. It would appear that COX-2 is the primary source of prostaglandins in such circumstances, and inhibition of this enzyme can lead to propagation of inflammatory responses. COX-2-derived prostaglandin D_2 may be a particularly important mediator in terms of down-regulating inflammation. Nitric oxide also contributes to the regulation of inflammatory responses in the gastrointestinal tract. The recent finding that a NO-releasing derivative of 5-ASA exhibits markedly enhanced anti-inflammatory effects over the parent drug illustrates the importance of NO in promoting tissue repair and in reducing leucocyte infiltration to sites of inflammation.

Acknowledgements

This work was supported by a grant from the Medical Research Council of Canada (MRC). Dr Ajuebor is supported by an Alberta Heritage Foundation for Medical Research (AHFMR) Fellowship. Dr Wallace is an MRC Senior Scientist and an AHFMR Senior Scientist and holds the Crohn's and Colitis Foundation of Canada Chair in Intestinal Disease Research.

References

1. Kuhn R, Lohler J, Rennick D, Rajewsky K, Muller W. Interleukin-10-deficient mice develop chronic enterocolitis. Cell. 1993;75:263–74.
2. Coleman RA, Smith WL, Narumiya S. VIII International Union of Pharmacology classification of prostanoids receptors: properties, distribution, and structure of the receptors and their subtypes. Pharmacol Rev. 1994;46:205–29.
3. Xie W, Chipman JG, Robertson DL, Erikson RL, Simmons DL. Expression of a mitogen-responsive gene encoding prostaglandin synthase is regulated by mRNA splicing. Proc Natl Acad Sci USA. 1991;88:2692–6.
4. Kargman S, Charleson S, Cartwright M et al. Characterization of prostaglandin G/H synthase 1 and 2 in rat, dog, monkey, and human gastrointestinal tract. Gastroenterology. 1996;111:445–54.
5. Reuter BK, Asfaha S, Buret A, Sharkey KA, Wallace JL. Exacerbation of inflammation-associated colonic injury in rat through inhibition of cyclooxygenase-2. J Clin Invest. 1996;98:2076–85.
6. Singer II, Kawka DW, Schloeman S, Tessner T, Riehl T, Stenson WF. COX-2 is induced in colonic epithelial cells in inflammatory bowel disease. Gastroenterology. 1998;115:297–306.
7. Gould SR, Brash AR, Conolly ME. Increased prostaglandin production in ulcerative colitis. Lancet. 1977;2:98.
8. Sharon P, Ligumsky M, Rachmilewitz D, Zor U. Role of prostaglandins in ulcerative colitis: enhanced production during active disease and inhibition by sulfasalazine. Gastroenterology. 1978;75:638–40.

9. Rampton DS, Sladen GE, Youlten LJF. Rectal mucosal prostaglandin E_2 release and its relation to disease activity; electrical potential difference, and treatment in ulcerative colitis. Gut. 1980;21:591–6.
10. Smith DW, Smith PR, Swan CHJ. Determination of prostaglandin synthetase activity in rectal biopsy material and its significances in colonic disease. Gut. 1978;19:875–7.
11. Harris DW, Smith PR, Swan CHJ. Determination of prostaglandin synthetase activity in rectal biopsy material and its significance in colonic disease. Gut. 1978;19:875–7.
12. Rampton DS, McNeil NI, Sarner M. Analgesic ingestion and other factors preceding relapse in ulcerative colitis. Gut. 1983;24:187–9.
13. Kaufmann HJ, Taubin HL. Nonsteroidal anti-inflammatory drugs activate quiescent inflammatory bowel disease. Ann Intern Med. 1987;107:513–16.
14. Wallace JL, Keenan CM, Gale D, Shoupe TS. Exacerbation of experimental colitis by nonsteroidal anti-inflammatory drugs is not related to elevated leukotriene B_4 synthesis. Gastroenterology. 1992;102:18–27.
15. Wallace JL, Whittle BJR, Boughton-Smith NK. Prostaglandin protection of rat colonic mucosa from damage induced by ethanol. Dig Dis Sci. 1985;30:866–76.
16. Fedorak RN, Empey LR, MacArthur C, Jewell LD. Misoprostol provides a colonic mucosal protective effect during acetic acid-induced colitis in rats. Gastroenterology. 1990;98:615–25.
17. Allgayer H, Deschryver K, Stenson WF. Treatment with 16,16'-dimethylprostaglandin E_2 before and after induction of colitis with trinitrobenzenesulfonic acid in rats decreases inflammation. Gastroenterology. 1989;96:1290–300.
18. Asako H, Kubes P, Wallace J, Gaginella T, Wolf RE, Granger DN. Indomethacin-induced leukocyte adhesion in postcapillary venules: role of lipoxygenase products. Am J Physiol. 1992;262:G903–8.
19. Wong K, Freund F. Inhibition of n-formylmethionyl-leucylphenylalanine induced respiratory burst in human neutrophils by adrenergic agonists and prostaglandins of the E series. Can J Physiol Pharmacol. 1981;59:915–20.
20. Gryglewski RJ, Szczeklik A, Wandzilak M. The effect of six prostaglandins, prostacyclin and iloprost on the generation of superoxide anions by human polymorphonuclear leukocytes stimulated by zymosan or formyl-methionyl-leucyl-phenylalanine. Biochem Pharmacol. 1987;36:4209–12.
21. Wallace JL, Higa A, McKnight GW, MacIntyre DE. Prevention and reversal of experimental colitis by a monoclonal antibody which inhibits leukocyte adherence. Inflammation. 1992;16:343–54.
22. Wallace JL, McKnight W, Asfaha S, Liu DY. Reduction of acute and reactivated colitis in rats by an inhibitor of neutrophil activation. Am J Physiol. 1998;37:G802–8.
23. Yamada T, Grisham MB. Role of neutrophil-derived oxidants in the pathogenesis of intestinal inflammation. Klin Wochenschr. 1991;69:988–94.
24. Ham EA, Soderman DD, Zanetti ME, Dougherty HW, McCauley E, Kuehl FA. Inhibition by prostaglandins of leukotriene B_4 release from activated neutrophils. Proc Natl Acad Sci USA. 1983;80:4349–53.
25. Kainoh M, Imai R, Umetsu T, Hattori M, Nishio S. Prostacyclin and beraprost sodium as suppressors of activated rat polymorphonuclear leukocytes. Biochem Pharmacol. 1990;39:477–84.
26. Wertheim WA, Kunkel SL, Standiford TJ et al. Regulation of neutrophil-derived IL-8: the role of prostaglandin E_2, dexamethasone, and IL-4. J Immunol. 1993;151:2166–75.
27. Hogaboam CM, Bissonnette EY, Chin BC, Befus AD, Wallace JL. Prostaglandins inhibit inflammatory mediator release from rat mast cells. Gastroenterology. 1993;104:122–9.
28. Kunkel SL, Wiggins RC, Chensue SW, Larrick J. Regulation of macrophage tumour necrosis factor production by prostaglandin E2. Biochem Biophys Res Commun. 1986;137:404–10.
29. Kunkel SL, Chensue SW. Arachidonic acid metabolites regulate interleukin-1 production. Biochem Biophys Res Commun. 1985;128:892–7.
30. Morteau O, Morham S, Sellon S, Smithies O, Sarton RB. Genetic deficiency in cyclooxygenase-2 but not in cyclooxygenase-1 exacerbates DSS-induced acute colitis in mice. Gastroenterology. 1997;112:A1046.
31. Flannigan A. Pharmacological inhibition and cyclooxygenase (COX)-2 gene knockout intensifies dextran sulfate (DSS)-induced colitis in mice. Gastroenterology. 1999;116:A880.
32. Wallace JL, Bak A, McKnight W, Asfaha S, Sharkey KA, MacNaughton WK. Cyclooxygenase-1 contributes to inflammatory responses in rats and mice: implications for GI toxicity. Gastroenterology. 1998;115:101–9.

33. Gilroy D, Colville-Nash PR, Willis D, Chivers J, Paul-Clark MJ. Inducible cyclooxygenase may have anti-inflammatory properties. Nature Med. 1999;5: 698–701.
34. Beckman JS, Beckman TW, Chen J, Marshall PA, Freeman BA. Apparent hydroxyl radical production by peroxynitrite: implications for endothelial injury from nitric oxide and superoxide. Proc Natl Acad Sci USA. 1990;87:1620–4.
35. Boughton-Smith NK, Evans SM, Hawkey CJ *et al.* Nitric oxide synthase activity in ulcerative colitis and Crohn's disease. Lancet. 1993;342:338–40.
36. Rachmilewitz D, Stamler JS, Bachwich D, Karmeli F, Ackerman Z, Podolsky DK. Enhanced colonic nitric oxide generation and nitric oxide synthase activity in ulcerative colitis and Crohn's disease. Gut. 1995;36:718–23.
37. Miller MJS, Thompson JH, Zhang XJ *et al.* Role of inducible nitric oxide synthase expression and peroxynitrite formation in guinea pig ileitis. Gastroenterology. 1995;109:1475–83.
38. Kimura H, Hokari R, Miura S *et al.* Increased expression of an inducible isoform of nitric oxide synthase and the formation of peroxynitrite in colonic mucosa of patients with active ulcerative colitis. Gut. 1998;42:180–7.
39. Eiserich JP, Hristova M, Cross CE *et al.* Formation of nitric oxide-derived inflammatory oxidants by myeloperoxidase in neutrophils. Nature. 1998;391:393–7.
40. Hogaboam CM, Jacobson K, Collins SM, Blennerhassett MG. The selective beneficial effects of nitric oxide inhibition in experimental colitis. Am J Physiol. 1995;268:G673–84.
41. Rachmilewitz D, Karmeli F, Okon E, Bursztyn M. Experimental colitis is ameliorated by inhibition of nitric oxide synthase activity. Gut. 1995;37:247–55.
42. Rachmilewitz D, Karmeli F, Okon E. Sulfhydryl blocker-induced rat colonic inflammation is ameliorated by inhibition of nitric oxide synthase. Gastroenterology. 1995;109:98–106
43. Ribbons KA, Currie MG, Connor JR *et al.* The effect of inhibitors of inducible nitric oxide synthase on chronic colitis in the rhesus monkey. J Pharmacol Exp Ther. 1997;280:1008–15.
44. Southey A, Tanaka S, Murakami T *et al.* Pathophysiological role of nitric oxide in experimental colitis. Int J Immunopharmacol. 1997;19:669–76.
45. McCafferty DM, Mudgett JS, Swain MG, Kubes P. Inducible nitric oxide synthase plays a critical role in resolving intestinal inflammation. Gastroenterology. 1997;112:1022–7.
46. McCafferty DM, Muscara MN, Wallace JL, Kubes P. Role of inducible nitric oxide synthase in spontaneously developing colitis in mice. Gastroenterology. 1999;116:A773.
47. Kubes P, Suzuki M, Granger DN. Nitric oxide: an endogenous modulator of leukocyte adhesion. Proc Natl Acad Sci USA. 1991;88:4651–5.
48. Hogaboam CM, Befus AD, Wallace JL. Modulation of rat mast cell reactivity by IL-1 beta. Divergent effects on nitric oxide and platelet-activating factor release. J Immunol. 1993;151:3767–74.
49. Masini E, Salvemini D, Pistelli A, Mannaioni PF, Vane JR. Rat mast cells synthesize a nitric oxide like-factor which modulates the release of histamine. Agents Actions. 1991;33:61–3.
50. Radomski MW, Moncada S. Regulation of vascular homeostasis by nitric oxide. Thromb Haemost. 1993;70:36–41.
51. Elliott SN, McKnight W, Cirino G, Wallace JL. A nitric oxide-releasing nonsteroidal anti-inflammatory drug accelerates gastric ulcer healing in rats. Gastroenterology. 1995;109:524–30.
52. Lund JN, Scholefield JH. Glyceryl trinitrate is an effective treatment for anal fissure. Dis Colon Rectum. 1997;40:468–70.
53. Wallace JL, Reuter B, Cicala C, McKnight W, Grisham MB, Cirino G. Novel nonsteroidal anti-inflammatory drug derivatives with markedly reduced ulcerogenic properties in the rat. Gastroenterology. 1994;107:173–9.
54. Wallace JL, Vergnolle N, Muscará MN *et al.* Enhanced anti-inflammatory effects of a nitric oxide-releasing derivative of mesalamine in rats. Gastroenterology. 1999;117:557–66.

4
New cytokines and their impact in mucosal pathogenesis

M. F. NEURATH, C. BECKER, J. MUDTER, R. ATREYA,
K. HILDNER, S. WIRTZ and S. FINOTTO

The important role of cytokines produced by cells of the mucosal immune system in the pathogenesis of intestinal inflammation has been widely accepted[1,2]. This review focuses on the role of two novel immunoregulatory cytokines in mucosal inflammation, namely IL-12 and IL-18.

Although the aetiology of inflammatory bowel diseases (IBD) remains unknown, recent studies in mice and humans have led to clear progress in our understanding of the pathogenesis of chronic intestinal inflammation. For instance, there is now increasing evidence for changes of mucosal immuno-regulation in patients with IBD[1]. One aspect of this altered immunoregulation is a hyperresponsiveness to mucosal antigens caused by a dysregulated immune response to otherwise less immunogenic or harmless products of the intestinal flora. Furthermore, it was shown that development of chronic intestinal inflammation in various animal models of IBD is abrogated when mice are kept under germfree conditions. Based on these results, loss of tolerance and hyper-responsiveness to mucosal antigens emerge as potential key events in the patho-genesis of IBD.

Furthermore, there is strong evidence to suggest that cells of the mucosal immune system (such as epithelial cells, B cells, macrophages and T lympho-cytes) and their products (e.g. growth factors, cytokines) play an important role in the pathogenesis of chronic intestinal inflammation[3-6]. For instance, it has been shown that a dysbalance between pro- and anti-inflammatory cytokines in various transgenic (e.g. IL-7) and knockout mice (e.g. IL-2, IL-10, STAT-3) can cause chronic intestinal inflammation. Furthermore, production of large amounts of Th1-type cytokines such as interferon-γ by CD4+ T cells and TNF by mono-cytes is a major feature of the inflammation in many Th1 colitis models[7,8]. In contrast, Th2 and Th3-type cytokines appear to mediate protection from Th1-initiated tissue injury[5,9]. However, two recent reports have shown that also Th2-type cytokines may mediate mucosal inflammation in two animal models of intestinal inflammation, namely colitis in T cell receptor (TCR) knockout mice and mice with oxazolone-induced colitis[10,11]. The pathogenic role of IL-4 in the former model was shown by the fact that IL-4 TCR double knockout mice, but not IFN-γ TCR knockout mice fail to develop colitis. In the latter model, antibodies to IL-4 have been successfully used to treat experimental colitis.

Based on the above data there was considerable interest to determine additional factors and cytokines that may modulate the Th1/Th2 pathway in the inflamed gut. In addition to IL-4, two important molecules that have been previously shown to modulate IFN-γ production by T cells consist of IL-12 and IL-18. IL-12 is a cytokine mainly produced by dendritic cells and macrophages that has been shown to induce Th1 T cell development *in vitro* and *in vivo* in various animal models of autoimmune diseases[12–14]. The molecular basis for this function is the activation of the transcription factor signal transducer and activator of transcription (STAT)-4 that *trans*-activates together with AP-1 the human IFN-γ promoter in primary T cells (Fig. 1)[15,16].

The essential role of IL-12 in chronic intestinal inflammation has been shown by studies in Th1 animal models using neutralizing anti-IL-12 antibodies that led to an abrogation or suppression of intestinal inflammation[7]. These data suggested that Th1 cytokine production in models of chronic intestinal inflammation is triggered by increased production of IL-12 heterodimer. The importance of IL-12 in TH1-mediated animal models is also demonstrated by the fact that STAT-4 transgenic mice develop Th1-dependent chronic intestinal inflammation and that anti-IL-12 antibodies lead to abrogation of such TH1-mediated colonic inflammation. The relevance of these findings to Crohn's disease in humans is underlined by recent studies showing that this disease is also associated with an excessive Th1 T-cell response driven by IL-12-producing lamina propria (LP) T cells[17]. Recent evidence suggests that IL-12 activates not only Th1 T cells but also matrix metalloproteinases in the gut (Monteleone and Pender, unpublished data), thus directly mediating tissue injury in the inflamed intestine.

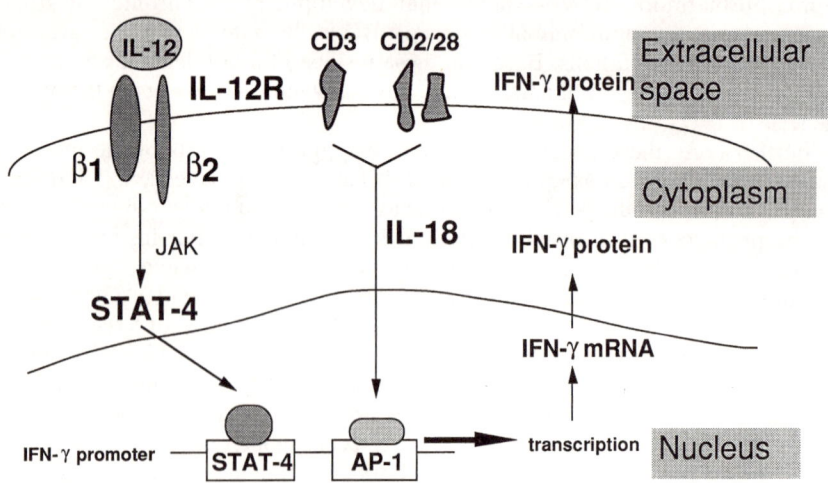

Figure 1   Function of IL-12 and IL-18 in mucosal Th1 T cells

The role of IL-18 in mucosal inflammation has only been preliminarily characterized. It is a pro-inflammatory cytokine mainly produced by monocytes and macrophages that activates IFN-γ production by Th1 T cells via a specific surface receptor. The molecular pathway that mediates this effect appears to be an activation of two transcription factors (NF-κB and AP-1) that in turn *trans*-activate the human IFN-γ promoter in primary T cells (Fig. 1)[15]. In mice with dextran sulphate colitis, antibodies to IL-18 have been used to suppress colitis activity. However, recent data (Finotto *et al.*, unpublished data) indicate that overexpression of IL-18 in a transgenic mouse model is not sufficient to cause mucosal immunopathology. However, the potentially potent function of IL-18 in human IBD has been shown by studies in which IL-18 expression was found to be up-regulated in lamina propria macrophages and intestinal epithelial cells in patients with Crohn's disease but not ulcerative colitis[18]. In addition, antisense DNA to IL-18 caused a marked suppression of IFN-γ protein production by human lamina propria cells in this disease. These data suggest a scenario in which IL-12 and IL-18 collaborate to induce and maintain an active Th1 cytokine profile by human lamina propria CD4+ T cells in Crohn's disease.

Taken together, IL-12 and IL-18 appear to play a predominant role in the regulation of mucosal Th1/Th2 pathways. Based on these observations it appears to be possible to design rational immunotherapeutic strategies for Crohn's disease patients, and one of these concepts (anti-IL-12) is currently approaching clinical phase II trials in this disease.

References

1. Duchmann R, Zeitz M. Crohn's disease. In: Ogra P, Strober J, editors. Handbook of Mucosal Immunology. New York: Academic Press; 1999:S1055.
2. Strober W, Neurath MF. Immunological diseases of the gastrointestinal tract. In: Rich RR, editor. Clinical Immunology. St Louis: Mosby; 1995:1401.
3. Autschbach F, Schurmann G, Qiao L et al. Cytokine messenger RNA expression and proliferation status of intestinal mononuclear cells in noninflamed gut and Crohn's disease. Virchows Arch. 1995;426:51.
4. Dullemen Hv, Deventer Sv, Hommes D et al. Treatment of Crohn's disease with anti-tumor necrosis factor chimeric monoclonal antibody (cA2). Gastroenterology. 1995;109:129.
5. Neurath MF, Fuss I, Kelsall BL et al. Experimental granulomatous colitis in mice is abrogated by induction of TGF-mediated oral tolerance. J Exp Med. 1996;183:2515.
6. Plevy SE, Landers CJ, Prehn J et al. A role for TNF-alpha and mucosal T helper-1 cytokines in the pathogenesis of Crohn's disease. J Immunol. 1997;159:6276.
7. Neurath MF, Fuss I, Kelsall BL, Stuber E, Strober W. Antibodies to IL-12 abrogate established experimental colitis in mice. J Exp Med. 1995;182:1280.
8. Powrie F, Leach MW, Mauze S et al. Inhibition of Th1 responses prevents inflammatory bowel disease in scid mice reconstituted with CD45RBhi CD4+ T cells. Immunity. 1994;2:553.
9. Powrie F, Carlino J, Leach MW, Mauze S, Coffman RL. A critical role for transforming growth factor-beta but not interleukin-4 in the suppression of T helper type 1-mediated colitis by CD45Rb(low) CD4+ T cells. J Exp Med. 1996;183:2669.
10. Boirivant M, Fuss IJ, Chu A, Strober W. Oxazolone colitis: a murine model of T helper cell type 2 colitis treatable with antibodies to interleukin 4. J Exp Med. 1998;188:1929.
11. Mizoguchi A, Mizoguchi E, Bhan AK. The critical role of interleukin 4 but not interferon gamma in the pathogenesis of colitis in T-cell receptor alpha mutant mice. Gastroenterology. 1999;116:320.
12. Kubin M, Kamoun M, Trinchieri G. Interleukin-12 synergizes with B7/CD28 interaction in inducing efficient proliferation and cytokine production of human T cells. J Exp Med. 1994;180:211.

13. Magram J, Connaughton SE, Warrier RR *et al*. IL-12-deficient mice are defective in IFN-gamma production and type 1 cytokine responses. Immunity. 1996;4:471.
14. Seder RA, Gazzinelli R, Sher A, Paul WE. IL-12 acts directly on CD4+ T cells to enhance priming for IFN-gamma production and diminishes IL-4 inhibition of such priming. Proc Natl Acad Sci USA. 1993;90:10188.
15. Barbulescu K, Becker C, Schlaak J *et al*. Cutting edge: interleukin-12 and interleukin-18 differentially regulate the transcriptional activity of the human IFN-gamma promoter in primary CD4+ T lymphocytes. J Immunol. 1998;160:3642.
16. Thierfelder WE, vanDeursen JM, Yamamoto K *et al*. Functional diversity of helper T lymphocytes. Nature. 1996;383:787.
17. Monteleone G, Biancone L, Marasco R *et al*. Interleukin-12 is expressed and actively released by Crohn's disease intestinal lamina propria mononuclear cells. Gastroenterology. 1997;112:1169.
18. Pizarro TT, Michie MH, Bentz M *et al*. IL-18, a novel immunoregulatory cytokine, is up-regulated in Crohn's disease: expression and localization in intestinal mucosal cells. J Immunol. 1999;162:6829.

5
Keratinocyte growth factor, activin and connective tissue growth factor: novel players in inflammatory bowel disease

H. STEILING, M. BRAUCHLE, W. FALK and S. WERNER

INTRODUCTION

Injury to adult tissues initiates a series of events including inflammation, new tissue formation and matrix remodelling which finally lead to repair of the lesion. However, in chronic inflammatory processes repair is often inhibited, and severe tissue destruction, fibrosis and finally loss of organ function can occur. The inflammatory reaction, the repair process, as well as the development of fibrosis are regulated by a wide variety of cytokines, growth and differentiation factors which have only partially been identified.

Recent studies from our laboratory have provided insight into the roles of keratinocyte growth factor, activin and connective tissue growth factor in cutaneous wound repair as well as in inflammatory bowel disease (IBD). The latter is a multifactorial disease of the gut and comprises two major forms of severe intestinal inflammation: Crohn's disease (CD) and ulcerative colitis (UC). Both chronic disorders are characterized by their unpredictable course with acute inflammatory phases followed by remission. Patients suffer from abdominal pain, weight loss, recurrent fever and diarrhoea. In CD, segments of inflamed tissue are adjacent to apparently non-affected gut and are mainly found in the terminal ileum, whereas UC is a disease of the colon with continuous inflammation usually extending from the rectum for a variable distance proximally. Histologically, damage of the mesenchyme and the intestinal epithelium is observed, accompanied by massive infiltration with various types of inflammatory cells. In addition, ulceration often occurs. Further complications of CD are the presence of granulomas, fissures and fistulas. Fibrosis, leading to stenosis and obstruction, is a major complication in CD but is seen only rarely in UC. Finally, UC patients have an increased risk of developing colon cancer (reviewed in ref. 1).

In spite of extensive clinical and experimental studies the aetiology of IBD is still unknown, and there is still no therapy apart from counteracting the symptoms using anti-inflammatory drugs or surgical resection of the affected part. However, recent molecular studies have provided some new insight into the roles of growth factors and cytokines in the pathogenesis of IBD. In our laboratory a role of keratinocyte growth factor (KGF), activin and connective tissue growth factor (CTGF) in cutaneous wound repair has recently been demonstrated[2–6]. Due to the similarities between cutaneous wound repair and inflammatory and repair processes in the intestine we speculated about a novel role of these factors in IBD. Indeed, we found a strong up-regulation of all of these factors in affected areas of patients suffering from UC and CD, and first results regarding their possible function in these disorders were recently obtained.

KERATINOCYTE GROWTH FACTOR

KGF was initially discovered by its mitogenicity for a lung fibroblast cell line[7]. It is a monomeric, glycosylated polypeptide which is produced by various types of mesenchymal cells *in vitro* and *in vivo* as well as by $\gamma\delta$T cells obtained from skin and intestine (reviewed in ref. 8). KGF expression has not yet been detected in cells of epithelial origin. However, most types of epithelial cells express FGFR2-IIIb, the only known high-affinity receptor for KGF[9], and these cells were shown to respond to KGF *in vitro* and *in vivo* (for review see ref. 8). These results suggested that KGF acts predominantly in a paracrine manner. Such a paracrine action of KGF seems to occur in various tissues and organs, particularly after injury. Thus increased expression of KGF in mesenchymal cells adjacent to the site of injury has frequently been observed (reviewed in ref. 8). The effects of this increased expression have been analysed in most detail in the skin. We and others demonstrated a weak expression of KGF in murine and human skin. However, expression of this mitogen was strikingly induced in dermal fibroblasts upon skin injury[2,10]. By contrast, the KGF receptor was exclusively expressed on keratinocytes of the epidermis and the hair follicles. This expression pattern of KGF and its receptor suggested that dermally derived KGF stimulates repair of the injured epidermis in a paracrine manner. This hypothesis was supported by the wound-healing phenotype seen in transgenic mice which express a dominant-negative KGF receptor in the basal keratinocytes of the epidermis and in the outer root sheath keratinocytes of the hair follicles. These mice were characterized by a severe delay in wound re-epithelialization[3], demonstrating the importance of KGF receptor signalling during cutaneous wound repair. Surprisingly, mice lacking KGF revealed no phenotypic abnormalities and even the healing process of incisional wounds appeared normal[11], suggesting that other KGF receptor ligands can compensate for the lack of KGF. The most likely candidate for such a compensatory effect is FGF-10, which is highly homologous to KGF[12] and which binds to the KGF receptor with high affinity[13]. Recent studies from our laboratory have provided new insight into the mechanisms of KGF action. We have identified a series of genes which are regulated by KGF in keratinocytes and these genes might help to explain how KGF regulates proliferation, differentiation and migration of keratinocytes during wound

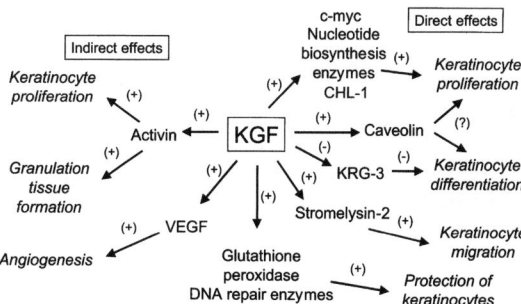

Figure 1 Overview of KGF-regulated genes. The products of the genes shown on the right-hand side are likely to mediate the direct effects of KGF, whereas those on the left-hand side could be responsible for the indirect effects of KGF on mesenchymal cells. VEGF: Vascular endothelial growth factor; CHL-1: human homologue of a yeast gene involved in chromosome segregation; KRG-3: KGF-regulated gene 3; putative transcription factor involved in keratinocyte differentiation

repair, and how it exerts indirect effects on mesenchymal cells (summarized in Fig. 1). Finally, the identification of a novel glutathione peroxidase as a KGF-regulated gene[14] is likely to provide an explanation for the protective effect of KGF for various types of epithelial cells (reviewed in ref. 8).

INCREASED EXPRESSION OF KGF IN IBD

Due to the strong overexpression of KGF after skin injury we speculated about a similar up-regulation of this growth factor in the injured gut. For this purpose we analysed the expression of KGF and its receptor in surgical specimens from control patients and from patients suffering from IBD. Interestingly, we and others found a strongly increased expression of KGF mRNA and protein in the mucosa and submucosa of the affected areas of CD and UC patients, whereby the degree of KGF overexpression showed a strong correlation with the degree of inflammation[15,16] (Figs 2 and 3). By *in-situ* hybridization and immuno-histochemical staining we found particularly high levels of KGF mRNA and protein in mesenchymal cells of the lamina propria, particularly in close proximity to inflammatory cells. Since these cells produce high levels of pro-inflammatory cytokines in IBD[17], and since KGF expression is strongly stimulated by interleukin-1 (IL-1) and tumour necrosis factor alpha (TNF-α)[18,19], inflammatory cell-derived cytokines are likely to be responsible for the increased expression of KGF in patients suffering from CD and UC. In addition, serum growth factors which are released in the inflamed bowel upon haemorrhage, a process that is frequently seen in CD patients, might further enhance the expression of KGF in mucosal fibroblasts.

Whereas our studies and those of Finch *et al.*[16] did not compare the relative expression levels of KGF between CD and UC patients, Bajaj-Elliott *et al.*[20] demonstrated a significantly higher expression of KGF in CD patients compared to UC patients because of increased production of KGF by mucosal mesenchymal cells.

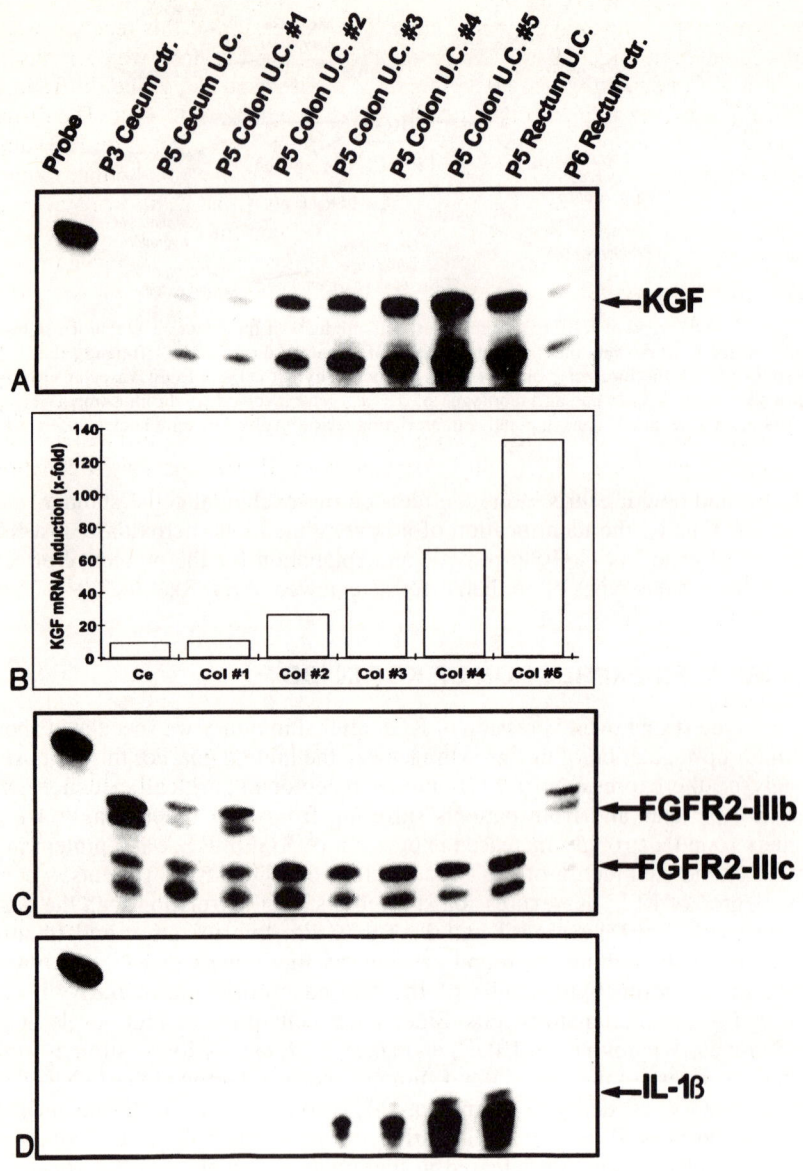

In contrast to KGF, its only known high-affinity receptor was exclusively present on the intestinal epithelial cells. The expression of this receptor was not up-regulated in affected areas, and in highly inflamed regions we even observed a strongly reduced expression[15] (Fig. 2). This is most likely due to the loss of FGFR2-IIIb-expressing epithelial cells in these regions of the gut. The distribution of KGF and its receptor in IBD is reminiscent of the situation in wounded skin. Therefore, KGF is likely to act in a paracrine manner to stimulate epithelial repair not only in the skin but also in the intestine. In addition to its mitogenic effect, KGF has also been shown to protect intestinal epithelial cells from chemotherapy- or radiation-induced damage[21], most likely by increasing intestinal epithelial stem cell survival[22]. Thus the increased levels of KGF in the inflamed gut might prevent additional loss of intestinal epithelial cells.

A role of KGF in the stimulation of intestinal epithelial cell proliferation might also be exploited therapeutically, since KGF has recently been shown to reduce the extent of intestinal injury in trinitrobenzene-sulphonic acid/ethanol-induced colitis in rats when administered intraperitoneally after induction of colitis[23]. Furthermore, KGF and its homologue FGF-10 were able to ameliorate dextran sodium sulphate-induced colitis in mice[24,25]. These data suggest a key role of KGF in the maintenance of the integrity of the colonic mucosa and its possible use in the treatment of IBD. Finally, the protective effect of KGF for intestinal stem cells suggests the use of this growth factor to lessen the intestinal side-effects of current cancer therapy regimens.

ACTIVIN

Activins, which belong to the TGF-β superfamily of growth and differentiation factors, are dimeric proteins, the monomeric polypeptides of which are connected by disulphide linkage. Three different forms of activin, activin A (βAβA), activin B (βBβB), as well as activin AB (βAβB) have been characterized (reviewed in refs 26 and 27). Furthermore, βC, βD, and βE chains have been discovered[28–30], although the function of the corresponding proteins is as yet unknown. Activins influence proliferation and differentiation of many different cell types (reviewed in ref. 27), but a role of activin in normal and wounded skin and in the gastrointestinal tract has only recently been demonstrated.

Figure 2 Increased expression of KGF and FGFR2 mRNA in the intestine of IBD patients. Surgical specimens from different areas of the caecum, colon, and rectum were obtained from a UC patient (P5). Tissue specimens from the caecum and rectum of control patients (P3 and P6) were used as controls; 30 μg total cellular RNA was analysed by RNase protection assay for expression of KGF (**A**), FGFR2 (**C**), and IL-1β (**D**). The degree of KGF overexpression in the caecum and in different areas of the colon of patient P5 (colon specimens 1–5) in comparison with the caecum of control patient P3 was assessed by laser scanning densitometry of the autoradiograms and is shown schematically in **B**. In **C**, transcripts encoding FGFR2-IIIb (KGF receptor splice variant) and FGFR2-IIIc (mesenchymal splice variant which does not bind KGF) give rise to different protected fragments as indicated on the right side of the figure. A total of 1000 cpm of the hybridization probes were loaded in the lanes labelled 'probe' and used as size markers. Reprinted from ref. 15, with permission from the American Society for Investigative Pathology

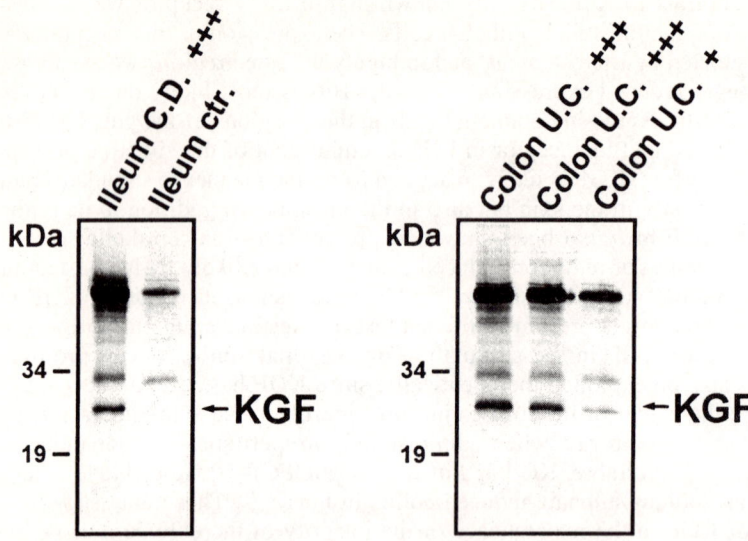

Figure 3 Increased expression of KGF protein in the intestine of UC and CD patients. Surgical specimens from the ileum of a CD patient and a control patient (left side) and from different areas of the colon of a UC patient (right side) were frozen in liquid nitrogen and homogenized. KGF proteins were enriched by their capacity to bind to heparin sepharose and analysed by Western-blotting using a KGF-specific polyclonal antiserum. The number of plus signs indicates the degree of inflammation: +, low degree of inflammation; +++, high degree of inflammation. Reprinted from ref. 15, with permission from the American Society for Investigative Pathology.

In the skin, activin is barely detectable under normal conditions, but we observed a strikingly increased expression of both the βA and the βB chain after cutaneous injury. Interestingly, activin transcripts were detectable in the granulation tissue as well as in the redifferentiating suprabasal cells of the hyperproliferative epithelium at the wound edge, indicating a role of activin in the repair of the mesenchyme and the epidermis[4]. To gain insight into the activities of activin in the skin we generated transgenic mice which overexpress activin in the basal keratinocytes of the epidermis and in hair follicle keratinocytes under the control of a keratin 14 promoter[6]. The transgenic mice were characterized by severe epidermal hyperthickening, abnormalities in keratinocyte organization and differentiation, and also by a replacement of fatty tissue by connective tissue. After skin injury a strong enhancement of the wound-healing process was observed in the transgenic mice, whereby the process of granulation tissue formation was particularly enhanced. Similar to non-wounded skin, the increased levels of activin stimulated extracellular matrix synthesis/deposition, indicating a role of activin in fibrotic processes. This hypothesis is supported by the detection of high levels of activin in fibrotic kidneys[31,32], cirrhotic livers[33,34], and in arteriosclerosis[35,36].

40

INCREASED EXPRESSION OF ACTIVIN A IN IBD

Due to the strong induction of activin expression after cutaneous injury we speculated about a role of activin in inflammatory processes of the intestine. Therefore, we analysed the expression of activin in the gut of control patients and of patients suffering from IBD. The activin βA chain was not detectable in the normal human gut. However, a strong expression was seen in surgical specimens obtained from affected areas of IBD patients. Interestingly, the levels of activin βA mRNA expression showed an outstanding correlation with the degree of inflammation as assessed by histological analysis of adjacent tissue and by expression analysis of the pro-inflammatory cytokine IL-1β[37] (Fig. 4). Since activin expression has been shown to be stimulated by pro-inflammatory cytokines in mesenchymal and epithelial cells[38], these factors are likely to be responsible for the increased expression of activin in IBD. In addition, serum growth factors are strong inducers of activin expression in fibroblasts[38]. Consistent with these observations, our *in-situ* hybridizations revealed the presence of particularly high levels of activin βA mRNA in fibroblasts adjacent to fibrin clots which result from local haemorrhage. Therefore, the release of serum growth factors upon haemorrhage could stimulate activin expression in adjacent fibroblasts. Strong *in-situ* hybridization signals were seen in regions where the intestinal epithelium was distorted and where a massive accumulation of inflammatory cells was observed (Fig. 5). Activated monocytes and macrophages are known to produce activin βA *in vitro* and *in vivo*[34,39]. These cells are abundant in the inflammatory infiltrate in both UC and CD[40] and may therefore contribute to the strong activin expression in IBD.

The role of activin in the pathogenesis of IBD is as yet unknown. The enhancement of the wound-healing process in our transgenic mice which express activin in the skin suggests a general role of activin in repair processes, particularly in the repair of the injured mesenchyme. Furthermore, activin could play a role in differentiation processes of gastrointestinal epithelial cells as recently demonstrated for the gastric epithelium[41]. Finally, the increased levels of activin might also lead to the development of fibrosis, as suggested by the dermal phenotype of the mice which overexpress activin in the skin and by the increased expression of this factor in various types of fibrotic disease (see above). Therefore, activin could also be involved in the fibrotic processes in the intestine, particularly in CD where fibrosis is a frequent complication. Thus the inhibition of activin action may represent a novel strategy for reducing fibrotic processes in this disease.

CONNECTIVE TISSUE GROWTH FACTOR (CTGF)

CTGF is a member of a rapidly growing protein family, now designated as the CNN (*CTGF*/*c*ysteine-rich 61/*n*ephroblastoma overexpressed) family (reviewed in ref. 42). It is expressed in a wide variety of tissues and organs[5,42]. It stimulates proliferation and chemotaxis of fibroblasts directly[43] and it enhances the mitogenic effect of other growth factors[44]. Most importantly, CTGF strongly stimulates expression of the extracellular matrix proteins collagen type I and fibronectin, as well as of integrin α5 by fibroblasts[45]. Due to these properties,

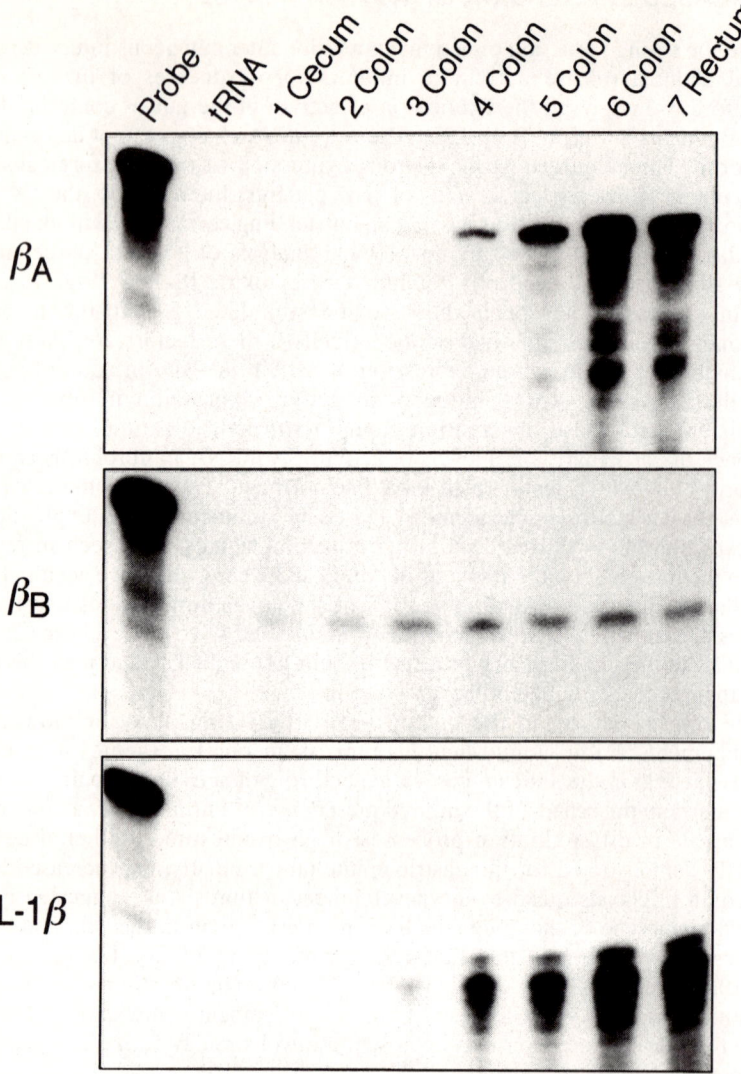

Figure 4 Expression of activin βA mRNA in the colon of a UC patient correlates with the degree of inflammation. RNA from the surgical specimens of UC patient 5 (Fig. 2) was used for the analysis of activin βA and βB expression. The IL-1β protection assay is shown for comparison; 50 μg tRNA were used as a negative control. A total of 1000 cpm of the hybridization probes were loaded in the lanes labelled 'probe' and used as a size marker. Note the high expression levels of both IL-1β and activin βA. Reprinted from ref. 37 with permission from Williams & Wilkins.

CTGF plays an important role in connective tissue cell proliferation and extra-cellular matrix deposition. Interestingly, it seems to act as a mediator of TGF-β_1 in these processes[46,47]. Various laboratories have shown a strong overexpression of CTGF in many types of fibrotic and inflammatory disease, including fibrotic

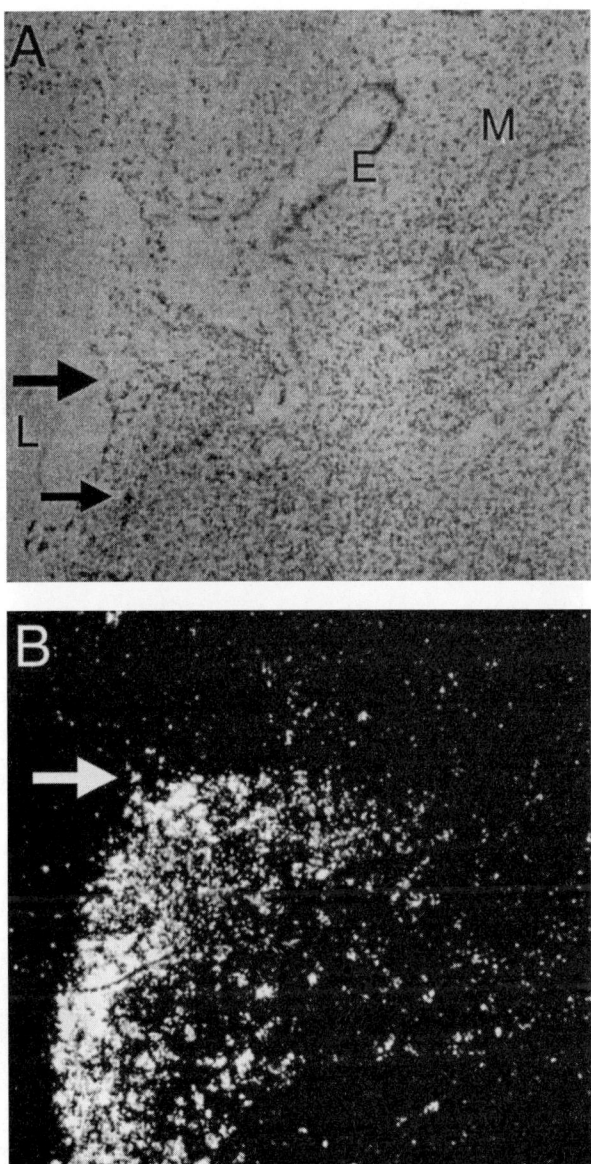

Figure 5 Detection of activin βA mRNA in the ileum of a CD patient by *in-situ* hybridization. Surgical specimens were fixed in 4% paraformaldehyde and frozen in tissue freezing medium. Frozen sections were hybridized with a ^{35}S-labelled riboprobe and counterstained with haematoxylin and eosin. The section was taken from a region of the ileum where highly inflamed tissue (tissue on the left side of the large arrow) could be clearly distinguished from relatively normal tissue (tissue on the right side of the large arrow). Activin βA-expressing cells are indicated by a thin arrow and appear white in the dark field (**B**). E, intestinal epithelium; M, mesenchyme; L, intestinal lumen. Original magnification ×400. Reprinted from ref. 37 with permission from Williams & Wilkins

skin disease[48,49], lung and kidney fibrosis[50,51], and advanced arteriosclerotic lesions[52]. In addition to these pathological situations, we and others found increased levels of CTGF mRNA and/or protein in normal repair processes of the skin[5,53].

INCREASED EXPRESSION OF CTGF IN IBD

The strong expression of CTGF in injured tissues, and its association with fibrotic disease, tempted us to speculate about a role of this growth factor in IBD. Indeed, we found a strong overexpression of CTGF in affected tissue from both CD and UC patients (Fig. 6). In most specimens we found a strong correlation of the levels of CTGF mRNA with the degree of inflammation, suggesting a role of CTGF in the normal repair process of the damaged tissue. Interestingly, specimens which were taken from highly fibrotic areas of CD patients where stenosis had occurred also revealed high levels of CTGF transcripts, even in the absence of a strong inflammatory infiltrate[54]. This result suggests the existence of a specific population of fibroblasts in CD patients which continues to express CTGF beyond the phase of acute inflammation. Such

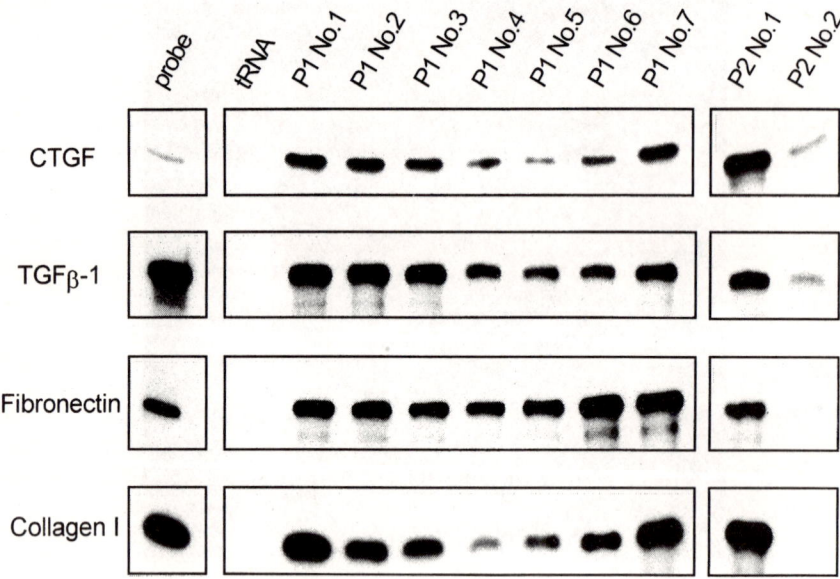

Figure 6 Expression of the CTGF-inducer TGF-β_1, as well as of its target genes collagen type I and fibronectin, correlates with CTGF mRNA expression in Crohn's disease. Surgical specimens from the ileum and caecum were obtained from two patients with CD (P4 and P5); 30 μg (CTGF and TGF-β_1) or 10 μg (collagen type I α chain and fibronectin) of total cellular RNA were analysed by RNase protection assay. The same set of RNAs was used for hybridization with the four different riboprobes; 20 μg tRNA were used as a negative control. A total of 1000 cpm of the hybridization probes were loaded in the lanes labelled 'probe' and used as size markers. Reprinted from ref. 54 with permission from Elsevier Science Ltd

a fibroblast population might be missing in UC patients who rarely develop fibrosis. In addition, differences in metalloproteinase expression between CD and UC patients could be important for the different scarring response in both types of disease as suggested by Matthes et al.[55].

The factors which stimulate CTGF expression in affected areas of IBD patients have as yet not been identified. However, the exclusive induction of CTGF expression by TGF-β_1 in vitro[53] suggests a role of this growth and differentiation factor in CTGF regulation in vivo. Consistent with this hypothesis we found a strong correlation between CTGF and TGF-β_1 expression in normal and affected areas of IBD patients by RNase protection assay (Fig. 6). Furthermore, co-localization of TGF-β_1-producing cells and CTGF-expressing fibroblasts was observed[54]. Finally, TGF-β_1 is present in large amounts in platelets from which it is released upon haemorrhage, a frequent event in IBD.

One of the most important features of CTGF is its potent stimulatory effect on extracellular matrix production. This biological activity might also be important in IBD, since we found a strong correlation between the expression of CTGF, fibronectin and collagen type I (Fig. 6). Therefore, these molecules might also be targets of CTGF action in vivo, indicating that CTGF stimulates extracellular matrix synthesis/deposition in the affected tissue. Although this is likely to be beneficial for the initial repair process, prolonged expression of CTGF could induce fibrosis. Therefore, the inhibition of CTGF action may slow down or even prevent fibrotic disease progression, as suggested by Grotendorst[56]. Thus CTGF could serve as a potential target for antifibrotic therapy in various types of fibrotic disease and also in CD.

Since IBD patients are frequently treated with anti-inflammatory steroids, we analysed the effect of glucocorticoids on the expression of CTGF in vitro and in vivo. Surprisingly, we found[5] a strong stimulation of CTGF mRNA and protein expression by dexamethasone in cultured fibroblasts which occurred independently of TGF-β_1. Most importantly, increased expression of CTGF was also observed in various mouse tissues and organs within 1–3 days of administration of pharmacological doses of glucocorticoids, demonstrating that this stimulatory effect of dexamethasone on CTGF expression is biologically important. This finding might at least partly explain the phenomenon that steroids can further increase the fibrotic condition in certain patients, as observed for the mineralocorticoid aldosterone in cardiac fibrosis. Aldosterone uses the same receptor as glucocorticoids in non-epithelial cells and therefore exerts the same effects as glucocorticoids in these cells[57]. By contrast, other types of fibrosis seem to benefit from glucocorticoid treatment; for example most forms of liver and lung fibrosis[58]. In addition, matrix deposition during cutaneous wound healing is strikingly reduced by dexamethasone[59], leading to a severe delay in wound repair. Therefore, we speculated that the CTGF induction by dexamethasone might be counteracted by other factors under these circumstances. Indeed, dexamethasone treatment of mice had no significant effect on the CTGF mRNA levels during wound repair, whereas the levels in non-wounded skin were significantly reduced. Because serum growth factors which are abundant in acute wounds have no effect on CTGF mRNA expression[53], pro-inflammatory cytokines such as IL-1α or TNF-α, which are present at high levels in wounded skin[60], might be the most likely candidates. Indeed, TNF-α but not IL-1β

suppressed the basal expression of CTGF in exponentially growing fibroblasts. Most importantly, it completely abolished the induction of CTGF mRNA expression by dexamethasone in these cells. These results suggest that dexamethasone up-regulates CTGF expression in various tissues and organs, although this increased expression is likely to be counteracted by TNF-α and possibly other cytokines in inflamed areas. Due to the strong effect of CTGF on extracellular matrix production, our finding might at least partially explain the phenomenon that glucocorticoid treatment can sometimes even aggravate the course of fibrotic disease, and indicates the use of a combination of anti-inflammatory steroids and CTGF inhibitors for the treatment of fibrotic disease, including IBD.

Acknowledgements

We thank Prof. Dr Michael Gregor, Dr D. Wagner and Dr H. Allgayer for providing surgical IBD specimens. Work in our laboratory is supported by the German Ministry for Education and Research, the Human Frontier Science Program and the Stiftung Verum.

References

1. Podolsky DK. Inflammatory bowel disease. N Engl J Med. 1991;325:928–37.
2. Werner S, Peters KG, Longaker MT, Fuller-Pace F, Banda M, Williams LT. Large induction of keratinocyte growth factor expression in the dermis during wound healing. Proc Natl Acad Sci USA. 1992;89:6896–900.
3. Werner S, Smola H, Liao X et al. The function of KGF in morphogenesis of epithelium and reepithelialization of wounds. Science. 1994;266:819–22.
4. Hübner G, Hu Q, Smola H, Werner S. Strong induction of activin expression after injury suggests an important role of activin in wound repair. Dev Biol. 1996;173:490–8.
5. Dammeier J, Beer H-D, Brauchle M, Werner S. Dexamethasone is a novel potent inducer of connective tissue growth factor expression: Implications for glucocorticoid therapy. J Biol Chem. 1998;273:18185–90.
6. Munz B, Smola H, Engelhardt F et al. Overexpression of activin A in the skin of transgenic mice reveals new activities of activin in epidermal morphogenesis, dermal fibrosis and wound repair. EMBO J. 1999;18:5205–15.
7. Rubin JS, Osada DP, Finch PW, Taylor WG, Rudikoff S, Aaronson SA. Purification and characterization of a newly identified growth factor specific for epithelial cells. Proc Natl Acad Sci USA. 1989;86:802–6.
8. Werner S. Keratinocyte growth factor: a unique player in epithelial repair processes. Cytokine Growth Factor Rev. 1998;9:153–65.
9. Miki T, Fleming TP, Bottaro DP, Rubin JS, Ron D, Aaronson SA. Expression cDNA cloning of the KGF receptor by creation of a transforming autocrine loop. Science. 1991;251:72–5.
10. Marchese C, Chedid M, Dirsch OR et al. Modulation of keratinocyte growth factor and its receptor in reepithelializing human skin. J Exp Med. 1995;182:1369–76.
11. Guo L, Degenstein L, Fuchs E. Keratinocyte growth factor is required for hair development but not for wound healing. Genes Dev. 1996;10:165–75.
12. Yamasaki M, Miyake A, Tagashira S, Itoh N. Structure and expression of the rat mRNA encoding a novel member of the fibroblast growth factor family. J Biol Chem. 1996;271:15918–21.
13. Igarashi M, Finch PW, Aaronson SA. Characterization of recombinant human fibroblast growth factor (FGF)-10 reveals functional similarities with keratinocyte growth factor (FGF-7). J Biol Chem. 1998;273:13230–5.
14. Frank S, Munz B, Werner S. The human homologue of a bovine non-selenium glutathione peroxidase is a novel keratinocyte growth factor-regulated gene. Oncogene. 1997;14:915–21.
15. Brauchle M, Madlener M, Wagner AD et al. Keratinocyte growth factor is highly overexpressed in inflammatory bowel disease. Am J Pathol. 1996;149:521–9.

16. Finch PW, Pricolo V, Wu A, Finkelstein SD. Increased expression of keratinocyte growth factor messenger RNA associated with inflammatory bowel disease. Gastroenterology. 1996;110:441–51.

17. Sartor RB. Pathogenic and clinical relevance of cytokines in inflammatory bowel disease. Immunol Res. 1991;10:465–71.

18. Brauchle M, Angermeyer K, Hübner G, Werner S. Large induction of keratinocyte growth factor expression by serum growth factors and pro-inflammatory cytokines. Oncogene. 1994;9:3199–204.

19. Chedid M, Rubin JS, Csaky KG, Aaronson SA. Regulation of keratinocyte growth factor gene expression by interleukin 1. J Biol Chem. 1994;269:10753–7.

20. Bajaj-Elliott M, Breese M, Poulsom R, Fairclough PD, MacDonald TT. Keratinocyte growth factor in inflammatory bowel disease. Increased mRNA transcripts in ulcerative colitis compared with Crohn's disease in biopsies and isolated mucosal myofibroblasts. Am J Pathol. 1997;151:1469–76.

21. Farrell CL, Bready JV, Rex KL *et al.* Keratinocyte growth factor protects mice from chemotherapy and radiation-induced gastrointestinal injury and mortality. Cancer Res. 1998;1:933–9.

22. Khan WB, Shui C, Ning S, Knox SJ. Enhancement of murine intestinal stem cell survival after irradiation by keratinocyte growth factor. Radiat Res. 1997;148:248–53.

23. Zeeh JM, Procaccino F, Hoffmann P *et al.* Keratinocyte growth factor ameliorates mucosal injury in an experimental model of colitis in rats. Gastroenterology. 1996;110:1077–83.

24. Egger B, Procaccino F, Sarosi I, Tolmos J, Buchler MW, Eysselein VE. Keratinocyte growth factor ameliorates dextran sodium sulfate colitis in mice. Dig Dis Sci. 1999;44:836–44.

25. Miceli R, Hubert M, Santiago G *et al.* Efficacy of keratinocyte growth factor-2 in dextran sulfate sodium-induced murine colitis. J Pharmacol Exp Ther. 1999;290:464–71.

26. Massagué J. The transforming growth factor-β family. Annu Rev Cell Biochem. 1990;6:597–641.

27. Vale W, Hsueh A, Rivier C, Yu J. The inhibin/activin family of hormones and growth factors. In: Sporn MB, Roberts AB, editors. Peptide Growth Factors and their Receptors. II. Berlin: Springer-Verlag; 1990:211–48.

28. Hötten G, Neidhardt H, Schneider C, Pohl J. Cloning of a new member of the TGF-β family: a putative new activin β_C chain. Biochem Biophys Res Commun. 1995;106:608–13.

29. Oda S, Nishimatsu S-I, Murakami K, Ueno N. Molecular cloning and functional analysis of a new activin β subunit: a dorsal mesoderm-inducing activity in *Xenopus*. Biochem Biophys Res Commun. 1995;210:581–8.

30. Fang J, Yin W, Smiley E, Wang SQ, Bonadio J. Molecular cloning of the mouse activin beta (E) subunit gene. Biochem Biophys Res Commun. 1996;228:669–74.

31. DeBleser PJ, Niki T, Xu G, Rogiers V, Geerts A. Localization and cellular sources of activins in normal and fibrotic rat liver. Hepatology. 1997;26:905–12.

32. Sugiyama M, Ichida T, Sato T, Ishikawa T, Matsuda Y, Asakura H. Expression of activin A is increased in cirrhotic and fibrotic rat livers. Gastroenterology. 1998;114:550–8.

33. Matsuse T, Fukuchi Y, Eto Y *et al.* Expression of immunoreactive and bioactive activin A protein in adult murine lung after bleomycin treatment. Am J Respir Cell Mol Biol. 1995;313:17–24.

34. Matsuse T, Ikegami A, Ohga E *et al.* Expression of immunoreactive activin A protein in remodeling lesions associated with intestitial pulmonary fibrosis. Am J Pathol. 1996;148:707–13.

35. Inoue S, Orimo A, Hosoi T *et al.* Demonstration of activin-A in arteriosclerotic lesions. Biochem Biophys Res Commun. 1994;205:441–8.

36. Pawlowski JE, Taylor DS, Valentine M *et al.* Stimulation of activin A expression in rat aortic smooth muscle cells by thrombin and angiotensin II correlates with neointimal formation *in vivo*. J Clin Invest. 1997;100:639–48.

37. Hübner G, Brauchle M, Gregor M, Werner S. Activin A: a novel player and inflammatory marker in inflammatory bowel disease? Lab Invest. 1997;77:311–18.

38. Hübner G, Werner S. Serum growth factors and proinflammatory cytokines are potent inducers of activin expression in cultured fibroblasts and keratinocytes. Exp Cell Res. 1996;228:106–13.

39. Erämaa M, Hurme M, Stenman U-H, Ritvos O. Activin A/erythroid differentiation factor is induced during human monocyte activation. J Exp Med. 1992;176:1449–52.

40. Allison MC, Cornwall S, Poulter LW, Dhillon AP, Pounder RE. Macrophage heterogeneity in normal colonic mucosa and in inflammatory bowel disease. Gut. 1998;29:1531–8.

41. Li Q, Karam SM, Coerver KA, Matzuk MM, Gordon JI. Stimulation of activin receptor II signaling pathways inhibits differentiation of multiple gastric epithelial lineages. Mol Endocrinol. 1998;12:181–92.
42. Brigstock DR. The connective tissue growth factor/cysteine-rich 61/nephroblastoma overexpressed (CCN) family. Endocrine Rev. 1999;20:189–206.
43. Bradham DM, Igarashi A, Potter RL Grotendorst GR. Connective tissue growth factor: a cysteine-rich mitogen secreted by human vascular endothelial cells is related to the SRC-induced immediate early gene product CEF-10. J Cell Biol. 1991;114:1285–94.
44. Kireeva ML, Latinki BV, Kolesnikova TV et al. Cyr61 and Fisp12 are both ECM-associated signaling molecules: activities, metabolism, and localization during development. Exp Cell Res. 1997;233:63–77.
45. Frazier K, Williams S, Kothapalli D, Klapper H, Grotendorst GR. Stimulation of fibroblast cell growth, matrix production, and granulation tissue formation by connective tissue growth factor. J Invest Dermatol. 1996;107:404–11.
46. Kothapalli D, Frazier KS, Welply A, Segarini PR, Grotendorst GR. Transforming growth factor β induces anchorage-independent growth of NRK fibroblasts via a connective tissue growth factor-dependent pathway. Cell Growth Differ. 1997;8:61–8.
47. Kothapalli D, Hayashi N, Grotendorst GR. Inhibition of TGF-β-stimulated CTGF gene expression and anchorage-independent growth by cAMP identifies a CTGF-dependent restriction point in the cell cycle. FASEB J. 1998;12:1151–61.
48. Igarashi A, Nashiro J, Kikuchi K et al. Significant correlation between connective tissue growth factor gene expression and skin sclerosis in tissue sections from patients with systemic sclerosis. J Invest Dermatol. 1995;105:280–4.
49. Igarashi A, Nashiro K et al. Connective tissue growth factor gene expression in tissue sections from localized scleroderma, keloid, and other fibrotic skin disorders. J Invest Dermatol. 1996;106:729–33.
50. Lasky JA, Ortiz LA, Tonthat B et al. Connective tissue growth factor mRNA expression is upregulated in bleomycin-induced lung fibrosis. Am J Physiol. 1998;275:L365–71.
51. Ito Y, Aten J, Bende RJ et al. Expression of connective tissue growth factor in human renal fibrosis. Kidney Int. 1998;53:853–61.
52. Oemar BS, Werner A, Garnier J-M et al. Human connective tissue growth factor is expressed in advanced atherosclerotic lesions. Circulation. 1997;95:831–9.
53. Igarashi A, Okochi H, Bradham DM, Grotendorst GR. Regulation of connective tissue growth factor gene expression in human skin fibroblasts and during wound repair. Mol Cell Biol. 1993;4:637–45.
54. Dammeier J, Brauchle M, Falk W, Grotendorst GR, Werner S. Connective tissue growth factor: a novel regulator of mucosal repair and fibrosis in inflammatory bowel disease? Int J Biochem Cell Biol. 1998;30:909–22.
55. Matthes H, Stallmach A, Matthes B, Herbst H, Schuppan D. Hinweise für einen differenten Kollagenmetabolismus bei Morbus Crohn und Colitis Ulcerosa. Med Klin. 1993;88:185–92.
56. Grotendorst GR. Identification and development of novel antifibrotic agents. Exp Opin Invest Drugs. 1997;6:777–81.
57. Lombes M, Alfaidy N, Eugene E, Lessana A, Farman N, Bonvalet JP. Prerequisite for cardiac aldosterone action. Mineralocorticoid receptor and 11 beta-hydroxysteroid dehydrogenase in the human heart. Circulation. 1995;92:175–82.
58. Franklin TJ. Therapeutic approaches to organ fibrosis. Int J Biochem Cell Biol. 1997;29:79–89.
59. Wahl SM. Glucocorticoids and wound healing. In: Schleimer RP, Claman HN, Oronsky AL, editors. Anti-inflammatory Steroid Action. Basic and Clinical Aspects. San Diego: Academic Press; 1989:280–302.
60. Hübner G, Brauchle M, Smola H, Madlener M, Fässler R, Werner S. Differential regulation of pro-inflammatory cytokines during wound healing in normal and glucocorticoid-treated mice. Cytokine. 1996;8:548–56.

6
Epithelial wound healing in the intestine: role of Erk-1/-2 MAP-kinase signalling

M. N. GÖKE and D. K. PODOLSKY

REGULATION OF INTESTINAL EPITHELIAL RESTITUTION AND PROLIFERATION

The epithelium of the intestinal tract is constantly confronted by many noxious luminal agents that can disrupt barrier function. Rapid resealing of the epithelium is essential after various forms of injury, e.g. gastric or duodenal erosions and ulcerations, inflammatory bowel disease, enteropathogenic infections, ischaemia, or radiation. A pivotal feature of the intestinal mucosa is the ability of epithelial cells to spread rapidly and migrate across the basement membrane to cover defects. This process, termed restitution, occurs over the course of hours and has been shown to be independent of proliferation[1–4]. Cell migration requires actin redistribution and coordinated extension of lamellipodia, formation and breaking of adhesive contacts at the leading edge as well as cytoskeletal-mediated retraction at the trailing edge of the cell[5,6]. Rho subfamily GTPase proteins are thought to play a critical role in cytoskeletal reorganization processes important for cell migration during the restitution phase after mucosal injury in the intestine[7]. Restitution is stimulated by various non-peptidyl factors such as polyamines, a slightly alkaline pH milieu, nitric oxide, prostaglandins, and short-chain fatty acids[1–4,8,9]. Furthermore, various peptide growth factors, including transforming growth factor (TGF)-β_1, TGF-α, epidermal growth factor (EGF), acidic and basic fibroblast growth factor (FGF), KGF, and hepatocyte growth factor (HGF), as well as the cytokines interleukin (IL)-1β, IL-2, and interferon (IFN)-γ present in the intestinal mucosa enhance intestinal epithelial restitution, presumably by mediating their effects through receptors at the basolateral pole of epithelial cells[2,4,10–12]. Some of the extracellular matrix molecules on which intestinal epithelial cells reside – in addition to their effects on cell adhesion, growth, differentiation, and spatial organization – also have the potential to stimulate intestinal epithelial cell migration[13–15]. The basement membrane components fibronectin and type IV collagen may be especially important[15]. Finally, trefoil factors, a recently identified family of protease-resistant peptides which are secreted onto the luminal surface where they form the viscoelastic mucus layer through interaction with mucin glycoproteins, also promote the important process of restitution acting at the apical cell surface[4,16-18].

Substantially later than restitution, cell proliferation contributes to wound healing by replacing lost intestinal epithelial cells. Proliferation of intestinal epithelial cells is stimulated by some of the same growth factors promoting cell migration such as TGF-α, EGF, HGF, IGF-I and IGF-II, FGFs, including KGF[1-4,19-28]. Among these growth factors, TGF-α appears to be essential for autocrine stimulation of intestinal epithelial cell proliferation, whereas HGF derived from subepithelial intestinal myofibroblasts may play a key role in paracrine stimulation of intestinal epithelial cell growth[26]. A recent report suggests that intestinal fibroblasts also promote intestinal epithelial cell proliferation in a paracrine fashion through IGF-II[29].

In contrast to accumulating knowledge about effects of peptide growth factors and cytokines on intestinal epithelial wound healing, little information exists about the intracellular events initiating these epithelial responses. However, recent studies yielded some insight into the intracellular signalling pathways controlling intestinal epithelial wound healing.

ACTIVATION OF ERK-1/ERK-2 MAP KINASES IN WOUNDED INTESTINAL EPITHELIUM

Over the past decade, mitogen-activated protein (MAP) kinase pathways have been recognized as a major signalling system by which cells transduce extracellular signals. Several distinct MAP kinase cascades have been identified[30-37]. Among the extracellular signal-regulated Erk-, c-Jun- and p38-kinase pathways, Erk-1 and Erk-2 are known to be activated by growth factors, including TGF-α, EGF, TGF-β, FGFs, and HGF. Erk-1/-2 kinases are activated by MAP kinase kinase 1 (MEK-1) through Ras or Raf dependent mechanisms[30,31,37]. Subsequently, Erk-1 and Erk-2 phosphorylate various downstream substrates, e.g. ternary complex factor-1/Elk, fos, or early growth response-1 (Egr-1) nuclear phosphoprotein resulting in activation of transcription factors that, for example, control cellular growth, differentiation, transformation and development.

Since some of the growth factors promoting epithelial wound repair, such as TGF-α, EGF, FGFs, HGF and also TGF-β, can activate both Erk-1 and Erk-2 MAP kinases, it was hypothesized that repair mechanisms after intestinal epithelial wounding may be mediated by activation of MAP kinase signal transduction pathways.

To assess the effect of intestinal epithelial wounding on MAP kinase pathway activation, an *in-vitro* wound assay was used[38]. Standard wounds in confluent monolayers of IEC-6 cells were created with a razor blade. Cell lysates were harvested for protein extraction at various time points after wounding. Proteins extracted from wounded and unwounded control IEC-6 lysates were analysed for Erk-1 tyrosine phosphorylation by immunoprecipitation and subsequent Western blotting using an anti-phosphotyrosine antibody. A marked increase in tyrosine phosphorylation of Erk-1 protein was observed within 5 min after wounding, whereas overall Erk-1 protein content before and after injury was virtually unchanged. Since the results of the phosphorylation studies suggested that the Erk MAP kinase signalling pathway might be involved in the signalling events after disruption of IEC-6 monolayers, activity of Erk-1, Erk-2 and Raf-1 MAP kinases was analysed by immune complex *in-vitro* kinase assays. Paralleling the tyrosine phosphorylation changes, a substantial increase of Erk-1 and Erk-2 kinase activity was observed within 5 min after wounding IEC-6 cells. Activation of the upstream Raf-1 kinase occurred in IEC-6 cells even within 1 min after wounding. In addition, conditioned medium collected from wounded IEC-6 monolayers stimulated Erk-1 and Erk-2 kinase activities suggesting a paracrine mechanism. To identify factors that might mediate this MAP kinase activation, the effect of wound-conditioned medium on Erk-1 and Erk-2 kinase activity was analysed in the presence of neutralizing anti-TGF-α or anti-TGF-β antibodies. In these experiments, neutralizing anti-TGF-α but not anti-TGF-β antibody reduced the stimulatory effect of wound-conditioned IEC-6 medium on Erk-1 and Erk-2 kinase activity. These results indicated that TGF-α is involved in activation of Erk-1 and Erk-2 MAP kinases after intestinal epithelial wounding. The findings were supplemented by increased Erk-1, Erk-2 and Raf-1 kinase activities in unwounded IEC-6 cells after stimulation with TGF-α found by us and others. Consistent with these observations, the TGF-α concentration in supernatants collected from wounded IEC-6 monolayers was significantly higher compared to control medium. Moreover, subconfluent IEC-6 cells incubated with wound-conditioned medium had a substantially higher proliferation rate as assessed by [^{3}H]thymidine incorporation compared to IEC-6 cells cultured with conditioned medium from unwounded cells. Addition of neutralizing anti-TGF-α antibody to wound-conditioned medium blocked the stimulatory effect on IEC-6 cell proliferation.

The concept that the rapid increase in Erk-1 and Erk-2 tyrosine phosphorylation and kinase activity in wounded IEC-6 cells is mediated by a paracrine mechanism in part by TGF-α is consistent with supplementary observations by other groups. It has recently been reported that wounding monolayers of immortalized mouse intestinal cells results in a rapid increase in tyrosine phosphorylation of the EGF-receptor (EGF-R), the receptor for EGF and TGF-α[39]. Furthermore, in this murine intestinal epithelial wound model an increased phosphorylation of phospholipase C-γ_1 was observed which appeared to be important for EGF-EGF-R-mediated signalling after injury[39]. Increased EGF-R phosphorylation and Erk-1/Erk-2 activity have recently also been observed in the mucosa during gastric ulcer healing in rats *in vivo*[40].

In addition to TGF-α-mediated Erk-1/-2 activation in association with increased proliferation of intestinal epithelial cells after wounding, MAP kinase activation may also be involved in effects of other protective peptide growth factors, including HGF. Recently, it has been shown that HGF, which is also called scatter factor, phosphorylates Erk-1 and Erk-2 MAP kinases in HT-29 colon epithelial cells, and that this increased Erk phosphorylation was blocked by an inhibitor of the Erk-1/-2 activating kinase MEK-1[41]. In addition, the same authors demonstrated that HGF-induced scattering of HT29 cells was also blocked by simultaneous addition of the same MEK-1 inhibitor. The hypothesis of the importance of Erk-1/-2 MAP kinases for epithelial wound healing in the intestine finds further support in a recent report that demonstrated increased Erk-1 and Erk-2 activation as well as increased fos and early growth response-1 (Egr-1) nuclear phosphoprotein mRNA expression in wounded IEC-6 cells[42]. Addition of the MAP kinase inhibitor PD98959 resulted in a dose-dependent strong inhibition of Erk activation as well as restitution. Moreover, restitution was inhibited after transfection of IEC-6 cells with a dominant negative Egr-1 mutant[42]. These data imply that MAP kinase activation and further downstream events are indeed important for cell migration in the restitution phase after intestinal epithelial injury *in vitro* (see Fig. 1).

In addition to Erk-1/Erk-2 activation, disruption of intestinal epithelial cell monolayers also activates c-Jun-N-terminal protein kinase-1 (JNK-1) and p38 MAP kinases[38,43]. The roles these signalling events may play for intestinal epithelial wound healing still need to be characterized.

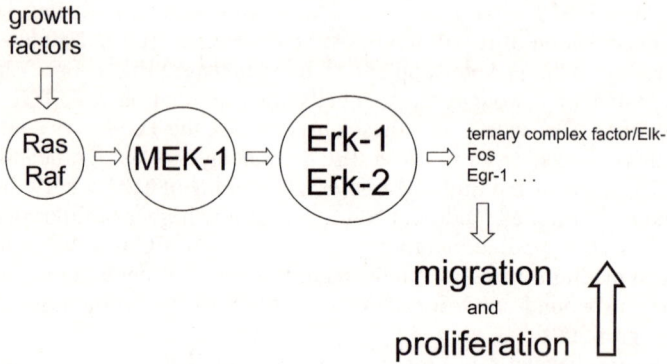

Figure 1   Role of Erk-1/-2 MAP kinases for intestinal epithelial wound healing

SUMMARY

Erk-1 and Erk-2 kinase activation by peptide growth factors appears to be a key mechanism for stimulation of proliferation but also migration in the restitution phase after epithelial injury. It is necessary to further elucidate the intracellular signalling and transcriptional events downstream of Erk MAP kinases after mucosal injury in the intestine. Better understanding of these processes may provide the basis for pharmacological modulation of intestinal epithelial restitution and proliferation.

Acknowledgements

Studies by the authors were supported by grants from the National Institutes of Health (DK-43351 and DK-46906), the Fritz Thyssen-Stiftung, and the Else Kröner Fresenius-Stiftung. M.N.G. thanks Prof. Dr Michael P. Manns for his support and advice.

References

1. Silen W. Gastric mucosal defense and repair. In: Johnson LR, editor. Physiology of the Gastrointestinal Tract. 2nd edn. New York: Raven Press; 1987:1055–69.
2. Göke M, Podolsky DK. Regulation of the mucosal epithelial barrier. Baillière's Clin Gastroenterol. 1996;10:393–405.
3. Wilson AJ, Gibson PR. Epithelial migration in the colon: filling in the gaps. Clin Sci. 1997;93:97–108.
4. Podolsky DK. Mucosal immunity and inflammation. Innate mechanisms of mucosal defense and repair: the best offense is a good defense. Am J Physiol. 1999;277:G495–9.
5. Gumbiner BM. Cell adhesion: the molecular basis of tissue architecture and morphogenesis. Cell. 1996;84:345–57.
6. Mitchison TJ, Cramer LP. Actin-based cell motility and cell locomotion. Cell. 1996;84:371–9.
7. Santos MF, McCormack SA, Guo Z et al. Rho proteins play a critical role in cell migration during the early phase of mucosal restitution. J Clin Invest. 1997;100:216–25.
8. McCormack SA, Viar MJ, Johnson LR. Migration of IEC-6 cells: a model for mucosal healing. Am J Physiol. 1992;263:G426–35.
9. Zushi S, Shinomura Y, Kiyohara T et al. Role of prostaglandins in intestinal epithelial restitution stimulated by growth factors. Am J Physiol. 1996;270:G757–62.
10. Ciacci C, Lind SE, Podolsky DK. Transforming growth factor β regulation of migration in wounded rat intestinal epithelial monolayers. Gastroenterology. 1993;105:93–101.
11. Dignass AU, Podolsky DK. Cytokine modulation of intestinal epithelial cell restitution: central role of transforming growth factor β. Gastroenterology. 1993;105:1323–32.
12. Beck PL, Podolsky DK. Growth factors in inflammatory bowel disease. Inflamm Bowel Dis. 1999;5:44–60.
13. Basson MD, Modlin IM, Madri JA. Human enterocyte (Caco-2) migration is modulated in vitro by extracellular matrix composition and epidermal growth factor. J Clin Invest. 1992;90:15–23.
14. Basson MD, Modlin IM, Flynn SD, Jena BP, Madri JA. Independent modulation of enterocyte migration and proliferation by growth factors, matrix proteins, and pharmacologic agents in an in vitro model of mucosal healing. Surgery. 1992;112:299–308.
15. Göke M, Zuk A, Podolsky DK. Regulation and function of extracellular matrix in intestinal epithelial restitution in vitro. Am J Physiol. 1996;271:G729–40.
16. Dignass A, Lynch-Devaney K, Kindon H, Thim L, Podolsky DK. Trefoil peptides promote epithelial migration through a transforming growth factor β-independent pathway. J Clin Invest. 1994;94:376–83.
17. Babyatsky MW, deBeaumont M, Thim L, Podolsky DK. Oral trefoil peptides protect against ethanol and indomethacin-induced gastric injury in rats. Gastroenterology. 1996;110:632–5.
18. Mashimo H, Wu DC, Podolsky DK, Fishman MC. Impaired defence of intestinal mucosa in mice lacking intestinal trefoil factor. Science. 1996;274:262–5.
19. Podolsky DK, Babyatsky MW. Growth and development of the gastrointestinal tract. In: Yamada T, editor. Textbook of Gastroenterology, 2nd edn. Philadelphia: JB Lippincott; 1995:546–77.
20. Koyama S, Podolsky DK. Differential expression of transforming growth factors α and β in rat intestinal epithelial cells. J Clin Invest. 1989;83:1768–73.
21. Suemori S, Ciacci C, Podolsky DK. Regulation of transforming growth factor expression in rat intestinal epithelial cell lines. J Clin Invest. 1991;87:2216–21.
22. Ohneda K, Ulshen MH, Fuller CR, D'Ercole AJ, Lund PK. Enhanced growth of small bowel in transgenic mice expressing human insulin-like growth factor I. Gastroenterology. 1997;112:444–54.
23. Park JHY, McCusker RH, Vanderhoof JA, Mohammadpour H, Harty RF, MacDonald RG. Secretion of insulin-like growth factor II (IGF-II) and IGF-binding protein-2 by intestinal epithelial (IEC-6) cells: implications for autocrine growth regulation. Endocrinology. 1992;131:1359–68.
24. Steeb CB, Trahair JF, Read LC. Administration of insulin-like growth factor-I (IGF-I) peptides for three days stimulates proliferation of the small intestinal epithelium in rats. Gut. 1995;37:630–8.

25. Fukamachi H, Ichinose M, Tsukada S *et al.* Hepatocyte growth factor region specifically stimulates gastro-intestinal epithelial growth in primary culture. Biochem Biophys Res Commun. 1994;205:1445–51.

26. Göke M, Kanai M, Podolsky DK. Intestinal fibroblasts regulate intestinal epithelial cell proliferation via hepatocyte growth factor. Am J Physiol. 1998;274:G809–18.

27. Housley RM, Morris CF, Boyle W *et al.* Keratinocyte growth factor induces proliferation of hepatocytes and epithelial cells throughout the rat gastrointestinal tract. J Clin Invest. 1994;94:1764–77.

28. Potten CS, Owen G, Hewitt D *et al.* Stimulation and inhibition of proliferation in the small intestinal crypts of the mouse after *in vivo* administration of growth factors. Gut. 1995;36:864–73.

29. Simmons JG, Pucilowska JB, Lund PK. Autocrine and paracrine actions of intestinal fibroblast-derived insulin-like growth factors. Am J Physiol. 1999;276:G817–27.

30. Boulton TG, Nye SH, Robins DJ *et al.* ERKs: a family of protein-serine/threonine kinases that are activated and tyrosine phosphorylated in response to insulin and NGF. Cell. 1991;65:663–75.

31. Bogoyevitch MA, Ketterman AJ, Sugden PH. Cellular stresses differentially activate c-Jun N-terminal protein kinases and extracellular signal-regulated protein kinases in cultured ventricular myocytes. J Biol Chem. 1995;270:29710–17.

32. Sanchez I, Hughes RT, Mayer BJ *et al.* Role of SAPK/ERK kinase-1 in the stress-activated pathway regulating transcription factor c-Jun. Nature. 1994;72:794–8.

33. Derijard B, Hibi M, Wu IH *et al.* JNK1. A protein kinase stimulated by UV light and Ha-Ras that binds and phosphorylates the c-Jun activation domain. Cell. 1994;76:1025–37.

34. Kyriakis JM, Banerjee P, Nikolakaki E *et al.* The stress-activated protein kinase subfamily of c-Jun kinases. Nature. 1994;369:156–60.

35. Rouse J, Cohen P, Trigon S *et al.* A novel kinase cascade triggered by stress and heat shock that stimulates MAPKAP kinase-2 and phosphorylation of the small heat shock proteins. Cell. 1994;78:1027–37.

36. Han J, Lee JD, Bibbs L, Ulevitch RJ. A MAP kinase targeted by endotoxin and hyperosmolarity in mammalian cells. Science. 1994;265:808–11.

37. Robinson MJ, Cobb MH. Mitogen-activated protein kinase pathways. Curr Opin Cell Biol. 1997;9:180–6.

38. Göke M, Kanai M, Lynch-Devaney K, Podolsky DK. Rapid mitogen-activated protein kinase activation by transforming growth factor alpha in wounded rat intestinal epithelial cells. Gastroenterology. 1998;114:697–705.

39. Polk DB. Epidermal growth factor receptor-stimulated intestinal epithelial cell migration requires phospholipase C activity. Gastroenterology. 1998;114:493–502.

40. Pai R, Ohta M, Itani RM, Safreh IJ, Tarnawski AS. Induction of mitogen-activated protein kinase signal transduction pathway during gastric ulcer healing in rats. Gastroenterology. 1998;114:706–13.

41. Sebolt-Leopold JS, Dudley DT, Herrera R *et al.* Blockade of the MAP kinase pathway suppresses growth of colon tumors in vivo. Nat Med. 1999;5:810–16.

42. Dieckgraefe BK, Weems DM. Epithelial injury induces Egr-1 and Fos expression by a pathway involving protein kinase C and ERK. Am J Physiol. 1999;276:G322–30.

43. Dieckgraefe BK, Weems DM, Santoro SA, Alpers DH. ERK and p38 MAP kinase pathways are mediators of intestinal epithelial wound-induced signal transduction. Biochem Biophys Res Commun. 1997;233:389–94.

7
Macrophage influence on epithelial cell function

G. ROGLER, T. SPÖTTL, M. HAUSMANN, K. SCHLOTTMANN, J. SCHÖLMERICH and T. ANDUS

INTRODUCTION

Intestinal macrophages play an important role during acute and chronic mucosal inflammation. They are able to secrete pro-inflammatory mediators, for example IL-1 and TNF, as well as oxygen radicals. The induction of most of these pro-inflammatory molecules is mediated by the actived transcription factor nuclear factor kappa B (NF-κB). Activated NF-κB could be demonstrated in macrophages and epithelial cells during mucosal inflammation *in situ*.

The study of macrophage influence on epithelial cell function was hampered by the lack of culture models for both cell types. Recently, a model for the primary culture of human intestinal epithelial cells was established. In addition a method for the isolation and purification of intestinal macrophages was described. With these models co-culture investigations are now possible.

The incubation of primary human intestinal epithelial cells (IEC) with the typical macrophage cytokine IL-1 (intestinal fibroblasts and IEC do not secrete IL-1) is followed by an induction of NF-κB activation (which has also been observed during inflammation *in situ*). Activated NF-κB induces IL-8 expression and secretion from the IEC which can be prevented by inhibitors of NF-κB activation.

Macrophages may also induce tissue damage by production of reactive oxygen metabolites. By subtractive mRNA screening methods subunits of NADPH oxidase, which is responsible for the oxidative burst reaction in macrophages, were found to be up-regulated in inflammation-associated macrophages. Whereas normal intestinal macrophages are areactive and anergic, inflammation-associated macrophages can damage IEC by NADPH oxidase-dependent oxygen metabolites.

Other new molecules found in intestinal macrophages, and their influence on epithelial cell function, are presently under investigation.

55

CULTURE MODELS FOR THE STUDY OF INTESTINAL MACROPHAGE–EPITHELIAL CELL INTERACTIONS

Intestinal macrophages represent one of the largest compartments of the mononuclear phagocyte system in the body[1,2]. They are localized preferentially at the sites of antigen entry, e.g. in the periepithelial region of the small intestine and in the subepithelial domes of Peyer's patches[3–8]. Macrophages constitute 10–20% of the mononuclear cells in the lamina propria, as determined by immunohistochemistry and tissue disaggregation experiments[2,6–9].

Recently we and others analysed the phenotype of colonic macrophages from normal and inflamed intestinal mucosa. Intestinal macrophages express CD44 and CD68, acid phosphatase and non-specific esterase[10–13]. CD33, a member of the sialoadhesin family of sialic acid-dependent cell adhesion molecules, could be identified as a useful recognition marker for intestinal macrophages in flow cytometric analysis[11,12]. Only very few macrophages from normal colonic mucosa express the typical MO/MAC-specific surface markers CD14, CD16, CD11b and CD11c[11]. The expression of the T cell costimulatory molecules B7-1 (CD80) and B7-2 (CD86) on intestinal macrophages is also low[11]. For other tissue macrophages, for example normal alveolar macrophages, a similar phenotype with low numbers of CD14- and CD16-positive cells was found[14–18].

Intestinal macrophages are able to secrete a high number of different mediators and these molecules may pass the basement membrane of the epithelium and influence epithelial cells of the intestinal mucosa. The investigation of direct interactions between intestinal macrophages and epithelial cells has been hampered by a lack of methods for the purification and culture of both cell types in the past. Recently, we could establish a technique for the purification and short-term culture of human intestinal macrophages[11]. LPMNC were isolated from normal and Crohn's disease mucosa specimens. Macrophages were labelled with immunomagnetic MicroBeads armed with CD33 antibody and purified twice using type AS separation columns (Miltenyi Biotec)[11]. LPMNC with magnetically labelled macrophages were passed through an AS separation column which was placed in the permanent magnet SuperMACS. The magnetically labelled cells were retained in the column and separated from the unlabelled cells, which pass through. After removal of the column from the magnetic field, the retained fraction could be eluted. Eluted cells were passed through a second AS separation column to increase purification of macrophages to a final purity of > 95%. The purified intestinal macrophages could be seeded on FALCON Primaria® plates and kept in culture for several days.

In addition we were able to establish a model for the culture of primary colonic or ileal epithelial cells[19]. Mucosa is stripped from submucosa within 30 min after bowel resection and rinsed with phosphate buffered saline several times. The mucus is removed by treatment with 1 mM dithiothreitol for 15 min. After washing with PBS the mucosa is placed in 1.5 mM EDTA in Hanks' balanced salt solution without calcium and magnesium, and tumbled for 10 min at 37°C. This supernatant, containing debris and mainly villus cells, is discarded. The mucosa is incubated again with EDTA for 10 min at 37°C. The supernatant is collected; it contains complete crypts, some single cells and a small amount of debris. To separate IEC (crypts) from contaminating non-epithelial cells the suspension is allowed to sediment for 15 min. The cells (mainly complete crypts) are collected and washed twice with PBS. The number and viability of the cells is determined by 0.1% trypan blue exclusion. The purity of the epithelial cell preparation is routinely checked by FACS analysis showing regularly more than 90% of EP4 positive cells. The amount of macrophages (CD33 positive) or lymphocytes (CD3 or CD19 positive) is less than 5% with this method.

For primary culture $1–5 \times 10^5$ of the isolated cells are resuspended in 400 μl minimal essential medium supplemented with Earle's salts, 20% FCS, ITS (5 μg/ml insulin, 5 μg/ml transferrin, 5 ng/ml selenious acid), 2 mM glutamine, 100 U/ml penicillin, 100 μg/ml streptomycin, 100 μg/ml gentamicin, 2.5 μg/ml fungizone. The IEC are then seeded onto collagen A coated Millicell-CM cell culture plate inserts suitable for 24-well culture plates with a translucent and permeable membrane at the bottom. The cells are incubated at 37°C in air[19] with 10% CO_2. With this method culture of viable primary human colonic or ileal epithelial cells is possible for several days, allowing study of the direct interaction between macrophages and epithelial cells.

MACROPHAGE-DERIVED MEDIATORS AND EPITHELIAL CELL ACTIVATION

During mucosal inflammation intestinal macrophages are activated. They are known to secrete pro-inflammatory mediators, for example IL-1 or TNF, which might be induced by the pro-inflammatory transcription factor NF-κB. A variety of genes has been shown to be induced in the inflamed mucosal, which have been shown to be regulated by NF-κB, including the genes encoding TNF-α, IL-1β, IL-6 and IL-8[20–36]. Some of these gene products, such as TNF-α and IL-1, are also able to activate NF-κB.

These pro-inflammatory cytokines secreted by activated macrophages could induce NF-κB activation in intestinal epithelial cells. With an antibody directed against the IκB binding site of p65 we demonstrated activation of NF-κB in IEC and macrophages from inflamed intestinal mucosa which was almost absent in non-inflamed mucosa[28]. In our study in IBD patients and inflammatory controls the number of cells showing NF-κB activation correlated with the degree of mucosal inflammation but was not significantly different between inflamed mucosa from patients with Crohn's disease, ulcerative colitis and non-specific colitis or diverticulitis[28].

In our primary culture model for human intestinal epithelial cells we could support the theory that macrophage-derived cytokines might be involved in activation of IEC. IL-1β and TNF are able to induce NF-κB activation in intestinal epithelial cells correlating with an increase in IL-8 secretion, which can be prevented by proteasome inhibitors such as ALLN.

IL-8 is an important cytokine for the host inflammatory response against bacterial invasion in the gastrointestinal tract. It is well known that different bacteria are able to activate NF-κB and induce secretion of pro-inflammatory mediators[29–33]. The up-regulation of IL-8 may lead to invasion of neutrophils and production of free oxygen radicals or the release of proteolytic enzymes from activated neutrophils.

IL-1ra, which is thought to be a major anti-inflammatory cytokine secreted by IEC, is not induced by macrophage-derived cytokines in our short-term culture model. Therefore it may be concluded that the lack of induction of this anti-inflammatory mediator is followed by an imbalance of the mucosal immune mediators, and that pro-inflammatory mediators predominate.

INDUCTION OF INTESTINAL MACROPHAGE DIFFERENTIATION BY INTESTINAL EPITHELIAL CELL LINES

The interaction of intestinal macrophages with intestinal macrophages is not a one-way street. If intestinal macrophages can influence functions of intestinal macrophages a reverse reaction may also take place.

The typical phenotype of intestinal macrophages from normal mucosa with a lack of CD14, CD16 and CD11b expression, as well as a lack of expression of co-stimulatory molecules, could not be induced *in vitro* in primary culture of peripheral blood monocytes. Intestinal epithelial cells are separated from these macrophages only by the basement membrane. We therefore assumed that intestinal epithelial cells could possibly influence the differentiation of intestinal macrophages. To investigate this possibility we used the technique of multi-cellular spheroids to allow close association of monocytes with intestinal epithelial cells in a three-dimensional environment similar to the lamina propria. In spheroids cells are forming cell-to-cell and cell-to-matrix contacts, which can also be found *in vivo*[34,35]. Epithelial cell lines especially secrete extracellular matrix, forming a milieu to invading cells that is similar to the *in-vivo* situation. Interaction with other cells, and contact with three-dimensional structures, may be crucial for tissue macrophage differentiation. Recently, Randolph and co-workers showed that monocytes can differentiate into CD14 negative dendritic cells in only 2 days when they migrate and remigrate across an endothelial model[36]. In contrast, monocytes that remained in the subendothelial matrix became macrophages retaining CD14 expression[36].

To investigate possible influences of three-dimensional structures and extra-cellular matrix on the specific differentiation of intestinal macrophages, MCS from IEC lines (HT-29, WiDr, LS174T) co-cultured with purified blood mono-cytes were used. The expression of CD14, CD11b, and CD68 was analysed by immunohistochemistry (APAAP technique) and flow cytometry after different time intervals. It could be shown that monocytes infiltrated the spheroids within 24 h of co-culture. During the 7 days of co-culture a significant change in the surface antigen expression of the macrophages could be observed. CD14 and CD11b, which had been detected after 24 h of co-culture, had disappeared after 7 days but were still present in the spheroids of non-intestinal origin. Flow cytometry showed a reduction of cells positive for both CD14 and CD68 from 81% of total CD68-positive cells at the 24 h time-point to 7.6% after 7 days. This was not observed with carcinoma cell lines from non-intestinal origin.

These results indicate that in the three-dimensional model of multicellular spheroids cell lines of intestinal epithelial cells induce an intestinal-like pheno-type in the invading macrophages. It may be concluded that intestinal epithelial cells play an important role in the differentiation process of intestinal macrophages.

The possibility to activate epithelial cells by macrophages may therefore be modulated by the epithelial cells themselves, giving them some control during that process. An interesting question arises from these findings: could there be a disturbed differentiation of intestinal macrophages during inflammatory bowel diseases? Could the inability of epithelial cells to induce the non-reactive normal intestinal macrophage phenotype be responsible for the presence of permanently activated macrophages in IBD? It will be interesting to find answers to these questions in the future.

References

1. Andus T, Rogler G, Daig R, Falk W, Schölmerich J, Groß V. The role of macrophages. In: Tytgat GNJ, Bartelsman JFWM, van Deventer SJH, editors. Inflammatory Bowel Disease. Dordrecht: Kluwer; 1995:281–97.
2. Lee SH, Starkey PM, Gordon S. Quantitative analysis of total macrophage content in adult mouse tissues. Immunochemical studies with monoclonal antibody F4/80. J Exp Med. 1985;161:475–89.
3. Rogler G, Andus T, Schölmerich J, Groß V. Intestinal macrophages. In: Emmrich J, Liebe S, Stange EF, editors. Innovative Concepts in Inflammatory Bowel Disease. Dordrecht: Kluwer; 1998:111–19.
4. Pavli P, Doe WF. Intestinal macrophages. In: Mac Dermott RP, Stenson WF, editors. Inflammatory Bowel Disease. New York: Elsevier; 1992:177–88.
5. Le Fevre M, Hammer R, Joel DD. Macrophages of the mammalian small intestine: a review. J Reticuloendothel Soc. 1979;26:553–73.
6. Bockman DE, Boydston WR, Beezhold DH. The role of epithelial cells in gut-associated immune reactivity. Ann NY Acad Sci. 1983;409:129–44.
7. Bull DM, Bookmann MA. Isolation and functional characterization of human intestinal mucosal lymphoid cells. J Clin Invest. 1987;59:966–74.
8. Donellan WL. The structure of the colonic mucosa. The epithelium and subepithelial reticulo-histiocytic complex. Gastroenterology. 1965;49:496–514.
9. Golder JP, Doe WF. Isolation and preliminary characterization of human intestinal macrophages. Gastroenterology. 1983;84:795–802.
10. Pavli P, Woodhaus CE, Doe WF, Hume DA. Isolation and characterization of antigen-presenting dendritic cells from the mouse intestinal lamina propria. Immunology. 1990;70:40–7.
11. Rogler G, Andus T, Aschenbrenner E et al. Phenotypic characterization of colonic macrophages. Clin Exp Immunol. 1998;112:205–15.
12. Rogler G, Andus T, Aschenbrenner E et al. Alterations of the phenotype of colonic macrophages in inflammatory bowel disease. Eur J Gastroenterol Hepatol. 1997;9:893–9.
13. Allison MC, Cornwall S, Poulter LW, Dhillon AP, Pounder RE. Macrophage heterogeneity in normal colonic mucosa and in inflammatory bowel disease. Gut. 1988;29:1531–8.
14. Stritz J, Wang YM, Teschler H et al. Phenotypic markers of alveolar macrophage maturation in pulmonary sarcoidosis. Lung. 1993;171:293–303.
15. Barbosa IL, Gant VA, Hamblin AS. Alveolar macrophages from patients with bronchogenic carcinoma and sarcoidosis similarly express monocyte antigens. Clin Exp Immunol. 1991;86:173–8.
16. Wasserman K, Subkleve M, Pothoff G et al. Expression of surface markers on alveolar macrophages from symptomatic patients with HIV-infection as detected by flow cytometry. Chest. 1994;105:1324–34.
17. Pforte A, Schiessler A, Gais P et al. Expression of CD14 correlates with lung function impairment in pulmonary sarcoidosis. Chest. 1994;105:349–54.
18. Pforte A, Schiessler A, Gais P et al. Increased expression of the monocyte differentiation antigen CD14 in extrinsic allergic alveolitis. Monaldi Arch Chest Dis. 1993;48:607–12.
19. Rogler G, Daig R, Aschenbrenner E et al. Establishment of long-term primary cultures of human small and large intestinal epithelial cells. Lab Invest. 1998;78:889–90.

20. McCabe RP, Dean P, Elson CO. Immunology of inflammatory bowel disease. Curr Opin Gastroenterol. 1996;12:340–4.
21. Stevens C, Walz G, Singaram C et al. Tumor necrosis factor-alpha, interleukin 1 beta, and interleukin 6 expression in inflammatory bowel disease. Dig Dis Sci. 1992;37:818–26.
22. MacDonald TT, Hutchings P, Choy MY, Murch S, Cooke A. Tumor necrosis factor-alpha and interferon gamma production measured at single cells level in normal and inflamed human intestine. Clin Exp Immunol. 1990;81:301–5.
23. Pullman WE, Elsbury S, Kobayashi M, Hapel AJ, Doe WF. Enhanced mucosal cytokine production in inflammatory bowel disease. Gastroenterology. 1992;102:529–37.
24. Reinecker HC, Steffen M, Witthoeft T et al. Enhanced secretion of tumor necrosis factor-alpha, IL-6 and IL-1 beta by isolated lamina propria mononuclear cells from patients with ulcerative colitis and Crohn's disease. Clin Exp Immunol. 1993;94:174–81.
25. Youngman KR, Simon PL, West GA et al. Localization of intestinal interleukin-1 activity and protein and gene expression to lamina propria cells. Gastroenterology. 1993;104:749–58.
26. Andus T, Daig R, Aschenbrenner E, Vogl D, Schölmerich J, Gross V. Pro- and antiinflammatory cytokines in the colonic mucosa. Gastroenterology. 1995;108:A770 (abstract).
27. Kusugami K, Fukatsu A, Tanimoto M et al. Elevation of interleukin-6 in inflammatory bowel disease is macrophage- and epithelial cell-dependent. Dig Dis Sci. 1995;40:949–59.
28. Rogler G, Vogl D, Brand K et al. Transcription factor NF-kappa B is activated in macrophages and epithelial cells of inflamed intestinal mucosa. Gastroenterology. 1998;115:1–13.
29. Masamune A, Shimosegawa T, Masamune O, Mukaida N, Koizumi M, Toyota T. *Helicobacter pylori*-dependent ceramide production may mediate increased interleukin 8 expression in human gastric cancer cell lines. Gastroenterology. 1999;116:1330–41.
30. Shimada T, Watanabe N, Hiraishi H, Terano A. Redox regulation of interleukin-8 expression in MKN28 cells. Dig Dis Sci. 1999;44:266–73.
31. Sharma SA, Tummuru MK, Blaser MJ, Kerr LD. Activation of IL-8 gene expression by *Helicobacter pylori* is regulated by transcription factor nuclear factor-kappa B in gastric epithelial cells. J Immunol. 1998;160:2401–7.
32. Li CK, Seth R, Gray T, Bayston R, Mahida YR, Wakelin D. Production of proinflammatory cytokines and inflammatory mediators in human intestinal epithelial cells after invasion by *Trichinella spiralis*. Infect Immun. 1998;66:2200–6.
33. Savkovic SD, Koutsouris A, Hecht G. Activation of NF-kappaB in intestinal epithelial cells by enteropathogenic *Escherichia coli*. Am J Physiol. 1997;273:C1160–7.
34. Sutherland RM. Cell and environment interactions in tumor microregions: the multicell spheroid model. Science. 1998;240:177–84.
35. Olive PL, Durand RE. Drug and radiation resistance in spheroids: cell contact and kinetics. Cancer Metastasis Rev. 1994;13:121–38.
36. Randolph GJ, Beaulieu S, Lebecque S, Steinman RM, Muller WA. Differentiation of monocytes into dendritic cells in a model of transendothelial trafficking. Science. 1998;282:480–3.

8
Influence of therapeutic intervention with interleukins on epithelial cell function

U. BÖCKER

INTRODUCTION

Intestinal epithelial cells (IEC) constitute a barrier between the toxic environment and the host. Increasing evidence impressively demonstrates that IEC actively participate in the initiation, abrogation and perpetuation of intestinal inflammation. IEC convey the initial response to adherence and invasion of viruses, bacteria and parasites by expressing and releasing inflammatory mediators. Conversely, IEC respond to cytokines, chemokines and growth factors produced by mucosal immune and non-immune cells. Accordingly, IEC are a potential target for exogenous intervention with interleukins in inflammatory bowel diseases (IBD).

INTESTINAL EPITHELIAL CELL FUNCTIONS

A population of intestinal epithelial stem cells in the crypts of the small and large intestine differentiates into distinct cell phenotypes, mainly mucus-secreting goblet and absorptive columnar cells. The IEC population undergoes a rapid turnover with a tightly regulated balance of proliferation and cell death. IEC serve multiple functions: the epithelial layer constitutes a barrier regulating absorption of nutrients, transport of electrolytes and exclusion of macro-molecules. Furthermore, IEC actively participate in the mucosal immune response. They are capable of presenting antigens to CD4+ and CD8+ lymphocytes[1], and they express the polymeric immunoglobulin receptor (pIgR)[2,3], eicosanoids[4], nitric oxide[5], complement factors[6,7], adhesion molecules[8,9] and peptide-regulatory factors (PRF) such as cytokines (IL-1α[10,11], IL-1β[12], IL-1Ra[13,14], IL-6[15–18], IL-7[19–22], IL-10[23,24], IL-15[25,26], IL-18[27,28], TNF-α[23]), chemokines (IL-8[29–31], ENA-78[32], RANTES[33], gro-α[30], MCP-1[30], MCP-3[34], MIP-1α[30], MIP-1β[30], MIP-2[35], IP-10[30]) and growth factors (TGF-α[36], TGF-β[36]).

Among the PRF produced are cytokines that are transcribed but not translated (e.g. IL-10), chemokines that are produced by both IEC and other mucosal cell populations (e.g. IL-8) and chemokines confined to IEC (e.g. ENA-78).

MODULATION OF INTESTINAL EPITHELIAL CELL FUNCTIONS

IEC functions are modulated from the luminal side by pathogens (bacteria, viruses, parasites), by resident bacteria, bacterial components (e.g. endotoxin) and bacterial products (e.g. short-chain fatty acids). From the basolateral side, IEC functions are altered by components of the extracellular matrix produced by IEC and lamina propria mesenchymal cells, by cell–cell interaction with lamina propria immune and non-immune cells and by inflammatory mediators. Pharmacological agents act upon IEC from both the luminal and the basolateral side. IEC are responsive to various cytokines, chemokines and growth factors (Table 1). Some of them (e.g. IL-1, IFN-γ) affect IEC morphology, proliferation and apoptosis, barrier function and expression of peptide-regulatory factors, others (e.g. IL-7, IL-9) induce early signalling events, but the consequences for IEC functions are incompletely understood.

POTENTIAL CANDIDATES FOR THERAPEUTIC INTERVENTION WITH INTERLEUKINS

Considering the data published on IEC responses to peptide-regulatory factors, there are two strategies to inhibit IEC activation: first, by inhibition of proinflammatory cytokines (IL-1, TNF-α, IFN-γ); secondly, by induction, up-regulation or delivery of anti-inflammatory or immunoregulatory cytokines (IL-4, IL-10, IL-11, IL-13).

TNF-α has a wide spectrum of effects on IEC, including regulation of pro-liferation and apoptosis[37,38], disruption of the barrier function[39], induction of complement factors, MHC molecules and chemokines[7,23,40–42]. Over-expression of TNF-α in mice due to enhanced TNF-α transcript stability results in the development of enterocolitis and arthritis similar to human Crohn's disease[43]. A monoclonal antibody to TNF-α is efficacious in Crohn's disease[44,45]. However, most of the *in-vitro* data on TNF-α effector functions have been obtained on transformed colonic epithelial cell lines (HT-29, Caco-2, T84), and there is conflicting data as to whether primary enterocytes express functional TNF-α receptors[46]. **INF-γ** is bound by IEC, and both experimental models of colitis and human Crohn's disease seem to be dominated by a Th1-type cytokine response[47,48]. Clinical trials aiming to inhibit IL-12, a main inducer of IFN-γ, are being performed. **IL-4** inhibits pro-inflammatory mediator expression of IEC and it modulates IEC barrier function[49]. Over-expression of IL-4 by gene trans-fer in an experimental model reduces severity of disease[50]. IL-4 has not been used in clinical trials. **IL-10** is bound by both IEC lines and primary entero-cytes[46]. In a specific-pathogen free environment, IL-10–/– mice develop sponta-neous colitis[51]. Furthermore, IL-10 seems to be beneficial in steroid-dependent Crohn's disease[52]. However, there are several *in-vitro* studies demonstrating lack

Table 1 IEC response to peptide-regulatory factors

IL-1	Induction of villous atrophy and crypt hyperplasia. Enhancement of proliferation. Induction of acute phase proteins, C3, factor B, DAF, IL-6, IL-8, MCP-1, ENA-78, gro-α, MIP-1α, MIP-1β, MIP-2.
IL-2	Regulation of proliferation. Up-regulation of MHC class II molecules.
IL-4	Inhibition of proliferation. Attenuation of barrier function. Inhibition of MCP-1, RANTES and iNOS expression. Enhancement of DAF and pIgR expression.
IL-6	Enhancement of proliferation. Induction of acute phase proteins, C4, factor B, CD44.
IL-7	Tyrosine phosphorylation.
IL-9	Tyrosine phosphorylation.
IL-10	Enhancement of barrier function.
IL-11	Inhibition of proliferation. Increase of the mitotic index of crypt cells. Suppression of apoptosis.
IL-13	Inhibition of MCP, RANTES and iNOS expression. Up-regulation of IL-8, lipoxin A4 receptor and CD44 expression.
IL-15	Enhancement of proliferation. Enhancement of transepithelial resistance. Activation of Stat3.
IL-17	Induction of chemokine expression.
TNF-α	Induction of villous atrophy and crypt hyperplasia. Modulation of proliferation, induction of apoptosis. Inhibition of proliferative response to growth factors. Disruption of barrier function. Induction of MHC class II molecules, IL-8 and MCP-1. Up-regulation of pIgR, DAF and complement.
IFN-γ	Induction of villous atrophy. Induction of apoptosis. Attenuation of barrier function. Inhibition of bacterial infection. Induction of RANTES, IL-8, MCP-1, MHC class II molecules Up-regulation of C4, pIgR, HLA-DR and ICAM-1.
MIP-1α	Induction of IL-8 and gro-α.
MIP-1β	Induction of IL-8 and gro-α.
TGF-α	Enhancement of restitution and proliferation.
TGF-β	Enhancement of migration and barrier function.
KGF	Enhancement of proliferation. Down-regulation of sucrase–isomaltase gene.
EGF	Enhancement of proliferation.
HGF	Enhancement of proliferation.
FGF	Enhancement of restitution.

of IL-10-mediated down-regulation of IEC expression of pro-inflammatory mediators[53–57]. Functional receptors for **IL-11** on IEC have not been described, but modulation of IEC proliferation and apoptosis by IL-11 has been reported[58–60]. A recently published paper on IL-11 treatment of patients with IBD demonstrated that rhIL-11 was safe and well tolerated, and it suggested reduction of clinical activity of the disease[61]. **IL-13** inhibits IEC chemokine expression *in vitro*[54]. Functional IL-13 receptors on IEC remain to be identified.

IL-1 MEDIATED ACTIVATION OF INTESTINAL EPITHELIAL CELLS

IL-1 is a pro-inflammatory cytokine with a pivotal role in the pathogenesis of IBD. Activated monocytes and macrophages in the lamina propria produce IL-1 that binds to primary enterocytes[46]. Several studies have demonstrated the importance of IL-1 in the concept of an imbalance of pro- and anti-inflammatory cytokines in IBD, although conflicting data exist as to whether the ratio of IL-1 to its natural antagonist, the IL-1 receptor antagonist (IL-1Ra), is specifically increased[13,62]. Neutralization of IL-1Ra exacerbates formalin-induced immune complex colitis in rabbits[63], while exogenous IL-1Ra reduces severity of the disease similar to its effects on intestinal and extraintestinal inflammation in rats with acute and chronic peptidoglycan–polysaccharide-induced enterocolitis[64]. Targeted deletion of IL-1Ra expression in mice increases susceptibility to endotoxaemia and mortality due to DSS-induced colitis[65]. Despite its impressive potential in experimental models of colitis, clinical trials with IL-1Ra have not been successfully conducted.

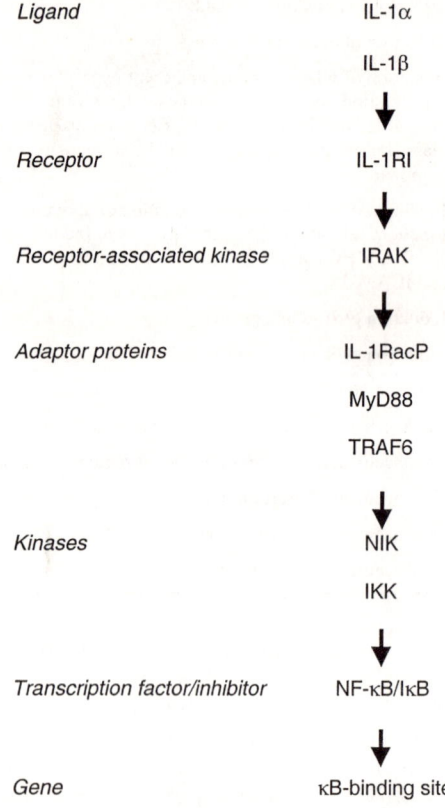

Ligand	IL-1α
	IL-1β
	↓
Receptor	IL-1RI
	↓
Receptor-associated kinase	IRAK
	↓
Adaptor proteins	IL-1RacP
	MyD88
	TRAF6
	↓
Kinases	NIK
	IKK
	↓
Transcription factor/inhibitor	NF-κB/IκB
	↓
Gene	κB-binding site

Figure 1 IL-1-mediated signal transduction

Binding of IL-1 to the IL-1 receptor type I initiates a cascade of signalling events (Fig. 1), most of which have recently been elucidated. The IL-1R-associated kinase (IRAK) is recruited to the receptor, rapidly phosphorylated and degraded[66,67]. IRAK activation depends on the association of adaptor proteins, such as the MyD88 and the IL-1R associated protein (IL-1RacP)[68–70]. IRAK activates the TNF-receptor associated factor 6 (TRAF6)[71], and the signal coming from IRAK and TRAF6 diverges towards the Jun-N-terminal kinase- and the NF-κB pathway[72–77]. Dissociation of the transcription factor NF-κB from its cytoplasmic inhibitor Iκ-B requires Iκ-B phosphorylation and ubiquination. TRAF6 activates a NF-κB-inducing kinase that activates the Iκ-B kinase complex. This complex contains two catalytic subunits, IKK-α and IKK-β and the regulatory subunit IKK-γ. IKK-α and IKK-β seem to be essential for NF-κB activation and cannot be substituted by each other. Dissociated NF-κB translocates to the nucleus and binds to κB-specific promoter sites initiating gene transcription. There are natural inhibitors to the IL-1-activated signal transduction pathway. First, a decoy receptor, the IL-1R type II, binds IL-1 without transmitting a signal[78]; furthermore IL-1RII is shed into the extracellular compartment and neutralizes IL-1. Secondly, the IL-1Ra is expressed. Three splice variants of the IL-1Ra gene product have been described[79–85]. Secretory IL-1Ra (sIL-1RA) is a glycoprotein secreted by activated monocytes and macrophages. Two intracellular forms, icIL-1Ra I and II, have been cloned. icIL-1Ra I protein and icIL-1Ra II mRNA are expressed in several types of epithelial cells as well as in fibroblasts and neutrophils. Although sIL-1Ra and icIL-1Ra I bind to the type-I IL-1 receptor with pure antagonistic activity, the function of icIL-1Ra I is not completely understood because of the spatial discrepancy between its cytoplasmic location and the IL-1 receptor on the external plasma membrane. There is evidence that icIL-1Ra I in its typical intracellular position alters the IL-1β-inducible immediate early gene expression and chemokine production[14,86]. Secretion into the extracellular compartment with subsequent competition with IL-1 for binding at the membrane IL-1 receptor, however, has been reported for keratinocytes and bronchial epithelial cells[87,88].

INHIBITION OF IL-1 EFFECTOR FUNCTIONS ON INTESTINAL EPITHELIAL CELLS

There are several strategies to inhibit IL-1-mediated IEC activation. First, by inhibition of IL-1 production and release, of IL-1R type I expression, of IL-1 binding to the signalling receptor and of IL-1-mediated activation of transcription factors. Secondly, by up-regulation of the decoy receptor IL-1R II and of the IL-1Ra.

Migration of IEC from the crypt base to the surface is accompanied by cellular differentiation that leads to fundamental morphological and functional changes. There are several models to study IEC differentiation *in vitro*[89–91]. Caco-2 cells spontaneously differentiate after reaching confluence in culture. Furthermore, transient differentiation can be obtained in both Caco-2 and HT-29 cell cultures by adding sodium butyrate at 5 mM for 24–48 h to the culture medium[92,93]. Parental HT-29 cells in culture represent a heterogeneous population of more or less differentiated cells. Exposure to methotrexate favours the emergence of a differentiated cell population that persists after withdrawal of methotrexate[94].

We compared the pro-inflammatory cytokine response of parental HT-29 cells and HT-29 cells permanently differentiated by exposure to methotrexate[95] (provided by Dr Lesuffleur, INSERM, Villejuif, France). While PMA and TNF-α induced similar levels of IL-8 in culture supernatants, the response of differentiated cells to IL-1β was blunted as compared to the parental cell line. As demonstrated by Northern blot analysis of total RNA probed for IL-8, the difference between the two cell lines was apparent at the transcriptional level. By using a competitive ligand-binding assay, we could show that the impaired IL-1 response in differentiated cells was not due to absent or reduced binding of IL-1β. Binding was specific, since excess of unlabelled IL-1β replaced iodinated IL-1β. As opposed to differentiated keratinocytes, overexpression of the decoy IL-1 receptor II was not responsible for the observed differences between the parental and the differentiated cell line. IRAK was only partially degraded in HT-29 cells, and IRAK steady-state levels were lower in differentiated cells. JNK activity was strongly induced in parental HT-29 cells as opposed to differentiated cells. Iκ-B was phosphorylated by IKK in HT-29, but not in differentiated cells. Steady-state levels of IKK-α were not significantly different between the two cell lines, suggesting that diminished IL-1β-mediated signalling was not due to an absence of IKK-α protein. NF-κB binding activity in nuclei from HT-29 cells was stimulated by IL-1β or TNF-α. No difference was detectable when TNF-α was used as a stimulus, while IL-1β failed to increase binding activity of the p50/p65 heterodimer in nuclei of differentiated cells. The data indicated differences downstream of the IL-1 receptor but up-stream of the NF-κB/IκB complex. Transient lipotransfection was performed on differentiated HT-29 cells and κB-promoter activity was assessed by using a κB-promoter–luciferase construct. Over-expression of the adapter protein TRAF-6 restored impaired IL-8 promoter activation, suggesting that the signalling cascade downstream of TRAF-6 is capable of responding in differentiated cells if appropriately activated. In summary, differentiation of HT-29 cells by exposure to methotrexate resulted in impairment of IL-1β-stimulated IL-8 expression due to differences downstream of the IL-1R, but upstream of the NIK.

By fractionated isolation of intestinal epithelial cells from the surface to the crypts of surgical specimens of the colon, we demonstrated that icIL-1RA I content was highest in surface epithelial cells[14]. Interestingly, differentiated HT-29 cells also contained significantly higher amounts of icIL-1Ra. To explore the function of icIL-1Ra, Caco-2 cells that are considered to be less differentiated than HT-29 cells, and that do not express IL-1Ra, were transfected and selected for permanent icIL-1Ra expression. IL-1β stimulation resulted in a significantly diminished IL-8 content in supernatants of IL-1Ra expressing cells as opposed to Caco-2 cells transfected with an empty control vector.

In summary the data suggest that diminished IL-8 expression in differentiated intestinal epithelial cells is due to at least two mechanisms. First, by abrogation of IKK activation and NF-κB nuclear translocation, and secondly by increased icIL-1Ra I expression.

CONCLUSION

Considering their immunoregulatory functions in gut homeostasis, and their responsiveness to various interleukins, intestinal epithelial cells are a potential therapeutic target in inflammatory bowel conditions such as Crohn's disease and ulcerative colitis. Blockade of pro-inflammatory cytokines and/or induction or delivery of anti-inflammatory cytokines are the strategies to prevent or abrogate IEC activation. Analysis of endogenous mechanisms by which IEC down-regulate their pro-inflammatory responses, e.g. reduced IL-1-mediated chemokine expression with cellular differentiation, can guide the therapeutic approach.

Acknowledgements

This work was supported by Deutsche Forschungsgemeinschaft (DFG), grants Bo 1340/1-1 and Bo 1340/2-1.

References

1. Mayer L, Shlien R. Evidence for function of La molecules on gut epithelial cells in man. J Exp Med. 1987;166:1471–83.
2. Brandtzaeg P, Bjerke K, Kett K et al. Production and secretion of immunoglobulins in the gastrointestinal tract. Ann Allergy. 1987;59:21–39.
3. Phillips JO, Everson MP, Moldoveanu Z, Lue C, Mestecky J. Synergistic effect of IL-4 and IFN-gamma on the expression of polymeric Ig receptor (secretory component) and IgA binding by human epithelial cells. J Immunol. 1990;145:1740–4.
4. Cohn SM, Schloemann S, Tessner T, Seibert K, Stenson WF. Crypt stem cell survival in the mouse intestinal epithelium is regulated by prostaglandins synthesized through cyclooxygenase-1. J Clin Invest. 1997;99:1367–79.
5. Kolios G, Brown Z, Robson RL, Robertson DA, Westwick J. Inducible nitric oxide synthase activity and expression in a human colonic epithelial cell line, HT-29. Br J Pharmacol. 1995;116:2866–72.
6. Molmenti EP, Ziambaras T, Perlmutter DH. Evidence for an acute phase response in human intestinal epithelial cells. J Biol Chem. 1993;268:14116–24.
7. Andoh A, Fujiyama Y, Bamba T, Hosoda S. Differential cytokine regulation of complement C3, C4, and factor B synthesis in human intestinal epithelial cell line, Caco-2. J Immunol. 1993;151:4239–47.
8. Kaiserlian D, Rigal D, Abello J, Revillard JP. Expression, function and regulation of the intercellular adhesion molecule-1 (ICAM-1) on human intestinal epithelial cell lines. Eur J Immunol. 1991;21:2415–21.
9. Kvale D, Krajci P, Brandtzaeg P. Expression and regulation of adhesion molecules ICAM-1 (CD54) and LFA-3 (CD58) in human intestinal epithelial cell lines. Scand J Immunol. 1992;35:669–76.
10. Stadnyk AW, Sisson GR, Waterhouse CC. IL-1 alpha is constitutively expressed in the rat intestinal epithelial cell line IEC-6. Exp Cell Res. 1995;220:298–303.
11. Vallette G, Jarry A, Lemarre P, Branka JE, Laboisse CL. NO-dependent and NO-independent IL-1 production by a human colonic epithelial cell line under inflammatory stress. Br J Pharmacol. 1997;121:187–92.
12. Waterhouse CC, Stadnyk AW. Rapid expression of IL-1beta by intestinal epithelial cells *in vitro*. Cell Immunol. 1999;193:1–8.
13. Casini-Raggi V, Kam L, Chong YJ, Fiocchi C, Pizarro TT, Cominelli F. Mucosal imbalance of IL-1 and IL-1 receptor antagonist in inflammatory bowel disease. A novel mechanism of chronic intestinal inflammation. J Immunol. 1995;154:2434–40.
14. Böcker U, Damiao A, Holt L et al. Differential expression of interleukin 1 receptor antagonist isoforms in human intestinal epithelial cells. Gastroenterology. 1998;115:1426–38.

15. Mascarenhas JO, Goodrich ME, Eichelberger H, McGee DW. Polarized secretion of IL-6 by IEC-6 intestinal epithelial cells: differential effects of IL-1 beta and TNF-alpha. Immunol Invest. 1996;25:333–40.
16. Parikh AA, Salzman AL, Fischer JE, Szabo C, Hasselgren PO. Interleukin-1 beta and interferon-gamma regulate interleukin-6 production in cultured human intestinal epithelial cells. Shock. 1997;8:249–55.
17. Goodrich ME, McGee DW. Regulation of mucosal B cell immunoglobulin secretion by intestinal epithelial cell-derived cytokines. Cytokine. 1998;10:948–55.
18. Goodrich ME, McGee DW. Effect of intestinal epithelial cell cytokines on mucosal B-cell IgA secretion: enhancing effect of epithelial-derived IL-6 but not TGF-beta on IgA+ B cells. Immunol Lett. 1999;67:11–14.
19. Watanabe M, Ueno Y, Yajima T et al. Interleukin 7 is produced by human intestinal epithelial cells and regulates the proliferation of intestinal mucosal lymphocytes. J Clin Invest. 1995;95:2945–53.
20. Madrigal-Estebas L, McManus R, Byrne B et al. Human small intestinal epithelial cells secrete interleukin-7 and differentially express two different interleukin-7 mRNA transcripts: implications for extrathymic T-cell differentiation. Hum Immunol. 1997;58:83–90.
21. Jiang Y, McGee DW. Regulation of human lymphocyte IL-4 secretion by intestinal epithelial cell-derived interleukin-7 and transforming growth factor-beta. Clin Immunol Immunopathol. 1998;88:287–96.
22. Watanabe M, Ueno Y, Yajima T et al. Interleukin 7 transgenic mice develop chronic colitis with decreased interleukin 7 protein accumulation in the colonic mucosa. J Exp Med. 1998;187:389–402.
23. Eckmann L, Jung HC, Schurer-Maly C, Panja A, Morzycka-Wroblewska E, Kagnoff MF. Differential cytokine expression by human intestinal epithelial cell lines: regulated expression of interleukin 8. Gastroenterology. 1993;105:1689–97.
24. Napolitano LM, Buzdon MM, Shi HJ, Bass BL. Intestinal epithelial cell regulation of macrophage and lymphocyte interleukin 10 expression. Arch Surg. 1997;132:1271–6.
25. Reinecker HC, MacDermott RP, Mirau S, Dignass A, Podolsky DK. Intestinal epithelial cells both express and respond to interleukin 15. Gastroenterology. 1996;111:1706–13.
26. Hirose K, Suzuki H, Nishimura H et al. Interleukin-15 may be responsible for early activation of intestinal intraepithelial lymphocytes after oral infection with Listeria monocytogenes in rats. Infect Immun. 1998;66:5677–83.
27. Pages F, Berger A, Henglein B et al. Modulation of interleukin-18 expression in human colon carcinoma: consequences for tumor immune surveillance. Int J Cancer. 1999;84:326–30.
28. Pizarro TT, Michie MH, Bentz M et al. IL-18, a novel immunoregulatory cytokine, is up-regulated in Crohn's disease: expression and localization in intestinal mucosal cells. J Immunol. 1999;162:6829–35.
29. Kolios G, Robertson DA, Jordan NJ et al. Interleukin-8 production by the human colon epithelial cell line HT-29: modulation by interleukin-13. Br J Pharmacol. 1996;119:351–9.
30. Yang SK, Eckmann L, Panja A, Kagnoff MF. Differential and regulated expression of C-X-C, C-C, and C-chemokines by human colon epithelial cells. Gastroenterology. 1997;113:1214–23.
31. Yu Y, Chadee K. Prostaglandin E2 stimulates IL-8 gene expression in human colonic epithelial cells by a posttranscriptional mechanism. J Immunol. 1998;161:3746–52.
32. Keates S, Keates AC, Mizoguchi E, Bhan A, Kelly CP. Enterocytes are the primary source of the chemokine ENA-78 in normal colon and ulcerative colitis. Am J Physiol. 1997;273:G75–82.
33. Casola A, Estes MK, Crawford SE et al. Rotavirus infection of cultured intestinal epithelial cells induces secretion of CXC and CC chemokines. Gastroenterology. 1998;114:947–55.
34. Wedemeyer J, Lorentz A, Goke M et al. Enhanced production of monocyte chemotactic protein 3 in inflammatory bowel disease mucosa. Gut. 1999;44:629–35.
35. Ohno Y, Lee J, Fusunyan RD, MacDermott RP, Sanderson IR. Macrophage inflammatory protein-2: chromosomal regulation in rat small intestinal epithelial cells. Proc Natl Acad Sci USA. 1997;94:10279–84.
36. Koyama SY, Podolsky DK. Differential expression of transforming growth factors alpha and beta in rat intestinal epithelial cells. J Clin Invest. 1989;83:1768–73.
37. Ruemmele FM, Gurbindo C, Mansour AM, Marchand R, Levy E, Seidman EG. Effects of interferon gamma on growth, apoptosis, and MHC class II expression of immature rat intestinal crypt (IEC-6) cells. J Cell Physiol. 1998;176:120–6.

38. Ruemmele FM, Dionne S, Levy E, Seidman EG. TNFalpha-induced IEC-6 cell apoptosis requires activation of IEC caspases whereas complete inhibition of the caspase cascade leads to necrotic cell death. Biochem Biophys Res Commun. 1999;260:159–66.

39. Schmitz H, From M, Bentzel CJ et al. Tumor necrosis factor-alpha (TNFalpha) regulates the epithelial barrier in the human intestinal cell line HT-29/B6. J Cell Sci. 1999;112:137–46.

40. Moon R, Parikh AA, Szabo C, Fischer JE, Salzman AL, Hasselgren PO. Complement C3 production in human intestinal epithelial cells is regulated by interleukin 1beta and tumor necrosis factor alpha. Arch Surg. 1997;132:1289–93.

41. Kvale D, Brandtzaeg P. Butyrate differentially affects constitutive and cytokine-induced expression of HLA molecules, secretory component, and ICAM-1 in a colonic epithelial cell line (HT-29, clone m3). Adv Exp Med Biol. 1993;371:183–8.

42. Nilsen EM, Johansen FE, Kvale D, Krajci P, Brandtzaeg P. Different regulatory pathways employed in cytokine-enhanced expression of secretory component and epithelial HLA class I genes. Eur J Immunol. 1999;29:168–79.

43. Kontoyiannis D, Pasparakis M, Pizarro TT, Cominelli F, Kolias G. Impaired on/off regulation of TNF biosynthesis in mice lacking TNF AU-rich elements: implications for joint and gut-associated immunopathogenesis. Immunity. 1999;10:387–98.

44. Van Dullemen HM, van Deventer SJ, Hommes DW et al. Treatment of Crohn's disease with anti-tumor necrosis factor chimeric monoclonal antibody (cA2). Gastroenterology. 1995;109:129–35.

45. Targan SR, Hanauer SB, van Deventer SJ et al. A short-term study of chimeric monoclonal antibody cA2 to tumor necrosis factor alpha for Crohn's disease. Crohn's Disease cA2 Study Group. N Engl J Med. 1997;337:1029–35.

46. Panja A, Goldberg S, Eckmann L, Krishen P, Mayer L. The regulation and functional consequence of proinflammatory cytokine binding on human intestinal epithelial cells. J Immunol. 1998;161:3675–84.

47. Niessner M, Volk BA. Altered Th1/Th2 cytokine profiles in the intestinal mucosa of patients with inflammatory bowel disease as assessed by quantitative reversed transcribed polymerase chain reaction (RT-PCR). Clin Exp Immunol. 1995;101:428–35.

48. Strober W, Ludviksson BR, Fuss IJ. The pathogenesis of mucosal inflammation in murine models of inflammatory bowel disease and Crohn's disease. Ann Intern Med. 1998;128:848–56.

49. Colgan SP, Resnick MB, Parkos CA et al. IL-4 directly modulates function of a model human intestinal epithelium. J Immunol. 1994;153:2122–9.

50. Hogaboam CM, Vallance BA, Kumar A et al. Therapeutic effects of interleukin-4 gene transfer in experimental inflammatory bowel disease. J Clin Invest. 1997;2766–76.

51. Kuhn R, Lohler J, Rennick D, Rajewsky K, Muller W. Interleukin-10-deficient mice develop chronic enterocolitis. Cell. 1993;75:263–74.

52. Van Deventer SJ, Elson CO, Fedorak RN. Multiple doses of intravenous interleukin 10 in steroid-refractory Crohn's disease. Crohn's Disease Study Group. Gastroenterology. 1997;113:383–9.

53. Bourreille A, Segain JP, Raingeard de la Bletiere D et al. Lack of interleukin 10 regulation of antigen presentation-associated molecules expressed on colonic epithelial cells. Eur J Clin Invest. 1999;29:48–55.

54. Lugering N, Kucharzik T, Kraft M et al. Interleukin (IL)-13 and IL-4 are potent inhibitors of IL-8 secretion by human intestinal epithelial cells. Dig Dis Sci. 1999;44:649–55.

55. Kolios G, Wright KL, Jordan NJ, Leithead JB, Robertson DA, Westwick. C-X-C and C-C chemokine expression and secretion by the human colonic epithelial cell line, HT-29: differential effect of T lymphocyte-derived cytokines. Eur J Immunol. 1999;29:530–6.

56. Kolios G, Rooney N, Murphy CT, Robertson DA, Westwick J. Expression of inducible nitric oxide synthase activity in human colon epithelial cells: modulation by T lymphocyte derived cytokines. Gut. 1998;43:56–63.

57. Paolieri F, Battifora M, Riccio AM, Pesce G, Canonica GW, Bagnasco M. Intercellular adhesion molecule-1 on cultured human epithelial cell lines: influence of proinflammatory cytokines. Allergy. 1997;52:521–31.

58. Orazi A, Du X, Yang Z, Kashai M, Williams DA. Interleukin-11 prevents apoptosis and accelerates recovery of small intestinal mucosa in mice treated with combined chemotherapy and radiation. Lab Invest. 1996;75:33–42.

59. Booth C, Potten CS. Effects of IL-11 on the growth of intestinal epithelial cells in vitro. Cell Prolif. 1995;28:581–94.

60. Qiu BS, Pfeiffer CJ, Keith JC, Jr. Protection by recombinant human interleukin-11 against experimental TNB-induced colitis in rats. Dig Dis Sci. 1996;41:1625–30.
61. Sands BE, Bank S, Sninsky CA *et al.* Preliminary evaluation of safety and activity of recombinant human interleukin 11 in patients with active Crohn's disease. Gastroenterology. 1999;117:58–64.
62. Andus T, Daig R, Vogl D *et al.* Imbalance of the interleukin 1 system in colonic mucosa – association with intestinal inflammation and interleukin 1 receptor antagonist [corrected] genotype 2. Gut. 1997;41:651–7.
63. Ferretti M, Casini Raggi V, Pizarro TT, Eisenberg SP, Nast CC, Cominelli F. Neutralization of endogenous IL-1 receptor antagonist exacerbates and prolongs inflammation in rabbit immune colitis. J Clin Invest. 1994;94:449–53.
64. McCall RD, Haskill S, Zimmermann EM, Lund PK, Thompson RC, Sartor RB. Tissue interleukin 1 and interleukin-1 receptor antagonist expression in enterocolitis in resistant and susceptible rats. Gastroenterology. 1994;106:960–72.
65. Hirsch E, Irikura VM, Paul SM, Hirsh D. Functions of interleukin 1 receptor antagonist in gene knockout and overproducing mice. Proc Natl Acad Sci USA. 1996;93:11008–13.
66. Cao Z, Henzel WJ, Gao X. IRAK: a kinase associated with the interleukin-1 receptor. Science. 1996;271:1128–31.
67. Yamin T-T, Miller DK. The interleukin-1 receptor-associated kinase is degraded by the proteasomes following its phosphorylation. J Biol Chem. 1997;272:21540–7.
68. Wesche H, Korherr C, Kracht M, Falk W, Resch K, Martin MU. The interleukin-1 receptor accessory protein (IL-1RAcP) is essential for IL-1-induced activation of interleukin-1 receptor-associated kinase (IRAK) and stress-activated protein kinases (SAP kinases). J Biol Chem. 1997;272:7727–31.
69. Volpe F, Clatworthy J, Kaptein A, Maschera B, Griffin AM, Ray K. The IL1 receptor accessory protein is responsible for the recruitment of the interleukin-1 receptor associated kinase to the IL1/IL1 receptor I complex. FEBS Lett. 1997;419:41–4.
70. Wesche H, Henzel WJ, Shillinglaw W, Li S, Cao Z. MyD88: an adapter that recruits IRAK to the IL-1 receptor complex. Immunity. 1997;7:837–47.
71. Cao Z, Xiong J, Takeuchi M, Kurama T, Goeddel DV. TRAF6 is a signal transducer for interleukin-1. Nature. 1996.383:443–6.
72. Lin X, Mu Y, Cunningham ET, Marcu KB, Geleziunas R, Greene WC. Molecular determinants of NF-κB-inducing kinase action. Mol Cell Biol. 1998.18:5899–907.
73. Ling L, Cao Z, Goeddel DV. NF-κB-inducing kinase activates IKK-a by phosphorylation of Ser-176. Proc Natl Acad Sci USA. 1998;95:3792–7.
74. Natoli G, Costanzo A, Moretti F, Fulco M, Balsano C, Levrero M. Tumor necrosis factor (TNF) receptor 1 signaling downstream of TNF receptor-associated factor 2. J Biol Chem. 1997;272:26079–82.
75. DiDonato JA, Hayakawa M, Rothwarf DM, Zandi E, Karin M. A cytokine-responsive Ikappa B kinase that activates the transcription factor NF-kappaB. Nature. 1997;388:548–54.
76. Zandi E, Rothwarf DM, Delhase M, Hayakawa M, Karin M. The IkappaB kinase complex (IKK) contains two kinase subunits, IKKalpha and IKKbeta, necessary for IkappaB phosphorylation and NF-kappaB activation. Cell. 1997;91:243–52.
77. Mercurio F, Zhu H, Murray BW *et al.* IKK-1 and IKK-2: cytokine-activated IkappaB kinases essential for NF-kappaB activation. Science. 1997;278:860–6.
78. Colotta F, Dower SK, Sims JE, Mantovani A. The type II 'decoy' receptor: a novel regulatory pathway for interleukin 1. Immunol Today. 1994;15:562–6.
79. Arend WP, Joslin FG, Thompson RC, Hannum CH. An IL-1 inhibitor from human monocytes. Production and characterization of biologic properties. J Immunol. 1989;143:1851–8.
80. Hannum CH, Wilcox CJ, Arend WP *et al.* Interleukin-1 receptor antagonist activity of a human interleukin-1 inhibitor. Nature. 1990;343:336–40.
81. Eisenberg SP, Evans RJ, Arend WP *et al.* Primary structure and functional expression from complementary DNA of a human interleukin-1 receptor antagonist. Nature. 1990;343:341–6.
82. Carter DB, Deibel MR, Jr, Dunn CJ *et al.* Purification, cloning, expression and biological characterization of an interleukin-1 receptor antagonist protein. Nature. 1990;344:633–8.
83. Haskill S, Martin G, Van Le L *et al.* cDNA cloning of an intracellular form of the human interleukin 1 receptor antagonist associated with epithelium. Proc Natl Acad Sci USA. 1991;88:3681–5.

84. Cominelli F, Bortolami M, Pizarro TT *et al.* Rabbit interleukin-1 receptor antagonist. Cloning, expression, functional characterization, and regulation during intestinal inflammation. J Biol Chem. 1994;269:6962–71.
85. Muzio M, Polentarutti N, Sironi M *et al.* Cloning and characterization of a new isoform of the interleukin 1 receptor antagonist. J Exp Med. 1995;182:623–8.
86. Watson JM, Lofquist AK, Rinehart CA *et al.* The intracellular IL-1 receptor antagonist alters IL-1-inducible gene expression without blocking exogenous signaling by IL-1 beta. J Immunol. 1995;155:4467–75.
87. Corradi A, Franzi AT, Rubartelli A. Synthesis and secretion of interleukin-1 alpha and interleukin-1 receptor antagonist during differentiation of cultured keratinocytes. Exp Cell Res. 1995;217:355–62.
88. Levine SJ, Wu T, Shelhamer JH. Extracellular release of the type I intracellular IL-1 receptor antagonist from human airway epithelial cells: differential effects of IL-4, IL-13, IFN-gamma, and corticosteroids. J Immunol. 1997;158:5949–57.
89. Rousset M. The human colon carcinoma cell lines HT-29 and Caco-2: two *in vitro* models for the study of intestinal differentiation. Biochimie. 1986;68:1035–40.
90. Zweibaum A, Laburthe M, Grasset E, Louvard D. Use of cultured cell lines in studies of intestinal cell differentiation and function. In: Frizell RFH, editor. Handbook of Physiology: The Gastrointestinal System, IV. New York: Alan Liss; 1991:223–55.
91. Louvard D, Kedinger M, Hauri HP. The differentiating intestinal epithelial cells: establishment and maintenance of functions through interactions between cellular structures. Annu Rev Cell Biol. 1992;8:157–95.
92. Huang N, Katz JP, Martin DR, Wu GD. Inhibition of IL-8 gene expression in Caco-2 cells by compounds which induce histone hyperacetylation. Cytokine. 1997.9:27–36.
93. Huang N, Wu GD. Short chain fatty acids inhibit the expression of the neutrophil chemoattractant, interleukin 8, in the Caco-2 intestinal cell line. Adv Exp Med Biol. 1997;427:145–53.
94. Lesuffleur T, Barbat A, Dussaulx E, Zweibaum A. Growth adaptation to methotrexate of HT-29 human colon carcinoma cells is associated with their ability to differentiate into columnar absorptive and mucus-secreting cells. Cancer Res. 1990;50:6334–43.
95. Böcker U, Schottelius A, Watson YM et al. Cellular differentiation causes a selective down-regulation of interleukin (IL)-1β mediated NF-$\kappa\beta$ activation and IL-8 gene expression in intestinal epithelial cells. J Biol Chem. 2000;275:12207–13.

9
Homeobox genes and intestinal development

C. DOMON-DELL, I. DULUC, M. KEDINGER and J.-N. FREUND

INTRODUCTION

Cell proliferation and differentiation of the intestinal epithelium are complex processes that occur not only during development and organogenesis of the digestive tract, but also throughout adult life, as the epithelium is continuously renewed from stem cells. During fetal development the stratified and undifferentiated endoderm is associated to lateral plate-derived mesenchyme, and it progressively becomes single-layered while the epithelial cells lining the nascent protruding villi are committed into the differentiation pathway and express molecules specific of the four major cell lineages: the absorptive cells, the mucus-secreting cells, the entero-endocrine cells and the Paneth cells. Concomitantly, mitotic cells are restricted to the intervillus regions that eventually invaginate into the connective tissue to form the crypts. From birth onwards the intestinal epithelium is continuously renewed. This is sustained by pluripotent stem cells present in the monoclonal crypts that generate an intermediate population of highly proliferating cells to finally differentiate when cells migrate from the crypts to the villi[1-3]. Despite some differences between mammalian species (for a specific review on the human gastrointestinal tract, see ref. 4), the intestine is essentially specialized for the digestion of milk at birth; at weaning it undergoes a functional maturation that allows digestion of the complex food of adults. During fetal development, and up to weaning, a morphological and functional regionalization progressively takes place to define the consecutive parts along the antero-posterior axis of the small and large intestines.

Intestinal development and homeostasis are dependent on a hierarchy of information that determines epithelial cell fate and behaviour as a function of the developmental stage, of the longitudinal localization along the intestinal tract, of the progression into the proliferation to differentiation path, and of the final cell differentiation type. During recent years, three major questions have been addressed in this field, yet the answers remain largely incomplete: (1) what are the molecular bases of the intrinsic imprints that determine epithelial cell fate and behaviour, (2) what are the extrinsic factors delivered locally or at long-range that regulate these imprints to co-ordinate intestinal functions, (3) what are the intracellular transducing pathways used to transmit extrinsic signals to the nucleus of epithelial cells? An increasing amount of data has accumulated recently in this area upon a specific class of genes: the homeobox genes. These studies have identified homeobox genes as molecular components of the intrinsic imprints that regulate epithelial cells, and as nuclear targets of extrinsic factors known to control intestinal development and function.

HOMEOBOX GENES IN THE INTESTINE

Homeobox genes belong to a large family of genes encoding nuclear *trans-acting* factors that bind DNA via a conserved helix-loop-helix basic-rich domain. Pioneer studies conducted in *Drosophila melanogaster* have demonstrated that these genes play a major role in morphogenesis, in cell identity and in cell differentiation[5]. Their function has principally been elucidated in segmented tissues derived from the mesoderm and from the neurectoderm owing to the dramatic phenotypes exhibited by mutants at homeobox loci. Indeed, the embryos show loss of some parts of the body, or transformation of one part of the body into another one. Consistent with their role in early development, homeobox genes are mostly expressed during embryonic and fetal life. However, active expression is retained throughout adulthood in a series of organs that display continuous cell renewal and differentiation, like the endodermally derived digestive epithelium[6].

During intestinal morphogenesis, homeobox genes – in particular genes of the *Hox* clusters – are expressed in both embryonic anlagen that associate to form the presumptive gastrointestinal tract: the lateral plate mesoderm and the visceral endoderm[7]. Only scarce and incomplete data are available relating to these genes in the intestinal mesenchyme. In chickens several genes of the *Hox* clusters exhibit specific and restricted patterns along the longitudinal axis of the intestinal mesenchyme, consistent with the *Hox* code and suggesting a role in the regionalization of the gut as a result of mesenchyme to epithelium signalling[8,9]. Moreover, in *Drosophila*, mesenchymal homeobox genes have been shown to provide the longitudinal information to the endoderm by controlling the expression of diffusible factors of the TGF-β and Wnt families[10]. In turn the mesenchymal homeobox genes are themselves controlled by Shh originating from the endoderm[8]. Studies conducted on transgenic and knockout mice confirm the primary role played by mesenchymal homeobox genes of the *Hox* clusters in the developing digestive tract. Indeed, *Hoxc-4* disruption causes disorganization of the oesophageal musculature and blockage of the oesophageal lumen, *Hoxc-8* ectopic misexpression in the stomach results in harmatoma, *Hoxa-4* overexpression causes megacolon, and *Hoxd-12/Hoxd-13* deficiency provokes defects at the level of the anal sphincter[11–14]. In addition, disruptions of mesenchymal homeobox genes outside the *Hox* clusters also result in intestinal phenotypes, as illustrated by the intestinal hypoplasia reported in *Hlx* knockout mice as well as in *Nkx2–3*-deficient mice[15,16].

In the endoderm, homeobox genes are also expressed during fetal development. However, unlike the mesenchyme, a high expression is maintained in the digestive epithelium throughout life[6,7]. Some of the homeobox genes exhibit a very specific and restricted expression in defined regions of the intestinal tract, i.e. genes of the *Hox* clusters, whereas others are expressed all along the intestinal length, i.e. the *Cdx* genes. These patterns are determined early during intestinal morphogenesis[7]. As the role of *Hox* genes in the intestinal epithelium has not been investigated so far in detail, we will focus on the *Cdx* genes in the remaining part of this chapter.

THE *Cdx* GENES ARE COMPONENTS OF THE INTRINSIC IMPRINTS THAT SPECIFY INTESTINAL EPITHELIAL CELLS

The *Cdx* genes belong to the *caudal* family of homeobox genes that comprises three members in vertebrates. The three genes are expressed in a wide series of tissues during embryonic and fetal life; two of them, *Cdx-1* and *Cdx-2*, become progressively restricted to the endoderm during gut organogenesis and remain active throughout adulthood in the intestinal epithelium. *Cdx-2*, at least, seems to belong to a *ParaHox* cluster[17]. A detailed review on these genes is beyond the scope of this chapter and can be found elsewhere (see ref. 18 and refs therein).

Cdx-1 and *Cdx-2* exhibit an increasing gradient from the anterior part of the duodenum to the colon. In addition, the CDX-1 gene product is essentially restricted to the crypt cells, whereas CDX-2 is present predominantly in the villus cells and at a lower level in the crypts.

Cdx genes and anteroposterior axis

The longitudinal pattern of the *Cdx* genes along the anteroposterior axis of gut is reminiscent of the cephalocaudal gradient of expression exhibited by the *caudal* gene in the *Drosophila* embryos. Evidence has been provided that this gradient constitutes a major component of the intrinsic information used by all nuclei to determine their longitudinal position. Thus, the question arose whether the *Cdx* genes also participate in the positional information along the intestinal length in mammals. A first indication of such an implication came from xenografts experiments in which the fate of fetal undifferentiated colonic endoderm can be modified depending on the origin of the mesenchyme. In this model, tissue recombinants comprising colonic endoderm associated to colonic mesenchyme follow a typical colonic development, whereas a structural and functional heterodifferentiation of the colonic endoderm towards a small intestinal phenotype occurs under the influence of small intestinal mesenchyme[19]. Correlated with this heterodifferentiation, we observed a decrease in *Cdx-1* and *Cdx-2* mRNAs levels in the colonic epithelial cells, which is consistent with the lower expression of these genes in the small intestine compared to the colon[7]. These data were further corroborated by differences in the level of *Cdx* gene expression in grafts of fetal endoderm associated either to an intestinal mesenchymal cell line that directs small intestinal-like differentiation, or to a mesenchymal cell line that directs a glandular colonic-like differentiation[7].

Definitive evidence that *Cdx* genes are involved in longitudinal patterning in mammals was provided by the phenotypes of knockout mice. Although the intestinal phenotype of homozygous *Cdx-1* –/– mice has not been described in detail, these mice show skeletal abnormalities consistent with a role of this gene in determining positional information during early development[20]. Homozygous *Cdx-2* –/– mice are lethal in early embryogenesis, whereas heterozygous *Cdx-2* +/– animals survive and have skeletal abnormalities like the *Cdx-1* –/– mice[21]. It is noteworthy that these mice also exhibit an interesting intestinal phenotype[22]. Indeed, the epithelium is essentially normal, indicating that a single dose of *Cdx-2* is compatible with proper intestinal development; however, areas of metaplasia in which the remaining wild-type copy of the gene is turned off, appear mainly in the colon. In these areas the colonic epithelium exhibits typical properties of the upper digestive tract, the stomach or the oesophagus, which normally fail to express *Cdx-2*. Moreover, a transitional epithelium showing typical characteristics of the anterior-to-posterior small intestine develops intercalated between the gastric-like areas and the surrounding regions of regular colonic phenotype, thus restoring the normal continuity of intestinal tissue types. Although the molecular basis of the transitional phenotype is not elucidated, these observations clearly demonstrate that *Cdx-2* is a major component of the intrinsic intestinal imprints that inform epithelial cells that they belong to the gut, and where they are located along the intestinal length. The data also indicate that loss of function of a homeobox gene in the non-segmented endoderm causes a typical homeotic transformation (anteriorization), consistent with the role attributed to these genes in segmented tissues.

The ways by which *Cdx* genes drive the endodermal cells towards the intestinal phenotype, and provide the positional information along the longitudinal axis of gut, are questions still under investigation. Interestingly, the skeletal phenotype resulting from the loss of *Cdx-1* in knockout mice is accompanied by changes in *Hox* gene patterns[20], and overexpression of *Cdx-2* in the human colonic Caco-2 cell line leads to up-regulation of the *Hoxc-8* gene[23]. This suggests that the function of the *Cdx* genes may be, at least in part, mediated by *Hox* genes. In addition, the CDX-2 homeoprotein directly interacts with *cis*-acting elements present in the promoters of several intestinal-specific genes including digestive enzymes, proteins involved in calcium metabolism and proteins required for vitamin absorption[18]. Taken together, these observations support the notion that the CDX proteins may participate to the transcriptional complex that dictates the tissue-specific expression of a specialized set of genes in the intestine and/or that they are at the head of a cascade of regulator genes including *Hox* genes whose function in determining cell identity has been demonstrated in other tissues.

Cdx genes and crypt–villus axis

Beside the role attributed to *Cdx* genes in positional information along the longitudinal axis of the gut, a role in controlling the progression of cells through the proliferation to differentiation path along the crypt–villus axis has been proposed, according to data obtained using intestinal cell lines transfected with expression plasmids engineered either to overexpress these genes or to inhibit their endogenous expression[23,24]. For instance, the growth of human colonic Caco-2 cells is reduced in culture by inhibition of *Cdx-1* with antisense RNA, suggesting that this gene, predominantly expressed in the crypts, may participate in the control of cell proliferation. Unlike the situation observed with *Cdx-1*, the proliferation of human Caco-2 cells and of rat intestinal IEC cells is reduced by *Cdx-2* overexpression. Moreover, *Cdx-2* overexpression triggers cell polarization and functional differentiation of the undifferentiated IEC cells, and it stimulates overall cell differentiation in the spontaneously differentiating Caco-2 cells. Indeed, the increase of *Cdx-2* in Caco-2 cells stimulates molecules that are preferentially expressed in villus epithelial cells as compared to crypt cells, like digestive enzymes (sucrase, lactase) and molecules involved in cell–cell or cell–matrix interactions (E-cadherin, APC, HD1/plectin, laminin-γ2 chain, the most prominent effect being the stimulation of integrin-β4). Thus, these data indicate that the *Cdx* genes are involved in regulation of the equilibrium between cell proliferation and differentiation that is crucial for homeostasis during the constant renewal of the intestinal epithelium. The two genes seem to play different roles in this process, consistent with their respective patterns along the crypt–villus axis. Except for the digestive enzymes lactase and sucrase, it is not yet known whether the CDX-1 and/or CDX-2 homeoproteins exert direct and/or indirect regulatory effects on the the downstream targets.

EXTRINSIC FACTORS REGULATE *Cdx* GENES IN THE INTESTINE

Short-range acting factors

As mentioned previously, a wide series of experiments has stressed the importance of epithelial–mesenchymal cell interactions in the developing intestine and later on for homeostasis of the adult intestine (see refs 3 and 25); these interactions are permissive, instructive and reciprocal. As development proceeds, the cellular environment of the epithelial cells becomes more complex and it additionally comprises cells of the lymphoid lineage as well as neuroendocrine terminations. It is also most likely that lateral interactions between neighbouring epithelial cells may influence their behaviour. There are as yet no data on the potential regulation of epithelial *Cdx* genes by lymphoid or neuroendocrine cell interactions. As far as interepithelial cell interactions are concerned, a possible effect on *Cdx* genes is suggested by the finding of a transitional phenotype in the metaplasia areas shown by *Cdx-2* +/– mice[22]. In addition, we have observed that a secretory peptide (neurotensin) produced by the N subtype of entero-endocrine epithelial cells can modulate the expression of *Cdx-2* in an intestinal epithelial cell line (unpublished data).

Epithelial–mesenchymal cell interaction is a common feature during organogenesis. A large number of studies performed during the past decade indicated that diffusible factors secreted locally are primary mediators of these interactions; in particular, molecules of the Wnt, TGF-β and FGF families have been implicated in the control of epithelial cells[26]. Although there are indications that some of these molecules regulate *Cdx* genes during early development (unpublished results), it is not known whether they also participate in the control of adult intestinal homeostasis.

The epithelial–mesenchymal cell interactions are also regulated by the extracellular matrix. In the intestine the extracellular matrix organizes at the epithelial–mesenchymal interface into a basement membrane mainly composed of different laminin isoforms, collagen IV, perlecan and nidogen; both epithelial and mesenchymal cells contribute to the production of basement membrane molecules[27]. Particular interest was directed to molecules of the laminin family, since the different isoforms are not evenly distributed along the crypt–villus axis; indeed, the laminin-1 and laminin-2 isoforms preferentially accumulate at the level of the crypt, whereas laminin-5 and laminin-10 concentrate in the villus basement membrane[28]. The use of several experimental models led to the conclusion that laminins, in particular the laminin-1 isoform, represent important regulators of intestinal cell behaviour and differentiation: these experiments used co-cultures of fetal endoderm and mesenchyme in the presence of anti-laminin antibodies, cultures of human colonic Caco-2 cells on laminin coatings, and inhibition of the endogenous production of laminin-1 in Caco-2 cells by antisense RNA directed against the $\alpha 1$ chain of this isoform. A compilation of these data suggests that laminin-1 stimulates intestinal epithelial cell differentiation[27]. It is noteworthy that the Caco-2 cell model allowed us to demonstrate that the differentiating effect of laminin-1 is correlated to a stimulation of Cdx-2[23]. This demonstrated for the first time that a homeobox gene can be regulated by a component of the extracellular matrix. Moreover, an overexpression of Cdx-2 modifies the production of extracellular matrix components by the epithelial cells themselves, as well as their cellular integrin repertoire (see above); this provides evidence for cross-talk between extracellular matrix components, integrins and the Cdx genes for the maintenance of an accurate equilibrium between cell proliferation and differentiation in the intestinal epithelium[23].

Long-range acting factors

Beside the cell interactions mediated locally by diffusible factors and basement membrane molecules, the epithelial–mesenchymal unit is also controlled by long-range acting factors including morphogens and hormones. Retinoic acids are general morphogenetic agents and major regulators of homeobox genes[29]. At the intestinal level, retinoic acid treatment of fetal intestinal explants cultured *in vitro* accelerates villus outgrowth and endoderm cell differentiation, and it stimulates crypt proliferation in grafted fetal intestines[30]. Interestingly, this is accompanied by an increase of Cdx-1 expression and by a less-pronounced effect on Cdx-2[31]. Unlike retinoic acids, which act on fetal development, thyroid hormones regulate intestinal functions postnatally. The role of these hormones has recently been approached using knockout mice for the T3Rα or T3Rβ subtypes of thyroid receptors[32]. Whereas the T3Rβ-deficient homozygotes only exhibit auditory defects, T3Rα–/– animals exhibit progressive defects in thyroid, bone and small intestinal development after birth, so that they stop growing and die around weaning. The strong intestinal phenotype is characterized by a reduced proliferation rate of the crypt cells and by a delayed differentiation of the villus enterocytes assessed by morphological and functional criteria. It is noteworthy that this phenotype is accompanied by a decrease in the expression of both Cdx-1 and Cdx-2 genes[33]. Two or three months rescue of the T3Rα–/– mice can be obtained by thyroxine injections; in the rescued animals intestinal morphology and functions is partially recovered, and concomitantly the level of *Cdx-1* expression is restored while that of *Cdx-2* is increased, but remained still lower than in wild-types. These data suggest that thyroid hormones, via the α subtype of receptors, participate in the network of extrinsic factors required for accurate intestinal functions and *Cdx* gene expression, and that T3Rβ, although dispensable, can substitute for T3Rα in the intestine[33].

EVIDENCE FOR AN INTRACELLULAR SIGNALLING PATHWAY THAT REGULATES THE TRANSCRIPTION OF *Cdx* GENES

The above results indicate that the *Cdx* genes are regulated by multiple extrinsic factors acting locally or at long range. This implies the involvement of intracellular signalling mediators to transmit the extracellular information to the nucleus of the epithelial cells. The molecular mechanisms by which retinoic acids or thyroid hormones control *Cdx* gene expression have not been investigated. Due to the complex expression patterns of the various subtypes of receptors for retinoic acids and thyroid hormones in the intestinal epithelium and mesenchyme, we cannot even rule out that the effects of these regulatory factors are, at least in part, indirect and mediated by the mesenchymal compartment, for instance via a regulatory effect on basement membrane molecules that subsequently control *Cdx* genes[30]. Yet a potential direct effect of retinoic acids on *Cdx* gene expression is supported by the fact that the level of *Cdx-1* is dependent on retinoic acids in the F9 embryonal carcinoma cells[34]. Further investigation of the *Cdx-1* and *Cdx-2* gene promoters will help to answer this question.

The signals provided locally by basement membrane molecules and by diffusible factors use distinct classes of membrane receptors, as well as several specific but interconnected transducing pathways that are still under investigation. Although the *Cdx* genes are good candidates for being nuclear targets of some of these intracellular signalling pathways, the data are sparse in this field as yet. However, we recently showed that the *Cdx* genes are targets of ras signalling, a major transducing pathway involved in normal and pathological processes[35]. These experiments were conducted on colonic Caco-2 cells stably transfected with a plasmid encoding oncogenic Val12 Ha-ras. In these cells, oncogenic ras activation has opposite effects on the two *Cdx* genes. Indeed it stimulates *Cdx-1* mRNA expression and the transcriptional activity of the *Cdx-1* promoter, whereas *Cdx-2* mRNA is reduced together with the promoter activity of the gene. We also reported that these effects use different signalling pathways, since the stimulatory effect on *Cdx-1* is mediated by Raf/MEK, whereas the inhibitory effect on *Cdx-2* is mediated by protein kinase C activation and consequently by a modification of the c-Jun/c-Fos balance that alters AP-1 binding at the level of the *Cdx-2* promoter. These data open the way for many investigations on other major intracellular signalling pathways, in particular those linked to extracellular matrix and growth factors.

CONCLUSION

The intestine for a long time represented a powerful model to study cell proliferation, differentiation and interactions during development, as well as during the continuous renewal of the digestive epithelium. The data collected during recent years have opened new insights into the molecular mechanisms involved in these processes. In particular, the finding of active homeobox gene expression in the intestinal epithelium beyond fetal life was the basis of an increasing number of studies in this field, according to the key role attributed to homeobox genes in controlling cell fate and behaviour in *Drosophila*.

The current data strongly support the view that the *Cdx* genes are major elements of the intrinsic imprints that inform epithelial cells about their position along the intestinal length (longitudinal axis), and that control the equilibrium between cell proliferation/differentiation along the crypt–villus axis (vertical axis). There is no evidence, however, as to whether they are involved in the cell commitment process that differentiates the four major cell types of the intestinal epithelium. The fact that the *Cdx* genes are regulated by a number of extrinsic factors via important intracellular signalling pathway(s) deserves the interest directed to these homeobox genes, to obtain a mechanistic view of how multiple signals delivered by extracellular factors are integrated to modulate the intrinsic imprints required for intestinal development and homeostasis. Moreover, according to the effects of oncogenic ras on the *Cdx* genes[35], and to the altered expression of these homeobox genes in several cancers of the digestive tract[36,37], it is tempting to speculate that changes in *Cdx* gene expression may participate in the defects in cell proliferation and/or differentiation related to intestinal pathology.

NOTE ADDED IN PROOF

Evidence has recently been provided that *Cdx1* is the first intestinal-specific target of growth/differentiation factors of the Wnt family, through activation of the β-catenin/Tcf pathway (Likert H, Domon C, Huls G, Wehrle C, Dulue I, Clevers H, Meyer B, Freund JN, Kemler R. Wnt/β-catenin signaling regulates the expression of the homeobox gene *Cdx1* in embryonic intestine. Development. 2000; in press).

References

1. Henning SJ, Rubin DC, Shulman JM. Ontogeny of the intestinal mucosa. In: Johnson LR, editor. Physiology of the Gastrointestinal Tract, 3rd edn. New York: Raven Press; 1994:571–601.
2. Hermiston ML, Simon TC, Crossman MW, Gordon JI. Model systems for studying cell fate specification and differentiation in the gut epithelium. From worms to flies to mice. In: Johnson LR, editor. Physiology of the Gastrointestinal Tract, 3rd edn. New York: Raven Press; 1994:521–68.
3. Kedinger M. Growth and development of intestinal mucosa. In: Campbell FC, editor. Small Bowel Enterocyte Culture and Transplantation. Austin, TX: R. G. Landes; 1994:1–31.
4. Montgomery RK, Mulberg AE, Grand RJ. Development of the human gastrointestinal tract: twenty years of progress. Gastroenterology. 1999;116:702–31.
5. McGinnis W, Krumlauf R. Homeobox genes and axial patterning. Cell. 1992;68:283–302.
6. James R, Kazenwadel J. Homeobox gene expression in the intestinal epithelium of adult mice. J Biol Chem. 1991;266:3246–51.

7. Duluc I, Lorentz O, Fritsch C, Leberquier C, Kedinger M, Freund JN. Changing intestinal connective tissue interactions alters homeobox gene expression in epithelial cells. J Cell Sci. 1997;110:1317–24.

8. Roberts DJ, Johnson RL, Burke AC, Nelson CE, Morgan BA, Tabin C. Sonic hedgehog is an endodermal signal inducing Bmp-4 and *Hox* genes during induction and regionalization of the chick hindgut. Development. 1995;121:3163–74.

9. Sekimoto T, Yoshinobu K, Yoshida M *et al.* Region-specific expression of murine *Hox* genes implies the *Hox* code-mediated patterning of the digestive tract. Genes Cells. 1998;3:51–64.

10. Bienz M. Homeotic genes and positional signalling in the *Drosophila* viscera. Trends Genet. 1994;10:22–6.

11. Boulet AM, Capecchi MR. Targeted disruption of *Hoxc-4* causes esophageal defects and vertebral transformations. Dev Biol. 1996;177:232–49.

12. Pollock RA, Jay G, Bieberich CJ. Altering the boundaries of *Hox3.1* expression: evidence for antipodal gene regulation. Cell. 1992;71:911–23.

13. Wolgemuth DJ, Behringer RR, Mostoller MP, Brinster RL, Palmiter RD. Transgenic mice overexpressing the mouse homoeobox-containing gene *Hox-1.4* exhibit abnormal gut development. Nature. 1989;337:464–7.

14. Kondo T, Dolle P, Zakany J, Duboule D. Function of posterior *HoxD* genes in the morphogenesis of the anal sphincter. Development. 1996;122:2651–9.

15. Hentsch B, Lyons I, Li R *et al.* *Hlx* homeo box gene is essential for an inductive tissue interaction that drives expansion of embryonic liver and gut. Genes Dev. 1996;10:70–9.

16. Pabst O, Zweigerdt R, Arnold HH. Targeted disruption of the homeobox transcription factor *Nkx2–3* in mice results in postnatal lethality and abnormal development of small intestine and spleen. Development. 1999;126:2215–25.

17. Brooke NM, Garcia-Fernandez J, Holland PW. The *ParaHox* gene cluster is an evolutionary sister of the *Hox* gene cluster. Nature. 1998;392:920–2.

18. Freund JN, Domon-Dell C, Kedinger M, Duluc I. The *Cdx-1* and *Cdx-2* homeobox genes in the intestine. Biochem Cell Biol. 1998;76:957–69.

19. Duluc I, Freund JN, Leberquier C, Kedinger M. Fetal endoderm primarily holds the temporal and positional information required for mammalian intestinal development. J Cell Biol. 1994;126:211–21.

20. Subramanian V, Meyer BI, Gruss P. Disruption of the murine homeobox gene *Cdx1* affects axial skeletal identities by altering the mesodermal expression domains of *Hox* genes. Cell. 1995;83:641–53.

21. Chawengsaksophak K, James R, Hammond VE, Kontgen F, Beck F. Homeosis and intestinal tumours in *Cdx2* mutant mice. Nature. 1997;385:84–7.

22. Beck F, Chawengsaksophak K, Waring P, Playford RJ, Furness JB. Reprogramming of intestinal differentiation and intercalary regeneration in *Cdx2* mutant mice. Proc Natl Acad Sci USA. 1999;96:7318–23.

23. Lorentz O, Duluc I, De Arcangelis A, Simon-Assmann P, Kedinger M, Freund JN. Key role of the *Cdx2* homeobox gene in extracellular matrix-mediated intestinal cell differentiation. J Cell Biol. 1997;139:1553–65.

24. Suh E, Traber PG. An intestine-specific homeobox gene regulates proliferation and differentiation. Mol Cell Biol. 1996;16:619–25.

25. Haffen K, Kedinger M, Simon-Assmann P. Cell-contact dependent regulation of enterocytic differentiation. In: Lebenthal E, editor. Human Gastrointestinal Development. New York: Raven Press; 1989:19–40.

26. Chuong CM. Molecular Basis of Epithelial Appendage Morphogenesis. Los Angeles: R. G. Landes; 1998.

27. Simon-Assmann P, Lefebvre O, Bellissent-Waydelich A, Olsen J, Orian-Rousseau V, De Arcangelis A. The laminins: role in intestinal morphogenesis and differentiation. Ann NY Acad Sci. 1998;859:46–64.

28. Beaulieu JF. Recent work with migration/patterns of expression: cell–matrix interactions in human intestinal cell differentiation. In: Halter F, Winton DJ, Wright N, editors. The Gut as a Model in Cell and Molecular Biology. London: Kluwer; 1997:149–64.

29. Marshall H, Morrison A, Studer M, Popperl H, Krumlauf R. Retinoids and *Hox* genes. FASEB J. 1996;10:969–78.

30. Plateroti M, Freund JN, Leberquier C, Kedinger M. Mesenchyme-mediated effects of retinoic acid during rat intestinal development. J Cell Sci. 1997;110:1227–38.

31. Kedinger M, Duluc I, Fritsch C, Lorentz O, Plateroti M, Freund JN. Intestinal epithelial–mesenchymal cell interactions. Ann NY Acad Sci. 1998;17:1–17.
32. Fraichard A, Chassande O, Plateroti M *et al.* The T3R alpha gene encoding a thyroid hormone receptor is essential for post-natal development and thyroid hormone production. EMBO J. 1997;16:4412–20.
33. Plateroti M, Chassande O, Fraichard A *et al.* Involvement of T3Ralpha- and beta-receptor subtypes in mediation of T3 functions during postnatal murine intestinal development. Gastroenterology. 1999;116:1367–78.
34. Taneja R, Bouillet P, Boylan JF *et al.* Reexpression of retinoic acid receptor (RAR) gamma or overexpression of RAR alpha or RAR beta in RAR gamma-null F9 cells reveals a partial functional redundancy between the three RAR types. Proc Natl Acad Sci USA. 1995;92:7854–8.
35. Lorentz O, Cadoret A, Duluc I *et al.* Downregulation of the colon tumour-suppressor homeobox gene *Cdx-2* by oncogenic ras. Oncogene. 1999;18:87–92.
36. Ee HC, Erler T, Bhathal PS, Young GP, James RJ. *Cdx-2* homeodomain protein expression in human and rat colorectal adenoma and carcinoma. Am J Pathol. 1995;147:586–92.
37. Silberg DG, Furth EE, Taylor JK, Schuck T, Chiou T, Traber PG. CDX1 protein expression in normal, metaplastic, and neoplastic human alimentary tract epithelium. Gastroenterology. 1997;113:478–86.

10
Regulation and significance of apoptosis in stem cells of the gastrointestinal epithelium

C. S. POTTEN

Cancer of the colorectal region of the gastrointestinal tract ranks third in terms of incidence and also mortality in the UK, with about 31 000 new cases a year and about 18 000 deaths a year, with virtually the same incidence and mortality levels in males and females. Worldwide there are approximately 700 000 new cases of colorectal cancer each year. (These data come from the UK Cancer Research Campaign factsheets and relate to the years 1985 for world values, 1988 for incidence and 1993 for mortality.) The surprising fact is that cancer of the small bowel is rare, the incidence and mortality figures being marginally over 1% of the figures for colorectal cancer. There have been many attempts to provide an explanation for why colorectal cancer is relatively common, but relatively few explanations as to why small intestine cancer is rare. Some of the data to be presented here allow the hypothesis to be raised that the small intestine is protected against cancer risk, at least in part, by the high propensity of its stem cells to undergo apoptosis following DNA damage induction.

The small intestine is a considerably larger organ than the large intestine, and the cells in the small intestinal crypt are proliferating nearly twice as fast as in the large bowel. The small intestine thus represents one of the most rapidly proliferating tissues of the body. In the mouse each proliferative unit, the crypt, contains about 150 rapidly dividing cells, which have a cell cycle of about half a day; as a consequence a cell enters mitosis every 5 min in each crypt. This high rate of proliferation results in about 300 cells being produced per day from each crypt and these emigrate from the crypt to the villus at a velocity of one or two cell diameters per hour. (About 10^9 cells are thus produced every 4.4 days in the mouse.) As a consequence of this cell proliferation rate and migration velocity, cells reach the tip of the villus between 2 and 3 days after birth by division in the upper regions of the crypt. Thus, most cells in the small intestinal epithelium have a functional life expectancy of only a few days. (Two to three days on the villus and perhaps another two to three days in the dividing transit compartment of the crypt.) The indications are that the cell cycle time in the large bowel is between $1\frac{1}{2}$ and 2 times longer than in the small intestine in both mouse and humans, and that the human cell cycle times, although poorly defined relative to the mouse, are about $3\frac{1}{2}$ times longer for all regions of the gastrointestinal tract. It can be estimated that in the human small intestine, with a possible cell cycle time of about 36 h and a total length of between 5 and 6 m, 10^9 cells are produced approximately every 3 h. In contrast, the mouse small intestine is about 20 cm in length. The human large intestine is about $1\frac{1}{2}$ m in length, compared to the 6–7 cm in the mouse (these data come from many sources and are summarized in ref. 1).

It is now generally accepted that cell proliferation in the crypts of both the small and large intestine is organized into a series of cell lineages of the sort illustrated in Fig. 1. The characteristics of these lineages are as follows: the entire lineage is ultimately dependent on a small number of self-maintaining lineage ancestor stem cells. In principle the removal or killing of a lineage ancestor stem cell will result within a short time in loss of the entire lineage. The

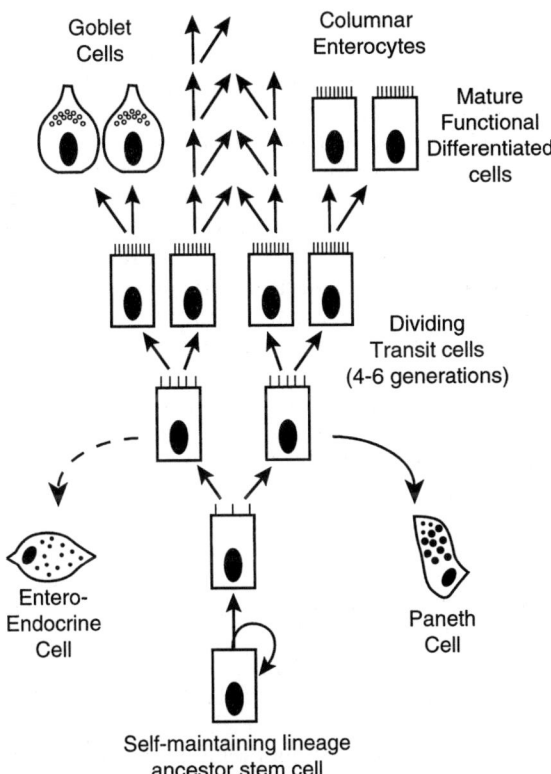

Figure 1 Cell lineage diagram showing the stem and transit cell divisions and the possible differentiation options for the murine small intestinal crypt. It is probable that about six cell generations exist in the transit population and about four to six such lineages exist in each crypt. A similar scheme operates in the murine large intestine but with different differentiation options and up to eight cell generations in the transit population. A similar number of lineages exist per crypt

lineage ancestor cells are the only permanent residents in the tissue, and for this reason it can be argued that it is only these cells that have any relevance in terms of carcinogenesis which requires a series of genetic changes which may take months in the mouse, or decades in humans to be completed (i.e. there is a long latent period between carcinogenic initiation and the ultimate appearance of a cancer). Within such lineages the stem cells are vastly outnumbered by the rapidly dividing cells in the amplifying dividing transit population. During passage through the dividing transit population, various differentiation events may occur, generating various differentiated cell lineages. Unfortunately, in the gastrointestinal system there are no markers as yet available that can be used to identify the stem cells. However, because of (1) its strict polarity, (2) the linear migration of cells from the crypt to the villus, and the fact that (3) various marker experiments and mutation studies have been undertaken, the intestinal crypt represents a biological model system where stem cells can be studied because they are located at very specific positions within the tissue. In the small intestine the relevant position is immediately above (cell position 4) or amongst (cell positions 1–3) the Paneth cells at the base of the crypt, while in the large intestine the relevant position is at the base of the crypt (cell positions 1–2).

Based on studies designed to investigate the origin of the cell migration pathways, as well as studies into long-lived mutant clones, and complex mathematical modelling of a range of cell kinetic experiments, it is believed that the small intestinal crypt of the mouse contains between four and six lineage ancestor stem cells[2,3].

As a consequence of a variety of studies into the radiobiological response of the tissue, for example (1) the levels of apoptosis (discussed below), together with (2) studies into the clonal regeneration ability of stem cells (also discussed below), (3) the patterns of p53 protein expression and (4) studies into the location of the proliferative response during crypt regeneration, we currently postulate a somewhat more complicated organization for the stem cells in the crypt, which is illustrated in Fig. 2. Here, it is suggested that the stem cells themselves make up a small part of the total lineage, i.e. are hierarchical themselves, and that the final commitment to differentiation does not occur until about the third division in the lineage, there being about six divisions or cell generations in total. Under normal steady-state circumstances the cells within cell generations two and three represent part of the dividing transit population. However, if all the ultimate stem cells die or are killed, cells within the first or second dividing transit population still possess the ability to repopulate the entire stem cell compartment and then the crypt. These cells should therefore be thought of as potential stem cells, and the data suggest that there are two tiers of such cells. The first tier represents the immediate daughters of the ultimate stem cell which would be present in the crypt in numbers equivalent to the ultimate stem cells, i.e. four to six. The second tier represents the second and perhaps part of the third transit generation, and may consist of up to about a further 24 cells per crypt. Beyond this, it would appear that there is no possibility for cells to repopulate the crypt, i.e. function as stem cells. It is important to realize that under normal circumstances it would be extremely unlikely that all six ultimate stem cells are killed. Thus, the concept and existence of the clonogenic potential stem cells is somewhat the consequence of laboratory experimentation. Under normal steady-state

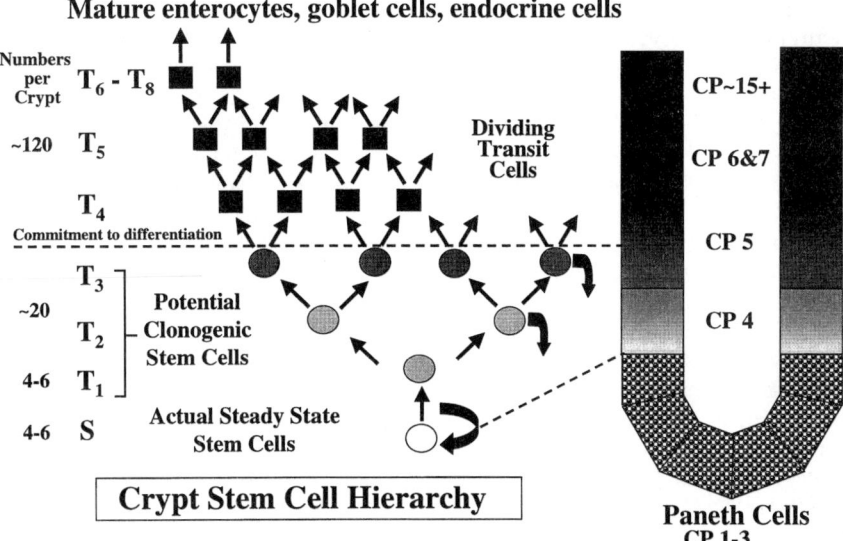

Figure 2 The current model for stem cell organization in the small and large intestinal crypts. Here the stem cell compartment is itself hierarchical with four to six actual steady-state stem cells and up to about 24 potential clonogenic (regenerative) stem cells. The latter are normally part of the transit population, but if the actual stem cells are killed they can replace the lost cells. In the large intestine the actual stem cells would be located at the crypt base (CP1-2).

conditions an occasional single ultimate stem cell may incur DNA damage and commit altruistic cell suicide (apoptosis); see below. This cell deletion could be easily compensated for by a single symmetric stem cell division or the assumption of ultimate stem cell attributes by one of the many potential stem cells. The proliferative organization of the crypt, including current models for the stem cell organization, have been reviewed extensively elsewhere[2,3].

Apoptosis is a form of programmed deletion of cells from tissues, and it characteristically involves isolated individual cells and absence of an inflammatory reaction. The dying cells undergo DNA degradation, via specific endonucleases resulting in characteristic chromatin condensation patterns in the nucleus. The final stages of cell death involve fragmentation of the nucleus and cytoplasm and the generation of apoptotic fragments or bodies. The process has been extensively described and documented for the intestinal mucosa[2,4–7] and the morphological changes can be readily detected in appropriately fixed and stained paraffin sections and the number of apoptotic fragments can be relatively easily quantitated[8]. The number of such fragments does not equal the number of dead cells, but is related to it. The levels of apoptosis can be dramatically raised by exposure to cytotoxic agents[6], and has been shown to be regulated by a variety of genes including the early-response gene *p53* and members of the *bcl-2* family of genes.

Normal healthy murine and human small intestinal crypts contain low levels of apoptosis. This *spontaneous apoptosis* can be seen in mouse small intestine, at a frequency of about one apoptotic fragment in every fifth crypt. When expressed as a proportion of the total epithelial cells in the crypt it represents an extremely low level of inferred spontaneous cell death. However, if this apoptosis is expressed as a percentage of the cells at cell position 4, the stem cell location, it represents about 5–10% of the stem cells dying at any given time. The frequency may be somewhat lower in human small intestine, perhaps because the spontaneous apoptosis in the mouse is associated with the stem cell position in the crypts, and this can only be seen in well-orientated longitudinal crypt sections and orientation is difficult to control in many human samples. The level of spontaneous apoptosis in the small intestine of *p53* knockout mice is essentially the same as in wild-type animals, suggesting that this cell death does not involve the damage-recognition response mechanisms associated with *p53*. Spontaneous apoptosis is extremely rare in the large intestine and is not associated with the stem cell location. The anti-apoptotic or cell survival gene *bcl-2* is not expressed at immunohistochemically detectable levels in the small intestine. However, it is expressed in the stem cell region of the large intestine, both in mouse and humans. The spontaneous apoptosis seen in the small intestine has been interpreted to be a reflection of the stem cell homeostatic mechanisms that maintain a constant stem cell number in every crypt. When occasional extra stem cells are produced, for example by the possible rare symmetric division amongst the otherwise asymmetrically dividing stem cells, one of the cells in the stem cell compartment, which would now contain one extra cell, is instructed, via the homeostatic regulatory mechanisms, to commit suicide via apoptosis. *bcl-2* would appear to compromise this homeostatic regulation in the large intestine, which may allow stem cell numbers per crypt to gradually drift upwards with the passage of time. Each large intestinal crypt containing an extra stem cell would become enlarged as a consequence of the stem cell-dependent lineage which could contain up to 128 cells, thus appearing hyperplastic[9–11]. Apoptosis is also involved in the removal of healthy undamaged cells at various critical stages during development of the embryo, when cells need to be deleted to allow for tissue organization and restructuring (e.g. the interdigital web on the hand). This type of naturally occurring apoptosis is also *p53* independent, since development occurs normally in *p53* knockout mice. However, the *p53* damage detection and response mechanism is also very important during embryogenesis for the detection of damage in embryonic cells and the prevention of embryo abnormalities[12].

There is some debate in the literature concerning the question of whether or not cells at the end of their natural functional lifespan, i.e. at the villus tip, undergo apoptosis. This type of apoptosis may be more associated with cell ageing, senescence, and functional impairment than DNA damage induction. Cells exhibiting the morphological changes characteristic of apoptosis are rarely observed at the villus tip. However, cell death-associated genes such as *bax* and *bak* appear to be up-regulated on the villus and intercrypt table in the colon, and techniques designed to detect DNA fragmentation, such as TUNEL staining, when optimized, show occasional positive cells at the villus tip. Such positive cells are also seen in *p53* null mice, and their frequency appears to vary considerably along the intestinal tract at any one time and also varies throughout the day (i.e. shows a circadian rhythm that is compatible with circadian variations in cell proliferation and cell migration) (Potten, unpublished data).

If mice are exposed to ionizing radiation the number of apoptotic fragments in the crypt rises rapidly and dramatically. Peak values tend to be observed within 3–6 h of exposure. Following low doses of radiation the apoptotic fragments disappear through cytoplasmic digestion after phagocytosis, and as a consequence of host cell migration, resulting in control values being reattained at about 24 h. When the spatial distribution of these radiation or DNA *damage-induced apoptotic cells* or bodies along the crypt axis is determined at the time of peak yield, it is very evident that the spatial distribution is centred around the fourth or fifth position from the bottom of the crypt, i.e. where the stem cells or early lineage cells are to be expected. Thus, it is not rapidly cycling cells that die via this rapid apoptosis, but a sub-compartment of the proliferative pool that occurs most frequently at around the fourth or fifth position. The dose response for the apoptotic yield at 3–6 h was unexpected in that the yield increased in a very dose-sensitive fashion up to doses of about 1 Gy when about six cells per crypt appear to be killed[4,13]; this representing the maximum number of cells per crypt that can die via apoptosis following exposure to ionizing radiation. The dose–response data show that these cells are exquisitely radiosensitive – doses of 0.01–0.05 Gy causing clearly detectable increases in the yield of apoptotic events per crypt. The dose–response data can be interpreted to provide survival curves for the apoptosis–susceptible cells which are exponential over their entire range and characteristically have a D_0 value (mean lethal dose see ref. 14) of about 0.25 Gy for low LET (linear energy transfer) radiation, and a D_0 of 0.06 Gy for 14 MeV neutrons[13]. The cells are so sensitive that tracer doses of tritiated thymidine raise the levels of apoptosis in the crypt. Figure 3

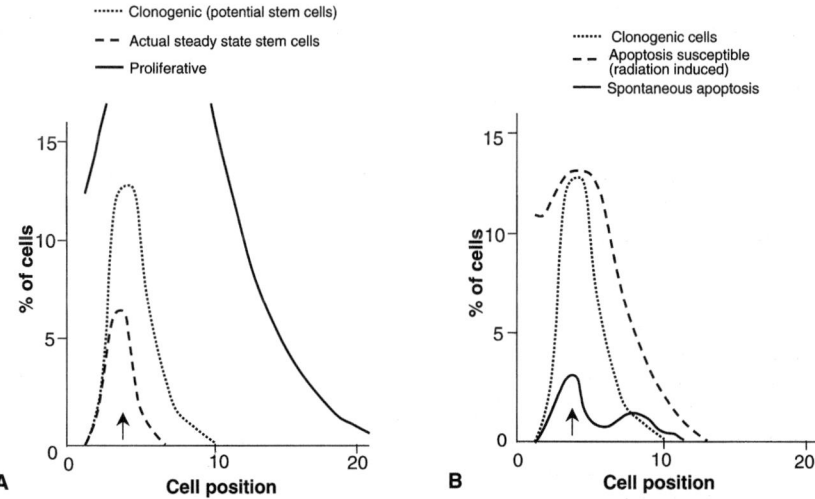

Figure 3 A: Diagram showing the proposed spatial distribution of actual and potential (clonogenic) stem cells based on mathematical modelling (Paulus *et al.*, unpublished) together with part of an actual cell positional distribution of proliferative cells (S phase cells). B: Spontaneous apoptosis yield at each cell position in the small intestinal crypt together with the spatial distribution of the apoptotic yield after low doses of radiation (less than 1 Gy) compared with the theoretical distribution of clonogenic stem cells from A

shows the spatial distribution deduced from mathematical modelling studies, for the presumptive actual steady-state stem cells, the potential clonogenic stem cells (assessed using the microcolony assay), compared with the measured distribution of DNA synthesizing cells (rapidly proliferating cells), and the measured distributions for the *spontaneous apoptosis* and small dose *radiation-induced apoptosis*. These observations suggest that up to six cells per crypt, located at the positions where stem cells are to be expected, are extremely radiosensitive. This implies that these cells have an extremely efficient damage-detection mechanism and little or no capacity to repair any DNA damage. Cells that incur damage activate an altruistic suicide apoptosis and in this way effectively remove the damage and protect the small intestinal tissue[2,11,15].

p53 has been implicated as an early-response gene involved in damage detection, cell cycle arrest, during which the downstream gene *p21* is up-regulated, and in the initiation of apoptosis. Studies with antibodies that recognize wild-type p53 protein show that nuclear protein levels are up-regulated over a time scale comparable to that seen for the apoptosis response, and that the cells expressing p53 protein have a cell positional distribution in the small intestine virtually identical to that for apoptosis, with particularly intensely staining cells distributed at cell positions 4 and 5 in the crypt[9]. However, the cells dying via apoptosis are negative for wild-type p53 protein expression 3–6 h after exposure to radiation. p21 protein is up-regulated over a similar time scale with a tendency for p21-positive cells to be distributed from the base of the crypt to slightly higher positions than were seen for p53-positive cells[16]. The fact that immunohistochemically detectable levels of wild-type p53 protein were not detected in apoptotic cells at the time points that have been studied does not imply that p53 plays no role in the triggering of apoptosis. The p53 protein may be up-regulated at other unstudied time points, or at functional levels that are below immunohistochemical detection. In fact it appears from the observation that radiation-induced apoptosis is completely absent in *p53* null mice and that *p53* does play a crucial role in some way in the apoptosis triggering process.

The hypothesis that we put forward to explain these observations is as follows: the crypt contains up to about six ultimate stem cells that have a high radiosensitivity and a high propensity for being triggered into apoptosis in a *p53*-dependent manner. These cells do not, however, within the time framework of our experiments, show immunologically detectable levels of p53 protein. They occur at about cell position 4 in the crypt. At the same position in the crypt there are up to about six clonogenic cells (the immediate daughters of the ultimate stem cells) that have a high radioresistance which means a good capacity for DNA damage repair. These cells express high levels of wild-type p53 protein and also express the downstream p21 protein. In the next annulus (cell position 5), there are yet other clonogenic cells with even better repair capacity and, therefore, higher radioresistance that express p53 protein and p21. At higher levels still, cells express declining levels of p53 and more constant levels of p21. The epithelial cells in the crypt appear to have an efficient G2/M checkpoint[17,18], but do not appear to operate a G1 checkpoint[17].

In the large intestine there are significantly lower levels of spontaneous apoptosis and fewer radiation-induced apoptoses per unit dose, particularly over the 0–6 Gy dose range[5]. Neither the spontaneous apoptosis nor the radiation-induced apoptosis seems to have any association with the stem cell position, which in the large intestine is at the base of the crypt, i.e. cell positions 1 to 2. As already mentioned, the survival gene *bcl-2* is expressed at the base of the crypt at low and somewhat variable levels in the mouse, but more consistently in the human. The expression of this gene compromises both the homeostatic regulatory processes controlling stem cell numbers (as mentioned above), but also the protective mechanism seen in the small intestine following exposure to DNA-damaging agents such as radiation. The compromisation of the spontaneous apoptosis associated with stem cell homeostasis may result in gradual age-dependent increases in a number of stem cells in a few crypts, i.e. the number of carcinogen target cells. Compromising the DNA damage protection mechanism may result in the perpetuation of DNA damage, either due to inefficient damage-detection mechanisms or misrepair. Either or both of these scenarios may provide an explanation for the increased risk of colorectal cancer.

The importance of the *bcl-2* gene is demonstrated by apoptosis studies in *bcl-2* knockout mice. The spontaneous and radiation-induced apoptosis in the small intestine of *bcl-2* knockout mice does not differ from that seen in the wild types, which is not surprising since no *bcl-2* expression was detected using immunohistochemistry in the small intestine. However, both the spontaneous and radiation-induced apoptosis in the colon of *bcl-2* knockout mice are dramatically increased[10]. *In-situ* hybridization studies suggest that *bcl-2* mRNA is present in the mouse small intestine but is apparently translationally regulated to largely prevent protein expression (Potten, Farrell and Scully unpublished observation). Tumours arising in the colon might be expected to arise from the stem cells which are inherently *bcl-2* expressing and therefore might be expected to continue to express *bcl-2* during the adenoma carcinoma development sequence[19]. The expression of *bcl-2* in these tumours would tend to render them resistant to cytotoxic drug or radiation treatment, as is often observed. We have noted that *bcl-2* expression tends to decrease as adenomas become more aggressive, at the same time that mutant p53 levels increase and that in adenocarcinomas of the colon another survival gene becomes up-regulated, namely *bcl-w*[20].

The only member of the *bcl-2* family of genes that we have detected that shows any association with the radiation-induced apoptosis response is *Bad* (Wilson and Potten, unpublished). *Bax*, which is commonly thought to be associated in a reciprocal fashion with *bcl-2*, is expressed at completely the opposite pole of the tissue in the gastrointestinal tract. *Bax* expression tends to be high on the intercrypt table at the top of the colonic crypts and on the villus in the small intestine.

These data are consistent with the concept that there is a complex set of interacting genes that determine whether cells die via apoptosis, differentiate, or survive and proliferate both in normal tissue and following DNA-damaging exposures. The genes involved are parts of complex families of genes with considerable redundancy and compensation, often making some of the interactions difficult to understand. However, some of the relevant players in this complex process are beginning to be identified and their temporal and cell lineage dependencies deduced.

Acknowledgements

This work has been supported by the Cancer Research Campaign (UK). I am grateful to Dr J. Wilson for helpful comments on this chapter, and to Dawn Booth for preparing Figure 2.

References

1. Potten CS. Structure, function and proliferative organisation of mammalian gut. In: Potten CS, Hendry JH, editors. Radiation and Gut. Amsterdam: Elsevier; 1995:1–31.
2. Potten CS, Booth C, Pritchard M. The intestinal epithelial stem cell: the mucosal governor. Int J Exp Pathol. 1997;78:219–43.
3. Potten CS. Stem cells in gastrointestinal epithelium: numbers, characteristics and death. Phil Trans Roy Soc Lond B. 1998;353:821–30.
4. Potten CS. Extreme sensitivity of some intestinal crypt cells to X and γ irradiation. Nature. 1977;269:518–21.
5. Potten CS, Grant H. The relationship between radiation-induced apoptosis and stem cells in the small and large intestine. Br J Cancer. 1998;78:993–1003.
6. Ijiri K, Potten CS. Further studies on the response of intestinal crypt cells of different hierarchical status to cytotoxic drugs. Br J Cancer. 1987;55:113–23.
7. Potten CS, Booth C, Wilson JW. Regulation and significance of apoptosis in the stem cells of the gastrointestinal epithelium. Stem Cells. 1997;15:82–93.
8. Potten CS. What is an apoptotic index measuring? A commentary. Br J Cancer. 1996;74:1743–8.
9. Merritt AJ, Potten CS, Hickman JA et al. The role of p53 in spontaneous and radiation-induced intestinal cell apoptosis in normal and p53 deficient mice. Cancer Res. 1994;54:614–17.
10. Merritt AJ, Potten CS, Watson AJM, Loh DY, Hickman JA. Differential expression of Bcl-2 in intestinal epithelia: correlation with attenuation of apoptosis in colonic crypts and the incidence of colonic neoplasia. J Cell Sci. 1995;108:2261–71.
11. Potten CS. The significance of spontaneous and induced apoptosis in the gastrointestinal tract of mice. Cancer Metast Rev. 1992;11:179–95.
12. Norimura T, Nomoto S, Katsuki M, Gondo Y, Kondo S. p53-dependent apoptosis suppresses radiation-induced teratogenesis. Nat Med. 1996;2:577–80.
13. Hendry JH, Potten CS, Chadwick C, Bianchi M. Cell death (apoptosis) in the mouse small intestine after low doses: effects of dose-rate 14.7 MeV neutrons and 600 MeV (maximum energy) neutrons. Int J Radiat Biol. 1982;42:611–20.
14. Hendry JH. Radiation sources, geometry, exposure schedules and effect quantitation for irradiation of the gut. In: Potten CS, Hendry JH, editors. Radiation and Gut. Amsterdam: Elsevier; 1995:31–44.
15. Potten CS, Li YQ, O'Connor PJ, Winton DG. Target cells for the cytotoxic effects of carcinogens in the murine large bowel and a possible explanation for the differential cancer incidence in the intestine. Carcinogenesis. 1992;13:2305–12.
16. Wilson JW, Pritchard DM, Hickman JA, Potten CS. Radiation induced p53 and p21[WAF-1/CIP1] expression in the murine intestinal epithelium: apoptosis and cell cycle arrest. Am J Pathol. 1998;153:899–909.
17. Lesher S, Bauman J. Cell kinetic studies of the intestinal epithelium: maintenance of the intestinal epithelium in normal and irradiated animals. Nat Cancer Inst. Monograph. 1969;30:185–98.
18. Chwalinski S, Potten CS. Radiation induced mitotic delay: duration, dose and cell position dependence in the crypts of the small intestine in the mouse. Int J Radiot Biol. 1986;49:809–19.
19. Watson AJM, Merritt AJ, Jones LS et al. Evidence of reciprocity of bcl-2 and p-53 expression in human colorectal adenomas and carcinomas. Br J Cancer. 1996;73:889–95.
20. Wilson JW, Nostro MC, Balzi M et al. Bcl-w expression in colorectal adenocarcinoma. Br J Cancer. 2000;82:178–85.

11
Non-mitogenic effects of growth factors and their receptors in the gastrointestinal tract

K. E. BARRETT

INTRODUCTION

It has long been recognized that a variety of peptide growth factors play a pivotal role in regulating the proliferative responses and differentiation of a variety of cell lineages in the gastrointestinal tract. This role is most clearly delineated for growth factors related to epidermal growth factor (EGF), a mitogen first identified in the 1960s[1,2]. EGF and related peptides, including transforming growth factor-α (TGF-α), heparin-binding EGF (HB-EGF), betacellulin, amphiregulin, and heregulins are widely expressed in the gastrointestinal system and in organs that drain into the intestinal tract[2]. Similarly, there is significant expression of the cognate receptors for these growth factors, known as the ErbB family of receptors (the EGF receptor (EGFr), also known as ErbB1, is the prototypic member of this receptor family)[3]. A significant body of data, including recent observations derived from mice genetically engineered to display selective deficiencies in members of these growth factor or receptor families, points to pivotal roles of such factors in maintaining the delicate balance of epithelial proliferation and differentiation that is required to subserve the normal function of the gastrointestinal tract without the uncontrolled proliferation that would lead to malignancy[2,4]. However, some paradoxical data also tend to contradict a mitogenic role for at least some of these factors. For example, the highest levels of TGF-α are found in the non-proliferative villus cell compartment of the small intestine, rather than in the crypt[5]. Similarly, tyrosine phosphorylation, a surrogate for growth factor activity, is highest in duodenal villus enterocytes[6]. Finally, Huang et al. reported that colonic epithelial cells lose their ability to proliferate in response to TGF-α as they mature, while retaining their ability to activate other EGFr-dependent signalling events[7]. Taken together, this latter body of data has led some authors to propose that growth factors of the EGF family (and probably others) may have roles in addition to their effects on mitogenesis in the gastrointestinal tract[3,8]. The goal of this chapter, therefore, is to review the spectrum of such non-mitogenic effects and their underlying mechanisms, as well as emerging evidence that the EGFr and other members of the ErbB family may be involved in transducing signalling initiated by non-peptide messengers in the gastrointestinal tract.

SOURCES OF EGF AND RELATED PEPTIDE GROWTH FACTORS IN THE GASTROINTESTINAL TRACT

It is pertinent to review briefly the sources of EGF-related peptides in the gastrointestinal system, as well as available information regarding the distribution of receptors for these factors, in that such information is useful in predicting targets of action of these substances. The EGF family of growth factors share broad structural homology and most members are capable of binding to the EGFr and thereby initiating similar (although not always wholly overlapping) cascades of signalling events[2,3,8]. The exception to this scenario are the hereglins, which are not ligands for EGFr but rather bind to and activate two other members of the ErbB family, ErbB3 and ErbB4[9]. Furthermore, ErbB2 is currently designated as an orphan receptor, with no known ligand[10,11].

EGF-like peptides share several features. All are synthesized as large, glycosylated transmembrane precursors, and the extracellular portion is cleaved by proteases to yield the mature, biologically active growth factor[11,12]. The mature forms of EGF, TGF-α, HB-EGF, amphiregulin, and betacellulin all contain a highly homologous motif, including six conserved cysteine residues, which contributes to the tertiary structure of the peptides via the formation of three disulphide bonds, and confers high-affinity binding to the EGFr. The hereglins also contain a highly related receptor binding motif, but subtle alterations in structure make these peptides specific for ErbB3 and ErbB4, with little or no affinity for EGFr[9].

EGF itself is frequently detected in gastrointestinal secretions, including those of salivary glands, Brunner's glands, and the pancreas[13]. In newborns the presence of EGF in breast milk also provides another source for this growth factor[14]. The location of EGF, therefore, is largely luminal, which contrasts with the localization of the EGFr, thought to be restricted to the basolateral pole of intestinal epithelial cells[15]. In the newborn, when the epithelium is relatively 'leaky', luminal EGF may in fact have access to these basolateral receptors, and thereby transduces effects on epithelial maturation[16]. However, under normal circumstances in the adult, this luminal source of EGF would not be expected to be biologically active (particularly since it is susceptible to processing and inactivation by luminal proteases)[3,16]. This paradox has prompted some authors to propose that EGF acts as a luminal 'surveillance' peptide, exerting effects on epithelial dynamics and other functions only in the setting of mucosal injury, where the barrier function of the epithelium is compromised[17].

In contrast to EGF, TGF-α expression and release is well positioned to exert biological effects even under normal circumstances. TGF-α is highly expressed by intestinal epithelial cells themselves, and is predominantly delivered to the basolateral poles of these cells where it can either be secreted following proteolytic cleavage, or exert effects on neighbouring cells via juxtacrine signalling without a requirement for cleavage[8,18]. These features of TGF-α synthesis and localization, as well as the numerical abundance of epithelial cells capable of synthesizing this ligand, suggest that TGF-α, rather than EGF, may be the predominant ligand for the EGFr in the normal intestine[8].

Other growth factors related to EGF (listed above) have been identified in various gastrointestinal tissues, although the precise cellular source of such factors, as well as their role in gastrointestinal function, have yet to be confirmed. It is felt, however, that these substances have at least the potential to regulate various aspects of gastrointestinal physiology and pathophysiology given their ability to bind to and activate the EGFr[3]. Likewise, the heregulins, which are predominantly of neural origin in other systems, have also been identified in various segments of the gastrointestinal tract but as yet have unknown functions secondary to their ability to activate members of the ErbB receptor family other than EGFr. In this regard all known ErbB family members do appear to be expressed in the human intestine (Keely and Barrett, unpublished observations), although only preliminary information is available as to the cell-specific patterns of expression of members other than EGFr.

Relatively little is known of the physiological signals that control the synthesis and release of EGF-related molecules under normal circumstances. Feeding and endurance exercise both induce modest increases in plasma EGF, though by unknown mechanisms[3,19]. However, there is a significant body of data to suggest that expression of several members of this growth factor family can be up-regulated more markedly under pathophysiological conditions. Thus, stress, mucosal injury, and administration of norepinephrine are associated with marked increases in blood, salivary and luminal levels of EGF[20-22]. Similarly, mucosal injury seen in models of gastric ulceration or intestinal inflammation, or in the setting of inflammatory bowel diseases, is associated with the development of cell lineages with up-regulated capacity for the synthesis and secretion of EGF and TGF-α[21,23]. These data suggest that this growth factor family probably contributes to intestinal homeostasis under both physiological and (perhaps more importantly) pathophysiological circumstances.

NON-MITOGENIC EFFECTS OF GROWTH FACTORS

The effects of EGF-related peptides in the gastrointestinal tract can broadly be categorized into three main classes (Fig. 1). The first class relates to the mitogenic actions of these substances, which are not the subject of this review. The second can be categorized as non-mitogenic effects of these substances that contribute to mucosal protection. Finally, there are non-mitogenic actions of EGF and related peptides that can most readily be considered as contributing to the normal intestinal processes of digestion and absorption. There is, however, some considerable overlap between these categories (Fig. 2).

Effects related to mucosal protection

EGF has long been known to exert effects on processes within the gastrointestinal system that could contribute to mucosal protection. For example, EGF

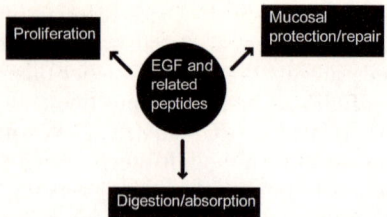

Figure 1 Overview of the different functions of epidermal growth factor (EGF) and EGF-like peptides in the gastrointestinal tract. Effects can be categorized broadly as mitogenic effects that promote epithelial proliferation and differentiation, or non-mitogenic effects that contribute to mucosal protection and repair or normal digestive and absorptive function. For further details, see text

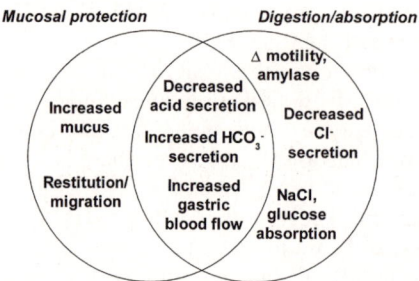

Figure 2 Non-mitogenic effects of EGF and related peptides in the gastrointestinal tract. Actions of these growth factors are categorized according to whether they probably contribute to mucosal protection and repair, or to normal digestion and absorption. As indicated by the overlap, some actions of these growth factors probably contribute to regulation in both areas

and TGF-α are potent inhibitors of gastric acid secretion in a variety of experimental models[3]. The mechanism of this effect appears to involve various points in parietal cell signal transduction pathways. For example, acid secretory responses that involve elevations in intracellular calcium are inhibited downstream of the rise in this messenger (perhaps via a mechanism involving the activity of protein kinase C)[24,25]. In contrast, the effect on secretion induced by agonists that stimulate increases in cAMP are apparently secondary to the activation of an inhibitory G protein (G_i) that reduces adenylate cyclase activity, and/or the activation of phosphodiesterases[24,26,27]. Both of these actions would limit the availability of cAMP in stimulated cells.

The ability of EGF to act as an inhibitor of gastric acid secretion is complemented by its stimulatory effects on defensive mechanisms in the gastroduodenal mucosa. For example, preliminary data imply that EGF can activate mucosal bicarbonate secretion *in vivo*, via a mechanism that may involve the stimulation of prostaglandin synthesis[28,29]. Similarly, a considerable body of data indicate that both EGF and TGF-α can stimulate both the synthesis and secretion of mucus from both gastric and small intestinal goblet cells[30–32]. Both of these effects of the growth factors would be expected to promote the ability of the mucosa to protect itself from acid-peptic damage[33]. Furthermore, both EGF and TGF-α have been shown to increase gastric blood flow, which could aid in mucosal protection during injurious conditions[34,35]. Finally, EGF and TGF-α both have profound effects on epithelial cell migration, a process that is central to the phenomenon of restitution[3,36]. This involves the rapid spreading and migration of epithelial cells across a denuded basement membrane to seal discontinuities in the epithelial barrier, and does not require cell proliferation[36]. Restitution is thought to be central to the early response to injurious agents, and presumably limits further mucosal penetration of noxious substances before cell proliferation can repair the barrier[36]. EGF and related factors are important mediators of this response. For example, EGF caused a rapid increase in the migration of both intestinal and gastric epithelial cells into artificial 'wounds' created *in vitro*[33,37,38]. The mechanism of these effects may differ depending on the tissue studied, with effects in the intestine being dependent, at least in part, on the autocrine activity of TGF-β, whereas the effect in the stomach may be independent of this cytokine[33,38].

Effects related to digestion and absorption

Other non-mitogenic effects of EGF and related peptides may underlie the normal function of the gastrointestinal tract in digesting and absorbing the products of a meal or other ingested substances. Some of the actions of these factors that fall under this category have already been alluded to above. For example, the ability of EGF and its relatives to control gastric acid secretion and duodenal bicarbonate secretion will impact on the pH of luminal contents, and in turn can influence digestive processes and the optimal activity of pancreatic enzymes. Similarly, the ability of EGF to stimulate increases in gastric blood flow would be expected to enhance the systemic absorption of substances that can be transported across the gastric mucosa, such as certain pharmaceutical agents.

In addition to these effects, EGF and related factors have other actions on gastrointestinal physiology that may contribute to digestion and absorption. For example, EGF delays gastric emptying and slows small intestinal transit in rats[39]. This would be expected to increase the contact time for digested components of the meal with the epithelium, and would thereby be expected to increase absorption. EGF has also been shown to modify pancreatic enzyme secretion, although here the effects are complex and both direct stimulatory and inhibitory effects have been reported, as well as an ability to potentiate amylase secretion from pancreatic acini that is stimulated by other agonists of this process[3]. Overall, the precise role for EGF or other related peptides in the control of pancreatic physiology is still a matter for some debate. Short-term stimulatory effects of EGF on amylase release may be related to the ability of the growth factor to elevate cAMP in pancreatic acini, whereas the more prolonged inhibitory actions could represent a negative feedback important in controlling the overall level of enzyme release[3,40].

EGF and related peptides are also potent modulators of the secretory and absorptive functions of the intestinal epithelium. In contrast to its ability to stimulate bicarbonate secretion, a wide range of peptide growth factors, including

EGF, TGF-α, heregulins, insulin and insulin-like growth factors, have been shown to inhibit intestinal epithelial chloride secretion (the mechanism of this effect will be discussed in greater detail below)[41–44]. Conversely, EGF acts to up-regulate electroneutral NaCl absorption in the small intestine as well as the coupled, electrogenic absorption of sodium and glucose[45–48]. Thus, the net effect of EGF and related peptides on solute transport processes, and correspondingly water flux, in the intestinal tract is pro-absorptive, both under fasting (via effects on NaCl absorption) and fed (via effects on sodium-glucose transport) states. The ability of EGF to stimulate NaCl absorption is dependent on the activity of the lipid kinase phosphatidylinositol (PI) 3-kinase, an enzyme known to be important in vesicular trafficking[48]. Accordingly, the up-regulation of transport may reflect the insertion of NHE sodium–hydrogen exchangers into the apical membrane of absorptive enterocytes, as well as direct activation of the turnover of these transporters. Similarly, the ability of EGF to induce a rapid increase in sodium–glucose absorption has been associated with a prompt increase in the surface area of intestinal microvilli[46]. Overall, growth factors such as EGF maximize the absorptive capacity of the epithelium (Fig. 3). Their activity in this regard may account for their ability to reduce secretory diarrhoea in the setting of mucosal injury or infection, both by up-regulating absorptive pathways and suppressing active secretion[49,50].

ROLE OF EGF AND EGFr IN REGULATION OF CHLORIDE SECRETION

Our laboratory has focused particularly on the mechanisms utilized by EGF to inhibit chloride secretion in intestinal epithelial cells[3,51]. This topic will be discussed in greater detail here, both because of its potential significance under

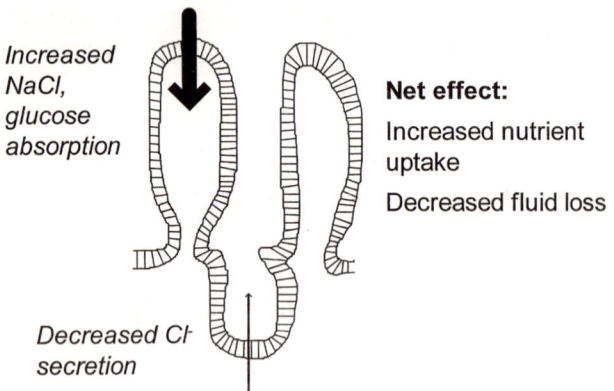

Increased NaCl, glucose absorption

Net effect:

Increased nutrient uptake

Decreased fluid loss

Decreased Cl⁻ secretion

Figure 3 Effect of EGF and related growth factors on intestinal solute transport mechanisms. EGF causes a marked up-regulation of electroneutral sodium chloride absorption, as well as the coupled absorption of sodium and glucose via SGLT1, in villus enterocytes. Simultaneously, EGF suppresses active chloride secretion across crypt epithelial cells. The net effect is more efficient nutrient uptake and decreased fluid loss. For further details, see text

both physiological and pathophysiological circumstances, and because of the insights this system provides into the ways in which the EGFr, and other ErbB family members, may also be involved in transducing signals from agonists that do not themselves bind to these receptors.

Regulation of chloride secretion by EGF

As noted above, EGF and related molecules are potent inhibitors of epithelial chloride secretion[41-44]. This is particularly apparent when studying secretion induced by agonists that exert their effects through an increase in intracellular calcium. However, EGF is probably also significant as an inhibitor of cAMP-dependent chloride secretion, although a different intracellular mechanism is likely to be involved (Maxion, Uribe and Barrett, unpublished observations).

The mechanism whereby EGF inhibits chloride secretion has been quite well elucidated at this point. The growth factor binds to its basolateral receptor and thereby induces activation of PI 3-kinase[52]. Via a pathway that is still the subject of ongoing investigation, but which appears to involve the recruitment of the epsilon isoform of protein kinase C by the lipid products of PI 3-kinase[52a], the ultimate target of the inhibitory mechanism is a basolateral potassium channel[53]. Because basolateral potassium recycling is required to sustain the driving force for chloride secretion, this inhibitory effect reduces the overall level of trans-epithelial chloride secretion. EGF also increases intracellular levels of another messenger that we have identified as an inhibitory modulator of chloride secretion: inositol 3,4,5,6-tetrakisphosphate $(Ins(3,4,5,6)P_4)$[41,54], via a mechanism that probably involves activation of phospholipase C-γ (Uribe and Barrett, submitted for publication). However, the levels of $Ins(3,4,5,6)P_4$ that are induced by EGF are relatively modest compared with those evoked by other, G-protein-coupled receptor ligands, and $Ins(3,4,5,6)P_4$ (an inhibitor of apical, calcium-activated chloride channels[55]) is not required for the full expression of the inhibitory effect of EGF on chloride secretion (Uribe and Barrett, submitted for publication).

Involvement of EGFr in response to unrelated ligands

We have also identified other substances that exert inhibitory actions on calcium-dependent chloride secretion. The prototypic agonist of this type, acetylcholine (or, as studied experimentally, carbachol) differs from EGF in that it first activates, then inhibits chloride secretion[54,56]. Moreover, the ability of carbachol to reduce subsequent calcium-activated chloride secretion is dependent on $Ins(3,4,5,6)P_4$, and targets an apical chloride conductance[53,55,56]. Nevertheless, our studies indicated some points of possible convergence of the carbachol- and EGF-stimulated inhibitory pathways. First, the inhibitory effect of carbachol was reversed by tyrosine kinase inhibitors, including one specific for the tyrosine kinase activity of the EGF receptor[56,57]. Second, we showed that carbachol, while binding to a G-protein coupled, m_3 muscarinic receptor linked to phospholipase C-β and the mobilization of intracellular calcium stores, also caused the transactivation and phosphorylation of the EGFr, with recruitment of downstream signalling components of the mitogen-activated protein kinase (MAPK) cascade[57]. Finally, inhibitors of MAPK activation can potentiate and prolong chloride secretory responses to carbachol, implicating MAPK as a component of an inhibitory signalling pathway that limits calcium-dependent chloride secretion[57]. Whether this pathway involves the downstream production of Ins(3,4,5,6)P$_4$, or other mechanisms for the inhibition of chloride secretion, remains a topic for investigation. In any event, however, the potential for recruitment of EGFr-related signalling pathways by neurohumoral agents that are not direct ligands for this receptor significantly expands the potential roles of this receptor family in the control of gastrointestinal physiology, in ways that are independent of mitogenesis.

Basis of signalling diversification

It should hopefully be apparent from the foregoing that carbachol and EGF induce convergent signalling in intestinal epithelial cells at the level of the EGFr[57]. However, the discussion above also indicates that the consequences of signalling through the EGFr are divergent, dependent on whether the receptor is activated by *bona-fide* ligand binding or transactivation by ligands for G-protein coupled receptors, such as carbachol. We have therefore sought an understanding of how this signalling diversification is controlled. At least part of the explanation may be derived from the knowledge that signal transduction through the ErbB family of receptors is dependent on the formation of receptor dimers, with both homodimers and heterodimers of all possible combinations of family members known to occur[58,59]. Thus, one possible explanation for the differences in signalling outcomes between EGF and carbachol in chloride secretory epithelial cells might be a differential recruitment of other ErbB family members to the EGFr. In fact, we established that only EGF, and not carbachol, causes the formation of EGFr/ErbB2 heterodimers in T$_{84}$ intestinal epithelial cells[43,44]. Similarly, EGF, but not carbachol, causes the recruitment of the regulatory subunit of PI 3-kinase to this receptor complex, and the presumed activation of this enzyme[43,44]. These findings suggest that differential regulation of ErbB receptors in the intestine will probably have implications for signalling outcomes evoked either by growth factors, or non-growth factor ligands capable of recruiting ErbB-dependent pathways. In this regard, preliminary evidence from other tissues suggests that ErbB receptors and their ligands may be subject to both up- and down-regulation under specific pathological conditions[60–62].

SUMMARY AND CONCLUSIONS

It is clear that peptide growth factors in the gastrointestinal tract, and particularly those related to EGF, are more than just growth factors in this system. As outlined above, growth factors can exert a variety of non-mitogenic actions that are potentially involved in both protection of the mucosa and recovery from injury, as well as in functions that underlie normal digestion and absorption. It is tempting to speculate that the integrated regulatory mechanisms that normally underlie the response to ingestion of a meal might also lead to the specific release of growth factors which in turn could provide for the short-term regulation of specific processes, such as secretion and absorption by the intestinal epithelium.

Moreover, the emerging role for growth factor receptors in mediating signalling by unrelated ligands, via a process of transactivation, provides an ever-widening scope for the involvement of such receptors in intestinal function[63,64].

Additional exploration of the mechanisms whereby growth factor ligands and receptors are involved in gastrointestinal physiology and pathophysiology may enhance our ability to intervene when intestinal function is compromised, such as in the setting of inflammation. For example, the ability of EGF to down-regulate active secretory processes, such as those for acid and chloride, may conserve cellular energy for other processes such as migration and restitution. Similarly, up-regulation of NaCl and glucose absorption would limit diarrhoea and enhance the efficiency of nutrient uptake, even under circumstances where the absorptive surface area or functional capacity is decreased. The efficacy of such an approach has already been demonstrated in an experimental model of bacterial enteritis[49]. Ultimately, stable analogues of EGF and related peptides, or peptidomimetic drugs (perhaps lacking mitogenic actions), could be considered as possible adjuncts or even replacements for more conventional anti-inflammatory, anti-ulcer, anti-diarrhoeal or prokinetic therapies.

Acknowledgements

I thank Ms Glenda Wheeler-Loessel for assistance with manuscript preparation. I am also grateful to the following colleagues for their contributions to some of the studies described in this chapter, and for stimulating discussions of this subject matter: Lone Bertelsen, PhD, Jimmy Yip Chuen Chow, PhD, Stephen Keely, PhD, Silvia Resta-Lenert, MD, PhD, Jane Smitham, and Jorge Uribe, MD, PhD. Studies from the author's laboratory pertinent to this chapter have been supported by the National Institutes of Health (USA) (grant numbers DK28305, DK35108 (Project 5) and DK53480).

References

1. Cohen S. Isolation of a mouse submaxilliary gland protein accelerating incisor eruption and eyelid opening in the new-born animal. J Biol Chem. 1962;237:1555–62.
2. Murphy MS. Growth factors and the gastrointestinal tract. Nutrition. 1998;14:771–4.
3. Uribe JM, Barrett KE. Non-mitogenic actions of growth factors: an integrated view of their role in intestinal physiology and pathophysiology. Gastroenterology. 1997;112:255–68.
4. Miettinen PJ. Epidermal growth factor receptor in mice and men – any applications to clinical practice? Ann Med. 1997;29:531–4.
5. Koyama S, Podolsky DK. Differential expression of transforming growth factors alpha and beta in rat intestinal epithelial cells. J Clin Invest. 1989;83:1768–73.
6. Kelleher D, Murphy A, Sheils O, Long A, McDevitt J. Tyrosine phosphorylation in the human duodenum. Gut. 1995;36:34–8.
7. Huang F, Sauma S, Yan Z, Friedman E. Colon absorptive epithelial cells lose their proliferative response to TGF-alpha as they differentiate. Exp Cell Res. 1995;219:8–14.
8. Podolsky DK. Regulation of intestinal epithelial proliferation: a few answers, many questions. Am J Physiol. 1993;264:G179–86.
9. Harris A, Adler M, Brink J et al. Homologue scanning mutagenesis of heregulin reveals receptor specific binding epitopes. Biochem Biophys Res Commun. 1998;251:220–4.
10. Riese DJ 2nd, Stern DF. Specificity within the EGF family/ErbB receptor family signaling network. Bioessays. 1998;20:41–8.

11. Prigent SA, Lemoine NR. The type 1 (EGFR-related) family of growth factor receptors and their ligands. Prog Growth Factor Res. 1992;4:1–24.
12. Massagué J, Pandiella A. Membrane-anchored growth factors. Annu Rev Biochem. 1993;62:515–41.
13. Konturek JW, Bielanski W, Konturek SJ, Bogdal J, Oleksy J. Distribution and release of epidermal growth factor in man. Gut. 1989;30:1194–200.
14. Carpenter G, Wahl MI, editors. Peptide Growth Factors and their Receptors. New York: Springer-Verlag; 1991.
15. Scheving LA, Shiurba RA, Nguyen TD, Gray GM. Epidermal growth factor receptor of the intestinal enterocyte. Localization to laterobasal but not brush border membrane. J Biol Chem. 1989;264:1735–41.
16. Thompson JF, Van Den Berg M, Stokkers PCF. Developmental regulation of epidermal growth factor receptor kinase in rat intestine. Gastroenterology. 1994;107:1278–87.
17. Playford RJ, Wright NA. Why is epidermal growth factor present in the gut lumen? Gut. 1996;38:303–5.
18. Dempsey PJ, Coffey RJ. Basolateral targeting and efficient consumption of transforming growth factor alpha when expressed in Madin-Darby canine kidney cells. J Biol Chem. 1994;269: 16878–89.
19. Konturek SJ, Bielanski W, Konturek JW, Oleksy J, Yamazaki J. Release and action of epidermal growth factor on gastric secretion in humans. Scand J Gastroenterol. 1989;24:485–92.
20. Konturek SJ, Brzozowski T, Konturek PK, Majka J, Dembinski A. Role of salivary glands and epidermal growth factor (EGF) in gastric secretion and mucosal integrity in rats exposed to stress. Reg Peptides. 1991;32:203–15.
21. Wright NA, Pike C, Ella G. Induction of a novel epidermal growth factor-secreting cell lineage by mucosal ulceration in human gastrointestinal stem cells. Nature. 1990;343:82–5.
22. Olsen PS, Kirkegarrd P, Poulsen SS, Nexo E. Adrenergic effects on exocrine secretion of rat submandibular epidermal growth factor. Gut. 1984;25:1234–40.
23. Alison MR, Chinery R, Poulsom R, Ashwood P, Longcroft JM, Wright NA. Experimental ulceration leads to sequential expression of spasmolytic polypeptide, intestinal trefoil factor, epidermal growth factor, and transforming growth factor alpha mRNAs in rat stomach. J Pathol. 1995;175:405–14.
24. Lewis JJ, Goldenring JR, Asher VA, Modlin IM. Effects of epidermal growth factor on signal transduction in rabbit parietal cells. Am J Physiol. 1990;258:G476–83.
25. Wang L, Wilson EJ, Osburn J, DelValle J. Epidermal growth factor inhibits carbachol stimulated canine parietal cell function via protein kinase C. Gastroenterology. 1996;110:469–77.
26. Atwell MM, Hanson PJ. Effect of pertussis toxin on the inhibition of secretory activation by prostaglandin E2, somatostatin, epidermal growth factor and 12-O-tetradecanoylphorbol 13-acetate in parietal cells from rat stomach. Biochim Biophys Acta. 1988;971:282–8.
27. Wang L, Lucey MR, Fras AM, Wilson EJ, DelValle J. Epidermal growth factor and transforming growth factor-alpha directly inhibit parietal cell function through a similar pathway. J Pharmacol Exp Ther. 1993;265:308–13.
28. Marrota F, Chui DH, Zhong GG, Safran P. Effect of graded intravenous doses of urogastrone on duodenal bicarbonate secretion in concious rats: evidence of a dose–response pattern. Digestion. 1990;47:88–94.
29. Marrota F, Chui DH, Fesce E, Zhong GG, Gaetano I. Duodenal bicarbonate secretion induced by epidermal growth factor in rats is partially mediated by prostaglandins. Digestion. 1993;54:19–23.
30. Yoshida S, Kasuga S, Hirao Y, Fuwa T, Nakagawa S. Effect of biosynthetic human epidermal growth factor on the synthesis and secretion of mucin glycoprotein from primary culture of rabbit fundal epithelial cells. In Vitro Cell Dev Biol. 1987;23:460–4.
31. Kelly SM, Hunter JO. Epidermal growth factor stimulates synthesis and secretion of mucus glycoproteins in human gastric mucosa. Clin Sci. 1990;79:425–7.
32. Ishikawa S, Cepinskas G, Specian RD, Itoh M, Kvietys PR. Epidermal growth factor attenuates jejunal mucosal injury induced by oleic acid: role of mucus. Am J Physiol. 1994;267:G1067–77.
33. Podolsky DK. Healing the epithelium: solving the problem from two sides. J Gastroenterol. 1997;32:122–6.

NON-MITOGENIC EFFECTS OF GROWTH FACTORS

34. Tepperman BL, Soper BD. Effect of epidermal growth factor, transforming growth factor-alpha and nerve growth factor on gastric mucosal integrity and microcirculation in the rat. Reg Peptides. 1994;50:13–21.
35. Hui WM, Chen BW, Kung AW, Cho CH, Luk CT, Lam SK. Effect of epidermal growth factor on gastric blood flow in rats: possible role in mucosal protection. Gastroenterology. 1993;104:1605–10.
36. Feil W, Lacy ER, Wong YM et al. Rapid epithelial restitution of human and rabbit colonic mucosa. Gastroenterology. 1989;97:685–701.
37. Polk DB. Epidermal growth factor receptor-stimulated intestinal epithelial cell migration requires phospholipase C activity. Gastroenterology. 1998;114:493–502.
38. Kato K, Chen MC, Nguyen M, Lehmann FS, Podolsky DK, Soll AH. Effect of growth factors and trefoil peptides on migration and replication in primary oxyntic cultures. Am J Physiol. 1999;276:1105–16.
39. Shinohara H, Williams C, Yakabe T, Koldovsky O. Epidermal growth factor delays gastric emptying and small intestinal transit in suckling rats. Pediatr Res. 1996;39:281–6.
40. Stryjek-Kaminska D, Piiper A, Zeuzem S. EGF inhibits secretagogue-induced cAMP production and amylase secretion by G_i proteins in pancreatic acini. Am J Physiol. 1995;269:G676–82.
41. Uribe JM, Gelbmann CM, Traynor-Kaplan AE, Barrett KE. Epidermal growth factor inhibits calcium-dependent chloride secretion in T_{84} human colonic epithelial cells. Am J Physiol. 1996;271:C914–22.
42. Chang N, Uribe JM, Barrett KE. Inhibition of calcium-dependent chloride secretion by insulin and insulin-like growth factor. Gastroenterology. 1996;110:A317.
43. Keely SJ, Halvorsen MJ, Barrett KE. Colonic epithelial ErbB2 receptors: a possible role in diversification of inhibitory signaling via the EGF receptor. Gastroenterology. 1998;114:A385.
44. Keely SJ, Barrett KE. Heregulin inhibits calcium-dependent chloride secretion: a role for ErbB2 and ErbB3. Gastroenterology. 1998;114:A385.
45. Opleta-Madsen K, Hardin J, Gall DG. Epidermal growth factor upregulates intestinal electrolyte and nutrient transport. Am J Physiol. 1991;260:G807–14.
46. Hardin JA, Buret A, Meddings JB, Gall DG. Effect of epidermal growth factor on enterocyte brush-border surface area. Am J Physiol. 1993;264:G312–8.
47. Donowitz M, Montgomery JL, Walker MS, Cohen ME. Brush-border tyrosine phosphorylation stimulates ileal neutral NaCl absorption and brush-border Na^+/H^+ exchange. Am J Physiol. 1994;266:G647–56.
48. Khurana S, Nath SK, Levine SA et al. Brush border phosphatidylinositol 3-kinase mediates epidermal growth factor stimulation of intestinal NaCl absorption and Na^+/H^+ exchange. J Biol Chem. 1996;271:9919–27.
49. Buret A, Olsen ME, Gall DG, Hardin JA. Effects of orally administered epidermal growth factor on enteropathogenic *Escherichia coli* infection in rabbits. Infect Immun. 1998;66:4917–23.
50. Procaccino F, Reinshagen M, Hoffman P et al. Protective effect of epidermal growth factor in an experimental model of colitis in rats. Gastroenterology. 1994;107:12–17.
51. Barrett KE. Integrated regulation of intestinal epithelial transport: intercellular and intracellular pathways. 1996 Bowditch Lecture. Am J Physiol. 1997;272:C1069–76.
52. Uribe JM, Keely SJ, Traynor-Kaplan AE, Barrett KE. Phosphatidylinositol 3-kinase mediates the inhibitory effect of epidermal growth factor on calcium-dependent chloride secretion. J Biol Chem. 1996;271:26588–95.
52a. Chow JYC, Uribe J, Barrett KE. A role for protein kinase C-e in the inhibitory effect of EGF on calcium-stimulated chloride secretion in human colonic epithelial cells. J Biol Chem. 2000;275:21169–76.
53. Barrett KE, Smitham J, Traynor-Kaplan AE, Uribe JM. Inhibition of Ca^{2+} dependent Cl^- secretion in T_{84} cells: membrane target(s) of inhibition are agonist-specific. Am J Physiol. 1998;274:C958–65.
54. Kachintorn U, Vajanaphanich M, Barrett KE, Traynor-Kaplan AE. Elevation of inositol tetrakisphosphate parallels inhibition of calcium-dependent chloride secretion in T_{84} colonic epithelial cells. Am J Physiol. 1993;264:C671–6.
55. Ismailov II, Fuller CM, Berdiev BK, Shlyonsky VG, Benos DJ, Barrett KE. A biologic function for an 'orphan' messenger: D-*myo*-inositol (3,4,5,6) tetrakisphosphate selectively blocks epithelial calcium-activated chloride channels. Proc Natl Acad Sci USA. 1996;93:10505–9.

56. Vajanaphanich M, Schultz C, Rudolf MT *et al.* Long-term uncoupling of chloride secretion from intracellular calcium levels by Ins(3,4,5,6)P$_4$. Nature. 1994;371:711–14.
57. Keely SJ, Uribe JM, Barrett KE. Carbachol stimulates transactivation of epidermal growth factor receptor and MAP kinase in T$_{84}$ cells: implications for carbachol-stimulated chloride secretion. J Biol Chem. 1998;273:27111–17.
58. Sundaresan S, Roberts PE, King KL, Sliwkowski MW, Mather JP. Biologic response to ErbB ligands in nontransformed cell lines correlates with a specific pattern of receptor expression. Endocrinology. 1998;139:4756–64.
59. Jones JT, Akita RW, Sliwkowski MX. Binding specificities and affinities of egf domains for ErbB receptors. FEBS Lett. 1999;447:227–31.
60. Polosa R, Prosperini G, Leir S-H, Holgate ST, Lackie PM, Davies DE. Expression of c-erbB receptors and ligands in human bronchial mucosa. Am J Resp Cell Mol Biol. 1999;20:914–23.
61. Tesfaigzi J, Johnson NF, Lechner JF. Induction of EGF receptor and erbB-2 during endotoxin-induced alveolar type II cell proliferation in the rat lung. Int J Exp Pathol. 1996;77:143–54.
62. Woodworth CD, McMullin E, Iglesias M, Plowman GD. Interleukin 1 alpha and tumor necrosis factor alpha stimulate autocrine amphiregulin expression and proliferation of human papillomavirus-immortalized and carcinoma-derived cervical epithelial cells. Proc Natl Acad Sci USA. 1995;92:2840–4.
63. Luttrell LM, van Biesen T, Hawes BE *et al.* G-protein-coupled receptors and their regulation: activation of the MAP kinase signaling pathway by G-protein coupled receptors. Adv Second Mess Phosphoprotein Res. 1997;31:263–77.
64. Luttrell LM, Daaka Y, Lefkowitz RJ. Regulation of tyrosine kinase cascades by G-protein-coupled receptors. Curr Opinion Cell Biol. 1999;11:177–83.

12
The function of epithelial–stromal interactions in the intestine

G. S. EVANS, M. D. BAUGH, A. C. WHEATCROFT and
M. KEDINGER

INTRODUCTION

The intestinal epithelium has a complex organization but is capable of dynamic change and adaptation following changes to the diet, after exposure to infectious agents, or following physical injury. Adaptation is possible because this is a renewing epithelium in which most cells are replaced every 5–7 days in humans. The old cells are shed into the bowel lumen and replaced by migration of new cells that ultimately derive from a few stem cells that reside near the base of the epithelial crypts. These pluripotent stem cells give rise to, e.g., enterocytes, mucin-secreting goblet cells, entero-endocrine cells, and Paneth cells, but even among these types there are further specialized subsets. The complex patterns of epithelial differentiation along the proximal–distal and crypt to villus axes and the kinetic organization of cell renewal in this organ have been extensively reviewed elsewhere[1,2].

Tissue grafting studies have shown that connective tissue cells generally provide permissive signals for the development of the intestinal epithelium[3,4]. Suggesting a plasticity in the potential of this mesenchyme to support a programmed pattern of epithelial differentiation. However, instructive effects of mesenchyme have been reported where, for example, ileal mesoderm induced small intestinal differentiation when grafted with colonic endoderm[5].

Importance has been attached to the regulatory role of fibroblasts in close proximity to the intestinal epithelium[6]. Recent evidence that fibroblast specialization can influence the developmental programme of the intestinal epithelium[7] underlines the need to understand how this connective tissue is organized to support mucosal function.

Studies of intestinal development have demonstrated that epithelial differentiation requires support from the connective tissue, and that reciprocal interactions between these tissues influence the expression and deposition of extracellular matrix molecules[3,8]. The influence of particular extracellular matrix (ECM) constituents on epithelial differentiation has been demonstrated in cell culture, and also the temporal expression of these molecules related to the programme of epithelial differentiation (for a comprehensive review see refs 8 and 9). The expression by this epithelium of integrin receptors for basement membrane constituents such as laminin[10] varies along the crypt–villus axes in some species[3] but not all. A matrix receptor clearly associated with one cellular compartment is that for hyaluronic acid, which is expressed on the proliferating crypt cells[11]. Therefore interactions with ECM molecules alone cannot explain the complex gradients or cellular differentiation of this epithelium. Growth factors, chemokines and morphogens released by the mesenchyme and epithelium are other potential signals involved in these tissue interactions. Examples where a ligand and its receptor have been found to be expressed on juxtaposed epithelial cells and fibroblasts[12] or ligands inducing other local signalling events[13] indicate how a localized and specific signalling process can be achieved. That intestinal epithelial stem cells can be maintained *ex vivo* in culture[14,15] in the presence of mesenchyme is further evidence of the essential role of connective tissue.

Many of these areas of research have been comprehensively reviewed by others; consequently these developments will be summarized and the chapter will focus more on emerging evidence that mesenchymal cells can disrupt epithelial function in the diseased mucosa.

EPITHELIAL–MESENCHYMAL INTERACTIONS IN INTESTINAL DEVELOPMENT

There are numerous studies illustrating the essential requirement for mesenchymal–epithelial interactions during intestinal development. The evidence is based upon the failure of pure isolated endoderm to express brush-border enzymes *in vitro*, or to survive when grafted ectopically to the chick coelomic cavity. In contrast, endoderm survives and develops into typical intestinal epithelium when associated with mesoderm in these grafts.[4,16,17]. Association of pure endoderm with mesoderm derived from different regions of the fetal intestine usually results in epithelial differentiation consistent with its original proximal–distal position in the gut, and not with the origin of the mesenchyme[5]. This supports the notion of a mesenchyme permissive for a pre- programmed pattern of epithelial differentiation. There is evidence from studies using transgenic mice carrying a liver fatty acid binding protein/human growth hormone reporter gene that these promixal–distal gradients of gene expression are laid down as a pattern in the epithelial stem cell very early in embryonic development[18]. Mesenchyme derived from the skin also supports intestinal epithelial development in grafts and itself undergoes partial differentiation consistent with bowel mesenchyme[19]. This suggests that the intestinal endoderm can instruct changes in the differentiation of mesenchymal cells. However, there are heterotypic associations in which endodermal differentiation is altered by mesenchyme of a different origin[5]. The evidence for such reciprocal tissue interactions has been discussed at length by Kedinger *et al.*[8,20].

ECM DEPOSITION ARISING FROM EPITHELIAL–MESENCHYMAL INTERACTIONS

The synthesis of the basement membrane is a well-characterized example of how intestinal epithelial cells and fibroblasts participate in the deposition of ECM. The basement membrane separates the two tissue compartments and is laid down progressively by coordinated deposition of molecules such as type IV collagen, laminin, nidogen and heparan sulphate (Perlican), and other minor constituents. The cellular origin of these constituents has been defined most clearly in the animal intestine using cross-species grafting experiments with species-specific antibodies to the basement membrane constituents. This work has demonstrated that, whilst many of the basement membrane components such as type IV collagen, nidogen and laminin are deposited by the fibroblasts, there are specific constituents of the basement membrane exclusively of epithelial origin, for example Perilcan (for reviews see refs 3 and 9). In co-culture models of mesenchyme and endoderm it was also recognized that the deposition of the basement membrane constituents precedes the expression of epithelial brush-border enzymes[21,22]. Variations in the composition of the basement membrane may specify signals to support different programmes of epithelial differentiation. Examples of such heterogeneity in ECM deposition along the crypt–villus axis include laminin chains, fibronectin, and tenascin. Detailed studies of the temporal and spatial expression of the laminin chains $\alpha 1$, $\beta 1$ and $\gamma 1$ and other variant chains have also been reported (for reviews of this subject see refs 3, 9 and 10). However, in tenascin 'knockout' mice[23] and in a merosin (laminin variant chain) deficient dy mutant mouse[24] there are no significant changes to the formation of crypts and villi. Therefore, it is unlikely that these ECM components are fundamental to organization of the crypts and villi. Besides, the expression of numerous variants of basement membrane molecules and integrins in the gut could represent 'molecular redundancy' and an indication of potential rescue pathways.

ECM SIGNALLING IN EPITHELIAL–MESENCHYMAL INTERACTIONS

Integrin receptors for specific connective tissue molecules transduce signals from the ECM to epithelial cells[25]. The intestinal distribution of integrin receptors for attachment to laminin (e.g. $\alpha 6\beta 1$ and $\alpha 6\beta 4$) and fibronectin (e.g. $\alpha v\beta 6$) and collagens ($\alpha 1$; $\alpha 2$ and $\beta 1$) have been mapped during the development of the intestine. Differential expression along proximal–distal and crypt–villus axes has been observed for some of these α and β chains but not consistently between species (for reviews of this topic see refs 3 and 10). As for the BM molecules, the lack of clear phenotype in some integrin 'knockout' mice[26], including effects on intestinal development[27], demonstrates that the relationship between integrin expression and cell differentiation is complex.

TRANSCRIPTIONAL REGULATION OF EPITHELIAL–MESENCHYMAL INTERACTIONS

The elegant and extensive mapping of the promoter elements of the mouse ileal lipid binding protein (*Ilbp*) in transgenic mice has demonstrated the complex spatial and temporal patterns in the expression of this molecule in the developing intestinal epithelium (for review see ref. 28).

Underlying the signalling processes that mediate these developmental interactions between epithelium and mesenchyme are transcriptional controls. Along the proximal–distal and crypt–villus, the expression of the caudal-related genes *Cdx-1* and *Cdx-2* is distinctive with *Cdx-1* in the proliferating crypt cells and *Cdx-2* on the differentiated villus cells[29–32] which are maintained beyond the period of organogenesis. Several *Hox* genes show proximal–distal gradients of expression during development and are expressed by the mesenchyme and epithelium[33]. There is also evidence that the expression of *Cdx-2* in differentiated epithelial cells can be modified by contact with mesenchymal cells[8,33]. Overexpression of *Cdx-2* in intestinal epithelial cells also leads to altered extracellular matrix deposition and integrin expression (see Chapter 9 by Jean-Noel Freund in this book). The downstream consequences of altered regulation of ECM deposition were demonstrated by studies in which laminin 1 expression in Caco-2 line was disrupted using antisense RNA strategy which affected the polarity and differentiation of these cells[34].

The functional importance of transcription factors in the mesenchyme has also been shown for winged helix transcription factor *Fkh6*. This is specifically expressed by the mesenchyme adjacent to the endoderm in the developing bowel but *Fkh6* mutations result in abnormal proliferation, differentiation, and morphogenesis of the bowel which are associated with the reduced expression of bone morphogenic proteins Bmp-2 and Bmp-4[35]. A very similar phenotype has been reported for the targeted disruption of the homeobox transcription factor Nkx2–3 in mice[36].

CELL–CELL SIGNALLING IN EPITHELIAL–MESENCHYMAL INTERACTIONS

There are many cytokines that are reported to regulate the proliferation, movement, and differentiation of the intestinal epithelium[37], though this evidence is largely based upon *in-vitro* studies using epithelial cell lines. However, some of these cytokines have been administered *in vivo*, but usually to animals in which mucosal regeneration has been stimulated after injury[38]. Most cytokines are expressed by a diversity of cell types with no clear mechanism for a specific involvement in epithelial–mesenchymal signalling. However, there are some cytokines and their receptors which are implicated in localized signalling at the mesenchymal–epithelial interface in the developing intestine. Examples include members of the fibroblast growth factor (FGF) family which are reported to be mitogenic and motility factors for bowel epithelial cells[39,40]. The binding and stabilization of FGFs by heparan sulphate[41] represents a potential ECM 'reservoir' of these factors, and proteolysis of the ECM following damage and inflammation may release these signals more widely.

Cytokines also appear to change the programme of epithelial differentiation through effects upon fibroblasts. Different populations of fibroblasts have been isolated from cultures of developing rat intestinal mucosa and human bowel[7,42]. From cultures of rat mesenchyme, two phenotypically different lines were isolated by cloning (F1:G9 and A1:F1) and these exhibited different phenotypes and growth responses to transforming growth factor-β_1 (TGF-β_1) and interleukin-2 (IL-2). When grafted in association with pure fetal endoderm both cell lines support different programmes of mucosal development. Pretreatment of these lines with TGF-β_1 and IL-2 prior to their association, and grafting with fetal endoderm, changed the programme of mucosal development but without obvious effects upon the deposition of ECM molecules[7]. Similar differential properties have been found among two clonal cell lines of human lamina propria cells (C9 and C20)[42].

Localized expression at the epithelial–mesenchymal interface in intestinal development has been reported for some 'morphogens' and their receptors. Hepatocyte growth factor, a molecule that stimulates epithelial motility and tubulogenesis[43], is expressed by mesenchymal cells adjacent to the endoderm during the development of villi in the fetal mouse bowel[12]. Most significantly the c-Met receptor for HGF is localized on the basolateral surface of the intestinal epithelium[44]. A potential candidate mediator of endodermally derived signals to the mesenchyme in the mouse embryonic hindgut is the secreted protein Sonic hedgehog (Shh). The Shh gene is expressed throughout the embryonic gut endoderm but not in the pancreatic bud endoderm. Forced expression of Shh in the pancreatic endoderm resulted in the mesoderm developing smooth muscle and interstitial cells of Cajal that are characteristic of the intestine[45]. Other examples of localized signalling molecules, particularly those where the receptor for the ligand is expressed on epithelial cells, have been reviewed by Birchmeier et al.[46]. Whilst the expression of some of these molecules is restricted to intestinal development it is likely that others continue to play an important role, particularly during epithelial regeneration after injury[6,38] or in the spread of malignant epithelial cells[47].

MAINTENANCE OF THE EPITHELIAL STEM CELL BY MESENCHYME

Future developments in the genetic manipulation and grafting of intestinal mucosa are likely to benefit from a better understanding of how mesenchyme supports self-renewal of the epithelial stem cell. No markers allowing specific labelling of these stem cells have been found, but kinetic models of epithelial turnover and regeneration[2] and measurements of cell mutation rate[48] suggest that there are between one and four such cells per crypt.

It has proved difficult to culture normal intestinal epithelium such that the proliferation and differentiation properties of these cells are maintained. Improvements to culture methods for these cells have included their isolation as intact units of epithelium, i.e. crypts, and their culture in the direct presence of fibroblasts, or fibroblast-conditioned medium[49]. This has been demonstrated for the fetal[50], neonatal[51], and adult rodent bowel[52]. The differentiation, or proliferation, of these cells in culture is not evidence that the stem cells have been maintained within these cultures. However, co-cultures of mesoderm and endoderm do retain the capacity for organotypic regeneration when grafted[17]. Co-cultures from neonatal[14] and adult rat intestine[15], when grafted subcutaneously, also regenerate mucosa that is self-renewing.

FIBROBLAST HETEROGENEITY AND EPITHELIAL DIFFERENTIATION

Changes to the differentiation of fibroblast may be required for the mesenchyme to appropriately support the differentiation of this epithelium. The altered differentiation of skin fibroblasts to smooth-muscle cells when grafted together with fetal endoderm confirms that epithelial cells can 'instruct' such changes[19]. The myofibroblasts form a juxtaparenchymal layer surrounding the crypt and villus epithelium. Significantly, these myofibroblasts appear after the epithelial crypts and villi form, and not before[19]. These juxtaparenchymal cells form close associations with each other and local nerve terminals. They express distinct $\alpha\beta$ integrin complexes, cytoskeletal components including smooth muscle α-actin, myosin, desmin and filamin. In addition receptors for endothelin and atrial natriuretic peptide (ANP) are expressed by these cells and mRNA for insulin-like growth factor IGF-I (for an extensive review see ref. 6). Therefore the juxtaparenchymal cell has been viewed as regulating the immunophysiology of the intestinal epithelium.

The rat fibroblast lines F1:G9 and A1:F1 show differences in their morphology, growth regulation, surface antigen expression, and differentiation in response to TGF-β[7]. The F1:G9 line resembles primary cultures of intestinal fibroblasts, particularly its sensitivity to the induction of smooth muscle α-actin (a myofibroblast marker) in response to TGF-β and heparin. In contrast the A1:F1 line, when treated with TGF-β or heparin, does not express smooth muscle β-actin. Significantly when used as feeder layers for fetal bowel endoderm only F1:G9 supports the expression of brush-border enzymes. In tissue grafts formed between either of these two cell lines and fetal endoderm, only F1:G9 supports small intestinal morphogenesis with crypts and villi and the appearance of enterocyte brush-border enzymes. In contrast, in grafts composed with A1:F1 the endoderm forms deep 'colonic-like' crypts and does not express typical brush-border enzymes. More recently fibroblasts isolated from the human bowel have also been characterized and found to contain heterogeneous populations similar to those described for the rat bowel[42].

Further evidence of a proximal–distal gradient in the expression of signalling molecules by fibroblasts in the postnatal day 8 rat intestine has been reported. Fibroblast cultures isolated from different regions of the bowel all expressed the morphogenic factors TGF-β_1, epimorphin, and HGF/scatter factor. However, the expression of each factor varied, but in a way that was consistent with levels observed in intact mesenchyme from that particular region of bowel[53].

DEGRADATION OF ECM BY FIBROBLAST AND EPITHELIAL CELLS

In addition to active matrix synthesis fibroblasts have the capacity to degrade many constituents of the ECM. Remodelling of the ECM is a major activity of fibroblasts during organ development, and is thought to involve phagocytosis and intracellular degradation by lysosomal proteases[54]. In inflammatory tissue reactions, however, there are many stimuli that promote the secretion and activation of proteases by the fibroblast leading to extracellular matrix degradation. A major family of proteinases, the matrix metalloproteinases (MMPs), are Zn^{2+} containing endopeptidases which are capable of degrading most components of the extracellular matrix. MMPs are secreted as latent proenzymes that require proteolytic (or oxidative) activation. They are specifically regulated by tissue inhibitors of metalloproteinases (TIMPs). Four of the most widely studied MMPs include the type IV collagenases (MMP-2 and MMP-9) thought to degrade type IV collagen and denatured interstitial collagens; interstitial collagenase (MMP-1) which cleaves the triple helix of native fibrillar collagens; and stromelysin (MMP-3) which degrades type IV collagen, fibrillar collagens, proteoglycans, laminin and fibronectin (for review see ref. 55).

The degradative activity of fibroblasts in periodontal and inflammatory joint disease is well recognized, but only recently has the intestinal fibroblast been studied in this context. As epithelial cells are dependent upon the ECM, particularly the basement membrane, matrix destruction and remodelling could have significant consequences for epithelial function. Increases in extracellular protease activity are also likely to disrupt localized cell–cell signalling, promoting the release of cell surface bound cytokines by 'sheddase activity'[56]; or chemotactic fragments of, for example, fibronectin that can promote cell motility[57].

INTERACTIONS BETWEEN MESENCHYME AND EPITHELIAL TUMOUR CELLS

The capacity of malignant epithelial cells to cross the basement membrane and to enter the vascular supply demonstrates how regulatory influences at the epithelial–mesenchymal interface can break down. The genetic and cellular changes that lead to malignant cell behaviour have been an obvious focus for cancer research, including the mechanisms by which tumours can promote localized angiogenesis. However, the behaviour of fibroblasts can be specifically modified at the tumour interface in ways compatible with the 'recruitment' of these cells to the malignant process.

Adjacent to many epithelial tumours fibroblasts undergo a well-described 'desmoplastic' response with increased ECM deposition and many layers of myofibroblasts forming around the growing tumour[58]. Direct interaction of colorectal cancer cells with fibroblasts also alters the expression and deposition of ECM molecules[59], and other responses of the fibroblast to tumour cells may facilitate tumour spread. It has been shown that levels of several MMPs are increased in gastrointestinal cancer[60]. Careful examination, using *in-situ* hybridization and immunostaining, has shown that the connective tissue and not the tumour shows the largest increase in the expression of these proteases, particularly at the invasive margins[60,61]. Expression of MT1-MMP (which is involved in the cell surface activation of MMP-2) on the surface of cancer cells could explain why activated MMP-2 is found around invading pockets of tumour cells but not the non-invading regions[62]. In a similar example the urokinase plasminogen activator (uPA) receptor is expressed by invading colon adenocarcinoma cells and its ligand uPA on adjacent stromal cells[63]. In addition to secreting increased levels of cytokines that stimulate protease expression in the connective tissue[64], some tumour cells also express a novel cell surface antigen, termed extracellular matrix metalloproteinase inducer (EMMPRIN). This immuno-globulin-like molecule stimulates fibroblasts to increase their expression of MMP-1, -2 and -3[65]. The consequences of a dysregulation in MMP expression have been shown in a model of mammary tumorigenesis. Transgenic mice in which the expression of MMP-3 was auto-activated in the mammary gland showed progressive changes in the expression of other proteases, and eventually in the deposition and organization of the ECM and basement membrane[66].

EXPRESSION OF MATRIX-METALLOPROTEASES BY FIBROBLASTS

Studies of inflammatory bowel disease (IBD) and other forms of mucosal ulcera-tion have provided *in-situ* evidence that connective tissue cells increase their expression of MMPs. Increased stromelysin-1 (MMP-3) and gelatinase B (MMP-9) expression has been demonstrated by immunohistochemistry in regions of mucosal damage in IBD compared to normal tissue. Much of this expression was localized to the connective tissue adjacent to the epithelium[67]. Using *in-situ* hybridization and immunohistochemistry high expression of collagenase (MMP-1), MMP-3, and collagenase (MMP-13) by fibroblast-like cells in the edges of mucosal ulcers has been observed[68,69]. In contrast, little expression of these enzymes was shown in the healthy mucosa. An increased expression of MMP-1 and MMP-3 mRNA by fibroblasts in sections of inflamed mucosa in patients with coeliac disease has also been reported[70].

However, very few MMPs appear to be expressed in abundance by the intes-tinal epithelium, with the exception of matrilysin (MMP-7) and stromelysin-2 (MMP-10), whose mRNA has been localized at the wound margins of ulcers[68,69]. This selective expression of MMPs suggests a specific role in epithelial move-ment and interaction with the basement membrane. The involuting mammary gland is an excellent paradigm for this, in which increased expression of MMP-3 by epithelial cells is associated with basement membrane degradation, loss of epithelial cell function, and an increased level of epithelial apoptosis[71].

In-vitro studies have provided direct evidence of factors that stimulate, or regulate, the increased expression of MMPs by intestinal fibroblasts. The normal human colonic intestinal fibroblast line CCD18Co[72], cultured in the absence of inflammatory factors, constitutively expresses MMP-2 in its latent form, but levels of other MMPs are barely detectable by sensitive chemiluminescent Western immunoblotting. In contrast the pro-inflammatory cytokines TNF-α, IL-1α and IL1-β promote a dose-dependent increase in the expression of MMPs 1 and -3 by these fibroblasts[73,74]. In contrast, molecules with anti-inflammatory properties such as corticosteroids generally suppress the expression and activa-tion of these MMPs, as has been reported for intestinal smooth muscle cells[75]. The increased expression of MMP-1 and -3, and their activation along with that of gelatinase A (MMP-2), corresponds to what has been observed in IBD[68–70,76], in which elevated levels of TNF-α and IL-1 have also been measured[77,78].

Changes to the composition and organization of the ECM can also modify the expression and activation of MMPs by fibroblasts. MMP-2 is constitutively expressed in its latent ~72 kDa form by intestinal fibroblasts grown on plastic, but is activated to the ~60 kDa form within 24 h when the cells are grown on gels of native type I collagen. This activation is MMP-mediated since it can be specifically inhibited only by BB-94, a specific MMP inhibitor, and not by inhibitors of other classes of protease[73]. Other substratum and ECM molecules that affect the shape and motility of the fibroblast can also increase the expression of these MMPs[73]. ECM-dependent expression and activation of MMP-1 by fibroblasts has also been noted on type I collagen substratum and can be blocked by inhibitors of the $\alpha1\beta1$ and $\alpha2\beta1$ integrin collagen receptors[79]. These results suggest that changes to the ECM environment can stimulate fibroblasts to remodel the matrix consistent with the observed behaviour of these cells at sites of wound repair and inflammation in the mucosa[67,68].

To date there is very little information about changes to MMP expression resulting from epithelial–fibroblast interactions in the development of the intestine.

EVIDENCE OF ECM DEGRADATION IN BOWEL DISEASE

McAlindon et al.[80] have reported the presence of pores in the epithelial basement membrane in active IBD through which infiltrating immune cells pass. The frequency and size of these pores in the IBD mucosa suggested a destructive process, particularly by infiltrating neutrophils. Disruption of contact with the basement membrane increases epithelial apoptosis, a process known as 'anoikis'[81]. In mouse mammary epithelial cells engineered to overexpress MMP-3, an enhanced cleavage of basement membrane components also led to increased levels of anoikis[71]. Increased apoptosis has also been shown in crypt epithelial cells in ulcerative colitis compared to control tissue[82]. Such changes could lead to a loss of epithelial integrity with an increased entry of bacteria, their products, and other pro-inflammatory factors.

Other evidence of increased turnover/degradation of ECM in the inflamed bowel includes the following: an increased level of the C-telopeptide of type I collagen in Crohn's disease[83], a reduced deposition of collagen types I and III compared to an elevated level of RNA transcripts for these proteins, indicating increased degradation of collagen molecules in ulcerative colitis[84], and a significant loss of sulphated GAGs demonstrated by poly-L-lysine colloidal gold staining in sections of inflamed bowel compared to healthy mucosa[85]. Specific evidence supporting the involvement of fibroblasts in ECM remodelling has been reported. Using a human fetal gut explant culture system, Pender et al.[86] demonstrated that pokeweed mitogen (PWM) stimulation of T lymphocytes leads to the shedding and loss of the villus epithelium. This damage was specifically blocked by a synthetic MMP inhibitor most effective against MMP-3. Furthermore, only MMP-3, but not other purified MMPs, could reproduce this pattern of destruction when added to the cultures in the absence of PWM. Intestinal mesenchymal cells grown in culture were found to produce MMP-1 and -3 when stimulated with IL-1 and TNF-α implicating their involvement in this T cell-mediated destruction of the lamina propria.

To further investigate whether the localized release of MMPs at the juxta-parenchymal surface leads to degradation of the epithelial basement membrane, an antibody (AH10W1) has been raised against a synthetic peptide (AH10) corresponding to a sequence (aa 449–463) in the $\alpha 1$ chain of type IV collagen[87]. This peptide sequence corresponds to the putative cleavage site for MMP-2 and -9 in the triple helix of this molecule. The antibody reacted specifically with denatured type IV collagen but not with the intact molecule, and demonstrated *in-situ* proteolytic damage to this constituent of the basement membrane. This approach has been successfully employed previously to detect the degradation of type II collagen by MMP-1[88].

The AH10W1 antibody was found to react only with purified type IV collagen molecules after their reduction and heat denaturation, or following digestion with MMP-2 and -9 but not MMP-1 or -3. The antibody did not stain any tissue component in frozen sections of healthy bowel mucosa unless the specimens were reduced and heat-denatured first. The resulting staining in these sections was typical for basement membrane type IV collagen and was equivalent to the pattern observed using a type IV collagen polyclonal antibody (gift from Dr P. Simon-Assmann, Strasbourg) which reacts on untreated frozen sections. All of this evidence confirmed that the AH10W1 antibody reacted with type IV collagen in tissue sections, but only after disruption of the triple helix.

Like the healthy mucosa, in most frozen sections of 'inflamed' ulcerative colitis there was no staining with AH10W1, though typical basement membrane staining was observed in serial sections pretreated by reduction and heat denaturation prior to antibody staining. However, in some specimens characterized by pathological features of cryptitis AH10W1 staining was seen in untreated frozen sections. This was evidence of *in-situ* ECM degradation in IBD, but paradoxically the staining was localized to the lamina propria and not the basement membrane. These reactions were specific, since the staining was not seen by substituting pre-immune serum, or after pre-absorption of AH10W1 antibody with the AH10 peptide. These results suggest that MMP-2 and MMP-9 degradation of type IV collagen occurs, but not when the molecule is organized within the basement membrane. Frozen sections of 'non-inflamed' mucosa were also subjected to predigestion with 50 nM of purified and activated forms of MMP-1, -2, -3 and -9, then stained with AH10W1. No staining was observed, but if these digested sections were then reduced and denatured typical basement membrane staining was obtained[87]. These results are consistent with other reports that show that MMP-2 and -9 are not efficient type IV collagenases[89,90].

Whilst fibroblasts adjacent to the epithelial basement membrane produce MMP-2 it therefore seems unlikely that this protease is an effective 'type IV collagenase' which initiates the destruction of this molecule. Indeed evidence points to the gelatinases such as MMP-9 being able to attach to the type IV collagen chains once denatured, but not when intact[91]. In those samples with advanced cryptitis the AH10W1 antibody may therefore have detected 'downstream' degradation of type IV collagen by neutrophils and macrophages. Both of these inflammatory cells produce proteases which are reported to cleave type IV collagen elsewhere in the molecule, they also express MMP-9 (and MMP-2 in the case of macrophages)[55]. Furthermore these cells cross the vascular and epithelial basement membranes in large numbers in ulcerative colitis.

Measurement of protease expression in IBD mucosa also confirms that inflammatory cells, rather than fibroblasts, are the major source of degradative proteases. In patients with ulcerative colitis and Crohn's disease the expression of several MMPs is significantly increased, particularly in areas of active inflammation[76]. The most abundant MMP detectable in these situations is MMP-9 present in a form characteristic of that produced by neutrophils where it associates with lipocalin in the storage granules[92]. This form of the enzyme can be identified as an additional ~145 kDa band on gelatin zymographs[76]. The abundance of MMP-9 is consistent with the large influx of granulocytes in the IBD mucosa. Whilst neutrophils are recognized for their destructive role in airway disease[93], it remains to be demonstrated whether they are pivotal, or passive bystanders, in mucosal damage in IBD. Evidence from studies with cultured fetal mucosa also implicate T cells and macrophage-derived proteases in mucosal destruction[86].

CONCLUSIONS

There is a growing body of evidence to show that coordinated differentiation of the intestinal epithelium may require interactions with a heterogeneous population of fibroblasts. What are the specific characteristics of these fibroblasts that are essential for such interactions; what are the tissue signals and how are they controlled at the transcriptional level? From a clinical perspective there is the potential for such research to lead to new strategies for the management of injured and inflamed mucosa and gastrointestinal cancers.

Acknowledgements

We acknowledge our collaborators in these studies, the staff at Inserm Unité 381 Strasbourg, Dr A. Hollander, Division of Musculoskeletal Medicine, Royal Hallamshire Hospital Sheffield, and Dr Vasanta Subramanian (School of Biological Sciences, University of Bath). The financial support of the Children's Hospital Medical Research Trust, Special Trustees for Sheffield Hospitals, and Nuffield Foundation is also acknowledged (G.S.E.).

References

1. Gordon JI, Hermiston ML. Differentiation and self-renewal in the mouse gastrointestinal epithelium. Current Opin Cell Biol. 1994;6:795–803.
2. Potten CS, Loeffler M. Stem cells: attributes, cycles, spirals, pitfalls and uncertainties. Lessons for and from the crypt. Development. 1990;110:1001–20.
3. Simon-Assmann P, Kedinger M, De Arcangelis A, Rousseau V, Simo P. Extracellular matrix components in intestinal development. Experientia. 1995;51:883–900.
4. Kedinger M, Simon-Assmann PM, Lacroix B, Marxer A, Hauri HP, Haffen K. Fetal gut mesenchyme induces differentiation of cultured intestinal endodermal and crypt cells. Dev Biol. 1986;113:474–83.
5. Duluc I, Freund JN, Leberquier C, Kedinger M. Fetal endoderm primarily holds the temporal and positional information required for mammalian intestinal development. J Cell Biol. 1994;126:211–21.
6. Powell DW, Mifflin RC, Valentich J D, Crowe S E, Saada JI, West AB. Myofibroblasts. II. Intestinal subepithelial myofibroblasts. Am J Physiol. 1999;277:C183–201.

7. Fritsch C, Simon-Assmann P, Kedinger M, Evans GS. Cytokines modulate fibroblast phenotype and epithelial–stroma interactions in rat intestine. Gastroenterology. 1997;112:826–38.
8. Kedinger M, Lefebvre O, Duluc I, Freund JN, Simon-Assmann P. Cellular and molecular partners involved in gut morphogenesis and differentiation. Phil Trans R Soc Lond. 1998;353:847–56.
9. Simon-Assmann P, Lefebvre O, Bellissent-Waydelich A, Olsen J, Orian-Rousseau V, De Arcangelis A. The laminins: role in intestinal morphogenesis and differentiation. Ann NY Acad Sci. 1998;859:46–65.
10. Beaulieu J-F. Recent work with migration/patterns of expression: cell–matrix interactions in human intestinal cell differentiation. In: Halter F, Winton D, Wright NA, editors. The Gut as a Model in Cell and Molecular Biology. Falk Symposium 94. Lancaster: Kluwer; 1996:165–79.
11. Alho AM, Underhill CB. The hyaluronate receptor is preferentially expressed on proliferating epithelial cells. J Cell Biol. 1989;108:1557–65.
12. Sonnenberg E, Meyer D, Weidner KM, Birchmeier C. Scatter factor/hepatocyte growth factor and its receptor, the c-met tyrosine kinase, can mediate a signal exchange between mesenchyme and epithelia during mouse development. J Cell Biol. 1993;123:223–35.
13. Roberts DJ, Johnson RL, Burke AC, Nelson CE, Morgan BA, Tabin C. Sonic hedgehog is an endodermal signal inducing Bmp-4 and Hox genes during induction and regionalization of the chick hindgut. Development. 1995;12:3163–74.
14. Tait IS, Evans GS, Flint N, Campbell FC. Colonic mucosal replacement by syngeneic small intestinal stem cell transplantation: Am J Surg. 1994;167:67–72.
15. Booth C, O'Shea JA, Potten CS. Maintenance of functional stem cells in isolated and cultured adult intestinal epithelium. Exp Cell Res. 1999;249:359–66.
16. Haffen K, Lacroix B, Simon-Assmann PM. Inductive properties of fibroblastic cell cultures derived from rat intestinal mucosa on epithelial differentiation. Differentiation. 1983;23:226–33.
17. Kedinger M, Plateroti M, Orian-Rousseau V et al. Cellular and molecular mechanisms regulating intestinal development. In: Halter F, Winton D, Wright NA, editors. The Gut as a Model in Cell and Molecular Biology. Falk Symposium 94. Lancaster Kluwer; 1996;137–48.
18. Rubin DC, Swietlicki E, Gordon JI. Use of isografts to study proliferation and differentiation programs of mouse stomach epithelia. Am J Physiol. 1994;267:G27–39.
19. Kedinger M, Simon-Assmann P, Bouziges F, Arnold C, Alexandre E, Haffen K. Smooth muscle actin expression during rat gut development and induction in fetal skin fibroblastic cells associated with intestinal embryonic epithelium. Differentiation. 1990;43:87–97.
20. Kedinger M, Freund JN, Launay JF, Simon-Assmann P. Cell interactions through basement membrane in intestinal development and differentiation. In: Sanderson IR, Walker WA, editors. Development of Gastrointestinal Tract. New York: Marcel Dekker, 1999.
21. Simo P, Simon-Assmann P, Arnold C, Kedinger M. Mesenchyme-mediated effect of dexamethasone on laminin in cocultures of embryonic gut epithelial cells and mesenchyme-derived cells. J. Cell Sci. 1992;101:161–71.
22. Stallmach A, Hahn U, Merker HJ, Hahn EG, Riecken EO. Differentiation of rat intestinal epithelial cells is induced by organotypic mesenchymal cells in vitro. Gut. 1989;30:959–70.
23. Saga Y, Yagi T, Ikawa Y, Sakakura T, Aizawa S. Mice develop normally without tenascin. Genes Dev. 1992;6:1821–31.
24. Simon-Assmann P, Duclos B, Orian-Rousseau V et al. Differential expression of laminin isoforms and alpha 6-beta 4 integrin subunits in the developing human and mouse intestine. Dev. Dynam. 1994;201:71–85.
25. Boudreau N, Bissell MJ. Extracellular matrix signalling: integration of form and function in normal and malignant cells. Curr Opin Cell Biol. 1998;10:640–6.
26. Hynes RO, Wagner DD. Genetic manipulation of vascular adhesion molecules in mice. J Clin Invest. 1996;98:2193–5.
27. Fässler R, Georges-Labouesse E, Hirsch E. Genetic analyses of integrin function in mice. Curr Opin Cell Biol. 1996;8:641–6.
28. Gordon JI, Hermiston ML. Differentiation and self-renewal in the mouse gastrointestinal epithelium. Curr Opin Cell Biol 1994;6:795–803.
29. James R, Kazenwadel J. Homeobox gene expression in the intestinal epithelium of adult mice. J Biol Chem. 1991;266:3246–51.
30. James R, Erler T, Kazenwadel J. Structure of the murine homeobox gene cdx-2. Expression in embryonic and adult intestinal epithelium. J Biol Chem. 1994;269:15229–37.

31. Freund JN, Boukamel R, Benazzouz A. Gradient expression of Cdx along the rat intestine throughout postnatal development. FEBS Lett. 1992;314:163–6.
32. Subramanian V, Meyer B, Evans GS. The murine CDX-1 gene product localises to the proliferative compartment in the developing and regenerating intestinal epithelium. Differentiation. 1988;64:11–18.
33. Duluc I, Lorentz O, Fritsch C, Leberquier C, Kedinger M, Freund JN. Changing intestinal connective tissue interactions alters homeobox gene expression in epithelial cells. J Cell Sci. 1997;110:1317–24.
34. De Arcangelis A, Neuville P, Boukamel R, Lefebvre O, Kedinger M, Simon-Assmann P. Inhibition of laminin alpha 1-chain expression leads to alteration of basement membrane assembly and cell differentiation. J Cell Biol. 1996;133:417–30.
35. Kaestner KH, Silberg DG, Traber PG, Schutz G. The mesenchymal winged helix transcription factor Fkh6 is required for the control of gastrointestinal proliferation and differentiation. Genes Dev. 1997;11:1583–95.
36. Pabst O, Zweigerdt R, Arnold HH. Targeted disruption of the homeobox transcription factor Nkx2–3 in mice results in postnatal lethality and abnormal development of small intestine and spleen. Development. 1999;126:2215–25.
37. Burgess AW. Growth control mechanisms in normal and transformed intestinal cells. Phil Trans R Soc Lond. B: Biol Sci. 1998;353:903–9.
38. Potten CS, Owen G, Hewitt D et al. Stimulation and inhibition of proliferation in the small intestinal crypts of the mouse after in vivo administration of growth factors. Gut. 1995;36:864–73.
39. Bajaj-Elliott M, Poulsom R, Pender SL, Wathen NC, MacDonald TT. Interactions between stromal cell-derived keratinocyte growth factor and epithelial transforming growth factor in immune-mediated crypt cell hyperplasia. J Clin Invest. 1998;102:1473–80.
40. Dignass AU, Tsunekawa S, Podolsky DK. Fibroblast growth factors modulate intestinal epithelial cell growth and migration. Gastroenterology. 1994;106:1254–62.
41. Lyon M, Gallagher JT. Bio-specific sequences and domains in heparan sulphate and the regulation of cell growth and adhesion. Matrix Biol. 1998;17:485–93.
42. Fritsch C, Orian-Rousseaul V, Lefebvre O et al. Characterization of human intestinal stromal cell lines: response to cytokines and interactions with epithelial cells. Exp Cell Res. 1999;248: 391–406.
43. Rosen EM, Nigam SK, Goldberg ID. Scatter factor and the c-met receptor: a paradigm for mesenchymal/epithelial interaction. J Cell Biol. 1994;127:1783–7.
44. Nusrat A, Parkos CA, Bacarra AE et al. Hepatocyte growth factor/scatter factor effects on epithelia. Regulation of intercellular junctions in transformed and nontransformed cell lines, basolateral polarization of c-met receptor in transformed and natural intestinal epithelia, and induction of rapid wound repair in a transformed model epithelium. J Clin Invest. 1994;93:2056–65.
45. Apelqvist A, Ahlgren U, Edlund H. Sonic hedgehog directs specialised mesoderm differentiation in the intestine and pancreas. Curr Biol. 1997;7:801–4.
46. Birchmeier C, Meyer D, Riethmacher D. Factors controlling growth, motility, and morphogenesis of normal and malignant epithelial cells. Int Rev Cytol. 1995;160:221–66.
47. Lanzsus K, Jin L, Fuchs A et al. Scatter factor stimulates tumour growth and tumour angiogenesis in human breast cancers in the mammary fat pads of nude mice. Lab Invest. 1997;76:339–53.
48. Winton DJ, Blount MA, Ponder BA. A clonal marker induced by mutation in mouse intestinal epithelium. Nature. 1988;333:463–6.
49. Evans GS, Flint N, Potten CS. Application of primary cultures to the study of normal small bowel enterocytes. Ann Rev Physiol. 1994;56:399–417.
50. Kedinger M, Simon-Assmann P, Alexandre E, Haffen K. Importance of a fibroblastic support for in vitro differentiation of intestinal endodermal cells and for their response to glucocorticoids. Cell Diff. 1987;20:171–82.
51. Evans GS, Flint N, Somers AS, Eyden B, Potten CS. The development of a method for the preparation of rat intestinal epithelial cell primary cultures. J Cell Sci. 1992;101:219–31.
52. Booth C, Patel S, Bennion GR, Potten CS. The isolation and culture of adult mouse colonic epithelium. Epithel Cell Biol. 1995;4:76–86.
53. Plateroti M, Rubin DC, Duluc I et al. Subepithelial fibroblast cell lines from different levels of gut axis display regional characteristics. Am J Physiol. 1998;274:G945–54.

54. Everts V, van der Zee E, Creemers L, Beertsen W. Phagocytosis and intracellular digestion of collagen, its role in turnover and remodelling. Histochem J. 1996;28:229–45.
55. Birkedal-Hansen H, Moore WGI, Bodden MK et al. Matrix metalloproteinases: a review. Crit Rev Oral Biol Med. 1993;4:197–250.
56. Gearing AJH, Beckett P, Christodoulou M et al. Processing of tumour necrosis factor-α precursor by metalloproteinases. Nature. 1994;370:555–8.
57. Long MM, King VJ, Prasad KU, Urry DW. Cell attachment and chemotaxis can utilize the same peptide sequence of fibronectin. Biochim Biophys Acta. 1987;928:114–18.
58. Liotta LA, Rao CN, Barsky SH. Tumor invasion and the extracellular matrix. Lab Invest. 1983;49:636–49.
59. Bouziges F, Simo P, Simon-Assmann P, Haffen K, Kedinger M. Altered deposition of basement-membrane molecules in co-cultures of colonic cancer cells and fibroblasts. Int J Cancer. 1991;48:101–8.
60. Brown PD. Matrix metalloproteinases in gastrointestinal cancer: Gut. 1998;43:161–3.
61. Porte H, Chastre E, Prevot S et al. Neoplastic progression of human colorectal cancer is associated with overexpression of the stromelysin-3 and BM-40/SPARC genes. Int J Cancer. 1995;64:70–5.
62. Nomura H, Sato H, Seiki M, Mai M, Okada Y. Expression of membrane-type matrix metallo-proteinase in human gastric carcinomas. Cancer Res. 1995;55:3263–6.
63. Pyke C, Kristensen P, Ralfkiaer E et al. Urokinase-type plasminogen activator is expressed in stromal cells and its receptor in cancer cells at invasive foci in human colon adenocarcinomas. Am J Pathol. 1991;138:1059–67.
64. Mauviel A. Cytokine regulation of metalloproteinase gene expression. J Cell Biochem. 1993;53:288–95.
65. Biswas C, Zhang Y, DeCastro R et al. The human tumor cell-derived collagenase stimulatory factor (renamed EMMPRIN) is a member of the immunoglobulin superfamily. Cancer Res. 1995;55:434–9.
66. Thomasset N, Lochter A, Sympson CJ et al. Expression of autoactivated stromelysin-1 in mammary glands of transgenic mice leads to a reactive stroma during early development. Am J Pathol. 1998;153:457–67.
67. Bailey CJ, Hembry RM, Alexander A, Irving MH, Grant ME, Shuttleworth CA. Distribution of the matrix metalloproteinases stromelysin, gelatinases A and B, and collagenase in Crohn's disease and normal intestine. J Clin Pathol. 1994;47:113–16.
68. Saarialho-Kere UK, Vaalamo M, Puolakkainen P, Airola K, Parks WC, Karjalainen-Lindsberg ML. Enhanced expression of matrilysin, collagenase, and stromelysin-1 in gastrointestinal ulcers. Am J Pathol. 1996;148:519–26.
69. Vaalamo M, Karjalainen-Lindsberg ML, Puolakkainen P, Kere J, Saarialho-Kere U. Distinct expression profiles of stromelysin-2 (MMP-10), collagenase-3 (MMP-13), macrophage metal-loelastase (MMP-12), and tissue inhibitor of metalloproteinases-3 (TIMP-3) in intestinal ulcerations. Am J Pathol. 1998;152:1005–14.
70. Daum S, Bauer U, Foss HD et al. Increased expression of mRNA for matrix metalloproteinases-1 and -3 and tissue inhibitor of metalloproteinases-1 in intestinal biopsy specimens from patients with coeliac disease. Gut. 1999;44:17–25.
71. Alexander CM, Howard EW, Bissell MJ, Werb Z. Rescue of mammary epithelial cell apoptosis and entactin degradation by a tissue inhibitor of metalloproteinases-1 transgene. J Cell Biol. 1996;135:1669–77.
72. Valentich J D, Popov V, Saada JI, Powell DW. Phenotypic characterization of an intestinal subepithelial myo-fibroblast cell line. Am J Physiol. 1997;272 (Cell Physiol. 41):C1513–24.
73. Baugh MD, Hollander AP, Evans GS. The regulation of matrix metalloproteinase (MMP) production in human fibroblasts. Ann NY Acad Sci.1998;559:175–80.
74. Pender SL, MacDonald TT. Regulation of matrix metalloproteinase production in human fetal intestinal mesenchymal cells by cytokines and the bacterial superantigen Staphylococcus aureus enterotoxin B. Ann NY Acad Sci. 1998;859:188–91.
75. Graham MF, Willey A, Zhu YN, Yager DR, Sugerman HJ, Diegelmann RF. Corticosteroids repress the interleukin 1 beta-induced secretion of collagenase in human intestinal smooth muscle cells. Gastroenterology. 1997;113:1924–9.
76. Baugh MD, Perry MJ, Hollander AP et al. Matrix metalloproteinase levels are elevated in inflammatory bowel disease. Gastroenterology. 1999;117:1–11.

77. Reimund J, Wittersheim C, Dumont S *et al.* Mucosal inflammatory cytokine production by intestinal biopsies in patients with ulcerative colitis and Crohn's disease. J Clin Immunol. 1996;16:144–50.
78. Isaacs KL, Sartor RB, Haskill S. Cytokine messenger RNA profiles in inflammatory bowel disease mucosa detected by polymerase chain reaction amplification. Gastroenterology. 1992;103:1587–95.
79. Langholz O, Rockel D, Mauch C *et al.* Collagen and collagenase gene expression in three-dimensional collagen lattices are differentially regulated by alpha 1 beta 1 and alpha 2 beta 1 integrins. J Cell Biol. 1995;131:1903–15.
80. McAlindon ME, Gray T, Galvin A, Sewell HF, Podolsky DK, Mahida YR. Differential lamina propria cell migration via basement membrane pores of inflammatory bowel disease mucosa. Gastroenterology. 1998;115:841–8.
81. Frisch SM, Francis H. Disruption of epithelial cell–matrix interactions induces apoptosis. J Cell Biol. 1994;124:619–26.
82. Iwamoto M, Koji T, Makiyama K, Kobayashi N, Nakane PK. Apoptosis of crypt epithelial cells in ulcerative colitis. J Pathol. 1996;180:152–9.
83. Kjeldsen J, Schaffalitzky de Muckadell OB, Junker P. Seromarkers of collagen metabolism in active Crohn's disease. Relation to disease activity and response to therapy. Gut. 1995;37:805–10.
84. Matthes H, Herbst H, Schuppan D *et al.* Cellular localisation of procollagen gene transcripts in inflammatory bowel diseases. Gastroenterology. 1992;102:431–42.
85. Pender SL, Lionetti P, Murch SH, Wathan N, MacDonald TT. Proteolytic degradation of intestinal mucosal extracellular matrix after lamina propria T cell activation. Gut. 1996;39:284–90.
86. Pender SLF, Tickle SP, Docherty AJP, Howie D, Wathen NC, MacDonald TT. A major role for matrix metalloproteases in T cell injury in the gut. J Immunol. 1997;158:1582–90.
87. Wheatcroft C, Hollander AP, Croucher LJ, Jones A, Taylor CJ, Evans GS. Evidence of *in-situ* stability of the type IV collagen triple helix in human inflammatory bowel disease using a denaturation specific epitope antibody A.C. Matrix Biol. 1999;18:361–72.
88. Hollander AP, Heathfield TF, Webber C *et al.* Increased damage to type II collagen in osteoarthritic articular cartilage detected by a new immunoassay. J Clin Invest. 1994;93:1722–32.
89. Mackay AR, Hartzler JL, Pelina MD, Thorgeirsson UP. Studies on the ability of 65-kDa and 92-kDa tumor cell gelatinases to degrade type IV collagen. J Biol Chem. 1990;265:21929–34.
90. Eble JA, Ries A, Lichy A *et al.* The recognition sites of the integrins alpha1-beta1 and alpha2-beta1 within collagen IV are protected against gelatinase A attack in the native protein. J Biol Chem. 1996;271:30964–70.
91. Olson MW, Toth M, Gervasi DC, Sado Y, Ninomiya Y, Fridman R. High affinity binding of latent matrix metalloproteinase-9 to the a(IV) chain of collagen IV. J Biol Chem. 1998;273:10672–81.
92. Hibbs MS, Hasty KA, Seyer JM, Kang AH, Mainardi CL. Biochemical and immunological characterization of the secreted forms of human neutrophil gelatinase. J Biol Chem. 1985;260:2493–500.
93. Hiemstra PS, van Wetering S, Stolk J. Neutrophil serine proteinases and defensins in chronic obstructive pulmonary disease: effects on pulmonary epithelium. Eur Resp J. 1998;12:1200–8.

13
Expression and function of death receptors in the gut

J. STRÄTER and P. MÖLLER

INTRODUCTION

The tumour necrosis receptor (TNFR) family is a still-growing group of type I transmembrane proteins which are homologous to each other in two to four extracellular cystein-rich domains (Fig. 1). Being involved in the regulation of diverse biological processes, they act as growth factors or contribute to the activation/stimulation of cells, especially in the immune system[1]. Some family

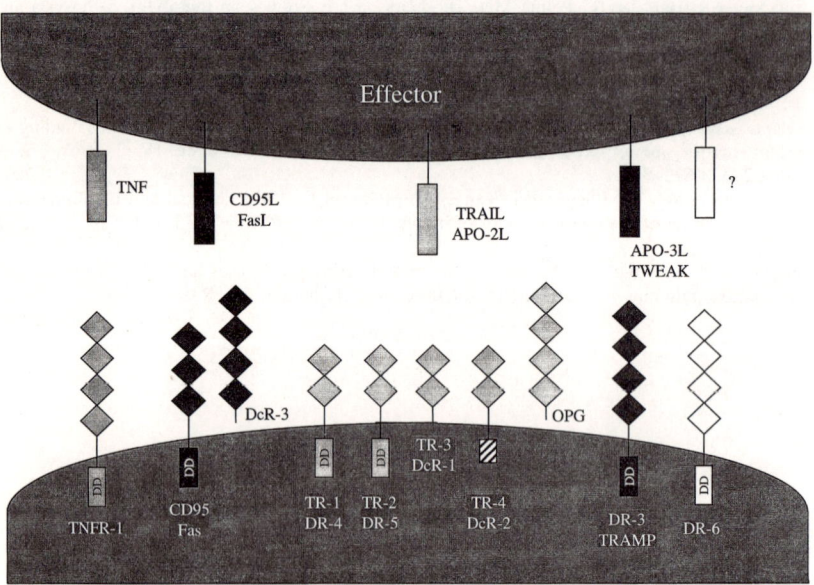

Figure 1 Apoptosis-inducing TNF family members (above) and their corresponding receptors of the TNFR family (below)

members are of special interest due to a particular property: they are directly able to induce apoptosis[2]. These apoptosis-mediating family members are characterized by a highly conserved intracellular signalling domain, the 'death domain', which recruits certain adapter molecules to the 'death-inducing signalling complex' (DISC), finally activating the apoptotic caspase cascade[3].

Their ligands, on the other hand, constitute a separate family of homologous type II transmembrane proteins, the TNF family[2] (Fig. 1). They typically exist in a trimeric form and it is by trimerizing their receptors that they perform their deadly work. Ligand binding may be simulated by agonistic anti-receptor antibodies *in vitro* and *in vivo*.

Why are these apoptosis-inducing TNF/TNFR systems of interest for gastroenterologists? In the normal situation senescent epithelial cells in the gut mucosa are eliminated by apoptosis, but it is not yet clear how apoptosis is induced in these cells[4,5]. Thus, death receptors present on gut epithelial cells may be involved in this elimination process. Next, apoptosis-inducing receptor/ligand systems are important regulators of inflammatory processes[6], making them potential players also in the pathogenesis of chronic inflammatory bowel diseases. Finally, some of them, such as the CD95/CD95L system, have been implicated in colorectal cancer[7].

In this chapter the possible function of two apoptosis-inducing receptor/ligand systems, the CD95/CD95L and the TRAIL/TRAIL receptor system, in the gastrointestinal tract will be discussed.

THE CD95/CD95L SYSTEM

Probably the best-studied apoptosis-inducing TNFR family member is CD95 (Fas/APO-1)[8,9]. CD95 is quite broadly expressed in a variety of normal organs and tissues[10]. It is also constitutively present on the basolateral surface of intestinal and colon epithelial cells all along the crypt(/villus) axis[11]. Moreover, isolated colonic crypt cells readily enter apoptosis when incubated with an agonistic CD95 antibody *in vitro*[12]. The biological significance of this functional CD95 expression in the normal gut, however, is not yet completely understood. Some clarification of this point was expected from addressing the question of where the CD95 ligand is expressed in the gut mucosa.

In contrast to CD95, the tissue distribution of its ligand, CD95L, is much more restricted. It was first detected in activated T cells[13-15] and natural killer cells[16], but also in B lymphocytes[17] and finally in plasma cells[18]. In the normal colon it is also exclusively found in a few scattered lamina propria cells, while gut epithelial cells do not express CD95L with the only, but remarkable, exception of Paneth cells[19]. Numbers and distribution of CD95L- expressing cells in the colon mucosa suggest that CD95-mediated apoptosis of epithelial cells is a rare event in the normal colon and not the way in which senescent epithelial cells are eliminated in the gut[12]. This view is further substantiated by studies on *lpr/lpr* and *gld/gld* mice having severe defects in CD95 function and CD95L expression, respectively. These mice do not show altered apoptotic rates in the colonic surface epithelium compared to wild-type animals (own unpublished data).

The predominant expression of CD95L in lymphatic cells, together with functional *in-vitro* data, have made clear that CD95L plays an important role in the regulation of immune processes and the elimination of virus-infected cells (for review cf. ref. 6). Thus, CD95L is crucially involved in the elimination of chronically activated T lymphocytes and the main cytotoxic effector of T helper type 1 cells. These findings drew attention to chronic inflammatory bowel diseases. CD95L is significantly up-regulated in lamina propria mononuclear cells in ulcerative colitis (UC)[12]. In parallel, the number of apoptotic lamina propria, but also epithelial, cells in UC is dramatically increased and a focal association of CD95L-expressing cells and epithelial apoptosis is observed. Although we do not yet completely understand the early processes leading to undue activation of inflammatory cells, the probable consequences are focally enhanced epithelial cell apoptosis via CD95 and the formation of epithelial microlesions. Epithelial damage may finally result in a breakdown of the mucosal barrier function, allowing the invasion of pathogenic microorganisms which, in turn, may aggravate the inflammatory process[12].

A particular role in the regulation of inflammatory responses was ascribed to the CD95 system when CD95L was detected in the testis[20] and some occular tissues[21]. In these organs, long known as 'immunoprivileged sites', immune processes may be cut down by CD95L expression in organ-constituting cells and induction of apoptosis in invading activated (CD95-expressing and sensitive) immune cells[22]. Thus, CD95L expression may act as a protective mechanism in organs in which inflammation would cause irreversible tissue damage and loss of function.

Recently, this concept was extended to malignant tumours when it was noticed that different tumour cell lines[23–25] express CD95L and are able to induce apoptosis in CD95-sensitive target cells *in vitro* (the 'CD95 counterattack' hypothesis; for review cf. ref. 7). In analogy to the concept of immunoprivileged sites, it has been proposed that tumour cells escape attack from tumour-infiltrating lymphocytes by expressing CD95L and inducing CD95-mediated apoptosis in the immune cells.

This concept of tumours as an immunoprivileged site implies that tumour cells themselves are resistant to CD95-mediated apoptosis. In contrast to the normal colonic epithelium, many colon carcinoma cell lines are relatively resistant to CD95 crosslink[26,27]. An important mechanism leading to CD95 resistance may be the loss of CD95 from the surface, which is seen immunohistochemically in most colorectal carcinomas compared to normal mucosa or adenomas[11]. It is probable that, apart from the 'CD95 counterattack theory', tumour cells profit from their CD95 down-regulation in that they become resistant to an important effector of cytotoxic immune cells.

Expression of CD95L, on the other hand, was detected not only in colon carcinoma cell lines, but also in primary colorectal carcinomas[28] and their metastases[29,30]. The latter observation is of particular interest since the formation of metastases in the liver may be facilitated by driving hepatocytes, which express and are highly sensitive to CD95, into apoptosis. However, most studies on CD95L expression in colorectal carcinomas rely on immunohistochemistry carried out with polyclonal antisera. We were not able to confirm these data using monoclonal antibodies (unpublished data). In addition, it is still an open question whether colon carcinoma cells express CD95L on their surface, or whether it is secreted in its soluble form. The mode of CD95L expression, however, may considerably influence its apoptosis-inducing activity[31,32]. Thus, although it seems very likely that development of CD95 resistance is an important step in the pathogenesis of colorectal cancer with respect to immune escape of tumour cells, the significance of CD95L expression in tumours has to be further substantiated.

THE TRAIL/TRAIL RECEPTOR SYSTEM

A recently described member of the TNF family is the 'TNF-related apoptosis inducing ligand', TRAIL[33], also called APO-2 ligand[34]. Similar to CD95L, TRAIL is able to induce apoptosis, but can also activate the transcription factor NF-κB. TRAIL exists in a membrane-bound form and, after proteolytic cleavage by cystein proteases, in a soluble form[35]. By Northern blot analysis, TRAIL was detected in a wide range of tissues including small intestine and colon[33].

So far, four homologous TRAIL receptors have been described (Fig. 1): TRAIL-R1[36] and TRAIL-R2[37-39] bear a cytoplasmic death domain and mediate apoptosis. TRAIL-R3 lacks a cytoplasmic domain and is linked to the cell membrane by a phosphatidyl inositol anchor[37,38,40]. TRAIL-R4, finally, has a defective death domain and is not able to transmit an apoptotic signal either[41,42]. The latter two are therefore thought to act as decoy receptors. Similar to TRAIL, TRAIL-R1[36] and TRAIL-R2[37-39], and TRAIL-R4[41] have been shown by Northern blot analyses to be widely expressed in normal tissues, the gut included. TRAIL-R3, though, is expressed in a much more restricted way, detectable on the transcriptional level mainly in peripheral blood cells and the spleen[37,40].

A possible fifth receptor for TRAIL is osteoprotegerin (OPG). Also a member of the TNFR family, its main function known so far is the inhibition of osteoclast differentiation and osteoclast-mediated bone resorption[43]. While Emery and co-workers[44] found OPG to bind to TRAIL *in vitro*, this was not confirmed by others[45]. OPG lacks a cytoplasmic domain and exists only in a dimeric soluble form. Thus, if OPG binding to TRAIL actually occurs *in vivo*, it should act as decoy receptor for TRAIL.

Although TRAIL, TRAIL-R1, TRAIL-R2, and TRAIL-R4 were shown to be expressed in the gut on the transcriptional level, their cellular distribution, as well as their physiological role, have not been determined. To address these open questions we studied the expression pattern of these apoptosis-mediating molecules in the gut and determined the *in-vitro* sensitivity of crypt epithelial cells to TRAIL.

Performing RT-PCR on isolated crypt cells, we revealed transcriptional expression of TRAIL as well as TRAIL-R1, TRAIL-R2, and TRAIL-R4, while a TRAIL-R3 message was not detected (Pukrop *et al.*, submitted). These findings were confirmed by immunohistochemistry. The apoptosis-inducing TRAIL-R1 showed a tissue distribution very similar to CD95: it was expressed in epithelial cells all along the crypt axis and in some interstitial mononuclear cells. Interestingly, TRAIL and TRAIL-R2 were co-expressed mainly in epithelial cells of the crypt mouths and the surface epithelium where senescent cells undergo apoptosis. Although this co-expression of TRAIL and TRAIL-R2 was very suggestive of a role in the physiological turnover of gut epithelial cells, isolated crypt cells turned out to be completely resistant to TRAIL *in vitro* (Pukrop *et al.*, submitted). This finding, however, may not necessarily exclude its involvement in the elimination of senescent cells. If the elimination of cells at the mucosal surface is in fact dependent on a signal directly inducing apoptosis, sensitivity towards this signal must be tightly regulated. Senescent cells may be prepared to die at the tips of the crypts by up-regulation of TRAIL and TRAIL-R2, but have to be ultimately sensitized towards TRAIL by additional factors not active *in vitro*. A knockout system may prove to be more appropriate to determine the role of TRAIL in enterocyte turnover.

Restriction of TRAIL and TRAIL-R2 expression to the upper parts of the crypts and the surface epithelium may indicate another possible function of this apoptosis-inducing system in the gastrointestinal tract. The surface epithelium is the first line of defence against pathogenic microorganisms invading from the gut lumen. Interestingly, there is evidence that apoptosis-mediating TRAIL-R1 and TRAIL-R2 are up-regulated in virus-infected cells while interferon-γ down-regulates the expression of TRAIL receptors in uninfected cells, rendering them more resistant to TRAIL[46]. It may be that epithelial cells at the mucosal surface, by co-expressing TRAIL and TRAIL-R2, dispose of a machinery that, upon infection, allows for their immediate elimination (together with their infectious load) by autocrine or T cell-derived TRAIL to avoid further spread of the infectious agent.

Another interesting point concerning the TRAIL system is the observation that TRAIL induces apoptosis in many cancer cell lines while untransformed cells are largely TRAIL-resistant[33,34,47,48]. This difference in TRAIL sensitivity has been ascribed to a selective expression of decoy receptors in untransformed cells[38,49]. Walczak and co-workers demonstrated that TRAIL induced regression of some mammary and colon cancer cell lines grown in SCID mice without causing detectable toxicity in the host[50]. This observation is in striking contrast to CD95 antibodies which lead to acute liver failure within a few hours following injection into mice[51]. Consequently, TRAIL has recently been attracting attention in cancer research as a possible anticancer therapy. We therefore wanted to test the TRAIL receptor expression pattern and *in-vitro* sensitivity of current colon carcinoma cell lines and isolated cells from sporadic colorectal carcinomas.

Interestingly, most cell lines tested (CaCo2, HT-29, Colo205, SW480, SW620) exhibit a very similar expression pattern on transcriptional and surface protein levels: with RT-PCR they co-express TRAIL and all four TRAIL receptors while, on the cell surface, they only bear TRAIL-R1 and TRAIL-R2. The only exception to this rule is Colo205, which also faintly expresses TRAIL-R3 protein on its surface. Thus, although colon carcinoma cell lines express TRAIL-R3 and TRAIL-R4 on the transcriptional and protein levels (own unpublished data) in the cytoplasm these 'decoy receptors' do not appear on the cell surface.

Despite the very similar TRAIL receptor expression pattern, colon carcinoma cell lines exhibit considerable differences in TRAIL sensitivity *in vitro*, ranging from resistant to highly sensitive (Pukrop *et al.*, submitted). Although expressing TRAIL-R3 on the surface, Colo205 is effectively killed by TRAIL.

When colon carcinoma cell lines are, at least in part, sensitive to TRAIL, does this also apply to sporadic colorectal carcinomas? To test this we isolated carcinoma cells from five colorectal cancer specimens, four of which were immuno-phenotyped by FACS analysis. Interestingly, only two out of four tumours showed the same surface expression pattern as cell lines, being positive for TRAIL-R1 and TRAIL-R2 while lacking the non-apoptosis receptors. The other two tumours analysed exhibited a complementary pattern, expressing TRAIL-R3 and TRAIL-R4 on their surface while lacking TRAIL-R1 and TRAIL-R2. All four tumours, as well as an additional fifth carcinoma which was not phenotyped, were completely resistant to TRAIL *in vitro*. These data led us to two conclusions:

1. TRAIL sensitivity is not regulated by expression of 'decoy receptors' alone. Griffith *et al.*[52] provided similar data on melanoma cell lines showing that TRAIL sensitivity in these cells did not depend on the TRAIL receptor status, and suggested FLICE as a critical regulator of TRAIL sensitivity.
2. Sporadic colorectal carcinomas may be more resistant to TRAIL than cell lines. This observation may not be surprising given the fact that TRAIL is expressed in activated T cells[53] and acts as one of the mediators of cytotoxic T-cell activity[54]. Thus, *in vivo*, carcinoma cells may be subjected to a strong selection due to TRAIL expression on tumour-infiltrating lymphocytes. Having examined only a limited number of carcinomas, further studies on TRAIL sensitivity of colorectal carcinomas are needed to assess the value of TRAIL as a potential anticancer therapy in colorectal cancers.

References

1. Baker SJ, Reddy EP. Modulation of life and death by the TNF receptor superfamily. Oncogene. 1998;17:3261–70.
2. Ashkenazi A, Dixit VM. Death receptors: signaling and modulation. Science. 1998;281:1305–8.
3. Medema JP, Scaffidi C, Kischkel FC *et al.* FLICE is activated by association with the CD95 death-inducing signaling complex (DISC). EMBO J. 1997;16:2794–804.
4. Hall PA, Coates PJ, Ansari B, Hopwood D. Regulation of cell number in the mammalian gastrointestinal tract: the importance of apoptosis. J Cell Sci. 1994;107:3569–77.
5. Sträter J, Koretz K, Günthert AR, Möller P. *In situ* detection of enterocytic apoptosis in normal colonic mucosa and in familial adenomatous polyposis. Gut. 1995;37:819–25.
6. Lynch DH, Ramsdell F, Alderson MR. Fas and FasL in the homeostatic regulation of immune responses. Immunol Today. 1995;16:569–74.
7. O'Connell J, Bennett MW, O'Sullivan GC, Collins JK, Shanahan F. The Fas counterattack: cancer as a site of immune privilege. Immunol Today. 1999;20:46–52.
8. Itoh N, Yonehara S, Ishii A *et al.* The polypeptide encoded by the cDNA for human cell surface Fas can mediate apoptosis. Cell. 1991;66:233–43.
9. Oehm A, Behrmann I, Falk W *et al.* Purification and molecular cloning of the APO-1 cell surface antigen, a member of the tumor necrosis/nerve growth factor receptor superfamily. J Biol Chem. 1992;267:10709–15.
10. Leithäuser F, Dhein J, Mechtersheimer G *et al.* Constitutive and induced expression of APO-1, a new member of the nerve growth factor/tumor necrosis factor receptor superfamily. Lab Invest. 1993;69:415–29.
11. Möller P, Koretz K, Leithäuser F *et al.* Expression of APO-1 (CD95), a member of the NGF/TNF receptor superfamily, in normal and neoplastic colon epithelium. Int J Cancer. 1994;57:371–7.
12. Sträter J, Wellisch I, Riedl S *et al.* CD95 (APO-1/Fas)-mediated apoptosis in colon epithelial cells: a possible role in ulcerative colitis. Gastroenterology. 1997;113:160–7.

13. Dhein J, Walczak H, Bäumle C, Debatin K-M, Krammer PH. Autocrine T-cell suicide mediated by APO-1/(Fas/CD95). Nature. 1995;373:438–40.
14. Ju S-T, Panka DJ, Cui H et al. Fas (CD95)/FasL interactions required for programmed cell death after T-cell activation. Nature. 1995;373:444–8.
15. Brunner T, Mogil RJ, LaFace D et al. Cell-autonomous Fas (CD95)/Fas-ligand interaction mediates activation-induced apoptosis in T-cell hybridomas. Nature. 1995;373:441–4.
16. Montel AH, Bochan MR, Hobbs JA, Lynch DH, Brahmi Z. Fas involvement in cytotoxicity mediated by human NK cells. Cell Immunol. 1995;166:236–46.
17. Hahne M, Renno T, Schröter M. Activated B cells express functional Fas ligand. Eur J Immunol. 1996;26:721–4.
18. Sträter J, Mariani SM, Walczak H et al. CD95 ligand (CD95L) in normal human lymphoid tissues: a subset of plasma cells are prominent producers of CD95L. Am J Pathol. 1999;154: 193–201.
19. Möller P, Walczak H, Riedl S, Sträter J, Krammer PH. Paneth cells express high levels of CD95 ligand transcripts. A unique property among gastrointestinal epithelia. Am J Pathol. 1996;149: 9–13.
20. Bellgrau D, Gold D, Selawry H, Moore J, Franzosoff A, Duke RC. A role for CD95 ligand in preventing graft rejection. Nature. 1995;377:630–2.
21. Griffith TS, Brunner T, Fletcher SM, Green DR, Ferguson TA. Fas ligand-induced apoptosis as a mechanism of immune privilege. Science. 1995;270:1189–92.
22. Griffith TS, Ferguson TA. The role of FasL-induced apoptosis in immune privilege. Immunol Today. 1997;18:240–4.
23. O'Connell J, O'Sullivan GC, Collins JK, Shanahan F. The Fas counter-attack: Fas-mediated T cell killing by colon carcinoma cells expressing Fas ligand. J Exp Med. 1996;184:1075–82.
24. Hahne M, Rimoldi D, Schröter M et al. Melanoma cell expression of Fas(Apo-1/CD95) ligand: implications for tumor immune escape. Science. 1996;274:1363–6.
25. Strand S, Hofmann WJ, Hug H et al. Lymphocyte apoptosis induced by CD95 (APO-1/Fas) ligand-expressing tumor cells – a mechanism of immune evasion? Nat Med. 1996;2:1361–6.
26. Owen-Schaub LB, Radinsky R, Kruzel E, Berry K, Yonehara S. Anti-Fas on nonhematopoietic tumors: levels of Fas/APO-1 and bcl-2 are not predictive of biological responsiveness. Cancer Res. 1994;54:1580–6.
27. Von Reyher U, Sträter J, Kittstein W, Gschwendt, Krammer PH, Möller P. Colon carcinoma cells use different mechanisms to escape CD95-mediated apoptosis. Cancer Res. 1998;58: 526–34.
28. O'Connell, Bennett MW, O'Sullivan GC et al. Fas ligand expression in primary colon adeno-carcinomas: evidence that the Fas counterattack is a prevalent mechanism of immune evasion in human colon cancer. J Pathol. 1998;186:240–6.
29. Shiraki K, Tsuji N, Shioda T, Isselbacher KJ, Takahashi H. Expression of Fas ligand in liver metastases of human colonic adenocarcinomas. Proc Natl Acad Sci USA. 1997;94:6420–5.
30. Yoong KF, Afford SC, Randhawa S, Hubscher SG, Adams DH. Fas/Fas ligand interaction in human colorectal hepatic metastases. A mechanism of hepatocyte destruction to facilitate local tumor invasion. Am J Pathol. 1999;154:693–703.
31. Suda T, Hashimoto H, Tanaka M, Ochi T, Nagata S. Membrane Fas ligand kills human peripheral blood T lymphocytes, and soluble Fas ligand blocks the killing. J Exp Med. 1997;186: 2045–50.
32. Tanaka M, Itai T, Adachi M, Nagata S. Downregulation of Fas ligand by shedding. Nat Med. 1998;4:31–6.
33. Wiley SR, Schooley K, Smolak PJ et al. Identification and characterization of a new member of the TNF family that induces apoptosis. Immunity. 1995;3:673–82.
34. Pitti RM, Marsters SA, Ruppert S, Donahue CJ, Moore A, Ashkenazi A. Induction of apoptosis by APO-2 ligand, a new member of the tumor necrosis factor cytokine family. J Biol Chem. 1996;271:12687–90.
35. Mariani SM, Krammer PH. Differential regulation of TRAIL and CD95 ligand in transformed cells of the T and B lymphocyte lineage. Eur J Immunol. 1998;28:973–82.
36. Pan G, O'Rourke K, Chinnaiyan AM et al. The receptor for the cytotoxic ligand TRAIL. Science. 1997;276:111–13.
37. Pan G, Ni J, Wei Y-F, Yu G-I, Gentz R, Dixit VM. An antagonist decoy receptor and a death domain-containing receptor for TRAIL. Science. 1997;277:815–18.

38. Sheridan JP, Marsters SA, Pitti PM *et al.* Control of TRAIL-induced apoptosis by a family of signaling and decoy receptors. Science. 1997;277:818–21.
39. Walczak H, Degli-Eposti MA, Johnson RS *et al.* TRAIL-R2: a novel apoptosis-mediating receptor for TRAIL. EMBO J. 1997;16:5386–97.
40. Degli-Eposti MA, Smolak PJ, Walczak H *et al.* Cloning and characterization of TRAIL-R3, a novel member of the emerging TRAIL receptor family. J Exp Med. 1997;186:1165–70.
41. Marsters SA, Sheridan JP, Ptti RM *et al.* A novel receptor for APO-2L/TRAIL contains a truncated death domain. Curr Biol. 1997;7:1003–6.
42. Degli-Eposti MA, Dougall WC, Smolak PJ, Waugh JY, Smith CA, Goodwin RG. The novel receptor TRAIL-R4 induces NF-κB and protects against TRAIL-mediated apoptosis, yet retains an incomplete death domain. Immunity. 1997;7:813–20.
43. Simonet WS, Lacey DL, Dunstan CR *et al.* Osteoprotegerin: a novel secreted protein involved in the regulation of bone density. Cell. 1997;89:309–19.
44. Emery JG, McDonnell P, Burke MB *et al.* Osteoprotegerin is a receptor for the cytotoxic ligand TRAIL. J Biol Chem. 1998;273:14363–7.
45. Lacey DL, Timms E, Tan TL *et al.* Osteoprotegerin ligand is a cytokine that regulates osteoclast differentiation and activation. Cell. 1998;93:165–76.
46. Sedger LM, Shows DM, Blanton RA *et al.* IFN-gamma mediates a novel antiviral activity through dynamic modulation of TRAIL and TRAIL receptor expression. J Immunol. 1999;163:920–6.
47. Mariani SM, Matiba B, Armandola EA, Krammer PH. Interleukin 1β-converting enzyme related proteases/caspases are involved in TRAIL-induced apoptosis of myeloma and leukemia cells. J Cell Biol. 1997;137:221–9.
48. Griffith TS, Chin WA, Jackson GC, Lynch DH, Kubin MZ. Intracellular regulation of TRAIL-induced apoptosis in human melanoma cells. J Immunol. 1998;161:2833–40.
49. MacFarlane M, Ahmad M, Srinivasula SM, Fernandes-Alnemri T, Cohen GM, Alnemri ES. Identification and molecular cloning of two novel receptors for the cytotoxic ligand TRAIL. J Biol Chem. 1997;272:25417–20.
50. Walczak H, Miller RE, Ariail K *et al.* Tumoricidal activity of tumor necrosis factor-related apoptosis-inducing ligand *in vitro*. Nature Med. 1999;5:157–62.
51. Ogasawara J, Watanabe-Fukunaga R, Adachi M *et al.* Lethal effect of the anti-Fas antibody in mice. Nature. 1993;364:806–9.
52. Griffith TS, Chin WA, Jackson GC, Lynch DH, Kubin MZ. Intracellular regulation of TRAIL-induced apoptosis in human melanoma cells. J Immunol. 1998;161:2833–40.
53. Jeremias I, Herr I, Boehler T, Debatin KM. TRAIL/Apo-2-ligand-induced apoptosis in human T cells. Eur J Immunol. 1998;28:143–52.
54. Kayagaki N, Yamaguchi N, Nakayama M *et al.* Involvement of TNF-related apoptosis-inducing ligand in human CD4+ T cell-mediated cytotoxicity. J Immunol. 1999;162:2639–47.

14
Bile acid-induced apoptosis in colon cancer cells

K. SCHLOTTMANN, F.-P. WACHS, G. ROGLER and J. SCHÖLMERICH

INTRODUCTION

Bile acids are involved in the pathogenesis of cholestatic diseases of the liver such as primary sclerosing cholangitis and primary biliary cirrhosis, and they are believed to play a role as a co-carcinogen in colorectal cancer. Scientific effort has increasingly clarified the mechanisms by which toxic bile acids exert their effects on hepatocytes and hepatic cancer cells[1]. While necrosis was believed to occur in hepatocytes exposed to high concentrations of toxic bile acids, in this way contributing to the pathophysiology of hepatic diseases, it is now well known that bile acids do not solely induce necrosis, but also lead to the fundamental biological process of programmed cell death or apoptosis. Hitherto, data on the molecular mechanisms of bile acid-induced apoptosis have been elucidated only in hepatocytes, while little is known about the important interaction of toxic bile acids with primary intestinal epithelial cells or colon cancer cell lines. The intracellular signal transduction cascades activated or inhibited by bile acids in the process of apoptosis in colon cancer cell lines have not yet been investigated. At present there is more speculation than information available on the significance of bile acid-induced intestinal epithelial cell or colon cancer cell apoptosis for the development of colorectal cancer. This review focuses on current knowledge concerning apoptotic signalling of bile acids in general, and on the data available regarding bile acid-mediated apoptosis in colon cancer cell lines.

BILE ACIDS CAN BE CYTOTOXIC

Bile acids are derivatives of cholesterol, synthesized in the liver via multistep pathways. The liver synthesises about 0.5–1 mM of bile acids daily. Twenty to 100 mM of bile acids are secreted into the duodenum daily. The primary conjugated bile acids taurocholate and glycocholate, as well as taurochenodeoxycholate and glycochenodeoxycholate, constitute about 95% of the total bile acids secreted. Upon ingestion of food bile acids are released into the duodenum via the common bile duct. In the small bowel bile acids play an important physiological role in the solubilization and resorption of fatty acids and vitamins. Upon their transport through the digestive tract about 95% of the bile acids are reabsorbed passively or actively in the terminal ileum. Only 2–5% of the total bile acids enter the colon where they are metabolized by bacteria. The most abundant bile acids in the colon are the 7α-dehydroxylated and deconjugated derivatives of taurocholate and glycocholate, deoxycholate and of taurochenodeoxycholate and glycochenodeoxycholate, lithocolate. Deoxycholate and lithocholate together form about 70–80% of all bile acids in the colon. While lithocholate can be found almost exclusively in the water-insoluble hydrophobic fraction of the faeces, deoxycholate is also found in faecal water which, at least theoretically, can come into direct contact with colon epithelial cells. Both bile salts, deoxycholate and lithocholate, have been shown to be cytotoxic for colon cancer cells as well as for intestinal epithelial cells[2-4].

Besides their physiological roles bile acids have been identified as toxic agents being causally related to various diseases. Cellular damage occurs when certain bile acids exceed concentrations which are supposed to be physiological, or if they affect cells for prolonged time periods. Cholestatic disorders coincide with prolonged action of bile acids on hepatocytes; indeed we can observe hepatocyte damage in diseases such as primary biliary cirrhosis or primary sclerosing cholangitis. Increased concentrations/amounts of bile acids in the (large) bowel have also been reported to be toxic for intestinal epithelial cells[4] and colon cancer cells[2]. Hence, how do bile acids cause cellular damage, what are the molecular mechanisms and in which context can bile acids cause a deterioration in cellular homeostasis in the colon?

Bile acids are amphipathic; therefore they adsorb to the lipid domains of cell membranes. Binding of bile acids correlates highly with hydrophobicity[5-8]. Conjugated with glycine and taurine residues, which contain sulphonic acid and carboxylic acid groups respectively, bile molecules are strong acids and fully ionized at physiological pH values. Such bile acids remain in the outer part of the lipid bilayer unless a transport system is present. Transporters for conjugated bile acids are found in hepatocytes, renal tubular epithelial cells and the ileal enterocytes. Unconjugated bile acids passively cross the lipid bilayer and thereby enter the cell. Diffusion of bile acids depends on the number of hydroxy groups: dihydroxy bile acids easily cross the cytoplasmic membrane, whereas trihydroxy bile acids such as cholic acid enter the cell much more slowly[9]. The two unconjugated dihydroxy bile acids chenodeoxycholic acid and deoxycholic acid enter the cell rapidly and are toxic at concentrations well below their critical micellar concentration[6]. Hence bile acids such as deoxycholate in the cell act in a toxic way, the mechanisms of which have yet to be unravelled. Differences in the physicochemical properties of bile acids should be kept in mind when bile acids are proposed to be used for experimental purposes, as will be discussed later. Since concentrations of unbound bile acids in plasma are well below 1 μM, circulating bile acids are not considered to interact significantly with the cells of peripheral tissues.

DIFFICULTIES IN THE INTERPRETATION OF BILE ACID EFFECTS ON INTESTINAL EPITHELIAL CELL LINES

Data concerning the effects of bile acids in intestinal epithelial cell lines have proved conflicting. Several factors are often not taken into account when studies with bile salts are performed. Due to a lack of standardization of the experimental design in the literature the following issues are mentioned as a cautionary note, at this point:

1. Colon cancer cell lines are not a primary colon epithelial cell: colon cancer cells such as HT-29 are a frequently used model for the investigation of bile effects on intestinal epithelial cells, or for the study of the co-carcinogenicity of bile acids in colorectal cancer. It should be kept in mind, however, that cell lines are already transformed. It is difficult to define the signalling pathways which have been affected by the transformation; therefore it is almost impossible to transfer features of such cells to primary colon epithelial cells. Results from the same cell line can often not be compared between laboratories, simply because they have been used and grown under many different conditions, with so many possible mutations that we cannot assume we are working with the same cells just because they have the same name (e.g. HT-29). Moreover the colonocyte is not one population of cells, it is a very heterogeneous population of different cell types in various states of differentiation along the crypt surface axis. Therefore we should be careful when interpreting differing results.

2. Bile acids vary in their physicochemical properties: every bile acid has specific sites where it can occur in the body, and according to the state of conjugation bile acids differ in their capacity to passively enter a cell. Furthermore, conjugated bile acids will not enter a cell unless the cell has a bile acid transporter for them. Thus a conjugated bile acid which can be toxic for a hepatocyte such as glycodeoxycholic acid will not be toxic for a colon cancer cell.

3. The concentration range of bile salts used is very broad in the published literature: it seems as if anyone who publishes work on bile acid effects in the colon justifies the concentrations used with some more or less reliable literature. In fact concentrations from 10 to 1000 μM seem to be 'physiological' in this way. Significantly, published cellular responses induced by deoxycholate in colon cancer cells are almost diametrically opposed: while some authors observe gene induction and activation of signalling pathways for cellular activation with low concentrations of deoxycholate, with high concentrations of deoxycholate cytotoxicity leading to rapid cell death has been described[1-3]. To our knowledge there is no publication which shows the actual concentration of bile acids to which primary colonocytes are exposed. Setchell and co-workers describe the problems of reliable and valid measurement of certain bile acids in the faeces in a review[10]. Even if the concentration of certain bile acids in a defined portion of faeces can be obtained, this concentration cannot reflect the conditions for a colonocyte. There is abundant mucus on the cells; the crypts are filled with this mucus. To what extent do bile acids penetrate the mucus, what is the final

concentration on the cell or in the cell? What is the effect of trefoil peptides on bile salts? What part of the colon comes into contact with most of the bile acids? Is there a constant exposure or does transient exposure to bile acids suffice to induce changes? Incubation of cells in a given concentration of bile acids may not reflect the physiological situation. The perfusion of the bowel transports bile acids to the liver and thereby removes bile acids from the enterocytes. The actual concentration in the colonic enterocytes might be much lower than in a tissue culture flask.

4. The incubation times with bile salts vary to a great extent: *in-vitro* studies have shown that bile acid effects vary with the time of incubation. It is impossible to state what time of exposure is normal, but the results of conflicting data should always be interpreted also in terms of the incubation conditions.

BILE ACIDS CAN CAUSE CELL DEATH BY APOPTOSIS

In the mid-1990s Hague *et al.* demonstrated that colon cancer cell lines incubated with deoxycholate showed signs of programmed cell death[2]. Payne *et al.* found that deoxycholate induces apoptosis in goblet cells from colonic biopsies[11]. Apoptosis resistance to deoxycholate in 'normal' colonic mucosa of patients with colorectal cancer, as compared to biopsies from control patients, was used to generate a model explaining the carcinogenicity of bile acids via induction of apoptosis resistance to bile acids[3,4]. On the other hand, we observed apoptosis in three different colon cancer cell lines and in one cell line derived from colon cancer metastasis after incubation with deoxycholate[1]. In all of these cell lines we were able to induce apoptosis with concentrations of sodium deoxycholate from 50 to 100 μM. Deoxycholate-induced apoptosis was specific, since glycodeoxycholate did not induce apoptosis. This is most likely due to a lack of a transporter for conjugated bile acids in these cells. Other bile acids, such as the primary bile acid chenodeoxycholate, also induced apoptosis, showing that hydrophobicity is important for this effect. The observation that all investigated colon cancer cell lines were highly sensitive to bile acids raises doubts as to the model established by Payne *et al.* In a later publication this group confirmed the apoptosis inducing capacity of deoxycholate in colon cancer cell lines[12].

Primary colonic epithelial cells from colon cancer patients undergo detachment-induced apoptotic cell death, also referred to as 'anoikis'[13,14]. Within minutes after detachment primary colonic crypt cells activate apoptotic signalling pathways, rapidly leading to apoptosis[15]. Data from Grossmann *et al.*[15] indicate that intestinal epithelial cells are not apoptosis resistant in general. We have used colonic crypt epithelial cells to determine the *ex-vivo* effect of deoxycholate. Concentrations from 50 to 1000 μM had no pro-apoptotic effect in these cells, detected by flow cytometry and DNA ladder. Caspase activation was not observed either in deoxycholate-treated colonic crypt enterocytes. As mentioned above, this indicates a marked capacity of colon crypt epithelial cells to resist bile acid-induced apoptosis. The lack of significant bile acid-induced colon epithelial apoptosis is in line with the physiological need of apoptosis resistance in order to prevent colonic mucosal damage by an abundant potentially cytotoxic chemical (deoxycholate) in the colon. The mechanisms by which crypt epithelial cells develop apoptosis resistance to deoxycholate are not yet clarified. One might speculate that the expression of the apoptosis inhibitor Bcl-2 in the colonic crypt could influence apoptosis induction[16]. We have some evidence for differentiation dependence of bile acid-induced apoptosis (Schlottmann *et al.* unpublished results) in colon cancer cell lines, indicating that the more differentiated an intestinal epithelial cell is, the stronger is its resistance to bile acid-induced apoptosis. Induction of mitogenic, under some conditions even contra-apoptotic, signalling pathways with PMA/ionomycin in colon cancer cells did not result in decreased bile acid-related apoptosis rates in our studies.

MOLECULAR MECHANISMS OF BILE ACID-INDUCED APOPTOSIS

After defining bile acids that are pro-apoptotic for colon cancer cells we tried to identify the signalling pathways involved for the execution of bile acid-mediated cellular death. Current literature describes a 'two-pathway model' in which, depending on the apoptosis inducer, receptor-mediated death or stress/drug-induced death is favoured. Some receptors which belong to the TNFRI family, such as Fas/CD95/Apo-1, are potent inducers of apoptosis. The signal transduction cascade of the CD95 receptor is well characterized (Fig. 1)[17]. The initiator caspase-8 is activated after docking to the adapter molecule Fas associated protein with a death domain (FADD), which binds to the death domain of the cytoplasmic tail of the CD95 receptor upon ligation. Caspase-8 cleaves and activates the pro-apoptotic Bcl-2 family member Bid (p22) generating an active subunit (p15) which then translocates to the mitochondrion. After binding to the outer mitochondrial membrane p15 induces dissipation of the mitochondrial

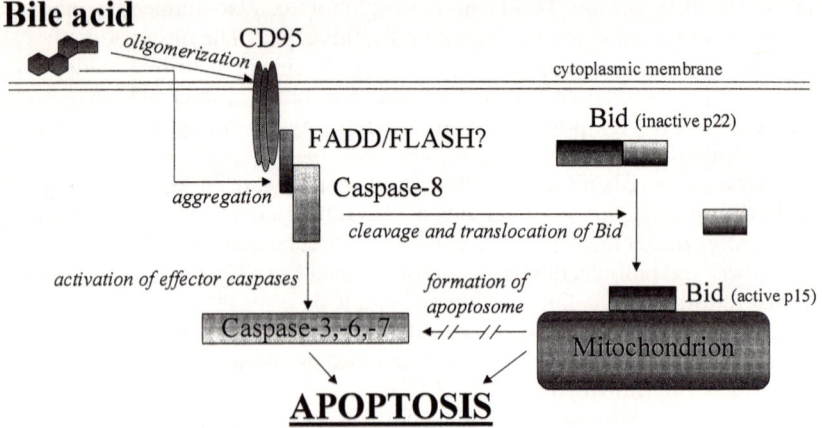

Figure 1 Current understanding of bile acid-mediated apoptosis via the CD95 pathway. This pathway is preferentially used by rodent hepatocytes[19]. The figure is described in the text in more detail

membrane potential $\Delta\Psi$ and releases cytochrome-c. The active subunit of Bid has channel-forming activity similar to other Bcl-2 family members[18]. Mitochondrial depolarization results in the release of pro-apoptotic factors such as cytochrome-c and apoptosis-inducing factor (AIF) from the intermembrane space into the cytosol. The cytoplasmic assembly of cytochrome-c, apoptosis protease activating factor-1 (apaf-1), (d)ATP and caspase-9 results in the formation of the apoptosome. Within the apoptosome caspase-9 is activated. Activated caspase-9 cleaves and activates downstream effector caspases such as caspase-3 or caspase-7. These effector caspases in turn cleave intracellular substrates, which finally culminates in apoptosis of the cell (Fig. 1).

As shown by Faubion *et al.* (see also Chapter 25 by M. E. Guicciardi in this book) CD95 is involved in bile acid-induced apoptosis in rodent hepatocytes and hepatic cancer cell lines[19], as well as in animal models of cholestasis[20]. Colon epithelial cells are highly positive for CD95 and colon enterocyte apoptosis can be induced by agonistic anti-CD95 antibodies[21-23]. This would potentially allow for bile acid-mediated colon epithelial cell death via CD95. However, since we did not observe apoptosis in the CD95-positive primary crypt epithelial cells it is unlikely that CD95 is recruited by bile acids in the colon. Furthermore, we have not observed apoptosis reduction when blocking CD95 by antagonistic anti-CD95 antibodies, and apoptosis of colon cancer cells exposed to deoxycholate did not correlate with the expression of CD95 on these cells. Cells devoid of CD95, as well as cells with high expression of CD95, all underwent deoxycholate-mediated apoptosis while these cells did not show an apoptotic response after addition of the agonistic anti-CD95 antibody CH-11[24]. It has been demonstrated that colon cancer cell lines need to be sensitized, e.g. with interferon-γ, before agonistic anti-CD95 antibodies can execute the CD95 pathway[25]. All of the latter data suggest a CD95 receptor-independent pathway for bile salt-induced apoptosis in colon cancer cells.

Another well-defined pathway for inducers of apoptosis which is not receptor dependent is the stress- or drug-mediated pathway (Fig. 2). This pathway directly induces the mitochondrial membrane permeability transition (MPT) by opening of a large pore designated as the permeability transition pore[28]. Opening of the pore is believed to result in large-scale membrane swelling leading to rupture of the outer mitochondrial membrane with consecutive release of the pro-apoptotic factor cytochrome-c which is necessary for the formation of the apoptosome. Again, caspase-9 cleaves and thereby activates downstream effector caspases such as caspase-3 and caspase-7.

We have investigated caspase cleavage and caspase activation in the colon cancer cell line HT-29[29]. Figure 3 shows the time-dependent cleavage of caspase-3 after exposure of HT-29 to deoxycholate in a Western blot. In other experiments we also detected the activation of caspase-2, -7, -8 and -9, while the rather pro-inflammatory caspase-1 was not cleaved in deoxycholate-treated cells. Data obtained with a dominant inhibitory FADD mutant suggest a FADD-dependent, CD95-independent activation of caspase-8. Whether other death receptors are involved in the apoptotic cell death after deoxycholate remains to be elucidated. Receptor-independent activation of caspase-8 has recently also been demonstrated by other groups[30-32].

Furthermore, we detected the deoxycholate-induced release of cytochrome-c into the cytoplasm in HT-29 cells. In recent publications by Rodrigues *et al.*

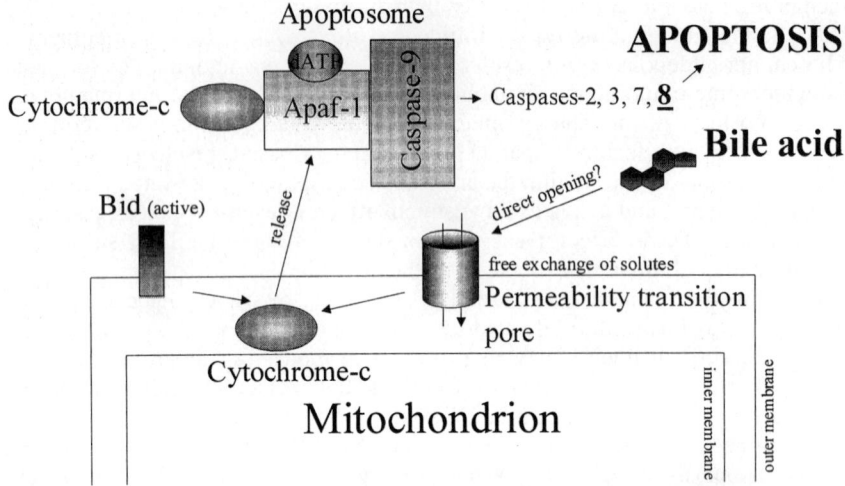

Figure 2 The stress/drug-activated pathway for apoptosis induction. This pathway does not recruit surface death receptors. In this scenario, which has been described by Rodrigues *et al.*[26,27], bile acids are able to directly dissipate mitochondrial $\Delta \Psi$ by opening the mitochondrial permeability transition pore. The downstream events are explained in the text

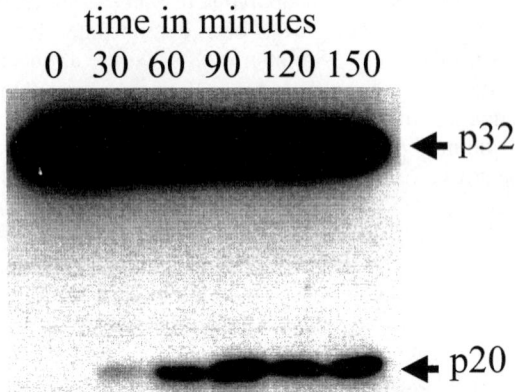

Figure 3 Western blot of caspase-3 from cytosol of deoxycholate-treated HT-29 colon cancer cells. The rapid induction of cleavage after 30 min can be detected. The p32 zymogen form decreases while the p20 fragment increases over time. Caspase cleavage is reminiscent of caspase activation

direct induction of the mitochondrial permeability transition in isolated hepatocyte mitochondria was demonstrated with toxic bile salts[26,27]. Hence, the stress/drug-induced pathway is an alternative pathway for bile acid-mediated cell death in hepatocytes.

The cytoprotective bile salt ursodeoxycholate directly inhibited the effect of toxic bile salts on mitochondrial permeability transition[27]. Ursodeoxycholate also inhibited apoptosis in hepatocytes treated with toxic bile salts, agonistic anti-CD95 and ethanol[26,33]. In our own studies we were not able to inhibit deoxycholate-mediated apoptosis in colon cancer cell lines with ursodeoxycholate. This might be explained by the fact that ursodeoxycholate is not conjugated by colon cancer cells as opposed to rapid conjugation of ursodeoxycholate in hepatocytes. However, ursodeoxycholate sufficiently maintained the mitochondrial transmembrane potential in isolated mitochondria[27]. In HT-29 conjugation of ursodeoxycholate is not expected. The situation in the cell might be more complicated; ursodeoxycholate suppressed ocadaic acid-mediated apoptosis in a sarcoma cell line which probably likely also does not conjugate ursodeoxycholate[26]. The fact that ursodeoxycholate influences the mitochondrial transmembrane potential makes it a broad apoptosis inhibitor. This would also suggest that colon cancer cell lines are an exception for their inability to respond to the cytoprotective effect of ursodeoxycholate. We are currently investigating this phenomenon.

SUMMARY

We were able to show that colon cancer cells exhibit an apoptotic response to toxic bile acids. The intracellular pathway is mediated by the release of cytochrome-c, activation of caspase-9 and further downstream caspases. The CD95 pathway is very unlikely to be involved in this scenario. In this regard, and in their inability to respond to ursodeoxycholate, colon cancer cells differ from hepatocytes and hepatic cancer cell lines. Primary colonic crypt cells do not undergo apoptosis after incubation with bile salts. The mechanism of this apoptosis resistance has not yet been elucidated. Further studies need to be performed in order to understand the role of bile acids in colonic enterocyte homeostasis.

References

1. Kullmann F, Schlottmann K, Schölmerich J. Bile acids and their role in colorectal cancer. In: Schmiegel W, Schölmerich J, editors. Colorectal Cancer – Molecular mechanisms, premalignant state and its prevention. Dordrecht: Kluwer; 1999:203–17.
2. Hague A, Elder DJ, Hicks DJ, Paraskeva C. Apoptosis in colorectal tumour cells: induction by the short chain fatty acids butyrate, propionate and acetate and by the bile salt deoxycholate. Int J Cancer. 1995;60:400–6.
3. Bernstein C, Bernstein H, Garewal H et al. A bile acid-induced apoptosis assay for colon cancer risk and associated quality control studies. Cancer Res. 1999;59:2353–7.
4. Garewal H, Bernstein H, Bernstein C, Sampliner R, Payne C. Reduced bile acid-induced apoptosis in 'normal' colorectal mucosa: a potential biological marker for cancer risk. Cancer Res. 1996;56:1480–3.
5. Schubert R, Jaroni H, Schölmerich J, Schmidt KH. Studies on the mechanism of bile salt-induced liposomal membrane damage. Digestion. 1983;28:181–90.
6. Schölmerich J, Becher MS, Schmidt K et al. Influence of hydroxylation and conjugation of bile salts on their membrane-damaging properties – studies on isolated hepatocytes and lipid membrane vesicles. Hepatology. 1984;4:661–6.
7. Heuman DM. Hepatoprotective properties of ursodeoxycholic acid. Gastroenterology. 1993;104:1865–70.
8. Baumgartner U, Schölmerich J, Sellinger M, Reinhardt M, Ruf G, Farthmann EH. Different protective effects of tauroursodeoxycholate, ursodeoxycholate, and 23-methyl-ursodeoxycholate against taurolithocholate-induced cholestasis. Dig Dis Sci. 1996;41:250–5.

9. Cabral DJ, Small DM, Lilly HS, Hamilton JA. Transbilayer movement of bile acids in model membranes. Biochemistry. 1987;26:1801–4.

10. Setchell KD, Ives JA, Cashmore GC, Lawson AM. On the homogeneity of stools with respect to bile acid composition and normal day-to-day variations: a detailed qualitative and quantitative study using capillary column gas chromatography-mass spectrometry. Clin Chim Acta. 1987;162:257–75.

11. Payne CM, Bernstein H, Bernstein C, Garewal H. Role of apoptosis in biology and pathology: resistance to apoptosis in colon carcinogenesis. Ultrastruct Pathol. 1995;19:221–48.

12. Martinez JD, Stratagoules ED, LaRue JM et al. Different bile acids exhibit distinct biological effects: the tumor promoter deoxycholic acid induces apoptosis and the chemopreventive agent ursodeoxycholic acid inhibits cell proliferation. Nutr Cancer. 1998;31:111–18.

13. Sträter J, Wedding U, Barth TF, Koretz K, Elsing C, Möller P. Rapid onset of apoptosis in vitro follows disruption of beta 1-integrin/matrix interactions in human colonic crypt cells. Gastroenterology. 1996;110:1776–84.

14. Grossmann J, Maxson JM, Whitacre CM et al. New isolation technique to study apoptosis in human intestinal epithelial cells. Am J Pathol. 1998;153:53–62.

15. Grossmann J, Mohr S, Lapetina EG, Fiocchi C, Levine AD. Sequential and rapid activation of select caspases during apoptosis of normal intestinal epithelial cells. Am J Physiol. 1998;274:G1117–24.

16. Merritt AJ, Potten CS, Watson AJ et al. Differential expression of bcl-2 in intestinal epithelia. Correlation with attenuation of apoptosis in colonic crypts and the incidence of colonic neoplasia. J Cell Sci. 1995;108:2261–71.

17. Schlottmann K, Coggeshall KM. CD95/Fas/Apo-1 mediated signal transduction. Cell Physiol Biochem. 1996;6:345–60.

18. Schendel SL, Azimov R, Pawlowski K et al. Ion channel activity of the BH3 only Bcl-2 family member, BID. J Biol Chem. 1999;274:21932–6.

19. Faubion WA, Guicciardi ME, Miyoshi H et al. Toxic bile salts induce rodent hepatocyte apoptosis via direct activation of Fas. J Clin Invest. 1999;103:137–45.

20. Miyoshi H, Rust C, Roberts PJ, Burgart LJ, Gores GJ. Hepatocyte apoptosis after bile duct ligation in the mouse involves Fas. Gastroenterology. 1999;117:669–77.

21. Leithauser F, Dhein J, Mechtersheimer G et al. Constitutive and induced expression of APO-1, a new member of the nerve growth factor/tumor necrosis factor receptor superfamily, in normal and neoplastic cells. Lab Invest. 1993;69:415–29.

22. Sträter J, Wellisch I, Riedl S et al. CD95 (APO-1/Fas)-mediated apoptosis in colon epithelial cells: a possible role in ulcerative colitis. Gastroenterology. 1997;113:160–7.

23. Sträter J, Walczak H, Wellisch I et al. Normal colon epithelium is highly sensitive to CD95-induced apoptosis. Indication for a role of cell death-induced CD95/CL95L systems under inflammatory conditions? Verh Dtsch Ges Pathol. 1996;80:217.

24. Wachs FP, Rogler G, Krieg RC, Schölmerich J, Messmann HCJ, Schlottmann K. Bile acid induced apoptosis in colon cancer cells is not CD95 dependent. 1999 (In preparation).

25. Möller P, Koretz K, Leithauser F et al. Expression of APO-1 (CD95), a member of the NGF/TNF receptor superfamily, in normal and neoplastic colon epithelium. Int J Cancer. 1994;57:371–7.

26. Rodrigues CM, Fan G, Ma X, Kren BT, Steer CJ. A novel role for ursodeoxycholic acid in inhibiting apoptosis by modulating mitochondrial membrane perturbation, J Clin Invest. 1998;101:2790–9.

27. Rodrigues CM, Fan G, Wong PY, Kren BT, Steer CJ. Ursodeoxycholic acid may inhibit deoxycholic acid-induced apoptosis by modulating mitochondrial transmembrane potential and reactive oxygen species production. Mol Med. 1998;4:165–78.

28. Susin SA, Zamzami N, Kroemer G. Mitochondria as regulators of apoptosis: doubt no more. Biochim Biophys Acta. 1998;1366:151–65.

29. Schlottmann K, Wachs F-P, Krieg RC, Kullmann F, Schölmerich J, Rogler G. Characterization of bile salt induced apoptosis in colon cancer cell lines. Cancer Res. 2000 (in press).

30. Nguyen M, Branton PE, Roy S et al. E1A-induced processing of procaspase-8 can occur independently of FADD and is inhibited by Bcl-2. J Biol Chem. 1998;273:33099–102.

31. Bitzer M, Prinz F, Bauer M et al. Sendai virus infection induces apoptosis through activation of caspase-8 (FLICE) and caspase-3 (CPP32). J Virol. 1999;73:702–8.

32. Granville DJ, Carthy CM, Jiang H *et al.* Rapid cytochrome c release, activation of caspases 3, 6, 7 and 8 followed by Bap31 cleavage in HeLa cells treated with photodynamic therapy. FEBS Lett. 1998;437:5–10.
33. Gores GJ, Miyoshi H, Botla R, Aguilar HI, Bronk SF. Induction of the mitochondrial permeability transition as a mechanism of liver injury during cholestasis: a potential role for mitochondrial proteases. Biochim Biophys Acta. 1998;1366:167–75.

15
Role of transcription factor NF-κB in intestinal inflammation

C. JOBIN

INTRODUCTION

There is mounting evidence that intestinal disorders such as inflammatory bowel disease (IBD) involve the dysregulated production of pro-inflammatory molecules. Many of these pro-inflammatory products, such as cytokines and chemokines, are transcriptionally controlled by a ubiquitous transcription factor named NF-κB. This chapter will address our current knowledge of the role of NF-κB in intestinal inflammation, and more specifically its regulation and impact on intestinal epithelial cell (IEC) gene expression.

IκB/NF-κB SYSTEM AND GENE REGULATION

NF-κB is a ubiquitous and inducible transcription factor member of the Rel protein family[1,2]. These proteins share a conserved region named the Rel-homology domain (RHD) responsible for DNA-binding activity, dimerization and nuclear translocation. Members of the NF-κB family include cRel, RelA, RelB, NF-κB1 (p50/p105) NF-κB2 (p52/p100) and bind DNA promoter element as dimer[1,2]. The classical NF-κB dimer, and also the strongest gene transactivator among the family, are the RelA (p65) and NF-κB1 (p50) subunits[3,4]. This heterodimer is also the predominant inducible NF-κB subunit found in the nucleus of cytokine-stimulated IEC[5,6].

A wide spectrum of agents such as cytokines and bacterial products induce NF-κB (see Table 1), which in turn transcriptionally activates many cellular genes implicated in early immune, acute-phase and inflammatory responses, including IL-1β, TNF-α, IL-2, IL-6, IL-8, IL-12, iNOS, COX-2, ICAM-1, VCAM-1, TCR-α and MHC class II molecules[1,2]. Consequently, the inducers and products of NF-κB activation are highly relevant to intestinal inflammation[7,8].

NF-κB activation is mainly regulated by its subcellular localization, a role assumed by the endogenous cytoplasmic inhibitors, IκBs. This protein associates with NF-κB and traps it in the cytoplasm. IκB molecules form a distinct family of

Table 1 Activators of NF-κB

Cytokines and growth factors	*Bacteria and bacteria products*
Interleukin-1β*	*Salmonella* and *Shigella**
Interleukin-2*	Enteropathogenic *E. coli**
Interleukin-17*	*Helicobacter pylori*
Interleukin-18*	*Listeria monocytogenes**
Lymphotoxin	PG-PS*
Leukotriene B4*	LPS*
Tumour necrosis factor α*	
Platelet-derived growth factor*	*Viruses*
	Adenovirus*
T cell mitogens	Epstein–Barr virus
Antigen	Human immunodeficiency virus type 1
Anti-CD2	Human T-cell leukaemia virus type 1
Anti-CD3	Hepatitis B virus
Anti-CD28	
Calcium ionophores	
Oxidative stress	
Hydrogen peroxide*	
Ozone	
Reactive oxygen intermediates (ROI)*	

* Stimuli documented to stimulate IEC

proteins that include IκB-α, IκB-β, IκB-ε, IκB-γ, Bcl3, p105 and p100[9,10]. Key structural features of IκB protein are responsible for its inhibitory ability. First, an N-terminal domain is involved in inducible phosphorylation at specific serine residues which lead to its destruction and cause the release of NF-κB; second, a central domain, formed by ankyrin repeat motifs, is necessary for its interaction with NF-κB; and finally a C-terminal domain (PEST domain) regulating basal protein turnover and also participating in DNA binding inhibition[11]. The most characterized and studied NF-κB inhibitor is IκB-α, and this chapter will focus on this protein.

IκB-α associates strongly with the p65 (RelA) subunit of NF-κB through the binding of the ankyrin repeat domains of IκB-α with the nuclear localization signal and the lg-like domain of p65[12,13]. During activation of NF-κB, numerous stimuli, including IL-1 and TNF-α, activate a complex of IκB kinases (IKK) which phosphorylate IκB-α on the N-terminus part of the molecules at serine residues 32 and 36[14] (Fig. 1). These two amino acids are critical in initiating the IκB degradation process[14-18]. Phosphorylated IκB-α is then selectively ubiquinated and rapidly degraded via a non-lysosomal, ATP-dependent 26S proteolytic complex composed of a 700 kDa proteasome[19-21]. This process exposes the NF-κB nuclear localization signal and causes its migration into the nucleus[11]. IκB-α is quickly resynthesized (60 min) in an NF-κB-dependent manner[22] (Fig. 1) and newly synthesized IκB-α complexes with both cytoplasmic and nuclear NF-κB to terminate gene transcription[11,23-25].

SIGNAL TRANSDUCTION LEADING TO NF-κB ACTIVATION

The proximal events leading to NF-κB activation were best characterized from cytokine receptors. These receptors utilize scaffolding and adaptor proteins to

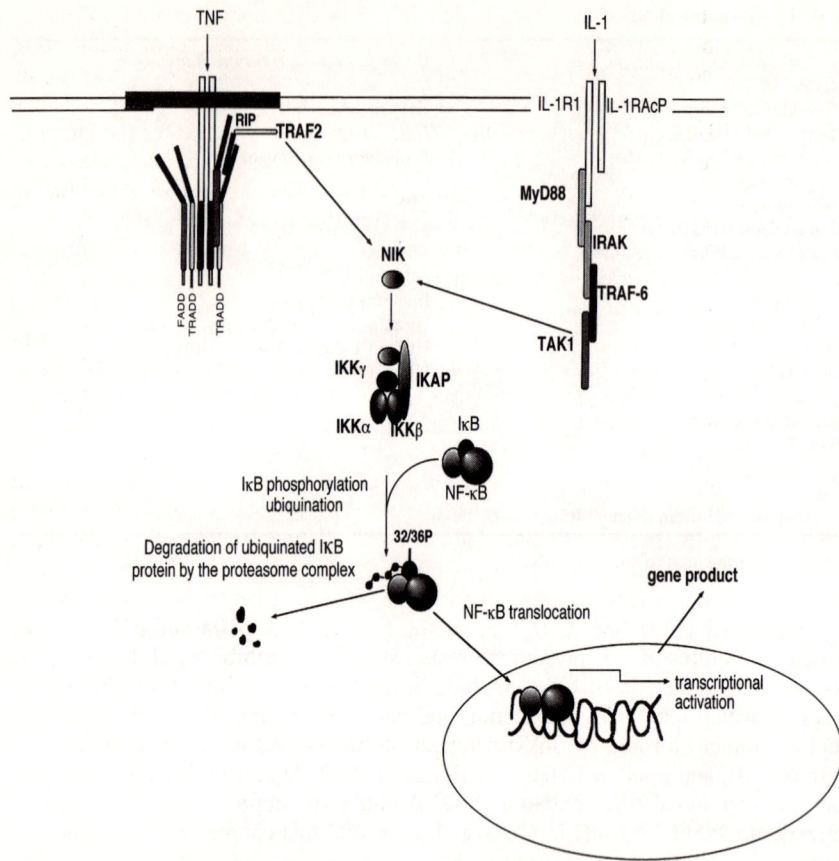

Figure 1   NF-κB is kept latent in the cytoplasm by the inhibitor protein IκB. IL-1 or TNF binding to their respective receptor and elicits a cascade of transductional signals that converge on NIK. NIK associates with the IKK complex via the action of IKAP, leading to phosphorylation of the IKKα and IKKβ subunits. Activated IKK then phosphorylates IκB which triggers the ubiquitination/degradation cascade and NF-κB release which migrates to the nucleus by virtue of its nuclear localization signal. NF-κB binds to multiple κB-dependent gene promoters and induces their transcriptional activation.

transmit their extracellular signal inside the cells. Upon ligand binding, cytokine receptors aggregate to form a platform necessary to the recruitment of specific downstream scaffolding and adaptor proteins to the cytoplasmic tail portion of the receptor (Fig. 1). In the case of TNF-α the TNF receptor-1 (TNFR1) trimerizes and recruits the TNF receptor-associated factor-2 (TRAF)-2 and the receptor interacting protein (RIP) to the cytoplasmic portion of the TNFR1 via the intermediate action of the TNFR1-associated death domain (TRADD)[26,27]. In another example, stimulation by the cytokine IL-1β initiates a signalling cascade that requires the participation of the IL-1 receptor accessory protein (IL-1RAcp), MyD88 and the IL-1 receptor-associated kinase (IRAK). This sequential action of these proteins leads to the activation of TRAF-6, which then recruits transforming growth factor β-activated kinase 1 (TAK1)[28–32]. The recruitment of a selective set of adaptor proteins may be necessary to ensure cytokine-specific responses. The signal coming from the respective TRAF/RIP or TAK1 protein is then transmitted to a molecule named NF-κB-inducing kinase (NIK)[33]. This kinase is believed to be the target of multiple upstream signals such as TNF-α, IL-1β and Fas[33]. NIK associates/activates the IKK complex (Fig. 1)[34–36], which then selectively phosphorylates IκB at the specific serine residues, signalling for its ubiquitination and degradation.

The IKK complex is formed by at least IKK-α, IKK-β, and IKK-γ/Nemo subunits and a scaffolding protein named IKK-complex-associated protein (IKAP)[37]. *In-vitro* studies using the dominant negative form of IKK-α and IKK-β suggest that both kinases are the functional core of the kinase complex mediating/controlling cytokine-induced IκB phosphorylation and NF-κB activation[38–42]. However, recent findings using gene deletion technology provide a different picture regarding the contribution of each kinase in NF-κB activation *in vivo*[43]. From these studies it appears that IKK-β is necessary for cytokine-induced NF-κB activation, whereas IKK-α is dispensable[44]. The latter seems to be involved in transmitting signals implicated in skeletal development and keratinocyte proliferation/differentiation[45,46]. Therefore, IKK-β appears to be a potential target for therapeutic intervention of the cytokine inflammatory cascade. Since NF-κB drives the expression of a number of genes involved in inflammation, its role in IBD was investigated.

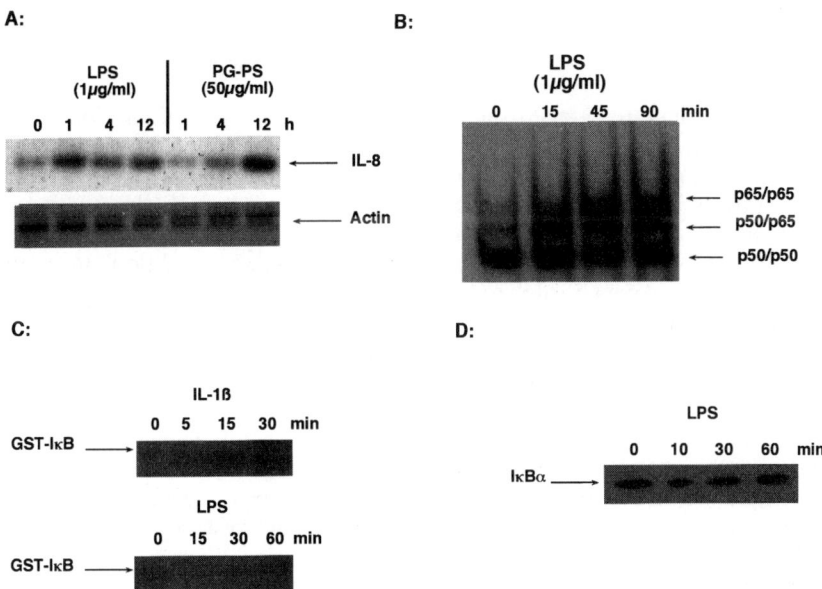

Figure 2 (A) High doses of LPS AND PG-PS induce IL-8 mRNA accumulation in HT-29 cells as seen by RT-PCR analysis. (B) LPS (5μg/ml) induced a rapid activation of NF-κB DNA binding activity in HT-29 cells. (B) IL-1β (2ng/ml), but not LPS (5μg/ml) induced IKK kinase activity in HT-29 cells as measured by in vitro phosphorylation of GST-IkBα (1-54). (D) IκBα is not degraded in LPS-stimulated HT-29 cells.

Table 2 Evidence for a role of NF-κB in intestinal inflammation

---

NF-κB is activated in patients with IBD
    Refs 47, 48
NF-κB-derived cytokines mediate experimental colitis
    TNF-α: ref. 69
    IL-12: ref. 70
Blocking NF-κB inhibits experimental colitis
    Refs 49, 50
IBD therapeutic drugs affect NF-κB activity
    Corticosteroids, sulphasalazine, mesalamine, cyclosporine A, IL-10: ref. 71

EVIDENCE FOR A ROLE OF NF-κB IN INTESTINAL DISORDERS

The transcription factor NF-κB was shown to have a strong relevance to IBD (Table 2). For example, activation of NF-κB in intestinal epithelial cells (IEC) and lamina propria mononuclear cells (LPMNC) has been demonstrated *in vivo*[47] in biopsies of patients with IBD. In addition, NF-κB DNA binding activity and p65 nuclear translocation is increased in the intestine of patients with Crohn's disease, ulcerative colitis and self-limited colitis[47–49], as well as in rodents with experimental colitis[49]. NF-κB activation plays a critical role in mediating intestinal inflammation since blockade of this transcription factor strongly inhibits experimental colitis[49,50]. In one study, local or systemic administration of p65 antisense oligonucleotides reversed chronic experimental colitis induced in mice by trinitrobenzene sulphonic acid[49]. In another study, administration of specific proteasome inhibitors markedly attenuated PG-PS-induced granulomatous colitis in rats, although NF-κB inhibition was not formally demonstrated[50].

Of considerable relevance to intestinal inflammation, several anti-inflammatory drugs used in the treatment of IBD mediate their effects in part through inhibition of the IκB/NF-κB pathway. Dexamethasone stimulates IκB-α synthesis, stabilizes IκB mRNA, and apparently interferes with IκB degradation in IEC-6 cells[51], and IBD patients treated *in vivo* with corticosteroids revealed a decrease of NF-κB activity in biopsy specimens[52]. In addition, the anti-inflammatory compound sulphasalazine blocks TNF-α and LPS-mediated IκB degradation and prevents NF-κB activation in transformed IEC[53].

Although these data indicate a role for NF-κB in intestinal inflammation, the cells origin where NF-κB exerts its inflammatory action is unclear. While lamina propria mononuclear cells may be predominantly responsible for chronic, immune-mediated inflammation, IEC are probably quite important in maintaining mucosal homeostasis and responding to environmental challenges which injure the intestine. Therefore, IEC not only represent the gut's first line of defence, but are also part of a complex and well-orchestrated mucosal immune system.

INTESTINAL EPITHELIAL CELLS PARTICIPATE IN THE MUCOSAL IMMUNE SYSTEM

A single layer of cells physically isolates the host from the hostile gut luminal environment. IEC can function as sensors of mucosal injury and actively participate in the mucosal response to intestinal inflammation and infection[54] in response to bacterial invasion[55], bacterial products[55,56] and pro-inflammatory cytokine stimulation[5]. Following appropriate stimulation, IEC produce a wide variety of chemokines, adhesion molecules, MHC class II molecules and inflammatory mediators which influence the adjacent immune and mesenchymal mucosal cells and recruit circulating inflammatory cells to the mucosa[54,57–59]. In turn, pro-inflammatory molecules such as IL-1β, TNF-α and IFN-γ, produced by recruited inflammatory and immune cells, reciprocally stimulate adjacent IEC. In addition, the interaction of IEC with both luminal antigens and resident intra-epithelial and lamina propria mononuclear cells creates a complex network of interrelated immunologically active cells that recognize and respond to mucosal infection, injury and inflammation. This cellular network might be critical for maintaining gut immune homeostasis[54]. Therefore there is a strong relevance for investigating the IκB-α/NF-κB system in IEC.

SIGNAL TRANSDUCTION LEADING TO NF-κB ACTIVATION IN IEC

We have shown that native colonic epithelial cells and most IEC lines have delayed and incomplete IκB-α degradation following IL-1β stimulation[5], which is preceded by a strong decrease in IKK activity and low IκB-α serine phosphorylation[60]. In addition, we have found that high doses of LPS or peptidoglycan-polysaccharide (PG-PS) are required to induce IL-8 gene expression (Fig. 2A) and NF-κB DNA binding activity (Fig. 2B). Interestingly, LPS failed to induce IKK activity in HT-29 cells (Fig. 2C). Accordingly, IκB-α is not degraded in LPS-stimulated HT-29 cells (Fig. 2D). This suggests that altered IκB-α degradation may be due to low IKK activity in HT-29 cells in response to various inducers. Surprisingly, a constitutively active NIK molecule delivered by adenoviral vector (Ad5wtNIK) induces a strong IκB-α phosphorylation and NF-κB-activated gene expression in HT-29 cells, without inducing significant IκB-α degradation[60]. By contrast, expression of constitutive active NIK and IKK-β induces almost complete IκB degradation in Caco-2 cells[60,61]. Recently we demonstrated that Ad5wtNIK and Ad5IKK-β totally restored IKK activity in HT-29 cells, and induced IκB degradation in cycloheximide-treated cells[62]. These data suggest that altered IκB degradation may be due to a malfunction of the NF-κB signalling pathway located upstream of the IKK complex in HT-29 cells. Interestingly, the IL-1β signalling kinase IRAK is rapidly and completely degraded in IL-1β-stimulated Caco-2 cells, but not in HT-29 cells[60,63].

It was reported that TRAF-2 protein is necessary to initiate TNF-α but not IL-1β signal transduction[26,29]. Interestingly, TRAF-2 was shown to be required for both IL-1β and TNF-α-mediated NF-κB activation and IL-8 gene expression in HT-29 cells[6]. This suggests that communication between TRAF proteins occurs with cytokine receptors, and that this may be a unique signalling feature of IEC.

The migration of IEC from the crypt to the surface of the colon is accompanied by cellular differentiation that leads to important morphological and functional changes. Interestingly, we have found that the IL-1β signalling pathway leading to IKK and NF-κB activation is down-regulated in differentiated compared to undifferentiated cells (crypt-like cells)[63]. In addition, Fas-mediated apoptosis is increased by cellular differentiation both *in vitro* and *in vivo*[64]. Therefore, IEC differentiation may represent a mechanism to maintain mucosal homeostasis.

Because the signalling cascade leading to NF-κB activation involves the participation of multiple proteins, this complex network provides many potential targets for therapeutic intervention. Recent studies have focused on the role of NF-κB in intestinal inflammation.

TARGETING THE IκB/NF-κB SYSTEM IN IEC

Various approaches have been tested to manipulate the NF-κB system in IEC. First, we used molecular interventions using dominant negative versions of individual components of the IκB/NF-κB pathway delivered by adenoviral vectors, and tested them in transformed and primary IEC. An adenoviral vector bearing a proteolysis-resistant IκB-α (Ad5IκB-αAA) strongly blocked cytokine-mediated IL-1, IL-8, iNOS and COX-2 gene expression[18,65]. Upstream of IκB-α, a dominant-negative TRAF-2 (Ad5dnTRAF-2) was partially effective in blocking TNF-α-induced gene expression of IL-8 and NF-κB nuclear transmigration[6,18]. Interestingly, Ad5dnNIK, but not Ad5dnIKK-β, failed to prevent IL-1β and TNF-α-mediated NF-κB activity and IL-8 gene expression in HT-29 cells[66]. This suggests that IKK-β, but not NIK or TRAF-2, represents a potential target for therapeutic intervention.

Adenoviral molecular approaches are a powerful tool to dissect the NF-κB signalling cascade, but their *in-vivo* application is limited. An alternative approach to adenoviral vectors to treat intestinal inflammation is the use of natural dietary products. We have shown that the natural dietary product curcumin is a potent inhibitor of cytokine-mediated NF-κB activation and IL-8 expression through IKK inhibition, suggesting a potential therapeutic application *in vivo*[61]. In addition, green tea inhibits NF-κB activation and TNF-α production in a monocytic cell line[67] and attenuates colitis in IL-2-deficient mice[68]. The complexity of the NF-κB activation pathway provides various potential targets for selective therapeutic intervention in IEC. The development of specific and safe NF-κB inhibitors delivered either locally or systemically could create a useful arsenal to complement the more globally acting drugs currently used to manage intestinal inflammation.

CONCLUSION

The IκB/NF-κB system controls many cellular functions such as immune and inflammatory responses. A complex network of adaptor proteins and kinases act in a well-regulated fashion to induce IκB phosphorylation/degradation, nuclear translocation of NF-κB and transcriptional activation of NF-κB-dependent genes. Many research groups have demonstrated the critical role of NF-κB in pro-inflammatory gene expression by IEC after cytokine or microbial stimulation. It has become evident that the NF-κB signalling cascade represents a target of choice for therapeutic intervention. However, to design an efficient, non-toxic blocking strategy, more data are needed to describe the precise mechanisms of bacterial and cytokine induction of the signalling cascade through the IκB/NF-κB system. This system represents a new and exciting era of research in intestinal inflammatory diseases that could potentially give rise to new targets for therapeutic intervention.

Acknowledgements

Grant support was provided by NIH DK 47700 and the Crohn's and Colitis Foundation of America.

References

1. Barnes PJ, Karin M. Nuclear factor-κB, a pivotal transcription factor in chronic inflammatory diseases. N Engl J Med. 1997;336:1066–71.
2. Baeuerle PA, Henkle T. Function and activation of NF-κB in the immune system. Annu Rev Immunol. 1994;12:141–79.
3. Ballard DW, Dixon EP, Peffer NJ et al. The 65-kDa subunit of human NF-κB functions as a potent transcriptional activator and a target for v-Rel-mediated repression. Proc Natl Acad Sci USA. 1992;89:1875–9.
4. Ruben SM, Narayanan ML, Klement JF, Chen C-H, Rosen CA. Functional characterization of the NF-κB p65 transcriptional activator and an alternatively spliced derivative. Mol Cell Biol. 1992;12:444–54.
5. Jobin C, Haskill S, Mayer L, Panja A, Sartor RB. Evidence for an altered regulation of IκB-α degradation in human colonic epithelial cells. J Immunol. 1997;158:226–34.
6. Jobin C, Holt L, Bradham CA, Streetz K, Brenner DA, Sartor RB. TRAF-2 is involved in both IL-1β and TNFa-signaling cascade leading to NF-κB activation and IL-8 expression in human intestinal epithelial cells. J Immunol. 1999;162:4447–54.
7. Fiocchi C. Inflammatory bowel disease: etiology and pathogenesis. Gastroenterology. 1998;115:182–205.
8. Sartor RB. Pathogenesis and immune mechanism of chronic inflammatory bowel diseases. Am J Gastroenterol. 1997;92:5–11S.
9. Thanos D, Maniatis T. NF-κB: a lesson in family values. Cell. 1995;80:529–32.
10. Gilmore TD, Morin PJ. The IκB protein: members of a multifunctional family. Trends Genet. 1993;9:427–33.
11. Baeuerle PA. IκB-NF-κB structures: at the interface of inflammation control. Cell. 1998;95:729–31.
12. Jacobs MD, Harrison SC. Structure of an IκB-α/NF-κB complex. Cell. 1998;95:749–58.
13. Huxford T, Huang D-B, Malek S, Ghosh G. The crystal structure of the IκB-αNF-κB complex reveals mechanisms of NF-κB inactivation. Cell. 1998;95:759–70.
14. Chen Z, Hagler J, Palombella VJ et al. Signal-induced site-specific phosphorylation targets IκB-α to the ubiquitin-proteasome pathway. Gene Dev. 1995;9:1586–97.
15. Brown K, Gersberger S, Carlson L, Franzoso G, Siebenlist U. Control of IκB-α proteolysis by site-specific, signal-induced phosphorylation. Science. 1995;267:1485–8.
16. Traenckner EB-M, Wilk S, Baeuerle PA. A proteasome inhibitor prevents activation of NF-κB and stabilizes a newly phosphorylated form of IκB-α that is still bound to NF-κB. EMBO J. 1994;13:5433–41.
17. Brockman JA, Scherer DC, McKinsey TA et al. Coupling of a signal response domain in IκB-α to multiple pathway for NF-κB activation. Mol Cell Biol. 1995;15:2809–18.
18. Jobin C, Panja A, Hellerbrand C et al. Inhibition of proinflammatory molecule production by adenovirus-mediated expression of an NF-κB superrepressor in human intestinal epithelial cells. J Immunol. 1998;160:410–18.
19. Li C-CH, Dai R-M, Longo DL. Inactivation of NF-κB inhibitor IκB-α: ubiquitin-dependent proteolysis and its degradation product. Biochem Biophys Res Commun. 1995;215:292–301.

20. Palombella VJ, Rando OJ, Goldberg AL, Maniatis T. The ubiquitin–proteasome pathway is required for processing the NF-κB1 precursor protein and the activation of NF-κB. Cell. 1994;78:773–85.
21. Scherer DC, Brockman JA, Chen Z, Maniatis T, Ballard DW. Signal-induced degradation of IκB-α requires site-specific ubiquitination. Proc Natl Acad Sci USA. 1995;92:11259–63.
22. Sun S-C, Ganchi PA, Ballard DW, Greene WC. NF-κB controls expression of inhibitor IκB-α: evidence for an inducible autoregulatory pathway. Science. 1993;259:1912–15.
23. Read MA, Neish AS, Gerritsen ME, Collins T. Postinduction transcriptional repression of E-selectin and vascular adhesion molecule-1. J Immunol. 1996;157:3472–9.
24. Arenzana-Seisdedos F, Thompson J, Rodriguez MS, Bachelerie F, Thomas D, Hay RT. Inducible nuclear expression of newly synthesized IκB-α negatively regulates DNA-binding and transcriptional activities of NF-κB. Mol Cell Biol. 1995;15:2689–96.
25. Turpin P, Hay RT, Dargemont C. Characterization of IκB-α nuclear import pathway. J Biol Chem. 1999;274:6804–12.
26. Hsu H, Shu H-B, Pan M-G, Goeddel DV. TRADD–TRAF-2 and TRADD–FADD interactions define two distinct TNF receptor 1 signal transduction pathways. Cell. 1996;84:299–308.
27. Hsu H, Huang J, Shu H-B, Baichwal V, Goeddel DV. TNF-dependent recruitment of the protein kinase RIP to the TNF receptor-1 signaling complex. Immunity. 1996;4:387–96.
28. Burns K, Martinon F, Esslinger C et al. MyD88, an adapter protein involved in interleukin-1 signaling. J Biol Chem. 1998;273:12203–9.
29. Cao Z, Xiong J, Takeuchi M, Kurama T, Goeddel DV. TRAF6 is a signal transducer for interleukin-1. Nature. 1996;383:443–6.
30. Cao Z, Henzel WJ, Gao X. IRAK: a kinase associated with the interleukin-1 receptor. Science. 1996;271:1128–31.
31. Wesche H, Henzel WJ, Shillinglaw W, Li S, Cao Z. MyD88: an adapter that recruits IRAK to the IL-1 receptor complex. Immunity. 1997;7:837–47.
32. Ninomiya-Tsuji J, Kishimoto K, Hiyama A, Inoue J-I, Cao Z, Matsumoto K. The kinase TAK1 can activate the NIK-IκB as well as the MAP kinase cascade in the IL-1 signaling. Nature. 1999;398:252–6.
33. Malinin NL, Boldin MP, Kovalenko AV, Wallach D. MAP3K-related kinase involved in NF-κB induction by TNF, CD95 and IL-1. Nature. 1997;385:540–4.
34. Stancovski I, Baltimore D. NF-κB activation: the IκB kinase revealed? Cell. 1997;91:299–302.
35. Verma IM, Stevenson J. IκB kinase, beginning, not the end. Proc Natl Acad Sci USA. 1997;94:11758–60.
36. Lin X, Mu Y, Cunningham ET, Marcu KB, Geleziunas R, Greene WC. Molecular determinants of NF-κB-inducing kinase action. Mol Cell Biol. 1998;18:5899–907.
37. Scheidereit C. Docking IκB kinase. Nature. 1998;395:225–6.
38. Woronicz JD, Gao X, Cao Z, Rothe M, Goeddel DV. IκB kinase-β: NF-κB activation and complex formation with IκB kinase-α and NIK. Science. 1997;278:866–9.
39. Zandi E, Rothwarf DM, Belhase M, Hayakama M, Karin M. The IκB kinase complex (IKK) contains two kinase subunits, IKK-α and IKK-β, necessary for IκB phosphorylation and NF-κB activation. Cell. 1997;91:243–52.
40. Mercurio F, Zhu H, Murray BW et al. IKK-1 and IKK-2: cytokine-activated IκB kinases essential for NF-κB activation. Science. 1997;278:860–6.
41. Rothwarf DM, Zandi E, Natoli G, Karin M. IKK-γ is an essential regulatory subunit of the IκB kinase complex. Nature. 1998;395:297–300.
42. Cohen L, Henzel WJ, Baeuerle PA. IKAP is a scaffold protein of the IκB kinase complex. Nature. 1998;395:292–6.
43. May MJ, Ghosh S. IκB kinases: kinsmen with different crafts. Science. 1999;284:271–3.
44. Li Q, Antwerp DV, Mercurio F, Lee K-F, Verma IM. Severe liver degeneration in mice lacking the IκB kinase 2 gene. Science. 1999;284:321–5.
45. Takeda K, Takeuchi O, Tsujimura T et al. Limb and skin abnormalities in mice lacking IKKα. Science. 1999;284:313–16.
46. Hu Y, Baud V, Delhasse M et al. Abnormal morphogenesis but intact IKK activation in mice lacking IKKα subunit of IKK kinase. Science. 1999;284:316–20.
47. Rogler G, Brand K, Vogl D et al. Nuclear factor κB is activated in macrophages and epithelial cells of inflamed intestinal mucosa. Gastroenterology. 1998;115:357–69.
48. Schreiber S, Nikolaus S, Hampe J. Activation of nuclear factor κB in inflammatory bowel disease. Gut. 1998;42:477–84.

49. Neurath M, Pettersson S, Meyer zum Büschenfelde K-H, Strober W. Local administration of antisense phosphothioate oligonucleotides to the p65 subunit of NF-κB abrogates established experimental colitis in mice. Nat Med. 1996;2:998–1004.

50. Conner EM, Brand S, Davis JM et al. Proteasome inhibition attenuates nitric oxide synthase expression, VCAM-1 transcription and the development of chronic colitis. J Pharmacol Exp Ther. 1997;283:1–8.

51. Jobin C, Herfarth HH, Sartor RB. Dexamethasone inhibits TNF-α gene expression through an IκB/NF-κB pathway in intestinal IEC-6 cells. Gastroenterology. 1996;110:A333.

52. Ardite E, Panes J, Miranda M et al. Effects of steroid treatment on activation of nuclear factor κB in patients with inflammatory bowel disease. Br J Pharmacol. 1998;124:431–3.

53. Wahl C, Liptay S, Adler G, Schmid RM. Sulfasalazine: a potent and specific inhibitor of nuclear factor kappa B. J Clin Invest. 1998;101:1163–74.

54. Kagnoff MF, Eckmann L. Epithelial cells as sensors for microbial infection. J Clin Invest. 1997;100:6–10.

55. Jung HC, Eckmann L, Yang S-K et al. A distinct array of proinflammatory cytokines is expressed in human colon epithelial cells in response to bacterial invasion. J Clin Invest. 1995;95:55–65.

56. Jobin C, Herfarth HH, Sartor RB. Bacterial products and cytokines upregulate IL-8 gene expression in human colonic epithelial cell lines. Gastroenterology. 1995;108:A–844.

57. Nathens AB, Rotstein OD, Dackiw APB, Marshall JC. Intestinal epithelial cells down-regulate macrophage tumor necrosis factor-alpha secretion: a mechanism for immune homeostasis in the gut-associated lymphoid tissue. Surgery. 1995;118:343–51.

58. Komano H, Fujiura Y, Kawaguchi M et al. Homeostatic regulation of intestinal epithelia by intraepithelial αγ T cells. Proc Natl Acad Sci USA. 1995;92:6147–51.

59. Boismenu R, Havran WL. Modulation of epithelial cell growth by intraepithelial αδ T cells. Science. 1994;266:1253–5.

60. Jobin C, Schottelius AJG, Holt L, Sartor RB. Mechanism of the IκB/NF-κB signaling pathway in Caco-2 and HT-29 cells. Lack of IRAK degradation and lower IKK activity is associated with decreased IκB degradation in IL-1β-stimulated HT-29 cells. Gastroenterology. 1999;116:A893.

61. Jobin C, Bradham CA, Russo MP et al. Curcumin blocks cytokine mediated NF-κB activation and proinflammatory gene expression by inhibiting IKK activity. J Immunol. 1999;163:3474–83.

62. Schwabe RF, Russo MP, Bennett BL et al. Adenoviral (Ad5) delivery of wild type IκB kinase β but not Ad5IKK-α restored the defective IκB/NF-κB signaling pathway in HT-29 cells. Gastroenterology. 2000;118:A614.

63. Bocker U, Schottelius AJG, Watson J et al. Cellular differentiation causes a selective down-regulation of IL-1β-mediated NF-κB activation and IL-8 gene expression in intestinal epithelial cells. J Biol Chem. 2000;275:12207–13.

64. Russo MP, Mehta NP, Keku TO, Sartor RB, Jobin C. Increased susceptibility to Fas-mediated apoptosis in differentiated HT-29 cells independent of its effects on NF-κB activation and IL-8 secretion. Gastroenterology. 2000;118:A820.

65. Jobin C, Morteau O, Han D-S, Sartor RB. Specific NF-κB blockade selectively inhibits TNF-a-induced COX-2 but not constitutive COX-1 gene expression in HT-29 cells. Immunology. 1998;95:537–43.

66. Russo MP, Bradham CA, Bennett BL, Manning AM, Brenner DA, Jobin C. IκB kinase β (IKK-β), but not NF-κB-inducing kinase (NIK) or IKK-α represent a therapeutic target for modulation of Fas, IL-1β and TNF-mediated NF-κB activation in intestinal epthelial cells. Gastroenterology. 2000;118:A587.

67. Yang F, de Villiers WJ, McClain CJ, Varilek GW. Green tea polyphenols block endotoxin-induced tumor necrosis factor-production and lethality in a murine model. J Nutr. 1998;128:2334–40.

68. Varilek GW, Yang F, Lee EY, Schweder D. Green tea attenuates inflammation and severity of colitis in IL-2 deficient mice. Gastroenterology. 1999;116:A836.

69. Kontoyiannis D, Pasparakis M, Pizarro TT, Cominelli F, Kollias G. Impaired on/off regulation of TNF biosynthesis in mice lacking TNF AU-rich elements: implications for joint and gut-associated immunopathologies. Immunity. 1999;10:387–98.

70. Neurath MF, Fuss I, Kelsall BL, Stuber E, Strober W. Antibodies to interleukin 12 abrogate established experimental colitis in mice. J Exp Med. 1995;185:1281–90.

71. Schottelius AJG, Baldwin AS. A role for transcription factor in intestinal inflammation. Int J Colorect Dis. 1999;14:18–28.

Section II
Liver

16
Role of cytokines in liver inflammation

A. M. DIEHL

INTRODUCTION

Because of its anatomical location and role in drug and xenobiotic detoxification, the healthy liver is confronted almost continuously with factors that induce injury-related, pro-inflammatory cytokines. For example, normal portal blood contains bacterial products, including lipopolysaccharide (LPS) endotoxin[1], which is a potent inducer of tumour necrosis factor alpha (TNF-α) production by macrophages and other mononuclear cells[2]. TNF induction is known to be one of the earliest events in hepatic inflammation, triggering a cascade of other cytokines that cooperate to kill hepatocytes, recruit inflammatory cells, and initiate a wound-healing response that includes fibrogenesis[3]. However, although the liver contains one of the largest populations of resident

Table 1 Cytokine mRNA expression in the healthy mouse liver

Not detectable
IL-4, 6, 10, 12 p40, 13, 15
IFN-β, γ
Inconsistently demonstrated
TNF-α, β
LT-β
Consistent, low-level expression
IL-1α, 1β, RA
IL-18

Total RNA was isolated from the livers of six healthy, male C57BL-6 mice and the expression of various cytokine mRNAs was evaluated by individual RNAase protection assays (i.e. a separate assay for each mouse) using commercial kits (Pharmingen) according to the manufacturer's instruction. The array of specific cytokine mRNAs were resolved by electrophoresis on agarose gels. Each of the six lanes on each gel contained RNA from a single animal. Duplicate gels were evaluated. Expression was quantified by phospho-imager analysis and results were normalized to GAPDH, a constitutively expressed mRNA that was measured in the same assays. Gels were then exposed to X-ray film to obtain autoradiograms. IL = interleukin, IFN = interferon, LT = lymphotoxin, TNF = tumour necrosis factor, RA = receptor antagonist

macrophages of any organ in the body, and these cells are routinely exposed to portal blood LPS, cytokine gene expression is barely detectable in the healthy liver. Table 1 lists all of the cytokine mRNAs that either cannot be detected at all, or are demonstrated only inconsistently or at very low levels, by RNAase protection analysis of total RNA from healthy mouse livers. It is evident that LPS is not a very effective inducer of either pro- or anti-inflammatory cytokines in the healthy liver. Furthermore, acute treatment with exogenous pro-inflammatory cytokines, e.g. TNF-α, is generally well tolerated by the liver. For example, several investigators have reported that TNF-α treatment induces hepatocytes in healthy rats to proliferate, rather than die[4,5]. The same response (i.e. hepatocyte proliferation) occurs when the healthy liver is confronted acutely by other insults, e.g. partial hepatectomy (PH), that acutely elicit hepatic production of pro-inflammatory cytokines[6]. Indeed, antibody neutralization studies[7] and experiments with type 1 TNF receptor-deficient mice[8] indicate that TNF-α must activate its receptor that contains a 'death domain', in order for the liver to regenerate after PH.

On the other hand, there is no question that, under some circumstances, hepatocytes become exquisitely vulnerable to TNF-mediated lethality. This vulnerability is manifested clinically by the evolution of serious liver injury following insults, such as lipopolysaccharide (LPS) exposure or ischaemia/reperfusion, that are relatively innocuous to normal livers. Several factors that sensitize hepatocytes to TNF-killing have been identified. Treatment with pharmacological agents, such as actinomycin D or d-galactosamine, which inhibit RNA and protein synthesis, are classical experimental tools that are used to sensitize hepatocytes to the lethal actions of TNF[9,10]. Other sensitizing factors (that may be more relevant to human pathophysiology) include infection with certain bacteria, such as *Propionibacterium acnes*[11], chronic ethanol ingestion[12], and obesity[13,14]. Study of experimental animal models with the latter conditions has provided important insights into the immunological mechanisms that regulate hepatic sensitivity to endotoxin.

IMMUNOLOGICAL MECHANISMS FOR *P. ACNES* SENSITIZATION TO LPS HEPATOTOXICITY

Careful work by a number of groups has delineated the immunological mechanisms that are believed to mediate the enhanced vulnerability of the liver to LPS-induced injury following infection with *P. acnes* (Fig. 1). Briefly, *P. acnes* infection activates hepatic macrophages, increasing the local production of IL-12 and IL-18[11]. These cytokines cooperate to selectively reduce hepatic CD4+NK1.1 T cells[11,15], which are normally the major source of IL-4 in the liver[16]. In the face of reduced IL-4 production, liver lymphocytes release decreased amounts of Th-2 cytokines, such as IL-10, and increased amounts of Th-1 cytokines, particularly interferon (IFN)-γ, when the animal is treated with LPS[11,16,17]. Subsequent increases in hepatocyte killing appear to require IL-18 and IFN-γ, because *P. acnes* does not sensitize transgenic mice that are deficient in either IL-18[18] or IFN-γ[19,20] to LPS hepatotoxicity. Furthermore, because the old name for IL-18 is IFN-γ inducing factor[21], it is presumed that IFN-γ is the

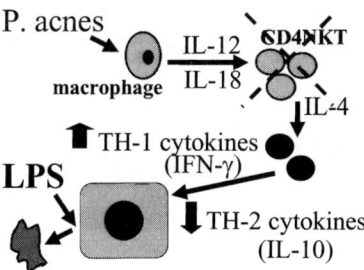

Figure 1 Immunological mechanisms involved in *P. acnes*-induced sensitization of the liver to lipopolysaccharide (LPS)-induced injury

proximate mediator of hepatocyte death in the *P. acnes* model[11]. However, the precise cellular and molecular mechanisms that cause IFN-γ-induced hepatocyte death remain uncertain. It is possible that perforin- and/or Fas-initiated signals may be involved, because there is some evidence that IL-18 sensitizes cells to lethality from these mediators[22,23].

MECHANISMS INVOLVED IN VULNERABILITY OF OBESITY-RELATED FATTY LIVERS

Fatty livers, in which large and small droplets of triglyceride accumulate within hepatocytes[24], are known to be particularly vulnerable to serious injury when challenged by small amounts of endotoxin[13] or transient ischaemia and reperfusion[25]. This hepatocyte sensitization has important clinical implications. For example, it is believed to play a fundamental role in the genesis of alcohol-related liver damage[26] and might also help to explain why fatty liver grafts are predisposed to primary non-function after transplantation[27]. A couple of years ago our group showed that genetically obese, ob/ob mice, which develop fatty livers spontaneously, are exquisitely vulnerable to injury by endotoxin[13] or ischaemia/reperfusion[25]. Thus, the obese ob/ob mouse provides a model that can be used to evaluate the mechanisms that sensitize fatty hepatocytes to killing.

Immunological abnormalities

Given the importance of hepatic CD4+NK1.1 T cells in the regulation of Th-1/ Th-2 responses in the liver[16], we recently performed experiments in collaboration with Dr Ursula Krytzch's group (Walter Reed Army Institute for Research, Washington, DC) to compare the distributions of liver lymphocyte subpopulations in the fatty livers of ob/ob, C57BL-6 mice and the normal livers of lean, C57BL-6 controls. Mononuclear cells were isolated from livers by collagenase digestion and centrifugation over Percoll gradients. Purified mononuclear cell fractions were incubated with antibodies to various murine mononuclear cell surface markers and FACS analysis was used to demonstrate the distribution of mononuclear cell populations. In each experiment, mononuclear cells were pooled from four to six obese and four to six lean mice. Experiments were

Table 2 Distribution of liver mononuclear cells in ob/ob and lean C57BL-6 mice

	ob/ob	Lean	p-value
NK(+) Cells	5.4 (0.4)	15 (4.3)	<0.05
CD3(+)			
CD4+	3.2 (1.1)	18.7 (5.8)	<0.05
CD8+	2.3 (0.3)	2.2 (0.4)	n.s.
CD3(–)	17.1 (2.2)	22.3 (6.4)	n.s.
NK (–) Cells			
CD3 (+)			
CD4+	13.2 (0.4)	23.6 (3.8)	<0.05
CD8+	23.6 (5.4)	18.5 (0.4)	n.s.
Mac3(+)	16.1 (9)	10.7 (1.5)	n.s.

Mononuclear cells were isolated from the livers of ob/ob mice and lean mice. FACS analysis was used to determine the relative distributions of mononuclear cell subpopulations in the two groups of mice. Results are shown as the mean (standard deviation) percentage of cells in each subpopulation in three experiments. In each experiment liver mononuclear cells from four to six mice/group were pooled for analysis

repeated three times to assure the reproducibility of our findings. As summarized in Table 2, the fatty livers have relatively reduced numbers of NK1.1 T cells. This is predominantly due to a selective reduction in CD4+NK1.1 T cells. Thus, the selective reduction of liver CD4+NK1.1 T cells in the fatty livers of otherwise healthy ob/ob mice resembles the depletion of this lymphocyte subpopulation that follows *P. acnes* infection in normal mice.

We have reported previously that hepatic macrophages of fa/fa rats and peritoneal macrophages of ob/ob mice are abnormal. These cells have impaired phagocytosis *in vivo*[13,28] and *in vitro*[28], release increased amounts of mitochondrially derived H_2O_2 *in vitro* and exhibit enhanced basal and LPS-induced production of IL-6, increased mRNA expression of cox-2, an IL-6-regulated gene, and increased release of Cox-2 prostanoid products[29]. Thus, macrophages from obese mice appear to be activated constitutively. Hence, similar to macrophages that have been activated by *P. acnes* infection[11], activated liver macrophages in ob/ob mice might produce increased amounts of IL-12 or IL-18, which are known to reduce CD4+NK1.1 T cells[11]. To evaluate this possibility the hepatic expression of these cytokine mRNAs was evaluated by RNAase protection assays. These studies demonstrated no difference in the basal expression of IL-12 p35, IL-12 p40, or IL-18 mRNAs in ob/ob mice and lean controls. However, following LPS treatment, the inductions of both IL-12 p40 and IL-18 mRNAs were greater and more sustained in the obese mice (Fig. 2). Although IL-12 expression is regulated predominantly at the level of transcription[30], post-transcriptional mechanisms play a key role in regulating IL-18 expression. Specifically, the production of biologically active IL-18 requires the cleavage of pro-IL-18 by caspase 1[21]. Thus, it is conceivable that basal IL-18 bioactivity may be greater in ob/ob mice than in lean controls despite apparent similarities in IL-18 mRNA expression in the two groups. To evaluate that possi-

IL-12 p40 mRNA

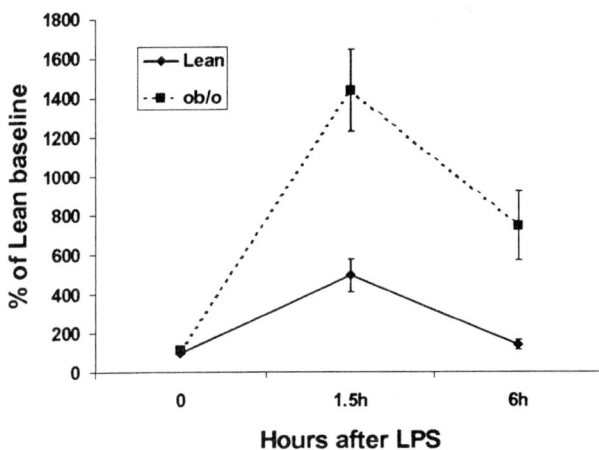

IL-18 mRNA

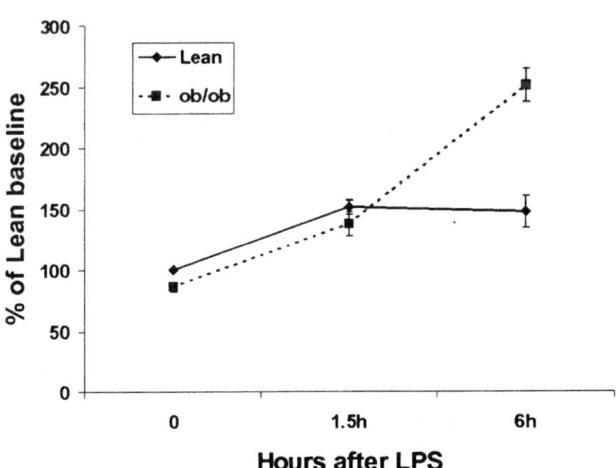

Figure 2 Expression of IL-12 p40, IL-12 p35, IL-18, and GAPDH mRNAs in the livers of obese, ob/ob C57BL-6 mice and lean C57BL-6 mice. As described in the legend to Table 1, cytokine gene expression was evaluated by RNAase protection assays and quantified by phospho-imager analysis. At each time point RNA from four mice/group were evaluated and results were normalized to GAPDH expression in the same sample. Data are shown as mean ± SD

bility, serum concentrations of IL-18 protein were quantified by ELISA. Interestingly, serum concentrations of IL-18 in ob/ob mice were twice that of lean controls even before LPS treatment. In addition, after LPS exposure, circulating levels of IL-18 were significantly more induced in ob/ob mice than in the control animals. However, it remains difficult to understand whether or not these differences in IL-18 production are responsible for the obesity-related decreases in hepatic CD4+NK1.1 T cells, because it is generally believed that IL-18 requires IL-12 to achieve this effect[11,17], and we could not detect IL-12 p40 expression in ob/ob livers. Thus, alternative mechanisms may be involved.

Pertinent in this regard is work which demonstrates that the adhesion molecule, leucocyte factor antigen (LFA)-1, and its receptor, ICAM-1, are required for CD4+NK1.1 T cells to accumulate in the liver. Transgenic mice that are deficient in either molecule develop selective reductions in this liver lymphocyte population[31,32]. In addition, both strains of transgenic mice become obese[33]. Given this curious association between obesity, adhesion molecule deficiency, and liver CD4+NK1.1 T cell depletion, we wondered if mononuclear cell expression of either LFA-1 or ICAM-1 might be reduced in spontaneously obese, ob/ob mice. Although ICAM-1 expression appears to be similar in mononuclear cell isolates from obese and lean mice, a 50% reduction in LFA-1 expression is observed in the obese group, raising the intriguing possibility that decreases in LFA-1 might contribute to the constitutive dearth of hepatic CD4+NK1.1 T cells in obesity-related fatty livers.

Because CD4+NK1.1 T cells are the predominant source of IL-4 in the liver[16], mononuclear cells from fatty livers are expected to produce less IL-4 than mononuclear cells from normal livers which contain the usual complement of CD4+NK1.1 T cells. To evaluate this possibility, ELISPOT assays were done to quantitate the number of IL-4-producing colonies in liver mononuclear cells isolated from fatty and normal livers. As expected, only about half as many IL-4-producing mononuclear cells were demonstrated in the isolates from the obese group compared to the lean controls.

Decreases in local production of IL-4 are believed to compromise the production of Th-2 cytokines, such as IL-10, while promoting overly exuberant production of Th-1 cytokines, such as IFN-γ, following LPS challenge[11,15,16]. Thus, after LPS treatment, the fatty livers of ob/ob mice are expected to produce less IL-10 and more IFN-γ than the normal livers of lean mice. To evaluate this possibility, total liver RNA was isolated from ob/ob mice and lean controls before or at two different time points after the animals were given 10 μg of LPS by introperitoneal injection. As expected, LPS up-regulated the mRNA expression of these cytokines in both groups. However, the induction of IL-10 mRNA was significantly inhibited, while the induction of IFN-γ mRNA was significantly enhanced, in the livers of the obese mice (Fig. 3). Thus, similar to P. acnes-infected mice[11], genetically obese mice with fatty livers have a disproportionately large Th-1 response to LPS.

Viable but vulnerable hepatocytes

Although similarities between the lymphocyte and cytokine profiles of two different animal models of hepatic sensitization (i.e. P. acnes-infection and obesity-

IL10 mRNA

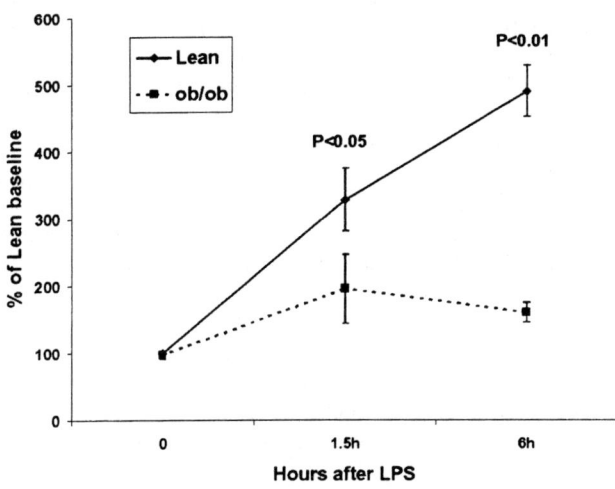

IFNγ mRNA

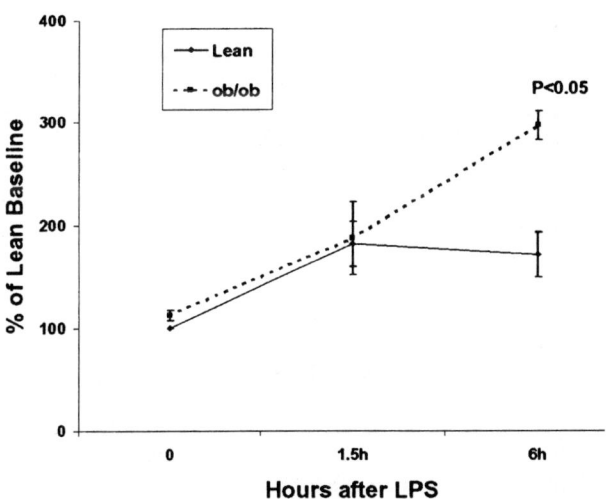

Figure 3 Expression of IL-10, IFN-γ, and GAPDH mRNAs in the livers of obese, ob/ob C57BL-6 mice and lean C57BL-6 mice. Gene expression was evaluated by RNAase protection assays as described in the legend to Fig. 2. Data are shown as the mean ± SD results from four mice/group per time point

related fatty liver) have been demonstrated, it remains difficult to understand how these immunological abnormalities promote hepatocyte lethality. Indeed, despite repeated efforts to demonstrate increased rates of hepatocyte death in ob/ob livers, we have been consistently unable to find constitutive increases in hepatocyte apoptosis or necrosis in these fatty livers[31]. However, we and others have noted several abnormalities in hepatocyte mitochondria of fatty livers. These include ultrastructural abnormalities[35], increased rates of O_2 consumption[25,36], enhanced H^+ ion permeability of the inner membrane[25], and up-regulated expression of both pro- and anti-apoptotic bcl-2 family members[34]. More recently our group has learned that mitochondria from fatty livers have decreased cytochrome-c content, increased production of superoxide anion and hydrogen peroxide, alterations in reduced glutathione, as well as in the activities of the antioxidant enzymes, manganese superoxide dismutase and glutathione peroxidase, and increased membrane content of the uncoupling protein (UCP)-2 (Diehl AM, Trush MA and colleagues, submitted). Taken together, these findings suggest that hepatocytes in fatty livers may be under increased apoptotic pressure but survive by inducing a number of adaptive responses in hepatocyte mitochondria. However, some of the adaptations might inadvertently make the hepatocyte more vulnerable to necrosis. For example, up-regulation of UCP-2 is predicted to partially depolarize the mitochondrial inner membrane and to decrease the efficiency of ATP synthesis[37]. Thus, increased UCP-2 might potentiate cellular necrosis if hepatocytes are challenged by secondary insults that further depolarize the mitochondrial membrane or deplete ATP stores.

AREAS FOR FUTURE STUDY

Many questions must be answered in order to completely clarify why obesity-related fatty livers are sensitized to LPS-induced lethality. Among the things that have yet to be discovered in the ob/ob mouse model are: (1) the mechanisms that mediate the activation of hepatic macrophages (or other non-parenchymal cells) in obesity, (2) the molecular events that affect selective reductions in hepatic CD4+NK1.1 T cells, (3) the extracellular signals that change the phenotype of hepatocyte mitochondria, (4) the intracellular signals that alter the expression of nuclear gene products which encode mitochondrial membrane components, and (5) the processes involved in functional regulation of obesity-adapted mitochondria.

POTENTIAL IMPLICATIONS OF FATTY LIVER ADAPTATIONS

Although many gaps in the knowledge base relating to fatty liver remain, the information that has been gained in the past few years has potentially important implications for other circumstances that result in liver damage. These insights can be summarized quite succinctly by a few famous quotations. First, 'what doesn't kill you, often makes you stronger' (i.e. adaptations to apoptotic pressure permit hepatocytes to survive in a pro-apoptotic environment). Second, 'never underestimate your own tendency to shoot yourself in the foot' (i.e.

adaptations to escape apoptosis might inadvertently enhance vulnerability to necrosis). Third, 'as usual, damned if you do, damned if you don't' (i.e. timing and luck determine survival – adaptation is beneficial unless the liver is unlucky enough to experience a sudden, unexpected secondary stress).

References

1. Trautwein C, Rakemann T, Niehof M, Rose-John S, Manns MP. Acute-phase response factor, increased binding, and target gene transcription during liver regeneration. Gastroenterology. 1996;110:1854–62.
2. Decker K. Biologically active products of stimulated liver macrophages (Kupffer cells). Eur J Biochem. 1990;192:245–61.
3. Tracey KJ, Cerami A. Tumor necrosis factor, other cytokines and disease. Annu Rev Cell Biol. 1993;9:317–43.
4. Feingold KR, Soued M, Grunfeld C. Tumor necrosis factor stimulates DNA synthesis in the liver of intact rats. Biochem Biophys Res Commun. 1988;153:576–82.
5. Beyer HS, Stanley M, Theologides A. Tumor necrosis factor-alpha increases hepatic DNA and RNA and hepatocyte mitosis. Biochem Int. 1990;22:405–10.
6. Diehl AM, Rai R. Regulation of signal transduction during liver regeneration. FASEB J. 1996;10:215–27.
7. Akerman P, Cote P, Yang SQ et al. Antibodies to tumor necrosis factor alpha inhibit liver regeneration after partial hepatectomy. Am J Physiol. 1992;263:G579–85.
8. Yamada Y, Kirillova I, Peschon JJ, Fausto N. Initiation of liver growth by tumor necrosis factor: deficient liver regeneration in mice lacking type I tumor necrosis factor receptor. Proc Natl Acad Sci. 1997;94:1441–46.
9. Hishinuma I, Nagakawa J, Hirota K et al. Tumor necrosis factor-alpha in galactosamine-induced hepatitis. Hepatology. 1990;12:1187–91.
10. Vassalli P. The pathophysiology of tumor necrosis factor. Annu Rev Immunol. 1992;10:411–52.
11. Matsui K, Yoshimoto T, Tsutsui H et al. Propionibacterium acnes treatment diminishes CD4+NK1.1+T cells but induces type 1 T cells in the liver by induction of IL-12 and IL-18 production from Kupffer cells. J Immunol. 1997;159:97–106.
12. Fernandez-Checa JC, Kaplowitz N, Garcia-Ruiz C et al. GSH transport in mitochondria: defense against TNF-induced oxidative stress and alcohol-induced defect. Am J Physiol. 1997;273:G7–17.
13. Yang SQ, Lin HZ, Lane MD, Clemens M, Diehl AM. Obesity increases sensitivity to endotoxin liver injury: implications for pathogenesis of steatohepatitis. Proc Natl Acad Sci USA. 1997;94:2557–62.
14. Faggioni R, Fantuzzi G, Gabay C et al. Leptin deficiency enhances sensitivity to endotoxin-induced lethality. Am J Physiol. 1999;276:R136–42.
15. Tanaka Y, Takahashi A, Watanabe K et al. A pivotal role of IL-12 in Th1-dependent mouse liver injury. Int Immunol. 1996;8:569–76.
16. Emoto M, Emoto Y, Kaufmann SH. IL-4 producing CD4+TCR alpha beta intermediate liver lymphocytes: influence of thymus, beta 2-microglobulin and NK1.1 expression. Int Immunol. 1995;7:1729–39.
17. Okamura H, Kashiwamura S, Tsutsui H, Yoshimoto T, Nakanishi K. Regulation of interferon-gamma production by IL-12 and IL-18. Curr Opin Immunol. 1998;10:259–64.
18. Sako Y, Takeda K, Tsutsui H et al. IL-18-deficient mice are resistant to endotoxin-induced liver injury but highly susceptible to endotoxin shock. Int Immunol. 1999;11:471–80.
19. Car BD, Eng VM, Schnyder B et al. Interferon gamma receptor deficient mice are resistant to endotoxic shock. J Exp Med. 1994;179:1437–44.
20. Car BD, Eng VM, Schnyder B et al. Role of interferon-gamma in interleukin 12-induced pathology in mice. Am J Pathol. 1995;147:1693–707.
21. Dinarello CA. IL-18: a TH1-inducing, proinflammatory cytokine and new member of the IL-1 family. J Allergy Clin Immunol. 1999;103:11–24.
22. Dao T, Mehal WZ, Crispe IN. IL-18 augments perforin-dependent cytotoxicity of liver NK-T cells. J Immunol. 1998;161:2217–22.

23. Ohtsuki T, Micallef MJ, Kohono K, Tanimoto T, Ikeda M, Kurimoto M. Interleukin 18 enhances Fas ligand expression and induces apoptosis in Fas-expressing human myelomonocytic KG-1 cells. Anticancer Res. 1997;17:3253–8.

24. Samazasinghe D, Tasman-Jones C. The clinical associations with hepatic steatosis: a retrospective study. NZ Med J. 1992;105:57–8.

25. Chavin K, Yang SQ, Lin HZ et al. Obesity induces expression of uncoupling protein-2 in hepatocytes and promotes liver ATP depletion. J Biol Chem. 1999;274:5692–5700.

26. Nanji AA, Khettry U, Sadrzadeh SMH, Tamanaka T. Severity of liver injury in experimental alcoholic liver disease. Am J Pathol. 1993;142:367–73.

27. D'Alessandro AM, Kalayoglu M, Sollinger HW et al. The predictive value of donor liver biopsy on the development of primary nonfunction after orthotopic liver transplantation. Transpl Proc. 1991;23:1536–7.

28. Loffreda S, Yang SQ, Lin HZ et al. Leptin regulates proinflammatory immune responses. FASEB J. 1998;12:57–65.

29. Lee F-Y, Li Y, Yang EK et al. Phenotypic abnormalities in macrophages from leptin-deficient, obese mice. Am J Physiol: Cell Physiol. 1999;276:C386–94.

30. Trinchieri G. Interleukin-12: a proinflammatory cytokine with immunoregulatory functions that bridge innate resistance and antigen-specific adaptive immunity. Annu Rev Immunol. 1995;13:251–76.

31. Emoto M, Mittrucker HW, Schmits R, Mak TW, Kaurmann SH. Critical role of leukocyte function-associated antigen-1 in liver accumulation of CD4+NKT cells. J Immunol. 1999;162:5094–98.

32. Marvin MR, Southall JC, Trokhan S, De Rosa C, Chabot J. Liver metastases are enhanced in homozygous deletionally mutant ICAM-1 or LFA-1 mice. J Surg Res. 1998;80:143–8.

33. Dong ZM, Gutierrez-Ramos JC, Coxon A, Mayadas TN, Wagner DD. A new class of obesity genes encodes leukocyte adhesion receptors. Proc Natl Acad Sci USA. 1997;94:7526–30.

34. Rashid A, Wu T-C, Huang CC et al. Mitochondrial proteins that regulate apoptosis and necrosis are induced in mouse fatty liver. Hepatology. 1999;29:1131–8.

35. Petersen P. Ultrastructure of periportal and centrilobular hepatocytes in human fatty liver of various etiologies. Acta Pathol Microbiol Scand. 1977;85:421–7.

36. Katyare S, Howland JL. Enhanced oxidative metabolism in liver mitochondria from genetically obese mice. Arch Biochem Biophys. 1978;188:15–20.

37. Boss O, Muzzin P, Giacobino JP. The uncoupling proteins, a review. Eur J Endocrinol. 1998;139:1–9.

17
Role of TNF-α-dependent pathways in models of acute liver failure

K. STREETZ, C. LIEDTKE, M. P. MANNS and C. TRAUTWEIN

INTRODUCTION

Tumour necrosis factor-α (TNF-α) is a cytokine mainly produced by activated macrophages and in smaller amounts by several other cell types. After its isolation during the 1980s, considerable efforts were made to understand the molecular mechanisms of the diverse biological effects of TNF-α[1,2]. In addition to its activity against transformed cells, TNF-α exerts various effects on different normal cell types[3,4], thereby implicating its role as an essential mediator in various physiological and pathophysiological conditions (i.e. septic shock, cerebral malaria and others)[5].

Additionally it has become clear that TNF-α is an important mediator of apoptosis (programmed cell death)[6]. In order to understand the pleiotropic effects mediated by TNF-α, much effort has been made to characterize the intracellular pathways which are involved in various biological processes such as cell proliferation, inflammation and apoptosis.

TNF LIGAND AND RECEPTOR FAMILIES

The cytokine TNF-α belongs to a family of nine known ligands (TNF-α, lymphotoxin-α, TNF-β, Fas-ligand, OX40L, CD40L, CD27L, CD30L, 4-1BBL and lymphotoxin-β) that activate structurally related receptor proteins known as the TNF-receptor superfamily[7]. So far 12 transmembrane proteins consisting of two identical subunits have been identified as members of the TNF-receptor superfamily: TNF receptor 1 (TNF-R1, p55), TNF-receptor 2 (TNF-R2, p75), TNF-RP, FAS, OX-40, 4-1BB, CD40, CD30, CD27, poxvirus PV-T2 and PV-A53R gene products, and p75 NGFR. TNF-α interacts with two receptors: TNF-R1 and TNF-R2[7,8]. Crystallographic studies of the 55-kDa TNF receptor indicated dimeric proteins arranged head to head to each other. From this observation the so-called molecular switch model has been developed to explain the interaction between TNF-α and its receptors. This is based on the hypothesis that a dimeric receptor protein is contacted by a trimeric ligand complex, leading to a rearrangement in receptor conformation that permits signal transduction through the plasma membrane (reviewed in ref. 7).

In addition to membrane-bound TNF-R1 and R2, soluble forms can be generated from both receptors by proteolytic cleavage of the extracellular domain[9]. The role of soluble TNF-R1 and TNF-R2 (sTNF-R1 and sTNF-R2) is not completely understood. However, there are reports which indicate that the interaction between TNF-α and sTNF-R1 or sTNF-R2 may increase the half-life of TNF-α in serum[10]. Additionally sTNF-R1 and -R2 block the interaction of TNF-α with the transmembrane forms and thus act as an antagonist of TNF-α[11].

INTRACELLULAR PATHWAYS ACTIVATED THROUGH THE TNF RECEPTORS

The intracellular regions of TNF-R1 and -R2 lack catalytic domains to phosphorylate downstream targets. Therefore receptor-associated proteins function as essential transducers in TNF-R-dependent signalling. The search for such molecules identified TNF receptor associated factor 1 and 2 (TRAF-1 and -2)[12]. Meanwhile a growing family of related molecules has been cloned which all share in the c-terminus the so-called TRAF domain. After TNF-R2 ligand binding TRAF-2 homodimers or TRAF-1 and TRAF-2 heterodimers bind to 78 amino acids at the c-terminal intracellular domain of TNF-R2 which results in NF-κB activation.

Further dissection of the TRAF-2 molecules showed that the N-terminal ring finger domain of TRAF-2 is necessary to mediate downstream signals which result in NF-κB activation. Therefore overexpression of a molecule which lacks the N-terminal ring finger domain acts as a dominant-negative TRAF-2 molecule which blocks NF-κB activation via TNF-R2[13–15]. However, recent results with TRAF-2 –/– mice show that activation of NF-κB is unchanged in these animals[16]. Another protein – TRIP (TRAF-interacting protein) – is able to associate with the TNF-R2 complex through its interaction with TRAF-2, thereby inhibiting the activation of NF-κB[16].

Besides its role in activating NF-κB, TRAF-2 is involved in mediating the activation of the SAPK/JNK pathway[17,18]. JNK phosphorylates the activation domain of c-Jun and ATF-2. A dominant-negative form of TRAF-2 also blocks SAPK/JNK[19]. In some cells it has been reported that SAPK/JNK activity is required for the induction of apoptosis in growth factor-deprived sympathetic neurons as well as in fibroblasts and leukaemia cells[20,21]. This is in contrast to lymphocytes, in which activation of JNK/SAPK through TRAF-2 seems to mediate anti-apoptotic mechanism[22]. Therefore the ultimate role of JNK/SAPK activation is not defined; cell-type-specific mechanisms could account for the differences which were found in different cells.

DEATH DOMAIN PROTEINS

The death domain is a conserved protein interaction motif of about 80 amino acids, first identified in the intracellular C-terminal regions of TNFR-1 and the

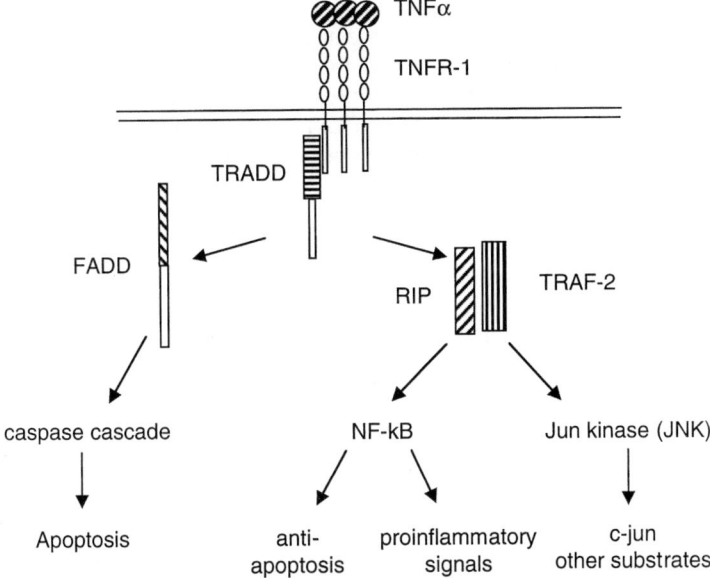

Figure 1 Intracellular pathways activated by TNF receptor 1. The intracellular molecules which bind to the intracellular domain of TNF-R1 are depicted. TRADD (TNF-R1-associated death domain protein) plays a central role, because most of the TNF-R1-dependent pathways diverge at this molecule

FAS receptor[23]. After ligand binding the death domain of the FAS receptor directly interacts with the death domain of FADD (FAS-associated death domain protein)[24,25].

In contrast to the FAS receptor the situation at the intracellular domain of TNF-R1 is more complex. FADD interacts with TNF-R1 via the intermediate protein called TRADD (TNFR-1-associated death domain protein) (Fig. 1). The association between the two molecules is mediated via the death domains of FADD and TRADD. The death domain of TRADD is located in the C-terminal part of the protein[26]. Additionally the N-terminal region of TRADD binds TRAF-2[14]. Therefore after binding of TNF-α to TNF-R1 the pathways which are activated by FADD or TRAF-2 diverge at a single molecule – TRADD – which binds at the intracellular domain of TNF-R1 (Fig. 1).

DOWNSTREAM TARGETS OF TNF-DEPENDENT SIGNALLING

In recent years the molecules which are involved in activating NF-κB or leading to apoptosis have been defined. The protein which directly interacts with FADD has been cloned and named FLICE/MACH/caspase 8. This interaction is mediated by the death effector domain in both proteins. The C-terminal part of caspase 8 contains a domain characteristic for the family of ICE proteases. Caspases are constitutively present in most cells and are located in the cytosol as a single-chain proenzyme. These are activated to fully functional proteases by a first proteolytic cleavage to divide the chain into large and small caspase subunits and a second cleavage to remove the N-terminal domain (prodomain). Two large and two small caspase subunits assemble into a tetramer with two catalytic sites. Cleavage of caspase-8 triggers apoptosis via a caspase cascade (Fig. 2). A dominant-negative form of FADD blocks TNF and FAS-induced apoptosis, indicating the functional role of this cascade for both receptor molecules[27,28].

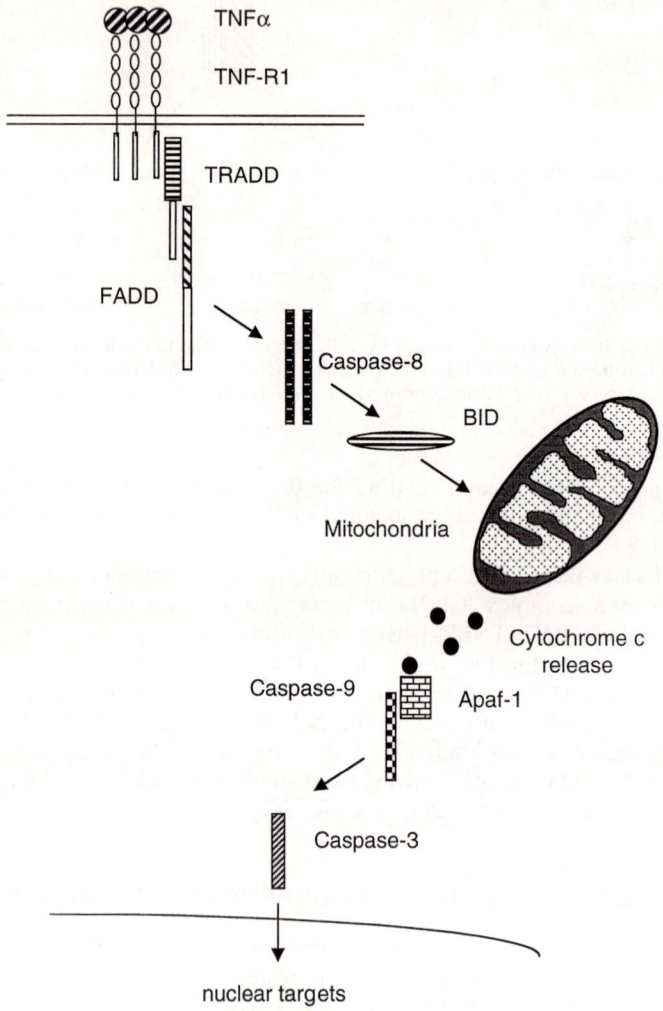

Figure 2 TNF receptor 1 mediates death via the FADD-dependent caspase cascade. After binding of TNF-α to TNF-R1 and FADD-dependent cascade is activated which induces apoptosis. In hepatocytes this pathway results in the activation of the mitochondrial permeability transfer. At the end of this process caspase-3 is activated, which cleaves several substrates involved in mediating mechanisms of apoptosis in the nucleus and the cytoplasm

The molecules and compartments of the cell which are located downstream of caspase-8 have been defined. From caspase-8 through BID is a direct link to mitochondria[29,30]. This interaction induces the mitochondrial permeability transfer which results in the release of cytochrome-c[31]. The association of cytochrome-c, Apaf-1 and procaspase-9 cleaves and thus activates caspase-9, a process which requires ATP[32,33]. Caspase-3, whose activity is induced by direct cleaving of its proenzyme by caspase-9, starts nuclear and cytoplasmic events leading to apoptosis.

The cascade which results in the activation of NF-κB consists of different kinases[34–36]. The serine/threonine kinase NIK directly binds to TRAF-2 and in turn recruits the I-κB kinase α (IKK-α) to this complex[35]. IKK-α phosphorylates I-κBa at serine 32 and 36, which results in its ubiquitination and rapid degrada-

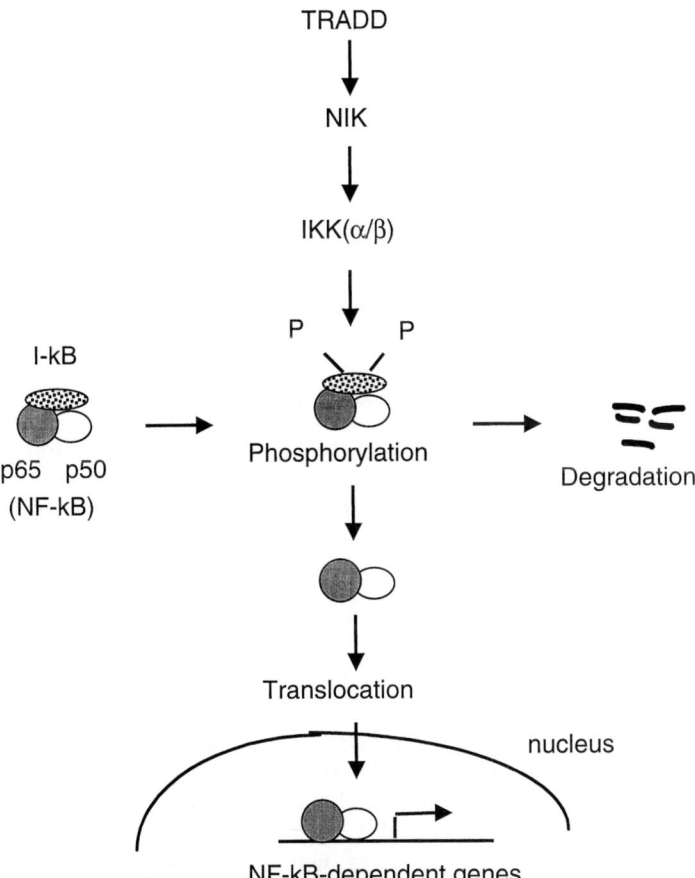

Figure 3 TNF-β-dependent activation of NF-κB via TNF receptor 1. TRADD activates the serine/threonine kinase NIK and as a result the IKKs. IKK phosphorylates I-κB which results in the degradation of I-κB through ubiquitination. NF-κB is released and translocates to the nucleus where it activates genes with NF-κB binding sites in its promoter region

tion by proteosomes[34,36]. In unstimulated cells I-κB complexes with NF-κB in the cytoplasm. After degradation of I-κB, NF-κB translocates to the nucleus and increases transcription of its target genes by binding to its cognitive DNA binding-site[37] (Fig. 3).

Activation of the NF-κB p65 (RelA) subunit increased the cells' ability to survive TNF cytotoxicity. In contrast, blocking NF-κB activation by use of a dominant-negative form of I-κb, or by agents that chemically inhibit NF-κB activation, significantly sensitized cells for TNF-induced apoptosis[38]. Furthermore cell lines derived from p65 knockout mice exhibited dramatically decreased viability after TNF-α treatment[39,40]. Thus TNF-α via NF-κB can induce proteins which render cells protective against TNF-α-induced apoptosis[40,41].

ROLE OF TNF-α IN ANIMAL MODELS OF ACUTE LIVER DAMAGE

The role of TNF-α for liver injury has been studied in several animal models. By using protective anti-TNF antibodies or knockout mice for TNF-α or TNF-R1 and R2, it has become evident that TNF-α triggers apoptosis and/or necrosis of hepatocytes *in vivo*. In this overview models in which TNF-α has a central role for the pathogenesis of acute liver cell damage will be discussed. Examples which will be covered are the endotoxin/galactosamine, the TNF-α/ galactosamine and the concanavalin A model. A striking example in which TNF-α has an important, but probably not a central, role for liver injury is alcohol-mediated liver toxicity. In this model anti-TNF antibodies clearly reduce, but do not prevent, liver cell damage[42,43].

ENDOTOXIN/GALACTOSAMINE MODEL

In the endotoxin/galactosamine model the bacterial cell wall constituent lipopolysaccharide (LPS) is used to initiate an inflammatory response. As rodents are less sensitive for LPS exposure than, for example, humans, LPS treatment is combined with the amino sugar D-galactosamine (GalN) to sensitize the animals[44]. GalN metabolism in the liver results in the selective depletion of uridine nucleotides which specifically inhibit transcription in hepatocytes[45]. The essential role of TNF in the LPS/GalN model can be shown by using C3H mice in comparison to the endotoxin-resistant strain C3H/FeJ. Wt C3H mice show a rise in TNF-α levels preceding liver failure, an event which is abolished in the C3H/FeJ mouse strain[46]. Additionally it has been demonstrated that TNF-R1 is essential to trigger the mechanism which results in liver damage[47].

During LPS/GalN-mediated liver injury TNF-α induces the transcription of several pro-inflammatory genes, e.g. chemokines, nitric oxide and adhesion molecules such as ICAM-1, VCAM-1 and P-selectin[4,48,49]. These changes are essential to trigger the extravasation of neutrophils into the liver parenchyme which results in cytotoxic liver cell damage. During this scenario a stepwise process has been described which consists of three events: (1) sequestration of neutrophils in the liver vasculature; (2) transendothelial migration, (3) adherence-dependent cytotoxicity against hepatocytes[46]. The initial sequestration step of neutrophils in the liver sinusoids seems to be a passive chemotactic process induced by a variety of pro-inflammatory mediators. The transendothelial migration process is controlled by adhesion molecules which are expressed on hepatocytes and non-parenchymal cells. The initial step in transmigration is mediated by VCAM-1, which is expressed only on sinu-endothelial and Kupffer cells[48]. ICAM-1 seems to be involved later in this process, because it is expressed on hepatocytes[49]. The adhesion molecules, responsible for neutrophil transmigration and interaction with VCAM-1 and ICAM-1, are β-integrins, e.g. VLA-4[48,49].

Two different periods can be differentiated during the step of hepatocyte cytotoxicity. The first period is characterized by apoptosis of hepatocytes, and in the later period liver cells become necrotic. Interestingly, apoptosis of hepatocytes is required for transmigration of neutrophils and consecutive necrosis[50]. Thus the induction of apoptosis in hepatocytes is an early and essential event in the LPS/GalN model of liver cell injury.

GALACTOSAMINE/TNF-α MODEL

The administration of galactosamine and TNF-α triggers apoptosis of hepatocytes *in vivo* and *in vitro*. The essential role of TNF-R1 in this model has been demonstrated by TNF-R1 knockout mice, which are resistant to TNF-α/GalN treatment[51]. As TNF-R1 is essential in this model, the transcriptional block induced by galactosamine directly inhibits synthesis of anti-apoptotic signals triggered by the TRAF-2 pathway.

Pretreatment of mice with either interleukin-1 or nitric oxide protects against GalN/TNF-α-mediated apoptosis[52]. These anti-apoptotic mechanisms are also dependent on gene transcription, which might indicate that, for example, IL-1 may activate similar anti-apoptotic genes as does TNF-α[53]. Interestingly, TNF-R2 mice are more susceptible to TNF-α/GalN treatment than wt mice. As transcriptional events are excluded to explain this phenomenon, other mechanisms must be responsible (Tiegs *et al.*, unpublished results). One mechanism could be the availability of TNF-α for activating TNF-R1. As TNF-R2 is deleted TNF might more readily bind to TNF-R1 and thus induce apoptosis. An alternative explanation could be the activation of additional protective pathways which are not related to gene transcription.

Our recent results indicate that the FADD pathway is essential to trigger apoptosis in this model, as adenoviruses expressing a dominant-negative form of FADD block liver cell damage after TNF-α/GalN treatment. These results also demonstrated that *in vivo* TNF-α induces apoptosis in this model by triggering mitochondrial permeability transfer and thus cytochrome-c release (Streetz *et al.*, unpublished results). Therefore these experiments offer an attractive new therapeutic approach.

CONCANAVALIN A MODEL

Concanavalin A (Con-A) is a leptin with high affinity towards the hepatic sinus[54]. Accumulation of Con-A in the hepatic sinus results in an increased influx of circulating lymphocytes into the hepatic sinus and their subsequent local proliferation via blastoid formation[55]. CD4-positive and polymorphonuclear cells are especially involved in this process[54,56]. The assembly of immune activated cells in the liver results in an increase of several cytokines which are essential to influence the degree of liver damage[54,56,57]. The important role of T-cell activation in this model can be deduced as selective immunosuppression by cyclosporin A or FK506 completely prevents liver injury after Con-A injection[56].

Interestingly the activated lymphocytes start to infiltrate into the liver tissue 8 h after Con-A injection at a time when liver damage has already started[58]. In contrast, the maximal serum level of most cytokines was found before infiltration of lymphocytes, showing that the early increase in cytokine levels is pivotal to trigger liver cell damage[56,59,60]. The role of some of these cytokines for Con-A-induced liver cell damage has been defined in more detail. Two cytokines – TNF-α and IFN-γ – directly contribute to liver cell damage, as anti-TNF and anti-IFN-γ antibodies protect from liver cell damage in this model[57,61]. Additionally it has been demonstrated that IFN and TNF-α –/– mice are protected from Con-A-induced liver cell damage, further supporting the role of these two cytokines for pathogenesis in this model[62,63]. Other cytokines have been defined to act in a protective way in the Con-A model. IL-6 and IL-10 directly inhibit liver cell damage by reducing the serum levels of IFN-γ and TNF-α[56,59].

Until now a stepwise process of liver damage, as shown for the endotoxin/LPS model, could not be defined for the Con-A model. Adhesion molecules such as ICAM-1 or VCAM-1 seem to play a minor role. Mice pretreated with antibodies against both adhesion molecules or ICAM-1 knockout mice are still undergoing liver cell injury[64,65]. However, ICAM-1 expression is clearly upregulated on hepatocytes, which correlates with the strong and immediate activation of NF-κB after Con-A injection[66] (Plümpe, Fregien and Trautwein, unpublished results). It seems possible that other NF-κB-dependent target genes might trigger mechanisms which are involved in contributing to liver injury.

The balance between the different cytokines seems to be essential in determining the extent of liver cell damage and recovery after Con-A injection. Recent studies have demonstrated that, following the initial period of liver cell damage, the liver starts to restore its original liver cell mass by hepatocyte proliferation[65]. During this process intracellular pathways activated by TNF-α and IL-6 seem necessary to control cell cycle progression of hepatocytes, as described in the classical partial hepatectomy model[60]. Additionally, our recent results indicate that IL6 –/– mice are hypersensitive against Con-A.

THERAPEUTIC IMPLICATIONS

TNF-α functions as a 'two-edged sword' in the liver. TNF-α is required for normal hepatocyte proliferation during liver regeneration; it functions both as a co-mitogen and as an inducer of NF-κB, which mediates anti-apoptotic effects. On the other hand, TNF-α is the mediator of hepatotoxicity in many animal models, including Con-A and LPS. TNF-α has also been proposed as an important mediator in patients with alcoholic liver disease and viral hepatitis. Blocking TNF-α, such as with neutralizing monoclonal antibodies, might have beneficial effects during hepatic inflammation, but might interfere with normal repair mechanisms. Therefore in the future it seems more promising to specifically inhibit intracellular TNF-α-dependent signalling pathways as a therapeutic approach.

SUMMARY

In recent years the intracellular pathways activated by TNF have been characterized in great detail. Adaptor molecules which bind to the intracellular domain of the TNF receptor 1 are able either to induce apoptosis or to activate signals which trigger cell proliferation, anti-apoptotic mechanisms or the inflammatory response. Recent results show that these pathways are relevant for hepatocytes *in vitro* and *in vivo*; for example during liver regeneration after partial hepatectomy or in models of acute liver failure. Knowledge of these mechanisms may have direct therapeutic implications.

Acknowledgement

This work was supported by DFG-grant Tr 285 4-3.

References

1. Aggarwal BB, Moffat B, Harkins RN. Human lymphotoxin: production by a lymphoblastoid cell line: purification, and initial characterisation. J Biol Chem. 1984;259:686–91.
2. Pennica D, Nedwin GE, Hayflick JS. Human tumor necrosis factor: precursor structure, expression and homology to lymphotoxin. Nature. 1984;312:724–9.
3. Dayer JM, Beutler B, Cerami A. Cachectin/tumor necrosis factor stimulates collagenase and prostaglandin E_2 production by human synovial cells and dermal fibroblasts. J Exp Med. 1985;162:2163–8.
4. Gamble JR, Harlan JM, Klebanoff SJ, Vadas MA. Stimulation of the adherence of neutrophils to umbilical vein endothelium by the human recombinant tumor necrosis factor. Proc Natl Acad Sci USA. 1985;82:8667–71.
5. Beutler B (editor). Tumor. Necrosis Factor: the molecules and their emerging role in medicine. New York: Raven Press, 1992.
6. Kerr JFR, Wyllie AH, Curie AR. Apoptosis: a basic biological phenomenon with wide-ranging implications in tissue kinetics. Br J Cancer. 1972;26:239–57.
7. Smith CA, Farrah T, Goodwin RG. The TNF receptor superfamily of cellular and viral proteins: activation, costimulation, and death. Cell. 1994;76:959–62.
8. Wong B, Choi Y. Pathways leading to cell death in T cells. Curr Opin Immunol. 1997;9:358–64.
9. Nophar Y, Kemper O, Brakebusch C et al. Soluble forms of tumour necrosis factors (TNF-Rs). The cDNA for the type 1 TNF-R, cloned using amino acid sequence data of its soluble form, encodes both the cell surface and a soluble form of the receptor. EMBO J. 1990;9:3269–74.
10. Aderka D, Engelmann H, Maor Y, Brakebusch C, Wallach D. Stabilization of the bioactivity of tumour necrosis factor by its soluble receptor. J Exp Med. 1992;175:323–9.
11. Van Zee, Kohno T, Fischer E, Rock CS, Moldawer LL, Lowry SF. Tumor necrosis factor soluble receptors circulate during experimental and clinical inflammation and can protect against excessive tumor necrosis factors α *in vitro* and *in vivo*. Proc Natl Acad Sci. 1992;89:4845–9.
12. Rothe M, Wong SC, Henzel WJ, Goedell DV. A novel family of putative signal transducers associated with the cytoplasmic domain of the 75 kDa tumor necrosis factor receptor. Cell. 1994;78:681–92.

13. Freemont PS. The RING finger: a novel protein sequence motif related to the zinc finger. Ann NY Acad Sci. 1993;684:174–92.
14. Hsu H, Shu HB, Pan MG, Goedell DV. TRADD-TRAF2 and TRADD-FADD interactions define two distinct TNF receptor 1 signal transduction pathways. Cell. 1996; 84:299–308.
15. Rothe M, Sarma V, Dixit VM, Goedell DV. TRAF2 mediated activation of NF-κB by TNF receptor 2 and CD40. Science. 1995;269:1424–7.
16. Lee SY, Lee SY, Choi Y. TRAF-interacting protein (TRIP): a novel component of the Tumor necrosis factor receptor (TNFR)-and CD30-TRAF signaling complexes that inhibit TRAF2-mediated NF-κB activation. J Exp Med. 1997;185:1275–85.
17. Natoli G, Costanzo A, Ianni A et al. Activation of SAPK/JNK by a noncytotoxic TRAF2-dependent pathway. Science. 1997;275:200–3.
18. Reinhard C, Shamoon B, Venkatakrishna S, Williams L. Tumor necrosis factor induced activation of c-jun N-terminal kinase is mediated by TRAF2. EMBO J. 1997;16:1080–92.
19. Liu ZG, Hsu H, Goedell DV, Karin M. Dissection of TNF receptor 1 effector functions. JNK activation is not linked to apoptosis while NF-κB activation prevents cell death. Cell. 1996;87:565–76.
20. Verheij M, Bose R, Lin XH et al. Requirement for ceramide initiated SAPK/JNK signalling in stress induced apoptosis. Nature. 1996;380:75–9.
21. Xia Z, Dickens M, Raingeaud J, Davis RJ, Greenberg ME. Opposing effects of ERK and JNK-p38 MAP kinases on apoptosis. Science. 1995;270:1326–31.
22. Yel, W-C, Shahinian A, Speiser D et al. Early lethality, functional NF-κB activation, and increased sensitivity to TNF-induced cell death in TRAF2-deficient mice. Immunity. 1997;7:715–25.
23. Tartaglia LA, Ayres TM, Wong GHW, Goeddel DV. A novel domain within the 55 kDa TNF receptor signals cell death. Cell. 1993;74:845–53.
24. Boldin MP, Varfolomeev EE, Pancer Z, Mett IL, Camonis JH, Wallach D. A novel protein that interacts with the death domain of Fas/APO1 contains a sequence motif related to the death domain. J Biol Chem. 1995;270:7795–8.
25. Chinnaiyan AM, O'Rourke K, Tewari M, Dixit VM. FADD, a novel death domain-containing protein, interacts with the death domain of Fas and initiates apoptosis. Cell. 1995;81:505–12.
26. Hsu H, Xiong J, Goedell DV. The TNF receptor 1-associated protein TRADD signals cell death and NF-κB activation. Cell. 1995;81:495–504.
27. Boldin MP, Goncharov TM, Golstev YV, Wallach D. Involvement of MACH, a novel MORT1/FADD-interacting protease in Fas/APO-1 and TNF receptor induced cell death. Cell. 1996;81:803–15.
28. Muzio M, Chinnaiyan AM, Kischkel FC et al. FLICE, a novel FADD homologous ICE/CED-3-like protease, is recruited to the CD95 (Fas/APO-1) death inducing signalling complex. Cell. 1996;85:817–27.
29. Li H, Zhu H, Xu C, Yuan J. Cleavage of BID by caspase 8 mediates the mitochondrial damage in the Fas pathway of apoptosis. Cell. 1998;94:491–501.
30. Luo X, Budihardjo I, Zhou H, Slaughter C, Wang X. Cleavage of BID by caspase 8 mediates the mitochondrial damage in the Fas pathway of apoptosis. Cell. 1998;94:481–90.
31. Bradham CA, Qian T, Streetz K, Trautwein C, Brenner DA, Lomaster, JL. The mitochondrial permeability transition is required for TNF-mediated apoptosis and cytochrome c release. Mol Cell Biol. 1998;18:819–27.
32. Cecconi F, Alvarez-Bolado G, Meyer B, Roth KA, Gruss P. Apaf1 (CED-4 homolog) regulates programmed cell death in mammalian development. Cell. 1998;94:727–37.
33. Yoshida H, Kong Y-Y, Elia AJ et al. Apaf1 is required for mitochondrial pathways of apoptosis and brain development. Cell. 1998;94:739–50.
34. DiDonato JA, Hayakawa M, Rothwarf DM, Zandi E, Karin M. A cytokine-responsive IκB kinase that activates the transcription factor NF-κB. Nature. 1997;388:548–54.
35. Malinin NL, Boldin MP, Kovalenko AV, Wallach D. MAP3K-related kinase involved in NF-κB induction by TNF, CD95 and IL-1. Nature. 1997;385:540–4.
36. Regnier CH, Yeong Song H, Gao X, Goeddel DV, Cao Z, Rothe M. Identification and characterisation of an IκB kinase. Cell. 1997;90:373–83.
37. Bauerle PA, Baltimore D. NF-κB: ten years after. Cell. 1996;87:13–20.
38. Wu M, Lee H, Bellas RE et al. Inhibition of NF-κB Rel induces apoptosis of murine B cells. EMBO J. 1996;15:4682–90.

39. Beg AA, Sha WC, Bronson RT, Ghosh S, Baltimore D. Embryonic lethality and liver degeneration in mice lacking the RelA component of NF-κB. Nature. 1995;376:167–70.
40. Beg AA, Baltimore D. An essential role for NF-κB in preventing TNF-alpha-induced cell death. Science. 1996;274:782–4.
41. Van Antwerp DJ, Martin SJ, Kafri T, Green DR, Verma IM. Suppression of TNF-α induced apoptosis by NF-κB. Science. 1996;274:787–9.
42. Iimuro Y, Gallucci RM, Luster MI, Kono H, Thurman RG. Antibodies to tumor necrosis factor alfa attenuate hepatic necrosis and inflammation caused by chronic exposure to ethanol in the rat. Hepatology. 1997;26:1530–7.
43. Nanji AA, Zakim D, Rathemulla A et al. Dietary saturated fatty acids down-regulate cyclooxygenase-2 and tumor necrosis factor alfa and reverse fibrosis in alcohol-induced liver disease in the rat. Hepatology. 1998;26:1538–45.
44. Galanos C, Freudenberg MA, Reutter, W. Galactosamine-induced sensitization to the lethal effects of endotoxin. Proc Natl Acad Sci. 1979;76:5939–43.
45. Decker K, Keppler D, Rudigier J, Domschke W. Cell damage by trapping of biosynthetic intermediates. The role of uracil nucleotides in experimental hepatitis. Hoppe-Seyler's Z Physiol Chem. 1971;352:412–18.
46. Jaeschke H, Smith CW, Clemens MG, Ganey PE, Roth RA. Mechanisms of inflammatory liver injury: adhesion molecules and cytotoxicity of neutrophils. Toxicol Appl Pharmacol. 1996;139:213–26.
47. Pfeffer K, Matsuyama T, Kündig TM et al. Mice deficient for the 55kd tumor necrosis factor receptor are resistant to endotoxic shock, yet succumb to L. monocytogenes infection. Cell. 1993;73:457–67.
48. Essani NA, Bajt ML, Farhood A, Vonderfecht SL, Jaeschke H. Transcriptional activation of vascular cell adhesion molecule-1 gene in vivo and its role in the pathophysiology of neutrophil-induced liver injury in murine endotoxin shock. J Immunol. 1997;158:5941–8.
49. Xu H, Gonzalo JA, Pierre YS et al. Leukocytosis and resistance to septic shock in intercellular adhesion molecule 1-deficient mice. J Exp Med. 1994;180:95–109.
50. Jaeschke H, Fisher MA, Lawson JA, Simmons CA, Farhood, A, Jones DA. Activation of caspase 3 (CPP32)-like proteases is essential for TNF-α-induced hepatic parenchymal cell apoptosis and neutrophil-mediated necrosis in a murine shock model. J Immunol. 1998;160:3480–6.
51. Leist M, Gantner F, Jilg S, Wendel A. Activation of the 55 kDa TNF receptor is necessary and sufficient for TNF-induced liver failure, hepatocyte apoptosis, and nitrite release. J Immunol. 1995;154:1307–16.
52. Bohlinger I, Leist M, Barsig J, Uhlig S, Tiegs G, Wendel A. Interleukin 1 and nitric oxide protect against tumor necrosis factor α-induced liver injury through distinct pathways. Hepatology. 1995;22:1829–37.
53. Cao Z, Xiong J, Takeuchi M, Kurama T, Goedell DV. TRAF6 is a signal transducer for interleukin-1. Nature. 1996;383:443–6.
54. Tiegs G, Hentschel J, Wendel A. A T cell-dependent experimental liver injury in mice inducible by concanavalin A. J Clin Invest. 1992;90:196–203.
55. Miyazawa Y, Tsutsui H, Mizuhara H, Fujiwara H, Kaneda K. Involvement of intrasinusoidal hemostasis in the development of concanavalin A-induced hepatic injury in mice. Hepatology. 1997;27:497–506.
56. Mizuhara H, O'Neill E, Seki N et al. T-cell activation-associated hepatic injury: mediation by tumor necrosis factor and protection by interleukin 6. J Exp Med. 1994;179:1529–37.
57. Gantner F, Leist M, Lohse AW, Germann PG, Tiegs A. Concanavalin A-induced T-cell-mediated hepatic injury in mice: the role of tumor necrosis factor. Hepatology. 1995;21:190–8.
58. Fujikura S, Mizuhara H, Miyazawa Y, Fujiwara H, Kaneda K. Kinetics and localisation of lymphoblasts that proliferate in the murine liver after concanavalin A administration. Biomed Res. 1996;17:129–39.
59. Louis H, Le Moine O, Peny M-O et al. Production and role of interleukin-10 in concanavalin A-induced hepatitis in mice. Hepatology. 1997;25:1382–9.
60. Trautwein C, Rakemann T, Malek, Plümpe J, Tiegs G, Manns MP. Concanavalin A-induced liver injury triggers hepatocyte proliferation. J Clin Invest. 1998;101:1960–9.
61. Küsters S, Gantner F, Künstle G, Tiegs G. Interferon gamma plays a critical role in T cell-dependent liver injury in mice initiated by concanavalin A. Gastroenterology. 1996;111:462–71.

62. Küsters S, Tiegs G, Alexopoulou L *et al. In vivo* evidence for a functional role of both tumor necrosis (TNF) receptors and transmembrane TNF in experimental hepatitis. Eur J Immunol. 1997;27:2870–5.
63. Tagawa Y-I, Sekikawa K, Iwakura Y. Suppression of concanavalin A-induced hepatitis in IFN-γ–/– mice, but not in TNF-α–/– mice. J Immunol. 1997;159:1418–28.
64. Watanabe Y, Morita M, Akaike T. Concanavalin A induces perforin-mediated but not Fas-mediated hepatic injury. Hepatology. 1996;24:702–10.
65. Wolf D, Hallmann R, Sass G *et al.* TNF α-induced expression of adhesion molecules in the liver is under the control of tumor necrosis factor receptor 1 – relevance for murine hepatitis. J Immunol. (in revision).
66. Trautwein C, Rakemann T, Brenner DA *et al.* Concanavalin A-induced liver cell damage: activation of intracellular pathways triggered by tumor necrosis factor. Gastroenterology. 1998;114:1035–45.

18
Role of cytokines in liver fibrosis

A. M. GRESSNER and S. SKRTIC

INTRODUCTION

Fibrotic tissue reactions accompany chronic inflammatory liver diseases and are a morphologically and clinically important life-threatening criterion of liver cirrhosis[1,2]. The evaluation of the pathomechanism of fibrosis is of great significance for a rational approach to the development of antifibrotic therapeutic trials and to the improvement of non-invasive devices for diagnostic monitoring of the dynamic process of fibrotic organ transition[3,4].

Fibrosis comprises not only (a) a 3–6-fold overall increase in extracellular matrix (ECM) (normally less than 0.6% of liver wet weight), but also (b) a disproportionate elevation of the five types of collagens, of various proteoglycans (preferentially increase in dermatan/chondroitin sulphate-bearing proteoglycans) and structural glycoproteins (tenascin, fibronectin, laminin, undulin, nidogen), (c) subtle changes in the microstructure of certain matrix molecules (modulation of hydroxylation of collagen α-chains and sulphation of glycosaminoglycans) and, clinically most important, (d) topographic redistribution of ECM with a preferential deposition in the perivenular and perisinusoidal space, where an incomplete basement membrane ('capillarization of sinusoids', according to Schaffner and Popper[5]) is developed. The latter is a diffusion barrier, which hinders the exchange processes between parenchymal cells and sinusoidal blood stream, and thus the systemic function of the liver, and interferes with hepatic microcirculation due to sinusoidal stenosis.

Fibrotic matrix changes in chronically injured liver are a consequence of a loss of homeostatic mechanisms controlling matrix formation (fibrogenesis) and matrix degradation (fibrolysis). Cell biological analyses of the past decade point clearly to a complex, direct or indirect interaction of parenchymal and non-parenchymal cell types in the process of fibrogenesis and fibrolysis[6,7].

All available data emphasize an outstanding role of hepatic stellate cells (HSC, formerly called fat-storing cells, vitamin A-storing cells, perisinusoidal lipocytes, Ito cells) as the main (precursor) cell type responsible for fibrogenesis and partially also for fibrolysis[8–11]. This cell type is localized in the space of Disse (perisinusoidal space) and has the perikaryon embedded in recesses between adjacent hepatocytes with cellular extensions embracing the endothelial cell layer (Fig. 1). Normally these cells have a low mitotic activity and are responsible for the storage of retinoids. They are present in a ratio of 3.6–6 cells per 100 hepatocytes (Ito cell index) and represent liver-specific pericytes, comparable with mesangial cells in the kidney. The pathogenetic significance of this cell type is based on its ability to be activated in an inflammatory tissue environment and spontaneously during culture on plain plastic surfaces to a morphologically and functionally different cell type. Full competency for fibrogenesis is reached by activation of HSC, which includes (a) stimulation of proliferation, (b) phenotypic transition (transformation, transdifferentiation) from the retinoid-storing to the ECM-secreting cell type (termed myofibroblast), (c) enhanced expression of almost all matrix protein genes and of hyaluronan, and (d) the acquisition of contractility[12]. The fully transformed counterpart of HSC, that is the myofibroblast (MFB), expresses characteristically smooth muscle α-actin filaments and a quite broad spectrum of growth factors and (pro-inflammatory) cytokines and chemokines (Fig. 2). In addition, these cells also express certain matrix metalloproteinases and their specific inhibitors (TIMP-1, -2) involved in fibrolysis. Although the pathogenetic key process of fibrogenesis, i.e. activation of HSC to MFB, is stimulated not only by peptide mediators, but also by re-

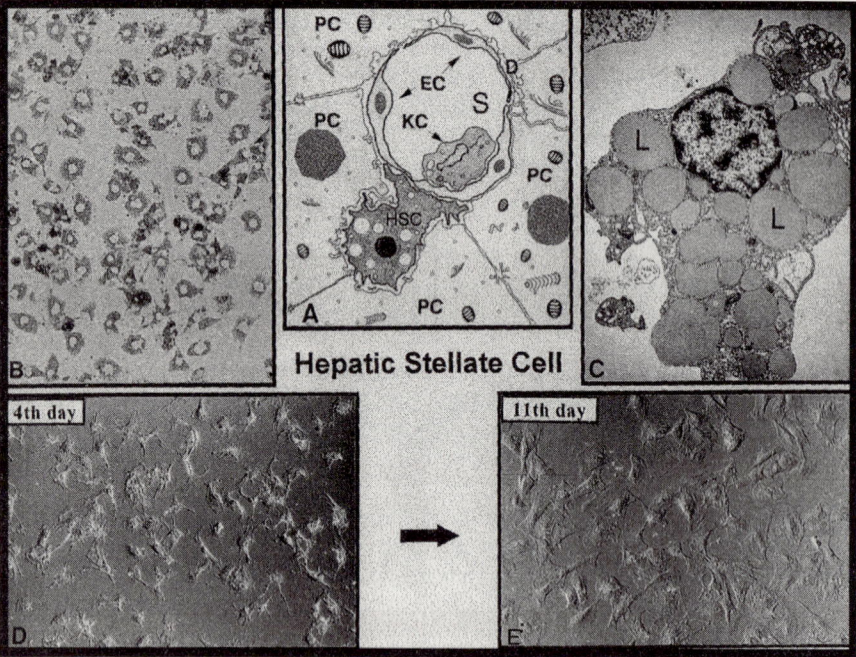

Figure 1 **A**: Schematic presentation of the topographical situation of hepatic stellate cells (HSC) in relation to parenchymal (PC), endothelial (EC) and Kupffer cells (KC) in liver; S = sinusoid. **B**: Light microscopic appearance of lipid-filled hepatic stellate cells in early culture. **C**: Electron micrograph of HSC having numerous lipid droplets (L) indenting the nucleus. Normarski micrographs of 4-day (**D**) and 11-day (**E**) old primary cultures of HSC in 10% fetal calf serum-supplemented medium

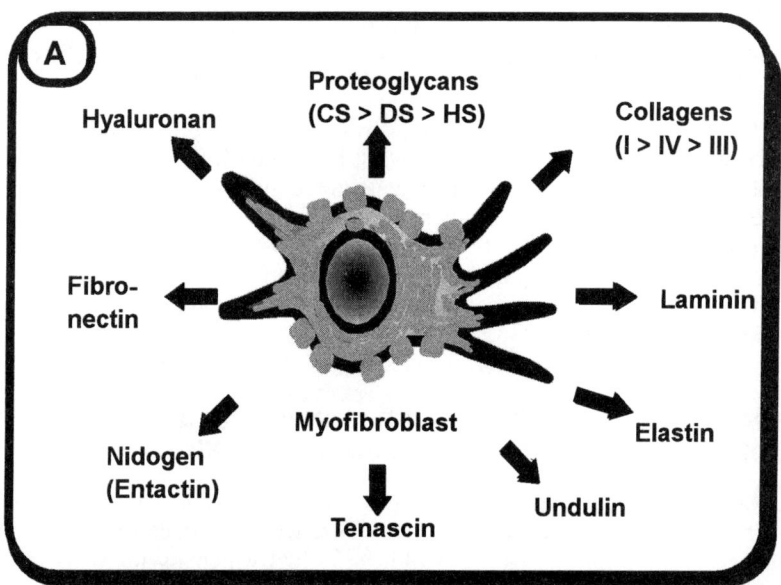

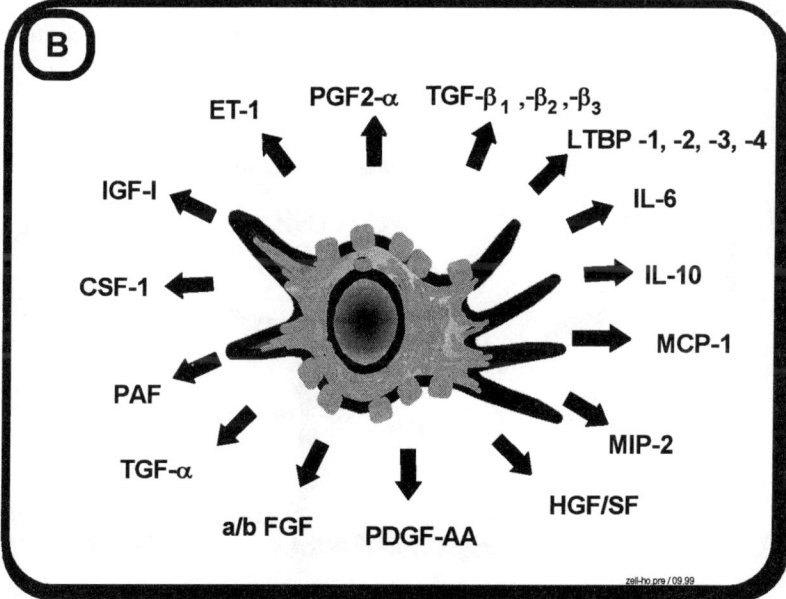

Figure 2 Synopsis of ECM components (**A**) and profibrogenic cytokines and chemokines (**B**) expressed and secreted by myofibroblasts (transformed HSC) in culture. The data are compiled from literature and are based on mRNA expression, immunological quantitation of matrix components and cytokines, and partially on the bioactivity of cytokines in the medium. For abbreviations see text

active oxygen species[13,14] and ethanol metabolites (acetaldehyde)[15-17] cytokines originating from resident liver cells and inflammatory immigrating cells are of significant relevance for:

1. The determination of the pool size of myofibroblasts regulated by the influx (mitogenesis) and efflux (apoptosis) of HSC and MFB[10].
2. The recruitment of inflammatory cells in the diseased liver tissue due to the expression and secretion of chemokines[18-21].
3. The transcriptional activation, secretion, deposition and remodelling of the individual components of the extracellular matrix[22,23].
4. The regulation of sinusoidal blood flow by modulation of the contractility of MFB[24-26].

HEPATIC STELLATE CELLS/LIVER MYOFIBROBLASTS SERVE AS SOURCE AND TARGET OF FIBROGENIC CYTOKINES

Activation of HSC is initiated by paracrine loops arising both from parenchymal, resident non-parenchymal and invaded cells, which synthesize and secrete a broad spectrum of profibrogenic cytokines[6,11,27], of which a synopsis is given in Fig. 2. Damaged hepatocytes in co-culture with HSC, or exposure of these cells to hepatocyte-conditioned medium, stimulates the proliferation of HSC without significantly affecting expression and secretion of extracellular matrix components and the transformation of HSC to MFB[28]. The mitogenic effect of hepato-

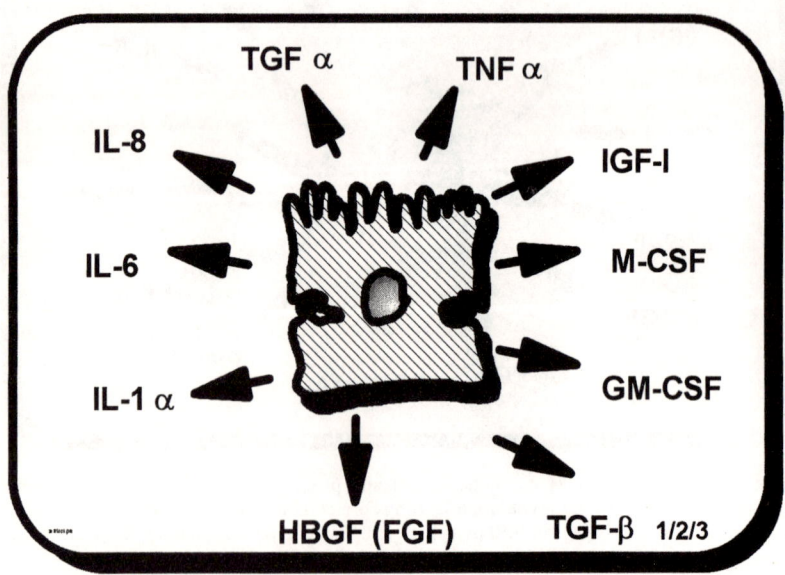

Figure 3 Compilation of cytokines/growth factors reported in the literature to be expressed by cultured hepatocytes. For abbreviations see text

cytes decreased with advanced transformation of HSC to MFB. The mitogen(s) of hepatocytes is (are) not yet identified, but preliminary data suggest a complex mixture of various mediators including insulin-like growth factor I (IGF-I) and IGF-binding proteins for which HSC express receptors[29]. Numerous mediators are identified in hepatocyte cultures (Fig. 3) but the possibility of contaminating HSC as a source of cytokines has to be considered[30]. The proliferative effect of these hepatocyte-derived mediators, which might be released by membrane damage of hepatocytes, is counteracted by the anti-mitogenic effect of trans-forming growth factor beta (TGF-β), which was recently discovered as a prominent cytokine within hepatocytes (see below)[31–33]. Thus, according to current knowledge, damaged hepatocytes might be able to modulate bidirectionally the proliferation of HSC, depending on the ratio of pro-mitogenic factors and anti-mitogenic TGF-β. From these findings we conclude that injury of hepatocytes initiates HSC proliferation and, via TGF-β, their transformation to MFB. This suggestion is compatible with the observations that parenchymal cell damage precedes fibrogenesis, that fibrosis and HSC activation are initiated where hepatocyte injury is prominent and that fibrogenesis can precede also without conspicuous inflammation, e.g. in haemochromatosis. The hepatocyte-directed activation of HSC forms the *pre-inflammatory* step of the previously proposed cascade model of HSC activation[11]. Activated Kupffer cells and invaded mono-cytes are well-known sources of cytokines/growth factors affecting activation of HSC and extracellular matrix synthesis[34–38]. Among them TGF-β_1, TGF-α, platelet-derived growth factor (PDGF), tumour necrosis factor alpha (TNF-α), interleukins IL-1 and IL-6 are mediators, which all affect proliferation, transfor-mation and matrix gene expression. Similarly, TGF-β, epidermal growth factor (EGF), PDGF, IGF-I released from the α-granules of disaggregating platelets can promote the activation of HSC[39]. These cells and their cytokines form the basis of the *inflammatory step* of HSC activation.

During phenotypic transformation of HSC to MFB these cells express and secrete among other cytokines TGF-α, TGF-β[40,41] and fibroblast growth factor (FGF)[42], which stimulate both proteoglycan and collagen synthesis and in a negative (TGF-β) and positive (TGF-α) manner the proliferation of HSC[43]. Consequently, neutralization of TGF-β has a stimulatory effect on HSC prolifer-ation, which indicates that these cells are able to activate in a paracrine way quiescent HSC. Furthermore, autocrine stimulatory mechanisms in MFB are suggested involving FGF, endothelium 1 (ET-1) and TGF-β, respectively[40,42,44]. This mechanism forms the *postinflammatory step* of HSC activation. However, the susceptibility of HSC to the cytokines is changed during transformation, depending on the expression status of the respective receptors[45]. This was shown for PDGF receptors[36], TGF-β receptors[46] and endothelin receptors[47].

Recently, MFB were also identified as an important signalling cell type for chemokines (macrophage inflammatory proteins MIP-1α, MIP-1β, MIP-2; monocyte chemotactic peptides MCP-1; MCP-2; and GRO-α) attracting neutro-philes and monocytes[18–21]. As a function of HSC transformation to MFB, TNF-α and lipolysaccharide (LPS) strongly increased expression and secretion of these chemoattractants, which greatly facilitates the influx of inflammatory cells forming the basis of a pathogenetic vicious circle. It is conceivable that LPS, of which the concentration in the portal vein is quite high and even increased in chronic alcoholics, is sufficient to stimulate MFB for the production of MIP-2 and MCP-1.

THE ROLE OF TGF-β AS FIBROGENIC MASTER CYTOKINE

TGF-β is a multifunctional protein that regulates cell proliferation, differentiation, migration, ECM formation and degradation and immunosuppression[48,49]. By binding to the high-affinity-receptor TβR2 (75 kDa) this receptor and TβR1 (53 kDa) form heterodimeric complexes leading to the activation of the intrinsic Ser/Thr-kinase of TβR1, which binds and phosphorylates certain pathway-restricted Smad proteins (Smad 2 and 3), which associate with common pathway SMAD 4 protein before translocation into the nucleus where, directly or indirectly, TGF-β-sensitive promoters are affected[50,51]. Antagonistic Smads 6 and 7 inhibit this signal transduction pathway by preventing the receptor interaction and phosphorylation of Smads 2 and 3. Interestingly, there are strong connections between TGF-β and the production of reactive oxygen intermediates (ROIs) in fibrotic livers and hepatic stellate cells[52]. Increased production of ROIs is associated with an up-regulation of TGF-β, and TGF-β induces the accumulation of H_2O_2. This oxidant is, in turn, directly involved in up-regulating the

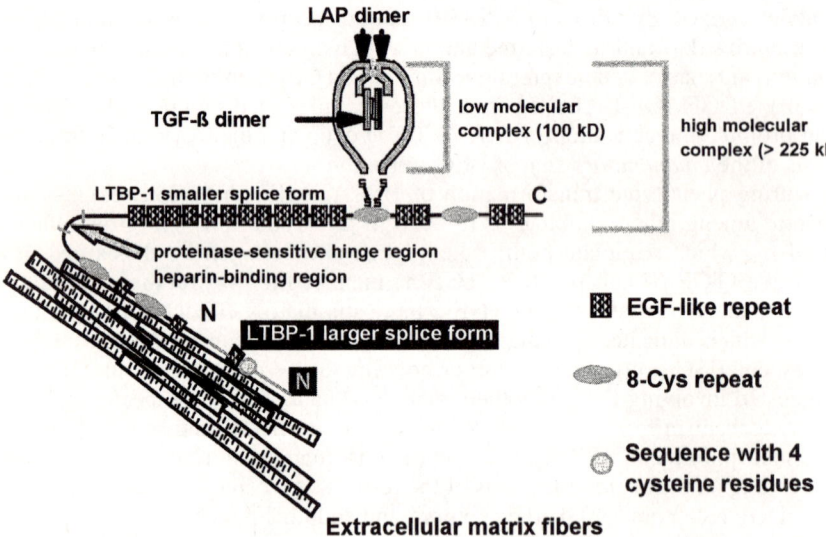

Figure 4 Schematic presentation of the structure of the large latent TGF-β complex bound to extracellular matrix components. The large complex consists of latent TGF-β-binding protein (LTBP), which has a domain structure with EGF-like repeats and three or four copies of repeats with eight cysteine residues, which enable the molecule for protein–protein interactions. Preferentially the N-terminal region is bound by transglutamination to matrix fibres. LTBP has sequence homologies to fibrillin-1 and fibrillin-2. The latency-associated peptide (LAP) is bound with two disulphide bridges to the second cysteine repeat of the molecule. The TGF-β homodimer is attached non-covalently to the LAP dimer. The latter two components form the low molecular latent TGF-β complex. For further details see ref. 120

expression of the collagen type I gene. Furthermore, this oxidant is also involved in TGF-β-mediated inhibition of cell proliferation. Catalase, an H_2O_2 enzyme scavenger, abrogates TGF-β-mediated gene expression. Presently, the connection of ROI metabolism with the activation of Smad proteins is not known.

MFB are an important source of all three isoforms of TGF-β, which are expressed increasingly during transformation of HSC to MFB. About 98% of secreted TGF-β (25 kDa) is biologically inactive, because it is integrated into a large latent complex (> 225 kDa) consisting of TGF-β, non-covalently associated latency-associated peptide (LAP) (75 kDa) and a covalently coupled latent TGF-β-binding protein (LTBP) (125–205 kDa)[53,54] (Fig. 4).

Four isoforms of LTBP [–1 bis –4] and several splice variants have been identified[53–55]. All these components can be visualized within HSC and MFB using confocal laser scanning microscopy (Fig. 5). The main function of LTBP is suggested to be covalent binding (via transglutamination) of its N-terminal region to the extracellular matrix from which the complex can be released by proteinases (e.g. elastase, plasmin, chymase), which cleave the molecule at its proteinase-sensitive hinge region[56]. The soluble complex is transferred to the cell surface, where it is bound to the mannose-6-phosphate/IGF-II-receptor via the mannose-6-phosphate residues of the LAP molecule[57]. Activated HSC increasingly express the receptor[58]. Cell surface-associated plasmin releases the active TGF-β homodimer for binding to the signalling receptors. Although all components of the TGF-β complex are now identified in rat and human liver, and their respective myofibro-

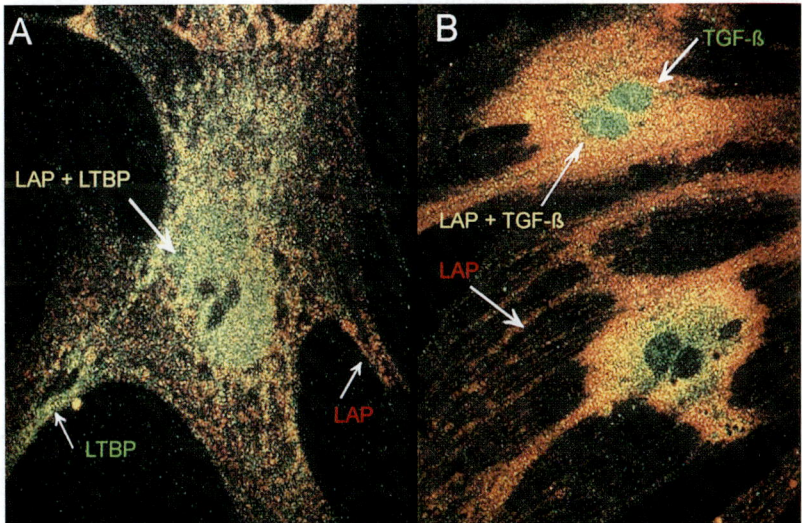

Figure 5 Confocal laser scanning micrographs of double-immunofluorescent stainings of TGF-β, LAP, and LTBP-1 in cultured rat HSC (**A**) and MFB (**B**). HSC were kept for 3 days in primary culture in medium with low fetal calf serum supplementation. MFB were cultured for 3 days in secondary culture. For immunostaining a mixture of polyclonal anti-LTBP-1 antiserum (Ab39) and monoclonal anti-LAP antibody or polyclonal anti-pan TGF-β antibody were used. Red fluorescence indicates LAP, green fluorescence indicates LTBP-1 and TGF-β, respectively. The overlay of green and red fluorescences leads to a yellow staining of respective structures. For details see ref. 121

blasts, the detailed physiological mechanism of TGF-β activation is still unknown. Available data from non-hepatic tissue, however, suggest an important role of LTBP in the process, because extracellular fixation of the complex is an important prerequisite of its activation[59]. Available data indicate that several mechanisms of latent TGF-β activation seem to exist which may partially substitute each other. Interaction of specific amino acid sequences of LAP with a defined region of the multifunctional platelet and matrix protein thrombospondin-1 results in partial activation of TGF-β and blocks re-inactivation by induction of conformational changes[60]. Alternatively, RGD sequences of LAP mediate the binding to integrin $\alpha v \beta 6$ followed by activation of latent TGF-β[61]. Reactive oxygen species can activate TGF-β *in vitro*[62]. It is likely that these and other mechanisms are relevant for the regulation of TGF-β bioavailability because mice deficient for one of these pathways do not show the phenotype of TGF-β knockouts.

TGF-β is a potent antiproliferative cytokine for HSC[63], which lose their susceptibility during transformation to MFB (Fig. 6). Thus, in contrast to HSC, the proliferation of MFB is not suppressed by TGF-β and the extracellular matrix synthesis is stimulated only weakly by this cytokine (Table 1). This is exemplified by the expression of decorin and biglycan, which are stimulated in HSC but not in MFB by TGF-β and activated Kupffer cell (KCcM) and myofibroblast (MFBcM) conditioned media (Fig. 7). TGF-α showed the reverse effect. Cell surface expression of the signalling receptors is down-modulated in MFB, in comparison to HSC, but the mechanism is not yet understood. The previously proposed autocrine stimulatory mechanism of MFB via TGF-β (see above) has to be questioned and must be re-evaluated.

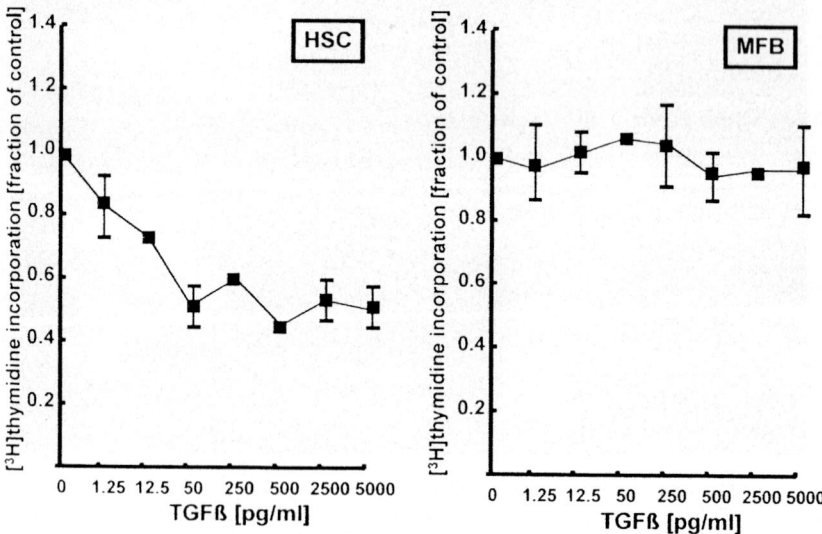

Figure 6 Dose–response of the TGF-β effect on the proliferation of untransformed hepatic stellate cells (HSC) on the 4th day of primary culture and transformed myofibroblasts (MFB) on the 3rd day of secondary culture. The results are expressed relative to the proliferation of the control not receiving TGF-β

Table 1 Effects of various agonists on proliferation, transformation, and proteoglycan synthesis of cultures of hepatic stellate cells and myofibroblasts

	Hepatic stellate cells			Myofibroblasts	
	Proliferation	Transformation	Matrix synthesis	Proliferation	Matrix synthesis
EGF/TGF-α	+	Φ	(+)	Φ	+
TGF-β_1	–	++	++	Φ	+
TNF-α	(+)	+	(+)	+	+
PDGF	(+)	Φ	Φ	++	Φ
FGF	(+)	Φ	Φ	(+)	Φ
IGF-I	+	Φ	(+)	+	Φ
IGF-II	+	Φ	Φ	+	Φ

+, Stimulation; Φ, no effect; –, inhibition.

Interestingly, TGF-β and the components of the small and latent TGF-β complex are also found in hepatocytes[31]. Under conditions of necrotic damage (latent) TGF-β is released from parenchymal cells, which can activate HSC in the immediate vicinity[32]. Under normal conditions TGF-β is masked within hepatocytes, and thus not available for immunological detection. Under injurious conditions (e.g. cell culture) it is activated by a calpain-dependent process[64,65]. If latent TGF-β secreted by myofibroblasts is activated, e.g. by transient acidification, it is very injurious to hepatocytes by induction of apoptosis[66]. Thus, in the microenvironment of liver tissue, TGF-β released by MFB, Kupffer cells, platelets and hepatocytes must be kept in a latent stage to avoid HSC activation, parenchymal cell apoptosis and suppression of PIT cells (Fig. 8).

TGF-β gene expression does not necessarily correlate with the amount of active TGF-β, because this cytokine undergoes extensive post-translational modification (activation, see above) and the half-life time of active TGF-β might be very short, since it binds avidly to scavengers, that is α_2-macroglobulin[67–69] and the extracellular matrix components fibronectin, betaglycan (identical with type III TGF-β receptor) and decorin[70] (Table 2). Because α_2-macroglobulin is secreted by stellate cells in increasing amounts during culture, a potential role of α_2-macroglobulin as a scavenger of active TGF-β at sites of liver injury is suggested. During HSC activation the α_2-macroglobulin receptor, which is identical with the low density lipoprotein (LDL) receptor-related protein is expressed and myofibroblasts internalize and degrade activated α_2-macroglobulin. Thus, these cells might also be involved in the clearance of TGF-β. In addition to the matrix binding property of TGF-β, TNF-α and PDGF isoforms and many other cytokines bind specifically to various types of collagens of liver, obviously using a consensus sequence[71]. Collagen-bound TNF-α and PDGF are biologically active, and thus can provide fixed signals for surrounding matrix-anchored cells[72]. Similarly, heparin/heparan sulphate is known to bind many growth factors and cytokines (Table 2). Potentially decorin or synthetic binding motifs of matrix molecules for TGF-β and other cytokines can be used for antifibrotic therapeutic trials. In experimental glomerulosclerosis fibrosis can be inhibited by the TGF-β binding proteoglycan decorin[73,74].

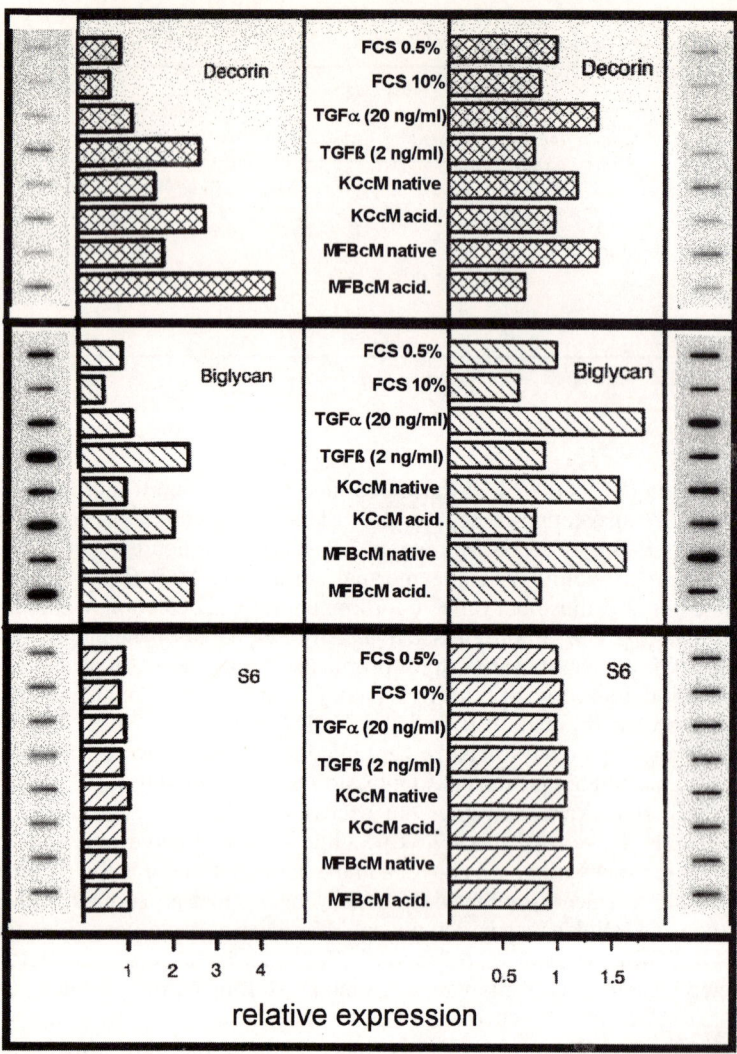

Figure 7 Steady-state levels of the proteoglycan core protein mRNAs of decorin and biglycan and of ribosomal protein S6 mRNA in HSC on the 4th day in primary culture (left side) and MFB on the 8th day of tertiary culture (right side) under various stimuli. TGF-α, TGF-β, 10% fetal calf serum (FCS), native and transiently acidified conditioned media of Kupffer cells (KCcM) and myofibroblasts (MFBcM) were added. The cells were grown for another 24 h before total RNA was extracted. Hybridization signals (bars) are expressed in relation to the signal intensity of HSC and MFB grown in 0.5% FCS after normalization to S6 expression

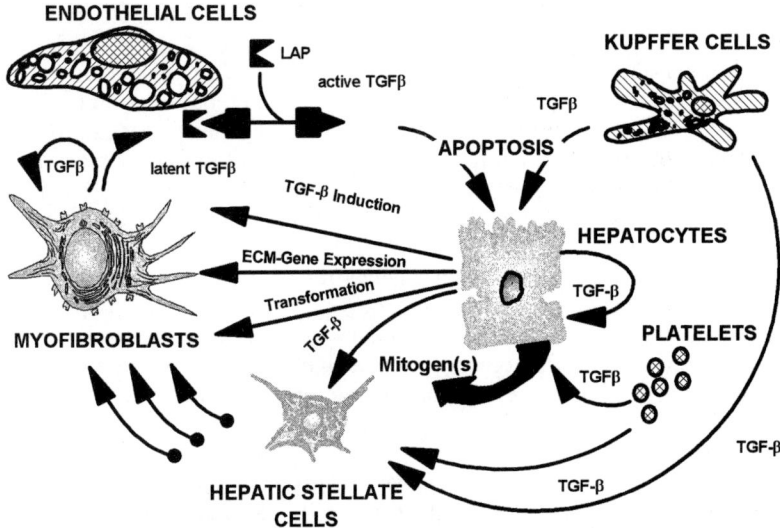

Figure 8 Schematic presentation of major pathobiochemical effects of active TGF-β on hepatic stellate cell transformation to myofibroblasts, parenchymal cell apoptosis and matrix gene expression. Latent TGF-β released by Kupffer cells, platelets, hepatocytes, and myofibroblasts is activated by sinusoidal endothelial cells and potentially inactivated by α_2-macroglobulin and extracellular matrix proteins. This must be kept in an inactive status to avoid detrimental effects

Table 2   Binding of growth factors to extracellular matrix components

---

Binding to heparin/heparan sulphate chains
FGFs (aFGF, bFGF and keratinocyte growth factor, KGF)
IL-1, -2, -3 and -6
HGF
Granulocyte/macrophage colony-stimulation factor (GM-CSF)
Schwann cell growth factor
Platelet factor 4
PDGF-A and -B
Heparin-binding epidermal growth factor (HBGF)

Binding to chondroitin sulphate chains
Platelet factor 4

Binding to proteoglycan core proteins
TGF-β ($\rightarrow$ betaglycan and decorin)

Binding to matrix glycoproteins
TGF-β ($\rightarrow$ fibronectin, $\rightarrow$ thrombospondin)
PDGF-A and -B ($\rightarrow$ SPARC)

Binding to collagens
HGF ($\rightarrow$ collagens I, III and IV)
PDGF ($\rightarrow$ collagens I, III, IV, V and VI)
FGF-7 (KGF)
IL-2 and -4
TNF-α and -β
Oncostatin M

HEPATOCYTE GROWTH FACTOR (HGF) IN LIVER FIBROGENESIS

HGF is synthesized in cells of mesodermal origin as a 728 amino acid long pro-peptide, structurally similar to plasminogen. The mature heterodimer is generated after proteolytic cleavage and consists of a heavy α-chain (69 kDa) containing four cringle structures, and a light β-chain (34 kDa) which has high homology to serine protease[75]. Its receptor (c-met) is a membrane-bound tyrosine kinase (approximately 190 kDa) of 1408 amino acids which is expressed on the surface of many cells of epithelial origin throughout the body[76]. Homozygous loss of either HGF or c-met genes results in embryological lethality, partly due to arrested hepatic development[77,78].

The adjacent location of the HGF-producing mesenchymal cells and the c-met-expressing epithelial cells suggests that the HGF/c-met system may have a role in paracrine epithelial–mesenchymal interactions. This has also been demonstrated in many organs, both during embryological development[79] and tissue regeneration in the adult animal.

HGF is secreted mainly as an inactive pro-peptide which binds to heparin in the ECM in the liver. After activation HGF can exert substantial mitogenic, motogenic and morphogenic effects on the nearby hepatocytes[80], but also on biliary epithelial cells[81]. HGF has been shown to be a very potent hepatocyte mitogen *in vivo*. HGF transgenic mice show a doubling of liver size[82].

In the intact liver HSC are the main producers of HGF[83–85]. In those studies it was shown that the expression of HGF mRNA was down-regulated during the transformation process. The fully transformed rat HSC, i.e. the myofibroblast, had a very low or unmeasurable amount of HGF mRNA. However, recent data from human myofibroblasts demonstrate that they express HGF mRNA and secrete HGF, which is bioactive and is able to increase the invasiveness of various human hepatocellular carcinoma cell (HCC) lines[86]. It has also been suggested that this HGF-mediated invasiveness is secondary to urokinase expression in HCC, which are able to activate HGF produced by myofibroblasts[87]. One further complexity of this system is that HSC *in vitro* during the transformation process start to express HGF receptors, and upon stimulation enhance their DNA synthesis and TGF-β_1 expression[88].

There are few previous reports on factors that can regulate HGF production in HSC. It has been shown that TGF-β_1 decreases the levels of HGF mRNA in HSC[84]. TGF-β inhibitory elements are present together with several other regulatory elements in the promoter sequence of the HGF gene[89]. In fibroblasts there are several as yet unidentified factors besides TGF-β_1 which influence HGF expression[90]. It has also been shown that HGF expression in fibroblasts is often regulated by cAMP-dependent pathways and respond to stimulation by prostaglandins[91]. However, it is uncertain to what extent these results apply to the liver. There are few reports so far about connections to IGF effects in the HGF gene promoter region[89]. It has been shown *in vitro*, with freshly isolated rat HSC, that IGFs are able to enhance both the expression of HGF mRNA and the levels of HGF protein[92]. Another interesting recent report has indicated that in cultured HSC TNF-α dose-dependently increases production of IL-6, which then in an autocrine fashion stimulates HGF production[93].

Little is known about the possible role of HGF production by HSC *in vivo*. The HGF produced by HSC of intact livers probably does not exert endocrine effects, since the levels of circulating HGF are very low in these animals[80]. *In vivo*, HGF has been shown to stimulate proliferation of hepatocytes in the intact liver and to accelerate liver regeneration. *In vitro*, mitogenic effects have been seen on cultured biliary epithelial cells[81] and myofibroblasts[88]. The bioactivity of HGF *in vivo* is regulated by binding to ECM, and by bioactivation of prepro-HGF by proteases. These enzymes may be produced by target cells of HGF action including the hepatocytes[94]. In addition, the responsiveness of the target cells may be modulated at the HGF receptor or postreceptor level. Some doubts have been raised recently about the correlation between hepatocyte proliferation and HGF levels *in vivo*. In HCC, proliferation seems to correlate better with expression of HGF receptor than with the expression of HGF itself[95]. Similarly, HGF does not correlate with the level of hepatocyte proliferation during liver regeneration, while there is such a correlation for TGF-α[96]. However, all studies must be interpreted with caution since the levels of HGF mRNA and HGF immunoreactivity may not reflect HGF bioactivity, which is probably regulated in a complex way *in vivo* by cleavage of prepro-HGF and detachment from ECM.

It is known that HGF increases the invasiveness of HCC[97], and recently the production of bioactive HGF in human myofibroblasts of liver carcinoma was demonstrated[86]. The IGF system has also been shown to be of importance for the development and progression of liver tumours[98]. Hence, it would be interesting to see whether the IGF–HGF regulation has any implications for liver tumour growth *in vivo*.

As mentioned above, transformed HSC both *in vitro* and *in vivo* express HGF receptors, and *in vitro* they respond by enhanced DNA synthesis and TGF-β_1 expression[88]. Thus, one could presume that exogenously administered HGF would be profibrotic. Instead, numerous *in-vivo* experiments have shown that HGF has an antifibrotic and hepatocyte-protective effect, thus antagonizing the initiating event in fibrogenesis.

Depending on the cell type and physiological conditions, HGF can exert both pro-apoptotic and anti-apoptotic effects. The pro-apoptotic actions are thought to be at least in part mediated via p53/bax-independent pathways activating JNK[99]. This effect is thought to be of importance for the inhibitory effect on liver tumour development that has been seen *in vivo* in combined c-myc/HGF transgenic mice[100]. HGF also has an anti-apoptotic effect in some *in-vivo* conditions, e.g. reducing the mortality in endotoxin-induced hepatic failure[101] and Fas-induced hepatic failure[102]. However, HGF also elicits direct cytoprotective effects by attenuating or preventing the onset of severe acute liver injury after the administration of hepatotoxins such as alpha-naphthylisothiocyanate[103].

Maybe one of the most interesting aspects of HGF in clinical practice is its effect in cirrhotic livers. In liver cirrhosis caused by dimethylnitrosamine (DMN) administration to rats, HGF was able to markedly suppress both the onset and progression of liver cirrhosis. Death caused by severe hepatic cirrhosis and dysfunction was also completely abrogated[104]. This has also been shown for rat liver cirrhosis caused by long-term administration of carbon tetrachloride (CCl$_4$)[105]. Recently, a promising gene therapy approach to suppress the pro-

Table 3 Antifibrotic cytokine antagonism

Antagonist	Organ fibrosis	Mode of action	Mode of application
IL-1-R antagonist	Liver	Inhibition of IL-1, inhibition of HSC activation	Protein supplement
IL-10	Liver	Anti-inflammatory (anti-Th1 cytokines)	Protein supplement
HGF	Liver	Suppression of TGF-β-mRNA	Gene transfer, protein supplement
Soluble TNF-α-R	Liver	Hepatocytoprotection	Protein supplement
Soluble TGF-β-R	Kidney	TGF-β scavenging	Gene transfer
Decorin	Kidney, lung	TGF-β scavenging	Gene transfer
Smad 7	Lung	Blockade of TGF-β signalling	Gene transfer
Interferon-gamma	Liver	Inhibition of Smads, inhibition of HSC activation	Protein supplement
Interferon-alpha	Liver	Increase of IL-1-R antagonist	Protein supplement

gression of DMN-induced liver cirrhosis in rats was demonstrated. This was accomplished by an intramuscular injection of an HVJ-liposome preparation with an HGF expression vector[95]. In the studies above, administration of HGF has led to suppression of TGF-β_1 expression, which plays an essential role in the fibrogenic process, thus inhibiting fibrogenesis and hepatic apoptosis caused by TGF-β_1.

It is well known that hepatic resection in patients with cirrhotic livers is accompanied by a markedly higher mortality than in patients with non-cirrhotic livers. There are promising animal experiments in which perioperative adminis-tration of rhHGF stimulates liver regeneration and function, thus preventing postoperative liver failure in rats with liver cirrhosis[106,107]. Even though there are many hopeful experimental data on the usage of HGF, more questions need to be answered until it can be used in a wider clinical practice.

CONCLUSION AND OUTLOOK

During fibrogenesis cytokines and growth factors function as important paracrine and autocrine mediators, which are focused on the activation of hepatic stellate cells, regulation of parenchymal cell proliferation and apoptosis, extracellular matrix synthesis and degradation and recruitment of inflammatory cell types. Although we begin to understand the effects of single cytokines on functions of specialized cells, the complex interaction of all these mediators is not yet known. Hopefully, with the use of organ-specific knockout mice, or over-expression of cytokines driven by tissue-specific promoters in transgenic mice, a more detailed insight into the cytokine network relevant for fibro-genesis may be obtained. A detailed knowledge of the intracellular signalling pathways forms a solid basis for therapeutic approaches based on cytokine antagonism[108].

This line has been pursued successfully in experiments with IL-10-deficient animals, which show that these mice are more susceptible to CCl_4-induced fibrosis, suggesting that administered IL-10 might be hepatoprotective[109] and antifibrogenic[110] (Table 3). Beneficial cytoprotective and antifibrotic effects were also obtained with TNF-α antagonists[111], IL-1 receptor antagonist[112,113] and with hepatocyte growth factor supplementation either by gene therapy[114] or infusions/injections[105,115]. The latter cytokine might act as a potent antagonist of TGF-β since HGF suppresses the elevated TGF-β_1-mRNA level in hepatic fibrosis[115]. HGF functions dominantly to block TGF-β effects, possibly by antagonism of Smad-signalling. Thus, the balance of TGF-β and HGF plays a role in control-ling fibrogenic and proliferative responses during liver repair, which can be exploited therapeutically. Alternatively, gene therapy with soluble TGF-β recep-tors[116] or scavenger proteoglycans such as decorin[117] offer a direct approach to therapeutic TGF-β antagonism. Recently, over-expression of the antagonistic Smad protein[7] in lung by adenoviral gene transfer has been shown to prevent bleomycin-induced lung fibrosis in mice[118]. The experimental data listed in Table 3, in combination with the pharmacological interference of specific intra-cellular signalling pathways[119], may offer useful clinical principles for effective antifibrotic therapeutic trials.

Acknowledgement

These studies were supported by grants Gr 463/9-3 and Gr 463/12-1 from the Deutsche Forschungsgemeinschaft (DFG).

References

1. Gressner AM, Schuppan D. Cellular and molecular pathobiology, pharmacological intervention, and biochemical assessment of liver fibrosis. In: Bircher J, Benhamou JP, McIntyre N, Rizzetto M, Rodés J, editors. Oxford Textbook of Clinical Hepatology. Oxford: Oxford Medical Publications; 1999:607–27.
2. Schuppan D, Gressner AM. Function and metabolism of collagens and other extracellular matrix proteins. In: Bircher J, Benhamou JP, McIntyre N, Rizzetto M, Rodés J, editors. Oxford Textbook of Clinical Hepatology. Oxford: Oxford Medical Publications; 1999:381–407.
3. Wu JA, Danielsson A. Detection of hepatic fibrogenesis: a review of available techniques. Scand J Gastroenterol. 1995;30:817–25.
4. Schuppan D, Stölzel U, Oesterling C, Somasundaram R. Serum assays for liver fibrosis. J Hepatol. 1995;22:82–8.
5. Schaffner F, Popper H. Capillarization of hepatic sinusoids in man. Gastroenterology. 1963;44:239–42.
6. Friedman SL. The cellular basis of hepatic fibrosis. N Engl J Med. 1993;328:1828–35.
7. Gressner AM. Cytokines and cellular crosstalk involved in the activation of fat-storing cells. J Hepatol. 1995;22 (Suppl.2):28–36.
8. Pinzani M. Hepatic stellate (Ito) cells: expanding roles for a liver-specific pericyte. J Hepatol. 1995;22:700–6.
9. Pinzani M. Novel insights into the biology and physiology of the Ito cell. Pharmacol Ther. 1995;66:387–412.
10. Gressner AM. The cell biology of liver fibrogenesis – an imbalance of proliferation, growth arrest and apoptosis of myofibroblasts. Cell Tissue Res. 1998;292:447–52.
11. Gressner AM, Bachem MG. Molecular mechanisms of liver fibrogenesis – a homage to the role of activated fat-storing cells. Digestion. 1995;56:335–46.
12. Gressner AM. Perisinusoidal lipocytes and fibrogenesis. Gut. 1994;35:1331–3.
13. Casini A, Ceni E, Salzano R et al. Neutrophil-derived superoxide anion induces lipid peroxidation and stimulates collagen synthesis in human hepatic stellate cells: role of nitric oxide. Hepatology. 1997;25:361–7.
14. Houglum K, Brenner DA, Chojkier M. D-alpha-Tocopherol inhibits collagen alpha 1 (I) gene expression in cultured human fibroblasts. J Clin Invest. 1991;87:2230–5.
15. Casini A, Galli G, Salzano R, Rotella CM, Surrenti C. Acetaldehyde–protein adducts, but not lactate and pyruvate, stimulate gene transcription of collagen and fibronectin in hepatic fat storing cells. J Hepatol. 1993;19:385–92.
16. Casini A, Cunningham M, Rojkind M, Lieber CS. Acetaldehyde increases procollagen type I and fibronectin gene transcription in cultured rat fat storing cells through a protein synthesis-dependent mechanism. Hepatology. 1991;13:758–65.
17. Maher JJ, Zia S, Tzagarakis C. Acetaldehyde-induced stimulation of collagen synthesis and gene expression is dependent on conditions of cell culture: studies with rat lipocytes and fibroblasts. Alcoholism Clin Exp Res. 1994;18:403–9.
18. Marra F, Defranco R, Grappone C et al. Increased expression of monocyte chemotactic protein-1 during active hepatic fibrogenesis: correlation with monocyte infiltration. Am J Pathol. 1998;152:423–30.
19. Marra F, Valente AJ, Pinzani M, Abboud HE. Cultured human liver fat storing cells produce monocyte chemotactic protein-1 – regulation by proinflammatory cytokines. J Clin Invest. 1993;92:1674–80.
20. Sprenger H, Kaufmann A, Garn H, Lahme B, Gemsa D, Gressner AM. Induction of neutrophil attracting chemokines in transforming hepatic stellate cells. Gastroenterology. 1997;113:277–85.
21. Sprenger H, Kaufmann A, Garn H, Lahme B, Gemsa D, Gressner AM. Differential expression of monocyte chemotactic protein-1 (MCP-1) in transforming rat hepatic stellate cells. J Hepatol. 1999;30:88–94.

22. Gressner AM. Activation of proteoglycan synthesis in injured liver – a brief review of molecular and cellular aspects. Eur J Clin Chem Clin Biochem. 1994;32:225–37.
23. Friedman SL. Cellular sources of collagen and regulation of collagen production in liver. Sem Liver Dis. 1990;10:20–9.
24. Rockey DC, Weisiger RA. Endothelin induced contractility of stellate cells from normal and cirrhotic rat liver: implication for regulation of portal pressure and resistance. Hepatology. 1996;24:233–40.
25. Kawada N, Tranthi TA, Klein H, Decker K. The contraction of hepatic stellate (Ito) cells stimulated with vasoactive substances – possible involvement of endothelin-1 and nitric oxide in the regulation of the sinusoidal tonus. Eur J Biochem. 1993;213:815–23.
26. Rockey D. The cellular pathogenesis of portal hypertension: stellate cell contractility, endothelin, and nitric oxide. Hepatology. 1997;25:2–5.
27. Gressner AM. Mediators of hepatic fibrogenesis. Hepato-Gastroenterology. 1996;43:92–103.
28. Gressner AM, Lotfi S, Gressner G, Lahme B. Identification and partial characterization of a hepatocyte-derived factor promoting proliferation of cultured fat storing cells (parasinusoidal lipocytes). Hepatology. 1992;16:1250–66.
29. Gressner AM, Lahme B, Brenzel A. Molecular dissection of the mitogenic effect of hepatocytes on cultured hepatic stellate cells. Hepatology. 1995;22:1507–18.
30. Maher JJ, Bissell DM, Roll FJ. Contaminating lipocytes contribute to collagen synthesis in hepatocyte cultures. Clin Res. 1987;35:591A.
31. Roth S, Schurek J, Gressner AM. Expression and release of the latent TGF-beta binding protein (LTBP) by hepatocytes from rat liver. Hepatology. 1997;25:1398–405.
32. Roth S, Michel K, Gressner AM. (Latent) transforming growth factor-beta in liver parenchymal cells, its injury-dependent release and paracrine effects on hepatic stellate cells. Hepatology. 1998;27:1003–12.
33. Chunfang Gao, Gressner G, Zoremba M, Gressner AM. Transforming growth factor-beta (TGF-beta) expression in isolated and cultured rat hepatocytes. J Cell Physiol. 1996;167:394–405.
34. Decker K. Biologically active products of stimulated liver macrophages (Kupffer cells). Eur J Biochem. 1990;192:245–61.
35. Zerbe O, Gressner AM. Proliferation of fat storing cells is stimulated by secretions of Kupffer cells from normal and injured liver. Exp Mol Pathol. 1988;49:87–101.
36. Friedman SL, Arthur JP. Activation of cultured rat hepatic lipocytes by Kupffer cell conditioned medium. J Clin Invest. 1989;84:1780–5.
37. Gressner AM, Haarmann R. Regulation of hyaluronate synthesis in rat liver fat storing cell cultures by Kupffer cells. J Hepatol. 1988;7:310–18.
38. Gressner AM, Zerbe O. Kupffer cell-mediated induction of synthesis and secretion of proteoglycans by rat liver fat storing cells in culture. J Hepatol. 1987;5:299–310.
39. Bachem MG, Melchior R, Gressner AM. The role of thrombocytes in liver fibrogenesis: effects of platelet lysate and thrombocyte-derived growth factors on the mitogenic activity and glycosaminoglycan synthesis of cultured rat liver fat storing cells. J Clin Chem Clin Biochem. 1989;27:555–65.
40. Bachem MG, Meyer DM, Melchior R, Sell KM, Gressner AM. Activation of rat liver perisinusoidal lipocytes by transforming growth factors derived from myofibroblast-like cells – a potential mechanism of self-perpetuation in liver fibrogenesis. J Clin Invest. 1992;89:19–27.
41. Deblesser PJ, Niki T, Rogiers V, Geerts A. Transforming growth factor-beta gene expression in normal and fibrotic rat liver. J Hepatol. 1997;26:886–93.
42. Rosenbaum J, Blazejewski S, Preaux AM, Mallat A, Dhumeaux D, Mavier P. Fibroblast growth factor 2 and transforming growth factor beta 1 interactions in human liver myofibroblasts. Gastroenterology. 1995;109:1986–96.
43. Bachem MG, Riess U, Gressner AM. Liver fat storing cell proliferation is stimulated by epidermal growth factor/transforming growth factor-alpha and inhibited by transforming growth factor-beta. Biochem Biophys Res Commun. 1989;162:708–14.
44. Reinehr RM, Kubitz R, Petersregehr T, Bode JG, Haussinger D. Activation of rat hepatic stellate cells in culture is associated with increased sensitivity to endothelin 1. Hepatology. 1998;28:1566–77.
45. Bachem MG, Meyer DH, Schäfer et al. The response of rat liver perisinusoidal lipocytes to polypeptide growth regulator changes with their transdifferentiation into myofibroblast-like cells in culture. J Hepatol. 1993;18:40–52.

46. Roulot D, Sevcsik AM, Coste T, Strosberg AD, Marullo S. Role of transforming growth factor-beta type II receptor in hepatic fibrosis: studies of human chronic hepatitis C and experimental fibrosis in rats. Hepatology. 1999;29:1730–8.

47. Housset C, Rockey DC, Bissell DM. Endothelin receptors in rat liver – lipocytes as a contractile target for endothelin-1. Proc Natl Acad Sci USA. 1993;90:9266–70.

48. Border WA, Noble NA. TGF-beta. Sci Am Sci Med. 1995;2:68–77.

49. Moses HL, Serra R. Regulation of differentiation by TGF-beta. Curr Opin Genet Develop. 1996;6:581–6.

50. Heldin CH, Miyazono K, Tendijke P. TGF-beta signalling from cell membrane to nucleus through SMAD proteins. Nature. 1997;390:465–71.

51. Massagué J. TGF-beta signal transduction. Annu Rev Biochem. 1998;67:753–91.

52. Garcia-Trevijano ER, Iraburu MJ, Fontana L et al. Transforming growth factor b1 induces the expression of a a1 (I) procollagen mRNA by a hydrogen peroxide-C/EBPb-dependent mechanism in rat hepatic stellate cells. Hepatology. 1999;29:960–70.

53. Sinha S, Nevett C, Shuttlerworth CA, Kielty CM. Cellular and extracellular biology of the latent transforming growth factor beta binding proteins. Matrix Biol. 1998;17:529–45.

54. Gong WR, Roth S, Michel K, Gressner AM. Isoforms of the latent transforming growth factor-beta binding protein in rat hepatic stellate cells. Gastroenterology. 1998;114:352–63.

55. Michel K, Roth S, Trautwein C, Gong WR, Gressner AM. Analysis of the expression pattern of the latent TGF-β binding protein (LTBP) isoforms in normal and diseased human liver reveals a new splice variant missing the proteinase sensitive hinge region. Hepatology. 1998;27:1592–9.

56. Taipale J, Lohi J, Saharinen J, Kovanen PT, Keski-Oja J. Human mast cell chymase and leukocyte elastase release latent transforming growth factor-beta1 from the extracellular matrix of cultured human epithelial and endothelial cells. J Biol Chem. 1995;270:4689–96.

57. Godár S, Horejsi V, Weidle UH, Binder BR, Hansmann C, Stockinger H. M6P/IGFII-receptor complexes urokinase receptor and plasminogen for activation of transforming growth factor-beta 1. Eur J Immunol. 1999;29:1004–13.

58. Debleser PJ, Jannes P, Buul-Offers van, SC et al. Insulin-like growth factor-II/mannose 6-phosphate receptor is expressed on CCl$_4$-exposed rat fat-storing cells and facilitates activation of latent transforming growth factor-beta in cocultures with sinusoidal endothelial cells. Hepatology. 1995;21:1429–37.

59. Hori Y, Katoh T, Hirakata M et al. Anti-latent TGF-beta binding protein-1 antibody or synthetic oligopeptides inhibit extracellular matrix expression induced by stretch in cultured rat mesangial cells. Kidney Int. 1998;53:1616–25.

60. Ribeiro SMF, Poczatek M, Schultzcherry S, Villain M, Murphyullrich JE. The activation sequence of thrombospondin-1 interacts with the latency-associated peptide to regulate activation of latent transforming growth factor-beta. J Biol Chem. 1999;274:13586–93.

61. Munger JS, Huang XZ, Kawakatsu H et al. The integrin alpha v beta 6 binds and activates latent TGF beta 1: a mechanism for regulating pulmonary inflammation and fibrosis. Cell. 1999;96:319–28.

62. Barcellos-Hoff MH, Dix TA. Redox-mediated activation of latent transforming growth factor-beta1. Mol Endocrinol. 1996;10:1077–83.

63. Saile B, Matthes N, Knittel T, Ramadori G. Transforming growth factor β and tumor necrosis factor a inhibit both apoptosis and proliferation of activated rat hepatic stellate cells. Hepatology. 1999;30:196–202.

64. Gressner AM, Wulbrand U. Variation of immunocytochemical expression of transforming growth factor (TGF)-beta hepatocytes in culture and liver slices. Cell Tissue Res. 1997;287:143–52.

65. Gressner AM, Lahme B, Roth S. Attenuation of TGF-beta-induced apoptosis in primary cultures of hepatocytes by calpain inhibitors. Biochem Biophys Res Commun. 1997;231:457–62.

66. Gressner AM, Polzar B, Lahme B, Mannherz HG. Induction of rat liver parenchymal cell apoptosis by hepatic myofibroblasts via transforming growth factor-beta. Hepatology. 1996;23:571–81.

67. LaMarre J, Wollenberg GK, Gonias SL, Hayes MA. Biology of disease: cytokine binding and clearance properties of proteinase-activated alpha2-macroglobulins. Lab Invest. 1991;65:3–14.

68. LaMarre J, Wollenberg GK, Gauldie J, Hayes MA. Alpha-macroglobulin and serum preferentially counteract the mitoinhibitory effect of transforming growth factor-beta2 in rat hepatocytes. Lab Invest. 1990;62:545–51.

69. Danielpour D, Sporn MB. Differential inhibition of transforming growth factor beta-1 and beta-2 activity by alpha2-macroglobulin. J Biol Chem. 1990;265:6973-7.
70. Yamaguchi Y, Mann DM, Ruoslahti E. Negative regulation of transforming growth factor-beta by the proteoglycan decorin. Nature. 1990;346:281-4.
71. Somasundaram R, Schuppan D. Type I, II, III, IV, V, and VI collagens serve as extracellular ligands for the isoforms of platelet-derived growth factor (AA, BB and AB). J Biol Chem. 1996;271:26884-91.
72. Taipale J, Keski-Oja J. Growth factors in the extracellular matrix. FASEB J. 1997;11:51-9.
73. Border WA, Noble NA, Yamamoto T et al. Natural inhibitor of transforming growth factor-beta protects against scarring in experimental kidney disease. Nature. 1992;360:361-4.
74. Isaka Y, Brees DK, Ikegaya K et al. Gene therapy by skeletal muscle expression of decorin prevents fibrotic disease in rat kidney. Nature Med. 1996;2:418-23.
75. Chirgadze DY, Hepple J, Byrd RA, Sowdhamini R, Blundell T, Gherardi E. Insights into the structure of hepatocyte growth factor/scatter factor (HGF/SF) and implications for receptor activation. FEBS Lett. 1998;430:126-9.
76. Comoglio PM, Boccaccio C. The HGF receptor family: unconventional signal transducers for invasive cell growth. Genes Cells. 1996;1:347-54.
77. Schmidt C, Bladt F, Goedecke S et al. Scatter factor/hepatocyte growth factor is essential for liver development. Nature. 1995;373:699-702.
78. Uehara Y, Minowa O, Mori C et al. Placental defect and embryonic lethality in mice lacking hepatocyte growth factor/scatter factor. Nature. 1995;373:702-5.
79. Birchmeir C, Gherardi E. Developmental roles of HGF/SF and its receptor, the c-Met tyrosine kinase. Trends Cell Biol. 1998;8:404-10.
80. Zarnegar R, Michalopoulos GK. The many faces of hepatocyte growth factor: from hepatopoiesis to hematopoiesis. J Cell Biol. 1995;129:1177-80.
81. Johnson M, Koukoulis G, Matsumoto K, Nakamura T, Iyer A. Hepatocyte growth factor induces proliferation and morphogenesis in nonparenchymal epithelial liver cells. Hepatology. 1993;17:1052-61.
82. Sakata H, Takayama H, Sharp R et al. Hepatocyte growth factor/scatter factor overexpression induces growth, abnormal development, and tumour formation in transgenic mouse livers. Cell Growth Differ. 1996;7:1513-23.
83. Schirmacher P, Geerts A, Pietrangelo A, Dienes HP, Rogler CE. Hepatocyte growth factor/hepatopoietin-A is expressed in fat storing cells from rat liver but not myofibroblast-like cells derived from fat storing cells. Hepatology. 1992;15:5-11.
84. Ramadori G, Neubauer K, Odenthal M et al. The gene of hepatocyte growth factor is expressed in fat storing cells of rat liver and is downregulated during cell growth and by transforming growth factor-beta. Biochem Biophys Res Commun. 1992;183:739-42.
85. Maher JJ. Cell-specific expression of hepatocyte growth factor in liver. Upregulation in sinusoidal endothelial cells after carbon tetrachloride. J Clin Invest. 1993;91:2244-52.
86. Neaud V, Faouzi S, Guirouilh J et al. Human hepatic myofibroblasts increase invasiveness of hepatocellular carcinoma cells: evidence for a role of hepatocyte growth factor. Hepatology. 1997;26:1458-66.
87. Monvoisin A, Neaud D, De Ledinghen V et al. Direct evidence that hepatocyte growth factor-induced invasion of hepatocellular carcinoma cells is mediated by urokinase. J Hepatol. 1999;30:511-18.
88. Ikeda H, Nagoshi S, Ohno A, Yanase M, Maekawa H, Fujiwara K. Activated rat stellate cells express c-met and respond to hepatocyte growth factor to enhance transforming growth factor beta 1 expression and DNA synthesis. Biochem Biophys Res Commun. 1998;250:769-75.
89. Liu Y, Michalopoulos GK, Zarnegar R. Structural and functional characterization of mouse hepatocyte growth factor gene promoter. J Biol Chem. 1994;269:4152-60.
90. Rubin JS, Bottaro DP, Aaronson SA. Hepatocyte growth factor/scatter factor and its receptor, the c-met proto-oncogene product. Biochim Biophys Acta. 1993;1155:357-71.
91. Matsunaga T, Gohda E, Takebe T et al. Expression of hepatocyte growth factor is up-regulated through activation of a cAMP-mediated pathway. Exp Cell Res. 1994;210:326-35.
92. Skrtic S, Wallenius S, Ekberg S, Brenzel A, Gressner AM, Jansson JO. Insulin-like growth factors stimulate expression of hepatocyte growth factor but not transforming growth factor $\beta1$ in cultured hepatic stellate cells. Endocrinology. 1997;138:4683-9.
93. Diehl AM. Roles of CCAAT/enhancer-binding proteins in regulation of liver regenerative growth. J Biol Chem. 1998;273:30843-6.

94. Miyazawa K, Shimomura T, Kitamura A, Kondo J, Morimoto A, Kitamura N. Molecular cloning and sequence analysis of the cDNA for a human serine protease responsible for activation of hepatocyte growth factor. Structural similarity of the protease precursor to blood coagulation factor XII. J Biol Chem. 1993;268:10024–8.

95. Ueki T, Fujimoto J, Suzuki T, Yamamoto H, Okamoto E. Expression of hepatocyte growth factor and its receptor c-met proto-oncogene in hepatocellular carcinoma. Hepatology. 1997;25:862–6.

96. Tomiya T, Ogata I, Fujiwara K. Transforming growth factor alpha levels in liver and blood correlate better than hepatocyte growth factor with hepatocyte proliferation during liver regeneration. Am J Pathol. 1998;153:955–61.

97. Vande Woude GF, Jeffers M, Cortner J, Alvord G, Tsarfaty, I, Resau J. Met-HGF/SF: tumorigenesis, invasion and metastasis. Ciba Found Symp. 1997;212:119–30.

98. LeRoith D, Baserga R, Helman L, Roberts Jr, CT. Insulin-like growth factors and cancer [see comments]. Ann Intern Med. 1995;122:54–9.

99. Connor E, Teramoto T, Wirth P, Kiss A, Garfield S, Thorgeirsson S. HGF-mediated apoptosis via p53/bax-independent pathway activating JNK1. Carcinogenesis. 1999;20:583–90.

100. Santoni-Rugiu E, Preisegger K, Kiss A et al. Inhibition of neoplastic development in the liver by hepatocyte growth factor in a transgenic mouse model. Proc Natl Acad Sci USA. 1996;93:9577–82.

101. Kosai K, Matsumoto K, Funakoshi H, Nakamura T. Hepatocyte growth factor prevents endotoxin-induced lethal hepatic failure in mice. Hepatology. 1999;30:151–9.

102. Kosai K, Matsumoto K, Nagata S, Tsujimoto Y, Nakamura T. Abrogation of Fas-induced fulminant hepatic failure in mice by hepatocyte growth factor. Biochem Biophys Res Commun. 1998;244:683–90.

103. Ishiki Y, Ohnishi H, Muto Y, Matsumoto K, Nakamura T. Direct evidence that hepatocyte growth factor is a hepatotrophic factor for liver regeneration and has a potent antihepatitis effect *in vivo*. Hepatology. 1992;16:1227–35.

104. Matsuda Y, Matsumoto K, Ichida T, Nakamura T. Hepatocyte growth factor suppresses the onset of liver cirrhosis and abrogates lethal hepatic dysfunction in rats. J Biochem Tokyo. 1995;118:643–9.

105. Matsuda Y, Matsumoto K, Yamada A et al. Preventive and therapeutic effects in rats of hepatocyte growth factor infusion on liver fibrosis/cirrhosis. Hepatology. 1997;26:81–9.

106. Kaibori M, Kwon A, Nakagawa M et al. Stimulation of liver regeneration and function after partial hepatectomy in cirrhotic rats by continuous infusion of recombinant human hepatocyte growth factor. J Hepatol. 1997;27:381–90.

107. Kaido T, Seto S, Yamaoka S, Yoshikawa A, Imamura M. Perioperative continuous hepatocyte growth factor supply prevents postoperative liver failure in rats with liver cirrhosis. J Surg Res. 1998;74:173–8.

108. Border WA, Noble NA. TGF-beta in kidney fibrosis: a target for gene therapy. Kidney Int. 1997;51:1388–96.

109. Louis H, Lemoine O, Peny MO et al. Hepatoprotective role of interleukin 10 in galactosamine/lipopolysaccharide mouse liver injury. Gastroenterology. 1997;112:935–42.

110. Louis H, Vanlaethem JL, Wu W et al. Interleukin-10 controls neutrophilic infiltration, hepatocyte proliferation, and liver fibrosis induced by carbon tetrachloride in mice. Hepatology. 1998;28:1607–15.

111. Czaja MJ, Xu J, Alt E. Prevention of carbon tetrachloride-induced rat liver injury by soluble tumor necrosis factor receptor. Gastroenterology. 1995;108:1849–54.

112. Mancini R, Benedetti A, Jezequel AM. An interleukin-1 receptor antagonist decreases fibrosis induced by dimethylnitrosamine in rat. Virchows Archiv. 1994;424:25–31.

113. Naveau S, Emilie D, Borotto E et al. Interleukin-1 receptor antagonist plasma concentration is specifically increased by alpha-2A-interferon treatment. J. Hepatol. 1997;27:272–5.

114. Ueki T, Kaneda Y, Tsutsui H et al. Hepatocyte growth factor gene therapy of liver cirrhosis in rats. Nature Med. 1999;5:226–30.

115. Yasuda H, Imai E, Shiota A, Fujise N, Morinaga T, Higashio K. Antifibrogenic effect of a deletion variant of hepatocyte growth factor on liver fibrosis in rats. Hepatology. 1996;24:636–42.

116. Isaka Y, Akagi Y, Ando Y et al. Gene therapy by transforming growth factor-beta receptor–IgG Fc chimera suppressed extracellular matrix accumulation in experimental glomerulonephritis. Kidney Int. 1999;55:465–75.

117. Border WA, Noble NA, Yamamoto T, Tomooka S, Kagami S. Antagonists of transforming growth factor-beta: a novel approach to treatment of glomerulonephritis and prevention of glomerulosclerosis. Kidney Int. 1992;41:566–70.
118. Nakao A, Fujii M, Matsumura R *et al.* Transient gene transfer and expression of Smad7 prevents bleomycin-induced lung fibrosis in mice. J Clin Invest. 1999;104:5–11.
119. Heimbrook DC, Oliff A. Therapeutic intervention and signaling. Curr Opin Cell Biol. 1998;10:284–8.
120. Sinha S, Nevett C, Shuttleworth CA, Kielty CM. Cellular and extracellular biology of the latent transforming growth factor-beta binding proteins. Matrix Biol. 1998;17:529–45.
121. Roth-Eichhorn S, Kühl K, Gressner AM. Subcellular localization of (latent) transforming growth factor β and the latent tgf-β binding protein in rat hepatocytes and hepatic stellate cells. Hepatology. 1998;28:1588–96.

19
Interferons and viral replication in the liver

D. MORADPOUR, M. H. HEIM and H. E. BLUM

INTRODUCTION

Infections with the hepatitis B virus (HBV) and hepatitis C virus (HCV) are leading causes of chronic hepatitis, liver cirrhosis, and hepatocellular carcinoma (HCC) worldwide. Therapeutic options are limited. For chronic hepatitis B, interferon-α (IFN-α) is the primary therapeutic option. Nucleoside analogues, i.e. lamivudine, famciclovir, penciclovir, and others are emerging alternatives. For chronic hepatitis C, current treatment modalities are IFN-α or IFN-α plus ribavirin combination therapy. IFN-α, therefore, is widely used to treat both chronic hepatitis B and C. Sustained response rates, however, are limited to 30–40% in chronic hepatitis B and 10–20% in chronic hepatitis C with IFN-α monotherapy and 30–40% with IFN-α plus ribavirin combination therapy[1-4].

IFNs are classified into type I IFNs, which comprise IFN-α and β, and type II IFN, or IFN-γ. Type I IFNs are produced by leucocytes, fibroblasts, epithelial cells and other cell types, and type II IFN by T lymphocytes and natural killer cells. During HBV infection IFN-α is produced in the liver by infiltrating mononuclear cells, sinusoidal cells, Kupffer cells and to a lesser extent by hepatocytes[5-8]. The antiviral effects of IFNs are mediated by several effector proteins, including double-stranded RNA-activated protein kinase (PKR), Mx, 2′–5′ oligoadenylate synthetase, and RNaseL[9]. The IFN-induced PKR phosphorylates the α-subunit of the eukaryotic translation initiation factor 2 (eIF-2α), thereby inhibiting protein synthesis[10]. IFNs also up-regulate MHC class I and II expression, which leads to enhanced antigen presentation and stimulation of acquired immunity. The mechanisms by which IFN-α inhibits replication of HBV and HCV are incompletely understood and may involve both direct antiviral and immunomodulatory effects. The investigation of these mechanisms has been hampered by the lack of efficient cell culture systems and small-animal models permissive for HBV and HCV infection and replication. Studies recently performed with the duck hepatitis B virus (DHBV), a virus closely related to HBV, have shown that recombinant duck IFN-α inhibits DHBV replication *in vitro* and *in vivo*[11,12]. This model allowed more detailed analyses of the IFN-sensitive steps of the viral life cycle[13]. Interestingly, recent studies performed in HBV transgenic mice suggested that inflammatory cytokines released in the context of a cellular immune response, namely tumour necrosis factor-α (TNF-α) and IFN-γ, can block HBV replication by a non-cytopathic mechanism[14]. HBV clearance without destruction of infected hepatocytes has also recently been documented in acutely infected chimpanzees, further supporting this concept[15]. The molecular mechanisms responsible for cytokine-mediated viral clearance are currently being investigated.

Viruses have evolved a number of strategies to escape the immune system[16,17]. The IFN-induced cellular antiviral response is the first line of innate defence against viral infection. In order to establish a productive infection, therefore, viruses must first overcome the IFN-induced mechanisms blocking viral replication. In the following, we will review the recent experimental data suggesting that both HBV and HCV have developed strategies to resist the antiviral effects of IFN-α.

INTERACTION OF HBV WITH THE IFN SYSTEM

Only a limited number of studies have addressed the interactions between HBV and the IFN system. In this context, expression of the HBV polymerase terminal protein has been reported to result in impaired activation of IFN-stimulated gene factor 3 (ISGF3)[18,19]. These findings, however, are still debated. More recently, studies performed in stably transfected HuH-7 human hepatoma cells suggested a selective inhibition of IFN-induced MxA protein expression by the HBV core protein[20].

INTERACTION OF HCV WITH THE IFN SYSTEM

Different mechanisms potentially underlying IFN resistance of HCV have recently been described. Viral proteins could interfere with IFN-induced intracellular signal transduction, thereby inhibiting induction of a number of antiviral effector proteins. Alternatively, the virus could have developed defence strategies against these cellular effector mechanisms. In this context a reduced basal and induced 2′–5′ oligoadenylate synthetase activity was found in peripheral blood lymphocytes from patients with persistent HCV viraemia[21]. In addition, repression of the catalytic activity of PKR by HCV proteins has recently been described in various experimental *in vitro* systems, as discussed in the following.

Interference of HCV with PKR

The HCV non-structural protein NS5A and the envelope glycoprotein E2 have recently been reported to interfere with PKR. NS5A is a serine phosphoprotein of as-yet-unknown function in the viral life cycle[22–25]. A role for NS5A in modulating the IFN response was first suggested by studies performed in Japan by Enomoto *et al.* These investigators found a correlation between mutations within a discrete region of NS5A (HCV amino acid positions 2209–2248), termed interferon sensitivity determining region (ISDR), and a favourable response to IFN-α therapy[26,27] (Fig. 1). These studies demonstrated that strains closely matching the prototype HCV genotype 1b (HCV-J) NS5A ISDR sequence correlated with IFN resistance. These findings were largely confirmed in Japan[28,29], but not in Europe or North America[30-36]. The reasons for this discrepancy are not understood but may involve both differences in doses and regimens of IFN treatment and the low prevalence of 'mutant-type' HCV genotype 1b isolates in Western countries[37,38]. Interestingly, however, an interaction with and repression of the catalytic activity of PKR by NS5A has been found by biochemical, transfection, and yeast functional analyses[39]. Mutations within the ISDR that were observed in clinically IFN-sensitive genotype 1b strains disrupted the ability of NS5A to interact with and repress PKR activity, supporting the notion that NS5A mediates HCV resistance to IFN through down-regulation of PKR[40]. In addition, disruption of PKR-dependent translational control and apoptotic programmes by NS5A has been suggested to confer oncogenic potential to HCV[41]. Finally, a recent study has provided evidence for a src homology 3 (SH3) domain-dependent interaction of NS5A with growth factor receptor-bound protein 2 (Grb2) adaptor protein which could interfere with mitogenic signal transduction pathways[42]. Since growth factor signalling may be linked to IFN signalling pathways[43] one could speculate that NS5A binding to Grb2 represents another mechanism by which HCV induces IFN resistance.

Expression of the NS5A protein in cultured cells resulted in a partial resistance to the effects of IFN-α against IFN-sensitive viruses[44,45]. Although these studies did not directly examine PKR function in these cells they provide further evidence for an interference of NS5A with IFN effector functions.

The HCV envelope glycoprotein E2 contains a sequence identical to phosphorylation sites of PKR and the PKR target eIF2α. Starting from this observation, a recent study described an interaction between E2 and PKR that resulted in an inhibition of the kinase activity of PKR and interference with its inhibitory effect on protein synthesis and cell growth[46]. The relevance of these observations for the natural history of HCV infection is not yet clear, but viral defence strategies targeting the effector mechanisms of IFN-induced antiviral activities could play an important role in viral pathogenesis.

Interference of HCV with signal transduction through the Jak-STAT pathway

HCV proteins could interfere with IFN-induced intracellular signal transduction and thereby prevent cellular antiviral responses at an early point. Indeed, examples of viral interference with IFN signal transduction have been reported. Vaccinia virus, for example, encodes a soluble type I IFN receptor which neutralizes IFN before it can bind to the cellular receptor[47]. More recently, human cytomegalovirus was reported to inhibit IFN-γ-induced Jak-STAT signalling, probably by enhancing Jak1 protein degradation[48]. Over the past several years the complete signal transduction pathway from the IFN receptors to the nucleus has been identified[49-52], and viral interference with IFN-induced signalling can now be studied in detail (Fig. 2). Type I IFNs bind to heterodimeric type I IFN receptors consisting of IFN-α receptor I (IFNARI) and IFNARII. Ligand binding

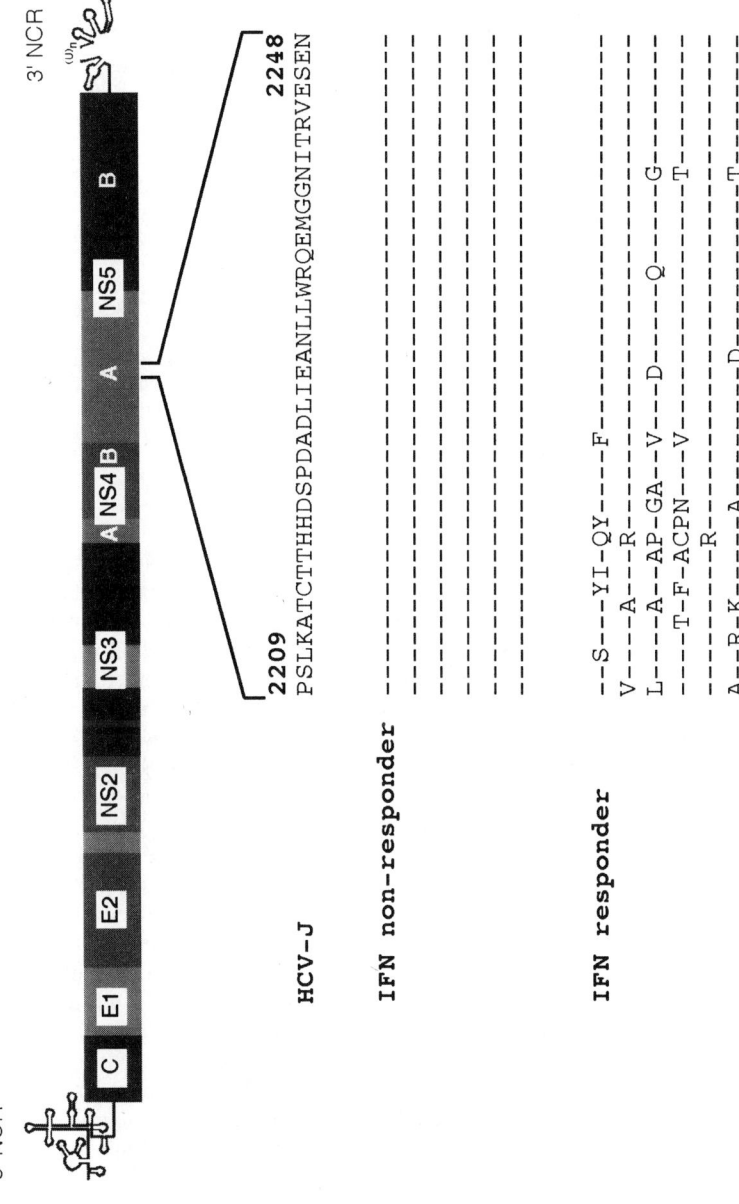

Figure 1 The HCV ISDR. Examples of sequences of HCV amino acid residues 2209–2248 within the NS5A protein in genotype 1b-infected IFN-α non-responders and responders. Amino acid residues are indicated by the standard single-letter codes and dashes indicate residues identical to those in the HCV-J prototype genotype 1b sequence. Patients with 'mutant-type' ISDR sequences (≥ 4 amino acid substitutions compared to the prototype sequence) showed a favourable response to IFN-α therapy whereas patients with 'wild-type' ISDR sequences did not respond[26,27].

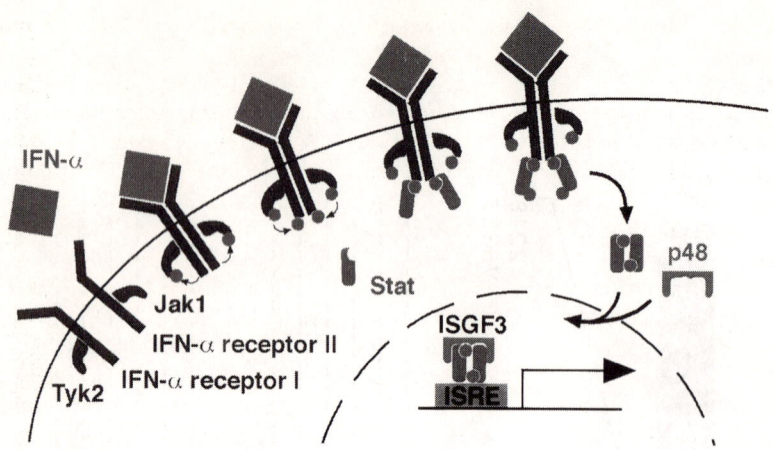

Figure 2   The Jak-STAT pathway. IFN-α binds to heterodimeric type I IFN receptors consisting of IFNARI and IFNARII. Ligand binding results in activation of the cytoplasmic receptor-associated protein tyrosine kinases Tyk2 and Jak1. The activated kinases then phosphorylate tyrosine residues of the receptors. These phosphotyrosines are consecutively bound by the SH2 domains of STATs. The STATs are then tyrosine phosphorylated and form hetero- or homodimers through mutual SH2 domain–phosphotyrosine interactions. Stat1–Stat2 heterodimers associate with a third DNA binding protein, ISGF3γ-p48, to form ISGF3. Binding of STAT factors to their cognate sequences in the promoter regions of target genes results in enhanced gene transcription

results in activation of two cytoplasmic protein tyrosine kinases associated with IFNARI and IFNARII, Tyk2 and Jak1. The activated kinases then phosphorylate tyrosine residues of the receptors. These phosphotyrosines are consecutively bound by the SH2 domains of signal transducer and activator of transcription 1 (Stat1), Stat2 and Stat3. The STATs are then tyrosine phosphorylated and form hetero- or homodimers through mutual SH2 domain– phosphotyrosine interactions. Stat3 and Stat1 form homodimers, designated serum inducible factor A (SIF-A) and SIF-C, respectively, and a Stat1–Stat3 heterodimer, SIF-B, that can be detected by electrophoretic mobility shift assays (EMSA) using the oligonucleotide probe m67 derived from the promoter of the c-fos gene. Stat1 can also dimerize with Stat2, and this Stat1–Stat2 heterodimer associates with a third DNA binding protein, ISGF3γ-p48, to form ISGF3. ISGF3 binds to a different response element and can be detected by EMSA with the oligonucleotide probe ISRE derived from the promoter of IFN-stimulated gene 15. Binding of these STAT factors to their cognate sequences in the promoter regions of target genes results in enhanced gene transcription. Among others, Stat1, Stat2, and ISGF3γ-p48 have been identified as IFN-α-induced target genes. A number of regulatory mechanisms of the Jak-STAT signal transduction pathway have recently been identified. The activity of the Jak kinases is controlled by receptor-associated phosphatases and by the newly discovered family of suppressors of cytokine signalling (SOCS). Binding of Stat3 dimers to DNA can be inhibited by PIAS3 (protein inhibitor of activated STATs). STATs are deactivated by an as yet unknown nuclear phosphatase and by protein degradation through the ubiquitin–proteasome pathway. At any of the steps outlined above, viral proteins could interfere with the Jak-STAT pathway and inhibit induction of antiviral effector proteins.

Given the lack of a suitable cell culture system for HCV to study viral interference with IFN signal transduction we employed a tetracycline-regulated gene expression system to establish a panel of continuous human cell lines inducibly expressing HCV structural and non-structural proteins[53] (Fig. 3). In these cell lines, termed UHCV, expression of the viral proteins can be tightly regulated by the concentration of tetracycline in the culture medium. HCV proteins are inducibly expressed in their biological context, faithfully processed by the cellular and viral proteolytic machineries, and posttranslationally modified. Using this well-characterized *in-vitro* system we investigated the effect of HCV protein expression on IFN-α-induced signalling through the Jak-STAT pathway[54].

To test for a possible interference of HCV proteins with IFN signal transduction, UHCV cells were analysed for IFN-α-induced ISGF3 formation. The founder cell line UTA-6[55], which constitutively expresses a tetracycline-controlled transactivator (tTA), but lacks the HCV transgene, and a UTA-6-derived cell line inducibly expressing the green fluorescent protein (GFP), termed UGFP-9, served as negative controls. Subconfluent cell monolayers were cultured for 24 h in the presence or absence of tetracycline and then either left untreated or stimulated for 30 min with 500 U/ml human IFN-α. Nuclear extracts were prepared and tested for ISGF3 DNA-binding activity by EMSA using the ISRE as an oligonucleotide probe, as shown in Fig. 4. ISGF3 induction after IFN-α treatment was detectable in UTA-6 and UGFP-9 cells irrespective of the culture conditions. In UHCV cells, however, ISGF3 induction was readily detectable only in cells cultured in the presence of tetracycline, i.e. in cells where viral protein expression has been repressed by tetracycline. If these cells were cultured in the absence of tetracycline, i.e. when they expressed HCV proteins, IFN-α-induced ISGF3 shift activity was inhibited. Likewise, a clear induction of SIF-A, SIF-B and SIF-C was observed in IFN-α-treated UTA-6 cells. In UHCV cells, however, expression of viral proteins inhibited the induction of SIF shifts, although to a somewhat lesser degree compared to ISGF3. A series of time-course and dose–response experiments, not illustrated here, demonstrated that HCV protein expression levels inversely correlated with the intensity of the ISGF3 gel shift and that inhibition of IFN-α-induced Jak-STAT signalling occurred already at low expression levels[54].

In order to exclude a general disturbance of cell homeostasis and intracellular signalling events by the expression of viral proteins we tested TNF-α-dependent NF-κB induction in UHCV cells as an example of a non-Jak-STAT signal transduction pathway. After binding to the 75 kDa TNF-receptor II, TNF-α allows rapid nuclear translocation of NF-κB through degradation of IκB inhibitory cytoplasmic retention proteins. In the nucleus, NF-κB binds to a decameric DNA sequence element in the promoter region of target genes. NF-κB activation as detected by EMSA with a consensus binding site oligonucleotide was not inhibited in UHCV cells expressing HCV proteins (Fig. 5).

Next, immunoprecipitation experiments were performed to examine at which step HCV proteins interfere with the Jak-STAT signal transduction pathway. As outlined above, STAT proteins are activated by tyrosine phosphorylation. To test whether the observed inhibition of DNA binding by STAT proteins is caused by

A + tet

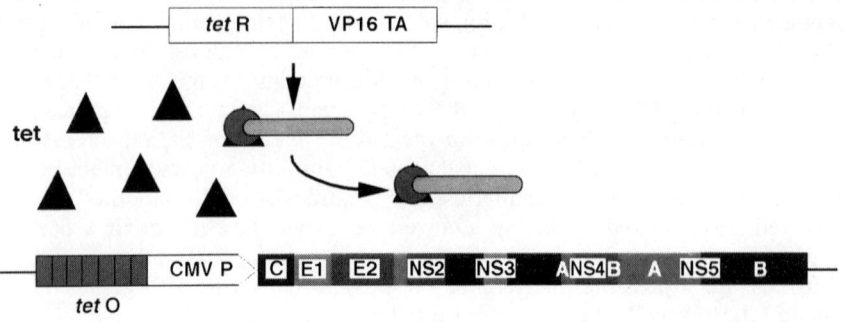

B - tet

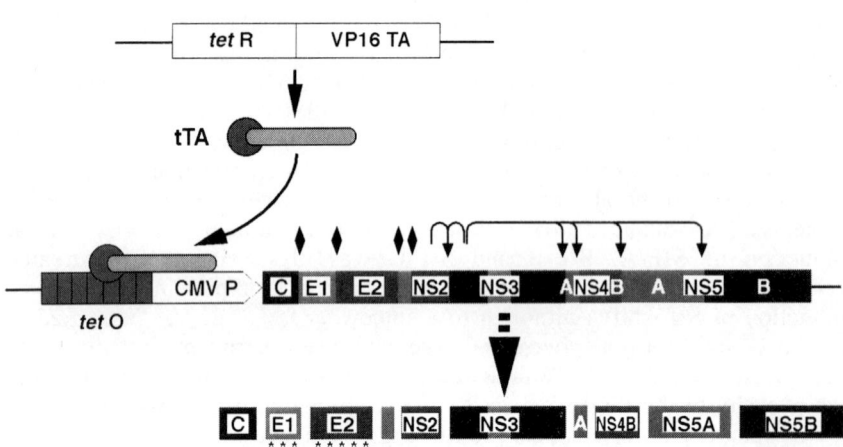

Figure 3 HCV-inducible cell lines. Schematic illustration of the tetracycline-regulated gene expression system and the HCV expression construct used to generate the UHCV cell lines. The system consists of a tetracycline-controlled transactivator (tTA), which is composed of the tetracycline repressor (*tet* R) fused to the activating domain of VP16 of herpex simplex virus, and of a tTA-dependent promoter, which is composed of a minimal sequence derived from the cytomegalovirus intermediate early promoter (CMV P) combined with heptameric tetracycline operator (*tet* O) sequences. When integrated into the proper genomic environment, the tTA-dependent promoter is virtually silent in many cell types in the presence of low concentrations of tetracycline (tet), which prevents the tTA from binding to *tet* O sequences (**A**). In the absence of tetracycline, the tTA binds to the *tet* O sequences to activate transcription from the minimal promoter (**B**). Asterisks in the E1 and E2 region indicate glycosylation of the envelope proteins. Diamonds denote cleavages of the HCV polyprotein precursor by the ER signal peptidase and arrows indicate cleavages by HCV NS2-3 and NS3 proteases

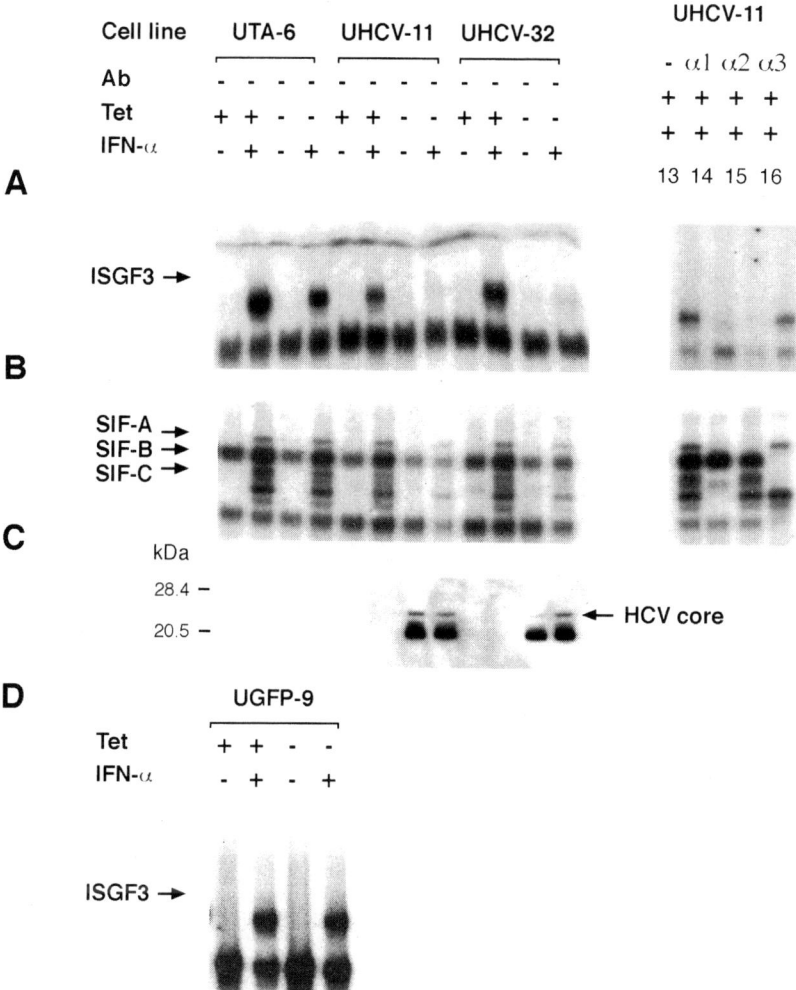

Figure 4 Inhibition of IFN signalling through the Jak-STAT pathway in UHCV cells expressing HCV proteins. UTA-6, UHCV-11 and UHCV-32 as well as UGFP-9 cells were cultured in the presence or absence of tetracycline and then either left untreated or stimulated for 30 min with 500 U/ml IFN-α, as indicated. **A** and **D**: EMSA with the ISRE oligonucleotide probe. The position of ISGF3 is indicated by an arrow. In UHCV cells expressing HCV proteins, the induction of ISGF3 by IFN-α is inhibited. Supershift experiments shown in (**A**) on the right confirmed the identity of the induced shift as ISGF3. Antibodies to Stat1 (α1) and Stat2 (α2) interfere with ISGF3, resulting in the disappearance of the gel shift signals. Stat3 specific serum (α3) has no effect. **B**: The same nuclear extracts were tested with an m67 oligonucleotide probe. The positions of SIF-A, SIF-B and SIF-C are indicated. IFN-α-induced formation of Stat1 and Stat3 complexes is impaired in cells expressing viral proteins. Antiserum to Stat1 (α1) supershifts SIF-B and SIF-C. Antiserum to Stat3 (α3) supershifts SIF-A and SIF-B. **C**: Western blot with the monoclonal antibody C7-50 against the HCV core protein with the corresponding cytoplasmic extracts. Viral proteins are expressed only in UHCV-11 and UHCV-32 cells cultured in the absence of tetracycline. Molecular weight markers in kDa are indicated on the left. From Heim MH *et al.* J Virol 1999;73:8469–75 with minor modifications. Reprinted with permission from the American Society for Microbiology.

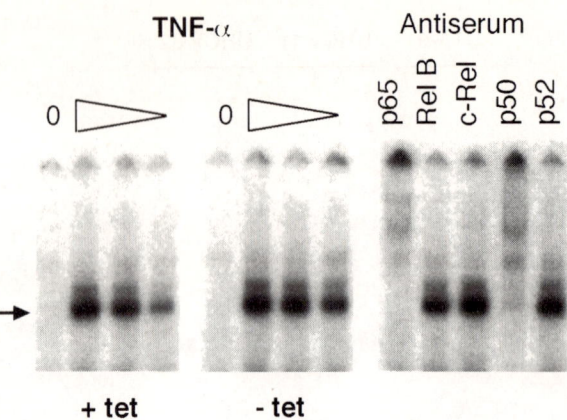

Figure 5 TNF-α-induced NF-κB activation is not inhibited by HCV protein expression. UHCV-32 cells were cultured in the presence or absence of tetracycline, as indicated at the bottom. Cells were left untreated or were stimulated for 15 min with 1000, 100, or 10 U/ml TNF-α, as indicated on top. EMSA was performed with nuclear extracts using the NF-κB consensus oligonucleotide. As shown in the right panel, antiserum specific for p65 and p50 can supershift the TNF-α-induced NF-κB shift. From Heim MH *et al.* J Virol 1999;73:8469–75 with minor modifications. Reprinted with permission from the American Society for Microbiology.

impaired STAT activation at the receptor–kinase complex, Stat1 was immuno-precipitated from whole-cell extracts of UHCV cells stimulated with IFN-α or left untreated after culture in the presence or absence of tetracycline. Phospho-Stat1-specific signals showed the same intensity in repressed and derepressed cells (Fig. 6). Stat2 phosphorylation was not inhibited either, as demonstrated by co-immunoprecipitation experiments. Co-immunoprecipitation is an indirect but reliable indicator of Stat2 phosphorylation, because Stat1–Stat2 heterodimers form only if both Stat1 and Stat2 are tyrosine phosphorylated. We concluded from these experiments that activation of STATs through tyrosine phosphoryla-tion at the receptor–kinase complex was not inhibited by HCV proteins. Viral protein expression could also diminish the cellular concentrations of STAT pro-teins or of ISGF3γ-p48 by either enhanced protein degradation or impaired gene expression. We could not, however, detect any quantitative difference for Stat1, Stat2, Stat3, or ISGF3γ-p48. Additional experiments, not shown here, suggest that viral proteins do not inhibit nuclear translocation of STATs. Since neither activation of STATs nor their nuclear translocation seems to be inhibited, we believe that HCV proteins or cellular proteins induced by the expression of viral proteins in an indirect way most likely interfere with DNA binding of STATs.

Finally, to examine the effect of HCV protein expression on the induction of IFN-α target genes, UGFP-9 and UHCV cells were cultured for 24 h in the presence or absence of tetracycline, stimulated for 8 h with IFN-α, and subse-quently examined for the expression of ISGF3γ-p48 and Stat1. As shown in Fig. 7, the inhibition of Jak-STAT signalling in UHCV cells resulted in reduced up-regulation of ISGF3γ-p48 and Stat1. Up-regulation of IFN-α-induced target genes was unaffected in UGFP-9 cells which inducibly express GFP as a non-relevant control protein. These observations indicate that the expression of HCV

A   IP with α-Stat1

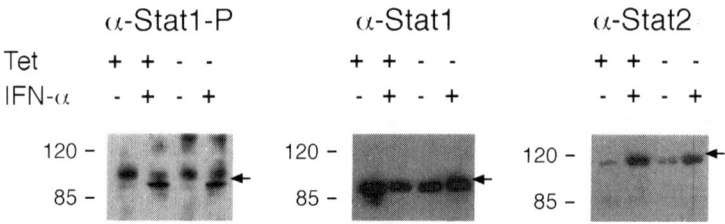

B   Supernatant

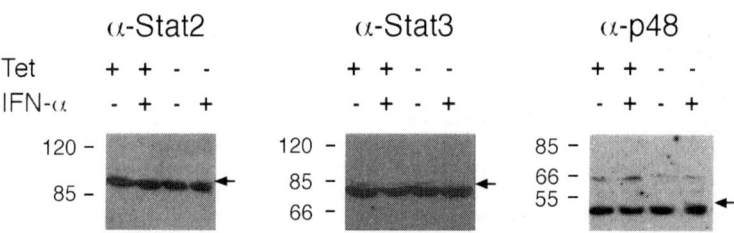

Figure 6   Phosphorylation of STAT proteins is not impaired by HCV protein expression. UHCV-32 cells were cultured for 24 h in the presence or absence of tetracycline and then left untreated or stimulated with IFN-α. Whole-cell lysates were prepared and used for immunoprecipitations with anti-Stat1-specific serum. **A**: The precipitated proteins were separated by SDS-Page, followed by Western blot analysis with antiserum to the phosphorylated form of Stat1 (α-Stat1-P), Stat1 in general (α-Stat1) and Stat2 (α-Stat2). Stat1 phosphorylation and heterodimerization with Stat2 were unaffected by HCV protein expression. **B**: Supernatants of the immunoprecipitation pellets were analysed by Western blot with antisera specific for Stat2 (α-Stat2), Stat3 (α-Stat3), and ISGF3γ-p48 (α-p48). The expression levels of these proteins were not influenced by viral protein expression. Molecular weight markers in kDa are indicated on the left. From Heim MH *et al.* J Virol 1999;73:8469–75. Reprinted with permission from the American Society for Microbiology.

proteins in UHCV cells affects not only IFN signalling but IFN effector functions as well.

In conclusion, expression of HCV proteins in UHCV cells inhibits IFN-α-induced signal transduction through the Jak-STAT pathway. Inhibition occurred downstream of STAT tyrosine phosphorylation and resulted in an impaired up-regulation of IFN target genes. In the context of a natural HCV infection, interference with IFN-induced signalling could be a strategy of HCV to escape natural host defence mechanisms. However, the biological and clinical relevance of these results clearly needs to be further addressed once a cell culture system is available, allowing productive HCV infection. In particular, it is presently unknown whether the inhibition of Jak-STAT signalling observed in our cell lines *in vitro* will be operative at the low levels of viral proteins expressed during natural HCV infection *in vivo*. In chronic HCV infection lasting for decades, however, even a slight impairment of IFN activity could contribute to viral persistence and pathogenesis. In addition, immunohistochemical analyses have shown that viral antigen expression in human liver in chronic hepatitis C is focal, with scattered hepatocytes

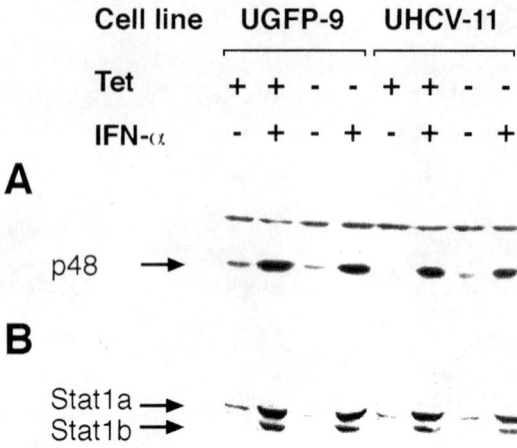

Figure 7 IFN-α-induced up-regulation of target genes is inhibited by the expression of HCV proteins. UGFP-9 and UHCV-11 cells were cultured for 24 h in the presence or absence of tetracycline as indicated and then stimulated for 8 h with 100 U/ml IFN-α. Expression levels of (**A**) ISGF3γ-p48 and (**B**) Stat1 were assessed by immunoblot following SDS-Page of whole-cell extracts. The non-specific band detected by the ISGF3γ-p48 antibody serves as an internal loading control. Stat1a and Stat1b are differentially spliced forms of Stat1. From Heim MH *et al*. J Virol 1999;73:8469–75 with minor modifications. Reprinted with permission from the American Society for Microbiology.

expressing higher levels of HCV antigens next to negative cells. It is possible, therefore, that in natural HCV infection in some hepatocytes viral antigen expression may reach levels similar to those in our *in vitro* system.

SUMMARY AND PERSPECTIVES

IFN-α is widely used for the treatment of chronic hepatitis B and C. The mode of action is incompletely understood and most likely involves both direct antiviral and immunomodulatory mechanisms. In chronic hepatitis B and C, however, a sustained response to IFN-α therapy is achieved in less than 40% of patients. Recent experimental data suggest that both HBV and HCV have developed strategies to resist the antiviral effects of IFN-α. In this context we have found that the expression of HCV proteins inhibits IFN-α-induced signalling from the cell surface receptor to the nucleus through the Jak-STAT pathway. Inhibition occurred downstream of STAT tyrosine phosphorylation and resulted in an impaired up-regulation of IFN target genes. In addition, others have found that the HCV envelope glycoprotein E2 and the non-structural protein NS5A may inhibit PKR. These mechanisms could contribute to the resistance to IFN-α observed in the majority of patients, and may represent a general escape strategy contributing to HCV persistence and pathogenesis of chronic liver disease. A better understanding of the interactions between HBV or HCV and the IFN system may ultimately result in more effective therapies against these viruses that are the leading cause of chronic hepatitis, liver cirrhosis, and HCC worldwide.

Acknowledgements

This work was supported by grants Mo 799/1-1 and Mo 799/1-2 from the Deutsche Forschungsgemeinschaft to D.M. and H.E.B., and grant 32-54973.98 from the Swiss National Science Foundation to M.H.H.

References

1. Hoofnagle JH, Di Bisceglie AM. The treatment of chronic viral hepatitis. N Engl J Med. 1997;336:347–56.
2. Lee WM. Hepatitis B virus infection. N Engl J Med. 1997;337:1733–45.
3. National Institutes of Health consensus development conference panel statement: management of hepatitis C. Hepatology. 1997;26(Suppl.1):2–10S.
4. Moradpour D, Blum HE. Current and evolving therapies for hepatitis C. Eur J Gastroenterol Hepatol. 1999;11:1199–202.
5. Jilbert AR, Burrell CJ, Gowans EJ, Hertzog PJ, Linnane AW, Marmion BP. Cellular localization of alpha-interferon in hepatitis B virus-infected liver tissue. Hepatology. 1986;6:957–61.
6. Dienes HP, Hess G, Woorsdorfer M et al. Ultrastructural localization of interferon-producing cells in the livers of patients with chronic hepatitis B. Hepatology. 1991;13:321–6.
7. Nouri-Aria KT, Arnold J, Davison F et al. Hepatic interferon-alpha gene transcripts and products in liver specimens from acute and chronic hepatitis B virus infection [published erratum appears in Hepatology. 1991;14:1308]. Hepatology. 1991;13:1029–34.
8. Greenway AL, Hertzog PJ, Devenish RJ, Dudley FJ, McMullen GL, Linnane AW. Immuno-localisation of interferon-alpha in hepatitis C patients and its correlation with response to interferon-alpha therapy. J Hepatol. 1994;21:842–52.
9. Stark GR, Kerr IM, Williams BR, Silverman RH, Schreiber RD. How cells respond to interferons. Annu Rev Biochem. 1998;67:227–64.
10. Meurs E, Chong K, Galabru J et al. Molecular cloning and characterization of the human double-stranded RNA-activated protein kinase induced by interferon. Cell. 1990;62:379–90.
11. Schultz U, Köck J, Schlicht HJ, Stäheli P. Recombinant duck interferon: a new reagent for studying the mode of interferon action against hepatitis B virus. Virology. 1995;212:641–9.
12. Heuss LT, Heim MH, Schultz U et al. Biological efficacy and signal transduction through STAT proteins of recombinant duck interferon in duck hepatitis B virus infection. J Gen Virol. 1998;79:2007–12.
13. Schultz U, Summers J, Stäheli P, Chisari FV. Elimination of duck hepatitis B virus RNA-containing capsids in duck interferon-alpha-treated hepatocytes. J Virol. 1999;73:5459–65.
14. Guidotti LG, Ishikawa T, Hobbs MV, Matzke B, Schreiber R, Chisari FV. Intracellular inactivation of the hepatitis B virus by cytotoxic T lymphocytes. Immunity. 1996;4:25–36.
15. Guidotti LG, Rochford R, Chung J, Shapiro M, Purcell R, Chisari FV. Viral clearance without destruction of infected cells during acute HBV infection. Science. 1999;284:825–9.
16. Ploegh HL. Viral strategies of immune evasion. Science. 1998;280:248–53.
17. Cerny A, Chisari FV. Pathogenesis of chronic hepatitis C: immunological features of hepatic injury and viral persistence. Hepatology. 1999;30:595–601.
18. Foster GR, Ackrill AM, Goldin RD, Kerr IM, Thomas HC, Stark GR. Expression of the terminal protein region of hepatitis B virus inhibits cellular responses to interferons alpha and gamma and double-stranded RNA [published erratum appears in Proc Natl Acad Sci USA. 1995;92:3632]. Proc Natl Acad Sci USA. 1991;88:2888–92.
19. Foster GR, Goldin RD, Hay A, McGarvey MJ, Stark GR, Thomas HC. Expression of the terminal protein of hepatitis B virus is associated with failure to respond to interferon therapy. Hepatology. 1993;17:757–62.
20. Rosmorduc O, Sirma H, Soussan P et al. Inhibition of interferon-inducible MxA protein expression by hepatitis B virus capsid protein. J Gen Virol. 1999;80:1253–62.
21. Podevin P, Guechot J, Serfaty L et al. Evidence for a deficiency of interferon response in mononuclear cells from hepatitis C viremic patients. J Hepatol. 1997;27:265–71.
22. Tanji Y, Kaneko T, Satoh S, Shimotohno K. Phosphorylation of hepatitis C virus-encoded nonstructural protein NS5A. J Virol. 1995;69:3980–6.
23. Reed KE, Xu J, Rice CM. Phosphorylation of the hepatitis C virus NS5A protein *in vitro* and *in vivo*: properties of the NS5A-associated kinase. J Virol. 1997;71:7187–97.

24. Reed KE, Gorbalenya AE, Rice CM. The NS5A/NS5 proteins of viruses from three genera of the family Flaviviridae are phosphorylated by associated serine/threonine kinases. J Virol. 1998;72:6199–206.
25. Koch JO, Bartenschlager R. Modulation of hepatitis C virus NS5A hyperphosphorylation by nonstructural proteins NS3, NS4A, and NS4B. J Virol. 1999;73:7138–46.
26. Enomoto N, Sakuma I, Asahina Y et al. Comparison of full-length sequences of interferon-sensitive and resistant hepatitis C virus 1b. J Clin Invest. 1995;96:224–30.
27. Enomoto N, Sakuma I, Asahina Y et al. Mutations in the nonstructural protein 5A gene and response to interferon in patients with chronic hepatitis C virus 1b infection. N Engl J Med. 1996;334:77–81.
28. Chayama K, Tsubota A, Kobayashi M et al. Pretreatment virus load and multiple amino acid substitutions in the interferon sensitivity-determining region predict the outcome of interferon treatment in patients with chronic genotype 1b hepatitis C virus infection. Hepatology. 1997;25:745–9.
29. Kurosaki M, Enomoto N, Murakami T et al. Analysis of genotypes and amino acid residues 2209 to 2248 of the NS5A region of hepatitis C virus in relation to the response to interferon-beta therapy. Hepatology. 1997;25:750–3.
30. Hofgärtner WT, Polyak SJ, Sullivan DG, Carithers RL, Jr, Gretch DR. Mutations in the NS5A gene of hepatitis C virus in North American patients infected with HCV genotype 1a or 1b. J Med Virol. 1997;53:118–26.
31. Khorsi H, Castelain S, Wyseur A et al. Mutations of hepatitis C virus 1b NS5A 2209–2248 amino acid sequence do not predict the response to recombinant interferon-alfa therapy in French patients. J Hepatol. 1997;27:72–7.
32. Squadrito G, Leone F, Sartori M et al. Mutations in the nonstructural 5A region of hepatitis C virus and response of chronic hepatitis C to interferon alfa. Gastroenterology. 1997;113:567–72.
33. Zeuzem S, Lee JH, Roth WK. Mutations in the nonstructural 5A gene of European hepatitis C virus isolates and response to interferon alfa. Hepatology. 1997;25:740–4.
34. Duverlie G, Khorsi H, Castelain S et al. Sequence analysis of the NS5A protein of European hepatitis C virus 1b isolates and relation to interferon sensitivity. J Gen Virol. 1998;79:1373–81.
35. Pawlotsky JM, Germanidis G, Neumann AU, Pellerin M, Frainais PO, Dhumeaux D. Interferon resistance of hepatitis C virus genotype 1b: relationship to nonstructural 5A gene quasispecies mutations. J Virol. 1998;72:2795–805.
36. Rispeter K, Lu M, Zibert A, Wiese M, de Oliveira JM, Roggendorf M. The 'interferon sensitivity determining region' of hepatitis C virus is a stable sequence element. J Hepatol. 1998;29: 352–61.
37. Bréchot C. The direct interplay between HCV NS5A protein and interferon transduction signal: from clinical to basic science. J Hepatol. 1999;30:1152–4.
38. Sarrazin C, Berg T, Lee JH et al. Improved correlation between multiple mutations within the NS5A region and virological response in European patients chronically infected with hepatitis C virus type 1b undergoing combination therapy. J Hepatol. 1999;30:1004–13.
39. Gale MJ, Jr., Korth MJ, Tang NM et al. Evidence that hepatitis C virus resistance to interferon is mediated through repression of the PKR protein kinase by the nonstructural 5A protein. Virology. 1997;230:217–27.
40. Gale M, Jr, Blakely CM, Kwieciszewski B et al. Control of PKR protein kinase by hepatitis C virus nonstructural 5A protein: molecular mechanisms of kinase regulation. Mol Cell Biol. 1998;18:5208–18.
41. Gale M, Jr, Kwieciszewski B, Dossett M, Nakao H, Katze MG. Antiapoptotic and oncogenic potentials of hepatitis C virus are linked to interferon resistance by viral repression of the PKR protein kinase. J Virol. 1999;73:6506–16.
42. Tan SL, Nakao H, He Y et al. NS5A, a nonstructural protein of hepatitis C virus, binds growth factor receptor-bound protein 2 adaptor protein in a Src homology 3 domain/ligand-dependent manner and perturbs mitogenic signaling. Proc Natl Acad Sci USA. 1999;96:5533–8.
43. David M, Petricoin ER, Benjamin C, Pine R, Weber MJ, Larner AC. Requirement for MAP kinase (ERK2) activity in interferon alpha- and interferon beta-stimulated gene expression through STAT proteins. Science. 1995;269:1721–3.
44. Polyak SJ, Paschal DM, McArdle S, Gale MJ, Jr, Moradpour D, Gretch DR. Characterization of the effects of hepatitis C virus nonstructural 5A protein expression in human cell lines and on interferon-sensitive virus replication. Hepatology. 1999;29:1262–71.

45. Song J, Fujii M, Wang F, Itoh M, Hotta H. The NS5A protein of hepatitis C virus partially inhibits the antiviral activity of interferon. J Gen Virol. 1999;80:879–86.
46. Taylor DR, Shi ST, Romano PR, Barber GN, Lai MMC. Inhibition of the interferon-inducible protein kinase PKR by HCV E2 protein. Science. 1999;285:107–10.
47. Symons JA, Alcami A, Smith GL. Vaccinia virus encodes a soluble type I interferon receptor of novel structure and broad species specificity. Cell. 1995;81:551–60.
48. Miller DM, Rahill BM, Boss JM et al. Human cytomegalovirus inhibits major histocompatibility complex class II expression by disruption of the Jak/Stat pathway. J Exp Med. 1998;187:675–83.
49. Darnell JE, Jr, Kerr IM, Stark GR. Jak-STAT pathways and transcriptional activation in response to IFNs and other extracellular signaling proteins. Science. 1994;264:1415–21.
50. Ihle JN. STATs: signal transducers and activators of transcription. Cell. 1996;84:331–4.
51. Ransohoff RM. Cellular responses to interferons and other cytokines: the JAK-STAT paradigm. N Engl J Med. 1998;338:616–18.
52. Heim MH. The Jak-STAT pathway: cytokine signalling from the receptor to the nucleus. J Recept Signal Transduct Res. 1999;19:75–120.
53. Moradpour D, Kary P, Rice CM, Blum HE. Continuous human cell lines inducibly expressing hepatitis C virus structural and nonstructural proteins. Hepatology. 1998;28:192–201.
54. Heim MH, Moradpour D, Blum HE. Expression of hepatitis C virus proteins inhibits signal transduction through the Jak-STAT pathway. J Virol. 1999;73:8469–75.
55. Englert C, Hou X, Maheswaran S et al. WT1 suppresses synthesis of the epidermal growth factor receptor and induces apoptosis. EMBO J. 1995;14:4662–75.

20
Termination and modulation of interleukin-6-type cytokine signalling through the gp130/Jak/STAT pathway

P. C. HEINRICH, I. BEHRMANN, J. G. BODE, P. GATSIOS,
L. GRAEVE, H. M. HERMANNS, G. MÜLLER-NEWEN,
A. NIMMESGERN, S. PFLANZ, S. RADTKE, F. SCHAPER,
J. SCHMITZ, E. SIEWERT, L. TERSTEGEN, S. THIEL and
M. WEISSENBACH

INTRODUCTION

Interleukin (IL)-6 and the related cytokines IL-11, leukaemia inhibitory factor (LIF), oncostatin M (OSM), cardiotrophin-1 and ciliary neurotrophic factor (CNTF) have been shown to induce acute-phase protein (APP) expression in liver cells. All these IL-6-type cytokines exert their action either through the homodimerization of gp130 (IL-6, IL-11) or the heterodimerization of gp130 and LIF receptor (LIF, OSM, CNTF, CT-1). Alternatively, OSM can also signal through heterodimers of gp130 and the OSM-receptor β. The dimerization of these signal transducers results in the activation of the Janus kinase (Jak)/signal transducer and activator of transcription (STAT) pathway characterized by a cascade of tyrosine phosphorylations, the translocation of STAT dimers into the nucleus and the activation of IL-6-type cytokine target genes[1] (Fig. 1).

In collaboration with the laboratory of Ian Kerr it has been shown that the tyrosine phosphorylation of gp130, STAT1 and STAT3 is greatly impaired in Jak1-deficient cells, indicating a central role of Jak1 in IL-6 signalling[2]. These findings have recently been confirmed by *in-vivo* experiments with Jak1 knock-out mice[3].

By the use of chimaeric gp130 receptors we have shown that STAT3 is the most important APP inducer in human hepatoma cells[4].

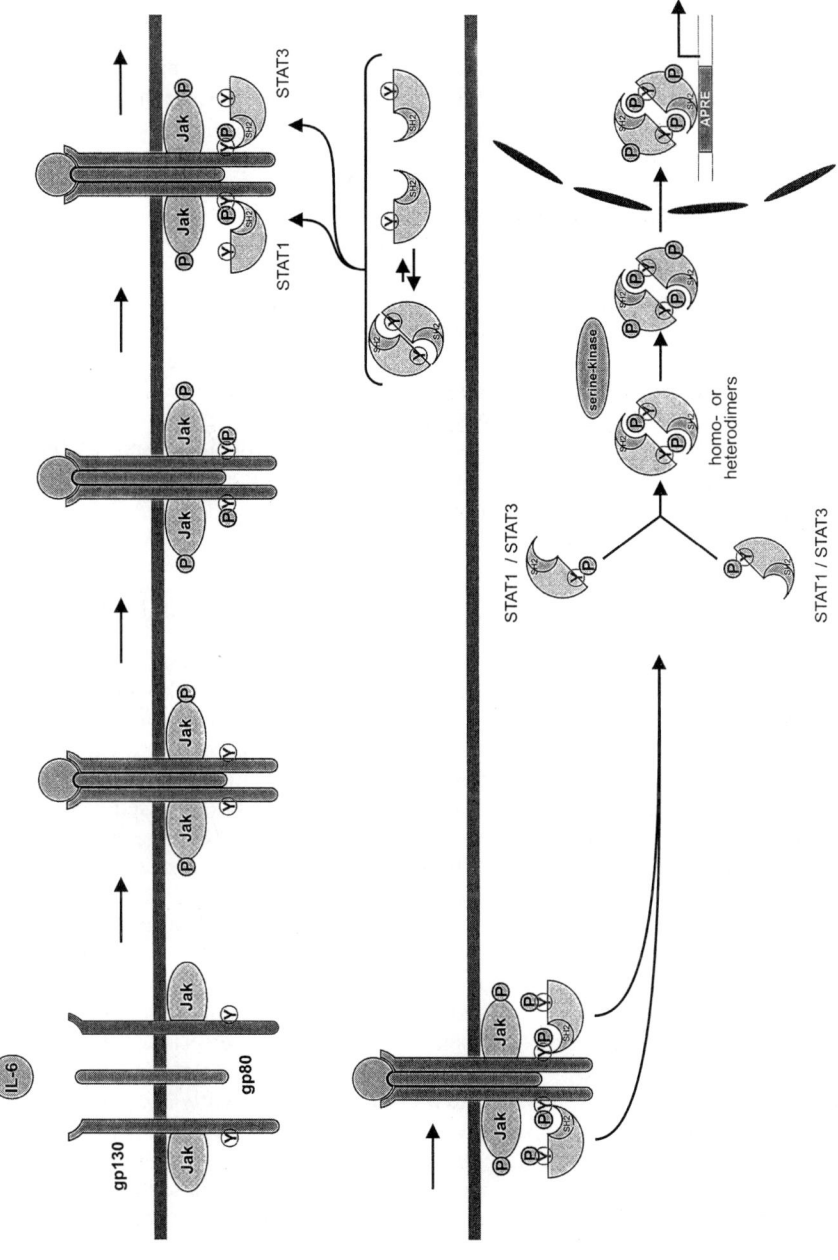

Figure 1 IL-6 signalling via the gp130/Jak/STAT pathway[1]

MOLECULAR MECHANISM OF gp130 ACTIVATION

The first molecular event in cytokine signal transduction is the activation of the receptor by its ligand. In this respect, receptors act like molecular switches that are turned on upon cytokine binding. To guarantee the highest reliability, receptors have to be silent in the absence of a stimulus and should trigger signal transduction only in the presence of the respective ligand. Thus, receptor activation is based on molecular recognition that provides specificity in receptor–ligand interaction and a molecular mechanism that couples ligand binding to signal transduction. The cyto-plasmic part of gp130 lacks any intrinsic kinase activity, but is constitutively associated with tyrosine kinases of the Jak family. The commonly accepted mechanism of receptor activation is ligand-induced dimerization of the receptor ectodomain leading to juxtaposition of the cytoplasmic parts and the associated kinases. As a consequence, the kinases are activated and phosphorylate downstream signalling molecules. A remaining question is whether receptor dimerization is necessary or even sufficient for receptor activation; i.e. are the receptors simply brought in spatial neighbourhood upon ligand binding or does the ligand induce a well-defined orientation and conformation of the receptor that could be a prerequisite for signal transduction. More provocative new findings on the erythropoietin (epo) receptor suggest that cytokine receptors may exist as preformed dimers that switch to an active conformation upon ligand binding[5].

ROLE OF THE MEMBRANE-DISTAL DOMAINS OF gp130 IN LIGAND BINDING

IL-6, IL-11 and CNTF must bind to specific α-receptor subunits (IL-6R, IL-11R, and CNTFR, respectively) before these cytokines are able to activate the signal-transducing receptor components gp130 or LIFR. These α-receptors can func-tionally be replaced by their soluble forms, since their cytoplasmic domains do not contribute to signal transduction. Gp130 is ubiquitously expressed, and tar-geted deletion of the gene in mice leads to embryonic lethality[6]. Responsiveness of cells to IL-6-type cytokines is tightly regulated by the more restricted expres-sion of IL-6R, IL-11R, CNTFR, LIFR and OSMR.

The ectodomain of gp130 is proposed to consist of an N-terminal Ig-like domain (D1) followed by a cytokine-binding module (CBM, D2–D3) and three fibronectin type III-like domains (D4–D6). The CBM is the hallmark of class I cytokine receptors and consists of two fibronectin type III-like domains. These conserved domains show a distinct pattern of four cysteine residues in the N-terminal domain and a WSXWS motif in the C-terminal domain. The structures of the CBM constituting domains 2 and 3 of gp130 have recently been solved by X-ray diffraction[7] as well as NMR spectroscopy[8]. In comparison to the ectodomains of short cytokine receptors such as epoR, IL-2R, IL-4R or GHR, that consist only of a single CBM, the architecture of gp130 is rather complex. Recent studies on the gp130 ectodomain have clarified the role of the individual domains in receptor activation. The Ig-like domain and the CBM of gp130 are required and sufficient to bind IL-6/IL-6R as well as IL-11/IL-11R complexes[9]. Inactive gp130 deletion mutants lacking D1 and gp130 muteins containing inactivating point mutations in the CBM complement each other (unpublished observations). Therefore, in contrast to the short cytokine receptors, gp130 binds its ligand non-symmetrically. In our current model the CBM of gp130 interacts with site II of the ligand whereas D1 binds site III.

ROLE OF THE MEMBRANE-PROXIMAL DOMAINS OF gp130 IN RECEPTOR ACTIVATION

Is high-affinity binding of the ligand to the membrane-distal part (D1–D3) of gp130 sufficient to transduce a signal, and what is the role of the membrane-proximal domains (D4–D6) of gp130 in receptor activation? A deletion mutant lacking D5 was stably transfected into Ba/F3 cells and analysed in respect to IL-6 binding and signal transduction in comparison with gp130 wild-type. In line with the above findings, deletion of D5 did not alter the affinity of the receptor to its ligand (Fig. 2, triangles). More surprisingly, however, this mutant was not able to transduce any signal in response to IL-6 or IL-11 stimulation (Fig. 3). Therefore, we argue that high-affinity ligand binding is not sufficient for receptor activation, but a defined active conformation has to be adjusted. If the corresponding domain of the related G-CSFR is added back to the above deletion

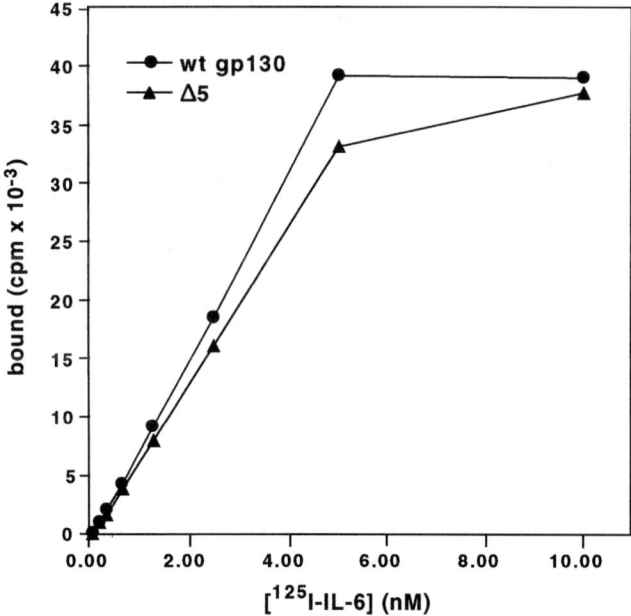

Figure 2 Binding of IL-6/sIL-6R complexes to membrane-bound gp130 wild-type and deletion mutant Δ5. 5×10^6 Ba/F3 cells stably transfected with gp130 or the deletion mutant Δ5, as well as untransfected cells, were incubated with 200 nM sIL-6R and different concentrations of [^{125}I]IL-6 (1340 cpm/fmol) for 16 h at 4°C. Radioactivity bound to untransfected cells was subtracted from radioactivity bound to transfected cells to obtain specific binding. Specifically bound radioactivity is presented as a function of [^{125}I]IL-6 concentration

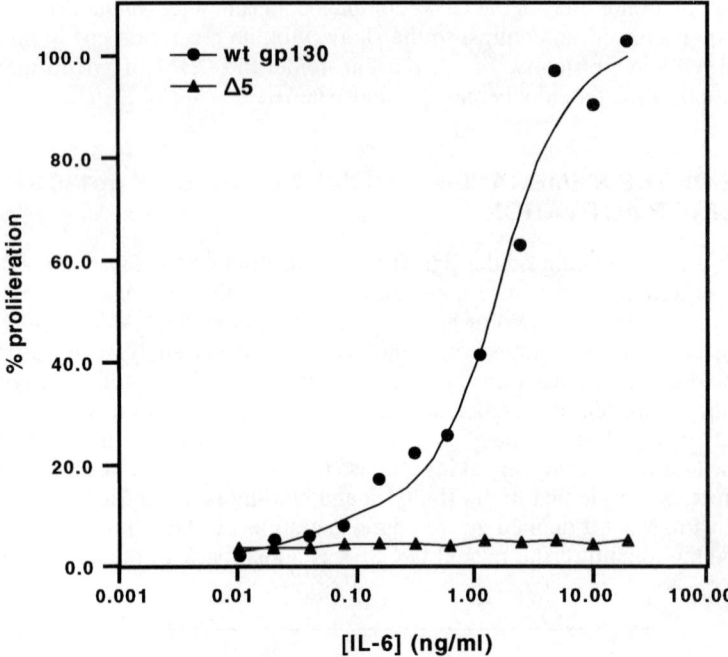

Figure 3 Biological activity of gp130 and the deletion mutant Δ5. Ba/F3 cells (4 × 10⁵/ml) stably transfected with gp130 or the deletion mutant Δ5 were seeded in a 96-well plate and incubated with 0.5 μg/ml sIL-6R and increasing amounts of IL-6 as indicated in the diagram. After 72 h a tetra-zolium compound was added as a substrate and incubated for 5 h at 37°C. Subsequently, the absorbance at 450 and 690 nm was measured. The difference of absorbances corresponds to the number of metabolically active cells (XTT proliferation assay)

mutant, functionality of the receptor is partially restored. Thus, we conclude that D5 of gp130 is required for adjustment of the correct spacing of the cytoplasmic parts of gp130. Therefore, a defined conformation of the gp130 dimer is a pre-requisite for signal transduction (Fig. 4).

Does the ligand actively dimerize the receptor, or is there a switch from an inactive to an active conformation in a preformed gp130 dimer induced? The fact that many cytokine receptors are activated by bivalent monoclonal anti-bodies served as an argument for the former possibility. We found that gp130 is not activated by a single monoclonal antibody, but that a specific combination of two different monoclonal antibodies against the gp130 ectodomain (B-S12-G7 and B-P8) is required to elicit a response comparable to IL-6 (unpublished observations). The individual antibodies do not induce signal transduction. In order to judge whether the antibodies activate gp130 by virtue of their bivalency, monovalent Fab fragments were prepared. Interestingly, the minimal require-ment for gp130 activation was found to be the combination of intact B-S12-G7 with a Fab fragment of B-P8. Neither the combination of B-P8 with the Fab fragment of B-S12-G7 nor the Fab fragments of both antibodies led to any receptor activation (unpublished observations). From these findings we conclude

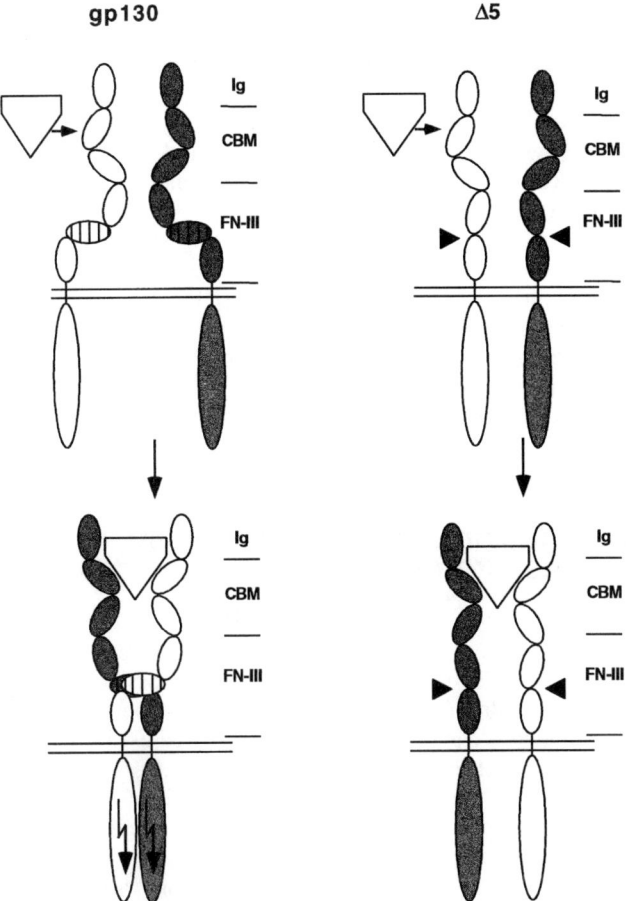

Figure 4 Proposed mechanism of gp130 activation. High-affinity binding of the ligand to the CBM and Ig-like domain of gp130 is not sufficient for receptor activation. The gp130 membrane-proximal domains are necessary for adjustment of the active dimer (left panel). The scheme highlights the functional role of domain 5 (striped) for productive spacing of the cytoplasmic part of gp130

that: (a) enforcement of receptor dimerization and (b) adjustment of a well-defined gp130 dimer conformation is required for gp130 activation and signal transduction.

FUNCTION OF THE INDIVIDUAL TYROSINE MOTIFS IN FULL-LENGTH gp130

Since there are six tyrosine residues in the cytoplasmic tail of gp130 we asked which tyrosine activates which STAT factor. Thus, we analysed the function of the individual cytoplasmic tyrosine residues of gp130 in the context of the full-length receptor protein in IL-6 signalling. Add-back receptor mutants containing only one cytoplasmic tyrosine were generated and tested for their efficiency in IL-6 signal transduction. Our studies have revealed that tyrosine motifs described to recruit STAT proteins[10] are not equivalent in respect to their potential to activate STAT factors and APP gene promoters: the two distal tyrosines Y905 and Y915 of gp130 were more potent than Y767 and Y814. Thus, the tyrosine residues in the cytoplasmic part of gp130 were found to contribute differentially to IL-6 signal transduction in the full-length gp130 protein. Surprisingly Y905 and Y915 mediate APP gene promoter activation stronger than the wild-type receptor containing all six cytoplasmic tyrosine residues. To elucidate the influence of the phosphotyrosine phosphatase SHP2 recruitment site in gp130 on STAT-mediated gene induction, chimaeric receptor add-back mutants containing tyrosine 759 plus one of the four membrane-distal cytoplasmic tyrosine residues were also analysed in the reporter gene assay with an α_2M-gene-promoter/luciferase construct. These experiments clearly demonstrate a negative influence of Y759 in gp130 on the α_2M-gene-promoter activation (Fig. 5).

CONTRIBUTIONS OF LIF RECEPTOR AND OSM RECEPTOR TO SIGNAL TRANSDUCTION IN HETERODIMERIC COMPLEXES WITH gp130

IL-6-type cytokines have in part overlapping functions, e.g. IL-6, LIF as well as OSM are able to induce the synthesis of APP in hepatocytes[1]. All three cytokines induce macrophage differentiation of mouse promyelocytic M1 cells[11–13]. This functional redundancy can be explained by the shared use of the receptor subunit gp130. Apart from exerting these redundant effects, each cytokine is additionally endowed with specific functions which can be explained in part by the restricted pattern of cytokine expression and the distribution of the ligand binding α-receptors. In addition, differences in signalling of gp130 homo- versus heterodimers have been noted, e.g. different preferences in STAT activation[14,15], differentiation of M1 transfectants, proliferation versus growth inhibition of breast carcinoma cells[16,17].

To study signalling of LIF and OSM we used a receptor system based on the extracellular parts of the IL-5Rα- and β-chains[18] which allows the directed formation of heterodimers, thereby mimicking the proposed natural receptor complexes (gp130/LIFR or gp130/OSMR). We investigated the contributions of LIFR and OSMR to signal transduction in human HepG2 hepatoma cells. In these cells LIF and OSM – as well as IL-6 – are able to induce the expression of genes encoding APP[19–21]. The cells were transfected with expression constructs encoding the receptor combinations, as indicated in Fig. 6, together with a luciferase reporter gene construct under the control of the α_2M promoter, an acute-phase response gene of the rat. Stimulation with IL-5 of both receptor combinations (α/gp130+β/LIFR, α/gp130+β/OSMR) led to a strong induction of luciferase activity which was comparable to that observed upon induced homodimerization of gp130 cytoplasmic tails (α/gp130+β/gp130). α/gp130 did not elicit luciferase expression when dimerized with β/Δcyt, a receptor chimaera devoid of a cytoplasmic region (Fig. 6). This indicates that the cytoplasmic parts

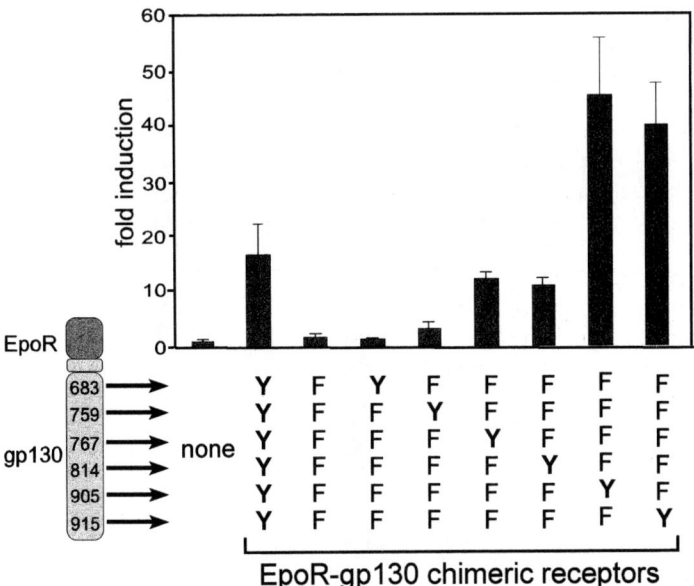

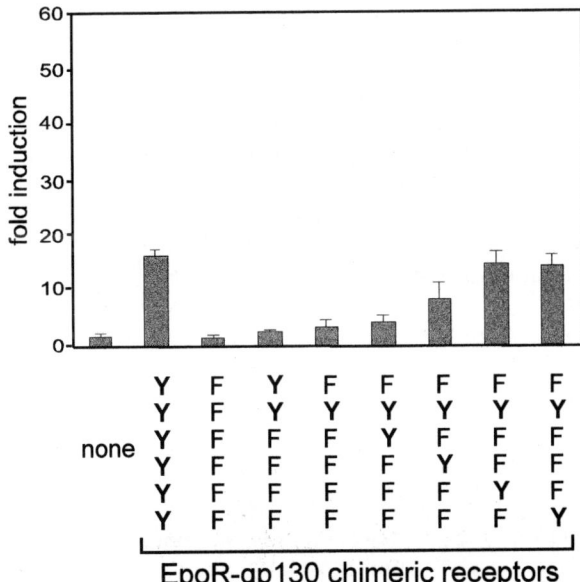

Figure 5 IL-6-stimulated gene induction via individual tyrosine motifs of gp130. HepG2 cells were transiently transfected with constructs coding for chimaeric receptor mutants containing the extracellular domain of the murine epoR, and the transmembrane and intracellular domains of gp130 Y→F mutants and an α_2M–promoter–luciferase gene reporter construct. Cells were untreated or stimulated with 7 U of epo/ml for 16 h. Luciferase activity was determined and related to the corresponding unstimulated cells

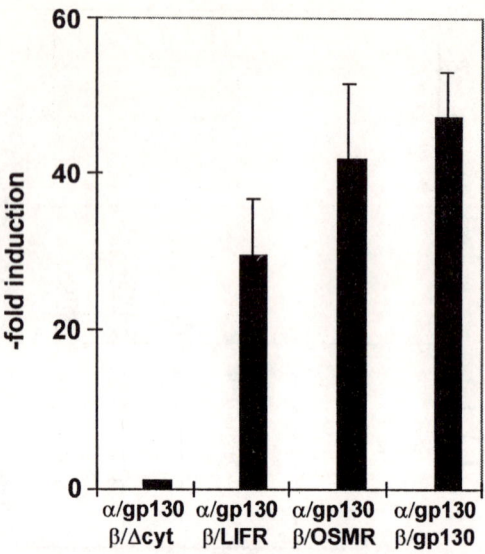

Figure 6 The cytoplasmic regions of LIFR and of OSMR contribute to signalling in heterodimeric complexes with gp130. HepG2 cells were transfected with expression plasmids encoding α/gp130 and the indicated β-chimaera together with an α_2M–promoter–luciferase reporter gene construct. One day after transfection cells were stimulated with IL-5 (80 ng/ml) for 24 h or left untreated. Luciferase activity of lysates was normalized to the activity of coexpressed β-galactosidase. The 'fold inductions' (relative to untreated cells) of three or four independent experiments (mean + SD) are presented

of LIFR and of OSMR contribute to signalling in heterodimeric complexes with α/gp130.

We then tested the ability of the heterodimeric receptor combinations to activate the transcription factor STAT3 in COS-7 cells. As indicated in the electrophoretic mobility shift assay (EMSA) in Fig. 7, the STAT signal of the heterodimer of gp130 and LIFR cytoplasmic parts (left panel) was somewhat weaker compared to that of the corresponding combination of gp130 cytoplasmic parts. The heterodimer of OSMR and gp130, however, turned out to be a stronger activator of STAT3 (right panel).

To further delineate the contributions of LIFR to signal transduction, we took advantage of chimaeras depicted in Fig. 8. Interestingly, a receptor combination of α/gp130-B1/2 (B1/2 = box 1/2) with full-length β/LIFR was able to induce a STAT signal, whereas a combination in which only the membrane-proximal parts of the LIFR and gp130 were present was not functional (Fig. 8, left panel). While a receptor combination in which only one gp130 cytoplasmic chain was present (α/gp130 + β/Δcyt) did not elicit STAT activation, the combination with the membrane-proximal region of the LIFR (α/gp130 + β/LIFR-B1/2) resulted in a STAT signal (Fig. 8, right panel). Analogous results were obtained for a heterodimeric combination of OSMR and gp130 parts (data not shown). Thus, membrane-proximal regions of LIFR or OSMR are crucial for signal transduction in the heterodimeric receptor complex. Only one cytoplasmic tail has to

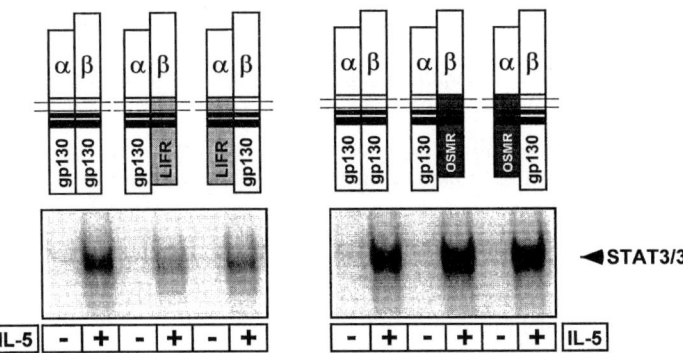

Figure 7   Induced heterodimerization of the cytoplasmic parts of the LIFR or OSMR with gp130 leads to STAT activation. COS-7 cells were cotransfected with expression plasmids encoding the IL-5Rα- and β-chimaeras as indicated, together with 5 μg of a STAT3 expression vector. Three days after transfection the cells were stimulated with IL-5 (80 ng/ml) for 30 min, or left untreated, before nuclear extracts were prepared. EMSAs were performed using the m67SIE probe. The bands resulting from STAT3 homodimers are marked

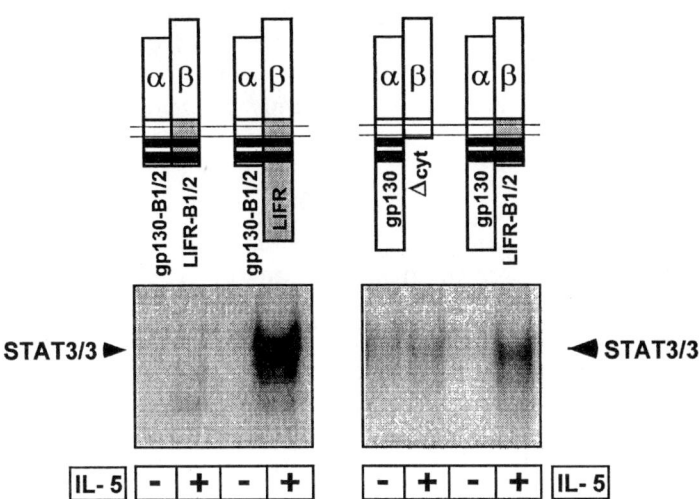

Figure 8   Both the membrane-proximal and -distal parts of the LIFR contribute to signalling in a heterodimeric complex with gp130. COS-7 cells were transfected with expression plasmids encoding STAT3, the IL-5Rα and β-chimaeras as indicated. Three days after transfection the cells were stimulated with IL-5 (80 ng/ml) for 30 min, or left untreated, before nuclear extracts were prepared. EMSAs were performed using the m67SIE probe. The bands resulting from STAT3 homodimers are marked

contain STAT recruitment sites and these can be contributed by either gp130, LIFR or OSMR[22].

The major part of this review deals with various mechanisms involved in the termination and modulation of IL-6 signalling:

1. tyrosine phosphatases – e.g. SHP2 – affects STAT and APP-promoter activation and
2. feedback inhibitors – suppressors of cytokine signalling (SOCS) – inhibit IL-6 signalling by inactivating Janus kinases.

In addition to these termination mechanisms, IL-6-type cytokine signalling is regulated by receptor internalization as well as by different half-lives of the signalling molecules.

In the last part of this review it is shown that activation of the MAP kinase ERK-2 – but not the JNK or p38 kinases – attenuates the IL-6-induced tyrosine phosphorylation of gp130, SHP2, STAT1 and STAT3 in HepG2 cells.

Finally, data will be presented on the inhibition of IL-6-induced STAT activation by tumour necrosis factor-α (TNF-α) in rat macrophages.

TERMINATION OF IL-6 SIGNALLING

SHP2 in IL-6 signal transduction

One immediate early effect of IL-6 stimulation is the tyrosine phosphorylation of the tyrosine phosphatase SHP2. SHP2 is able to bind grb2, and very probably links the Jak/STAT pathway to the ras/raf/MAPK pathway. When human fibrosarcoma cell lines deficient in Jak1, Jak2 or Tyk2 were stimulated with IL-6/sIL-6R complexes, it was found that only in Jak1 – but not in Jak2 – or Tyk2-deficient cells SHP2 activation was greatly impaired. We concluded that

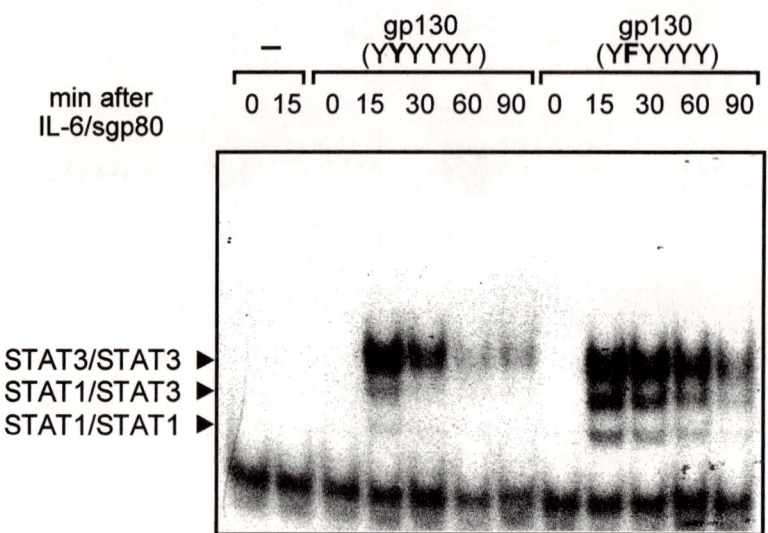

Figure 9 Prolonged STAT activation by the substitution of phenylalanine for tyrosine 759 of gp130. Wild-type and stably transfected Ba/F3 cells expressing native gp130 or the Y759→F receptor mutant were stimulated with IL-6/sIL-6R for the times indicated. Nuclear extracts of these cells were analysed for binding a STAT1/STAT3-specific DNA probe in EMSA

Jak1 is required for the tyrosine phosphorylation of SHP2[23]. This phosphorylation depends on tyrosine 759 in the cytoplasmic region of gp130, since a
Y759→F exchange abrogates SHP2 activation[24] and in turn leads to elevated
and prolonged STAT1 and STAT3 activation (Fig. 9), resulting in an enhanced
APP gene induction[23].

Feedback inhibitors: suppressors of cytokine signalling

Recently, a new family of inhibitors of cytokine signalling has been discovered
in three different laboratories. These proteins are referred to as suppressors of
cytokine signalling (SOCS)[25], Jak-binding proteins (JAB)[26] or STAT-induced
STAT inhibitors (SSI)[27]. Depending on the cell type examined, SOCS1, SOCS2,
and SOCS3 expression was found to be rapidly induced by IL-6[25]. Interestingly,
SOCS1, SOCS2 and SOCS3 differ in their potential to inhibit IL-6 signal transduction[28]. We found SOCS1 and SOCS3 to be potent inhibitors of IL-6-induced
activation of an α_2M promoter reporter construct. In contrast, the regulatory
potentials of SOCS2 and CIS (a formerly described member of the family of
SOCS proteins) are negligible (Fig. 10). There is at present no explanation for
the different specificities of the individual SOCS proteins.

Half-lives of signalling components

Whereas considerable information has been accumulated concerning the time-
course of activation for the individual signalling molecules, data on the availability of the proteins involved in IL-6-type cytokine signal transduction are scarce.
Nevertheless, the availability of these molecules, determined by the balance of

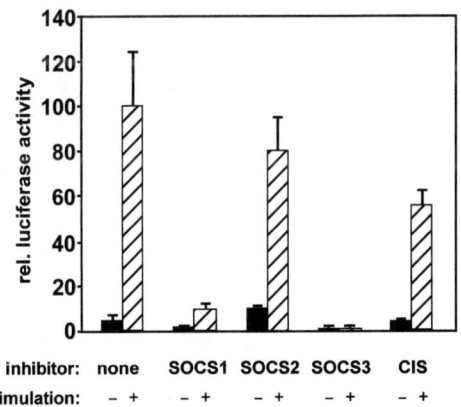

Figure 10 SOCS1 and SOCS3 are potent inhibitors of α_2M gene promoter activation. Human
hepatoma cells (HepG2) were transfected with expression vectors coding for the EpoR/gp130 chimaeric receptor proteins, and for the indicated SOCS/CIS proteins and an α_2M-gene promoter
luciferase reporter gene construct. The cells were stimulated for 16 h with 7 U/ml Epo where indicated, and cellular extracts were prepared for the determination of luciferase activity. Luciferase
expression was normalized to the luciferase activity in cell extracts from stimulated HepG2 cells
which were not transfected with SOCS-cDNAs

Table 1   Half-lives of the proteins involved in IL-6-type cytokine signalling[29]

Protein	Half-life (h)
gp130	2.5
Jak1	3.2
Jak2	1.9
Tyk2	2
SOCS-1	1.5
SOCS-2	1
SOCS-3	1.6
STAT3	8.5
STAT1	16
SHP2	18–20

protein synthesis and degradation, also influences IL-6-type cytokine signal transduction. We therefore analysed the half-lives of the key molecules involved in the IL-6 signal transduction pathway. The turnover rates for the various proteins differ substantially[29]. Three groups of signalling proteins can be discriminated: whereas the feedback inhibitors SOCS1, SOCS2 and SOCS3 are very short-lived (1–1.5 h), STAT1, STAT3 and SHP2 have an extremely low turnover (8.5–20 h). The Janus kinases Jak1, Jak2, Tyk2 and gp130 show intermediate half-lives (2–3 h). Our data (summarized in Table 1) imply that signalling components activated by post-translational modifications are long-lived, whereas the activity of very short-lived proteins is mainly regulated at the transcriptional level.

Endocytosis of the IL-6 receptor complex

Most cells escape from being overstimulated by surface receptor internalization. After binding to its receptor, IL-6 is efficiently internalized and the α-receptors/gp80 are down-regulated, resulting in a complete depletion of IL-6 surface binding sites within 30–60 min[30]. In order to replenish IL-6 binding sites, *de-novo* protein synthesis is required, suggesting that ligand and gp80 have been degraded after internalization, most likely in the lysosomal compartment. We have previously demonstrated that the IL-6 signal transducer gp130 contains a di-leucine internalization motif within its cytoplasmic tail necessary for the endocytosis of the IL-6 receptor complex[31]. Since gp80 *per se* is internalized very inefficiently, the observed down-regulation of gp80 can be explained by the formation of the ternary receptor complex in which gp130 not only mediates signal transduction but also promotes efficient endocytosis of the IL-6 receptor complex. Recently, we have demonstrated activation of the Jak/STAT pathway via the IL-6 receptor complex or agonistic antibodies against gp130 not to be required for efficient endocytosis to occur[32], suggesting that signalling and endocytosis are independent processes. Interestingly, the signal transducer gp130 undergoes constitutive endocytosis independent of the presence of a ligand. The constitutive internalization of gp130 occurs most probably via clathrin-coated pits, since a constitutive interaction between gp130 and the plasma membrane adaptor protein complex AP-2 has been observed[33].

Upon ligand binding, all IL-6-type cytokines recruit gp130 to their receptor complexes, forming homo- or heterodimeric signal-transducing receptor complexes. We therefore examined whether gp130 alone is responsible for mediating endocytosis of all receptor complexes formed. Using a chimaeric receptor system we found that the cytoplasmic domain of the LIF-R contains an autonomous di-leucine-based leucine–isoleucine internalization motif, which mediates efficient endocytosis of the LIFR independent of the IL-6 signal transducer gp130[34].

Preactivation of Erk1/2 inhibits IL-6-induced STAT signalling

Recently it became evident that signalling events induced by the binding of a mediator to its respective receptor experience remarkable modulations by crosstalks with other signal transduction pathways activated by parallel-acting cytokines, i.e. the response of an organism towards a single mediator depends largely on simultaneously acting factors.

A number of mediators have been reported to down-regulate Jak/STAT activation, e.g. transforming growth factor β, granulocyte/macrophage colony-stimulating factor and angiotensin II[35–37]. The protein kinase C activator phorbol 12-myristate 13-acetate (PMA) was recently shown to inhibit IL-6-induced STAT3 activation via the Erk/MAP kinases[38]. The mechanism of this inhibition, however, still remains to be elucidated. Therefore, inhibition of IL-6-induced STAT activation by PMA was studied in human hepatoma cells. HepG2 cells were pretreated with PMA for 45 min and subsequently stimulated with IL-6 (100 U/ml) for 15 min. Western blot analyses of nuclear extracts using specific antibodies against the tyrosine-phosphorylated forms of STAT1 and STAT3 were performed (Fig. 11A). Tyrosine phosphorylation of both STAT1 and STAT3 was induced by IL-6 and clearly decreased after PMA pretreatment. Electrophoretic mobility shift assays (EMSA) revealed that the reduced STAT phosphorylation results in a strongly diminished DNA binding of STAT1 and STAT3 which is partially reversed by the specific MEK inhibitor PD98059 (Fig. 11B). Furthermore, the tyrosine phosphorylation of the signal transducer gp130 and of the phosphotyrosine phosphatase SHP2 also underlie a negative regulation by MAP kinases (Fig. 11C). In addition, basic fibroblast growth factor, a physiological activator of MAP kinases (Erk2)[39], negatively regulates IL-6-induced STAT activation in a similar fashion in NIH-3T3 cells (Fig. 12).

Transient transfection studies in COS-7 cells with chimaeric receptor mutants consisting of the extracellular part of the erythropoietin (Epo) receptor and wild-type or mutant forms of the gp130 transmembrane and cytoplasmic domains (Fig. 13A)[10,15] show that tyrosine-759 of gp130 – the docking site for SHP2 – is crucial for the inhibitory effect of MAP kinases (Fig. 13B). Inhibition is also dependent on de novo mRNA and protein synthesis since preincubation of HepG2/NIH-3T3 cells with actinomycin D or cycloheximide leads to a partial reversal of the inhibitory PMA/bFGF effect. Both PMA and bFGF rapidly stimulate mRNA expression of the suppressor of cytokine signalling-3 (SOCS-3) (Fig. 14A). These results raise the intriguing possibility that pretreatment of cells with PMA or bFGF inhibits the subsequent stimulation of the Jak/STAT pathway via induction of its negative feedback inhibitor SOCS-3 (Fig. 14B).

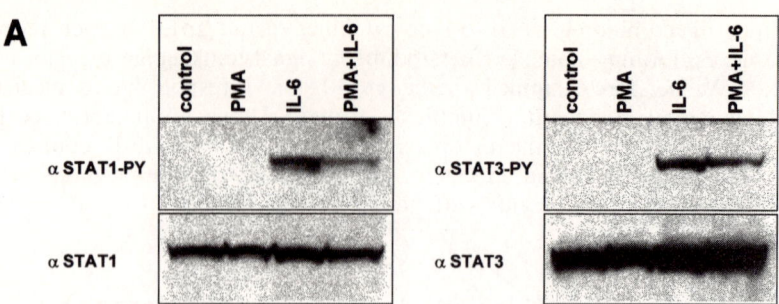

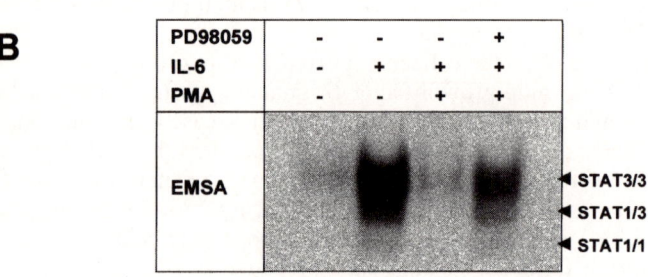

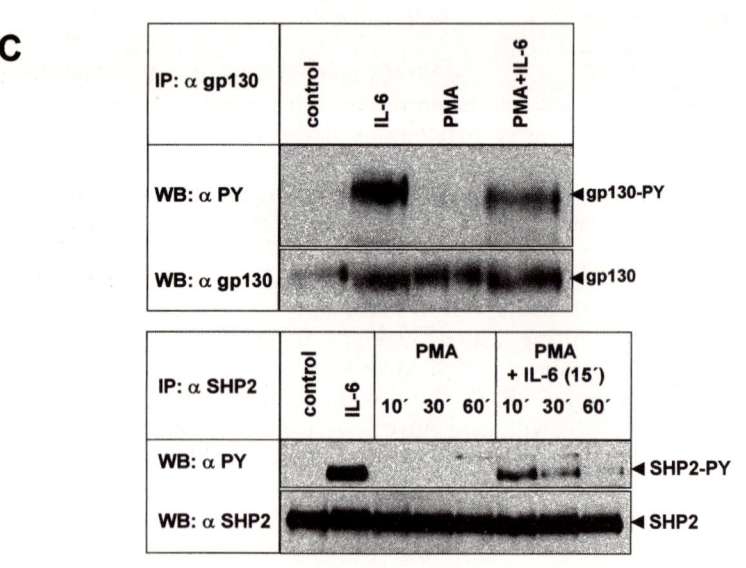

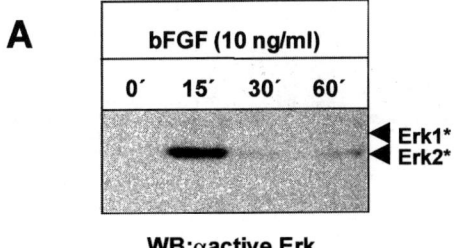

A

bFGF (10 ng/ml)			
0′	15′	30′	60′

◄ Erk1*
◄ Erk2*

WB:αactive Erk

B

PD98059	-	-	-	+
IL-6+sgp80	-	+	+	+
bFGF	-	-	+	+

EMSA

◄ STAT3/3
◄ STAT1/3
◄ STAT1/1

Figure 12 Inhibition of IL-6-induced STAT1 and STAT3 activation by bFGF. **A**: NIH-3T3 cells were stimulated with bFGF (10 ng/ml) for the times indicated. Whole cell lysates were prepared, 50 μg protein were separated by SDS-polyacrylamide (10%) gel electrophoresis and blotted onto a PVDF membrane. Membranes were incubated with anti-active MAP kinase Erk1/2 antibodies. **B**: NIH-3T3 cells were preincubated with the specific MKK1/2 inhibitor PD98059 (10 μM) for 45 min and incubated with bFGF (10 ng/ml) for 45 min followed by an exposure to IL-6 (100 U/ml) and sgp80 (0.5 μg/ml) for 15 min. Nuclear extracts were prepared and EMSAs performed as described in the legend to Fig. 11

Figure 11 Inhibition of IL-6-induced STAT1 and STAT3 activation by PMA. **A**: HepG2 cells were pretreated with PMA (10^{-7} M) for 45 min before stimulation with IL-6 (100 U/ml) for 15 min. Nuclear extracts were prepared and 50 μg of nuclear proteins were separated by SDS-PAGE and blotted onto PVDF membranes. Membranes were incubated with phosphospecific STAT1 (Tyr-701) (left panel) or phosphospecific STAT3 (Tyr-705) antibodies (right panel). Blots were stripped and reprobed with antibodies against STAT1 or STAT3. Immunogenic proteins were visualized with the ECL system. **B**: HepG2 cells were stimulated as described in **A**. Preincubation with the specific MKK1/2 inhibitor PD98059 (10 μM) was for 45 min; 10 μg of nuclear extracts were mixed with a ^{32}P-labelled oligonucleotide (mutated SIE probe of the c-fos promoter) and EMSAs were performed. The positions of the activated STAT homo- and heterodimers are indicated by arrow heads. **C**: HepG2 cells were pretreated with PMA (10^{-7} M) for 45 min before stimulation with IL-6 (100 U/ml) for 15 min or the times indicated. Cell lysates were prepared and immunoprecipitations with anti-gp130 (upper panel) or anti-SHP2 (lower panel) antibodies were performed. Precipitated proteins were separated by SDS-polyacrylamide (10%) gel electrophoresis, blotted onto a PVDF membrane and analysed by immunodetection with a specific anti-phosphotyrosine antibody (4G10) (upper panels). Blots were stripped and reprobed with anti-gp130 or anti-SHP2 (**C**, lower panels) antibodies for verification of equal loading

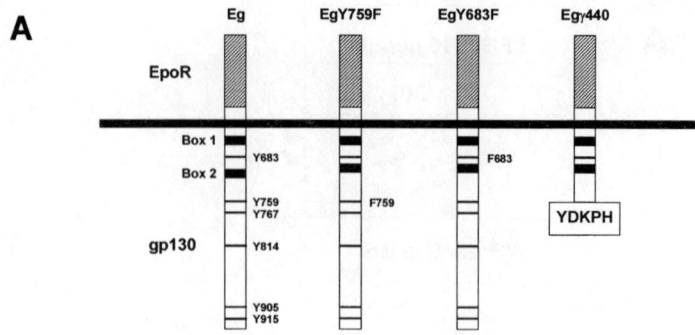

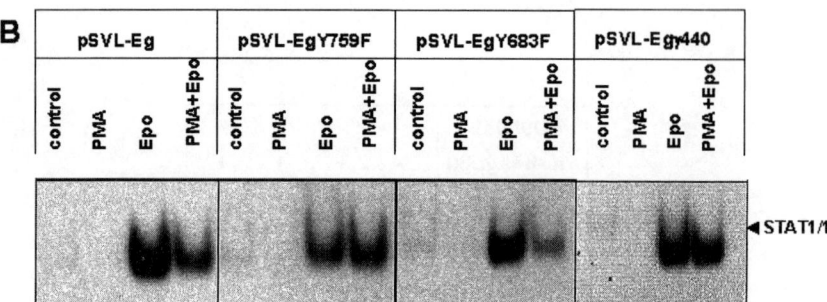

Figure 13 Role of the cytoplasmic part of gp130. **A**: Schematic representation of receptor chimaeras. **B**: COS-7 cells were transiently transfected with expression vectors for the chimaeric receptors depicted in **A**. Cells were preincubated with PMA (10^{-7} M) for 45 min followed by stimulation with Epo (7 U/ml) for 15 min. Nuclear extracts were prepared and EMSAs performed as described in the legend to Fig. 11

MODULATION OF IL-6 SIGNALLING

TNF-α preincubation inhibits STAT3 activation in rat liver macrophages (Kupffer cells)

We have shown in rat liver macrophages (Kupffer cells) (Fig. 15A) and in the mouse macrophage cell line RAW 264.7 (Fig. 15B) – but not in human hepatoma cells (HepG2) (Fig. 15C) – that IL-6-induced STAT3 activation is dose-dependently inhibited by pretreatment with TNF-α.

Moreover, in RAW 264.7 cells the inhibitory effect of TNF-α on IL-6-induced STAT3 activation is restored by pretreatment of the cells with the p38-specific inhibitor SB 202190 (Fig. 16), indicating that the p38-mitogen-activated protein kinase (MAP-kinase) is very probably involved in the inhibition of IL-6-induced STAT3 activation by TNF-α in macrophages.

Furthermore, we discovered that TNF-α induces the expression of SOCS3-mRNA in mouse macrophages, but not in HepG2 cells (Fig. 17). As mentioned above, SOCS proteins represent a family of inhibitory molecules, which are

A

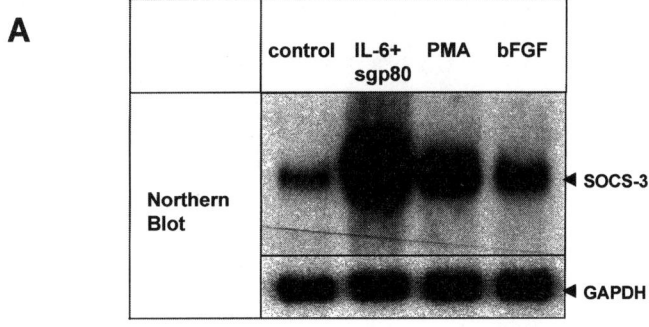

B

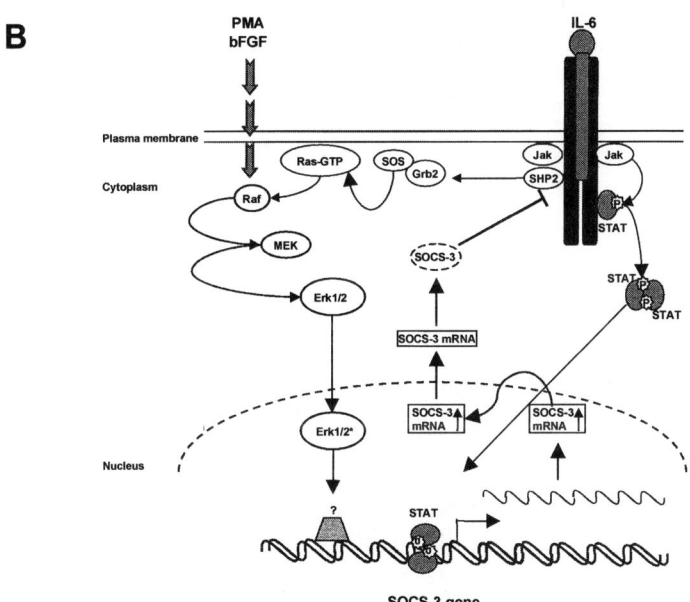

Figure 14 SOCS-3 mRNA is rapidly up-regulated upon PMA and bFGF treatment. **A**: Total RNA (15 μg/lane) isolated from NIH-3T3 cells stimulated with IL-6 (100 U/ml) plus sgp80 (0.5 μg/ml), PMA (10^{-7} M) or bFGF (10 ng/ml) for 30 min was hybridized with the ^{32}P-labelled cDNA probe for the murine SOCS-3 gene and the glyceraldehyde 3-phosphate dehydrogenase (GAPDH) as a loading control. **B**: Proposed mechanism of the PMA/bFGF-induced inhibition of the IL-6-induced STAT activation

A

| TNFα (ng/ml) | – | – | 1 | 5 | 10 | 30′ pre-incubation |
| IL-6 (200 U/ml) | – | + | + | + | + | 30′ |

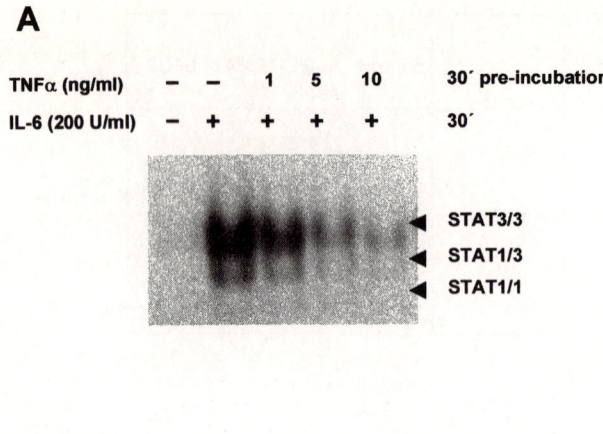

STAT3/3
STAT1/3
STAT1/1

B

| TNFα (ng/ml) | – | – | 1 | 5 | 10 | 20′ pre-incubation |
| IL-6 (200 U/ml) | – | + | + | + | + | 30′ |

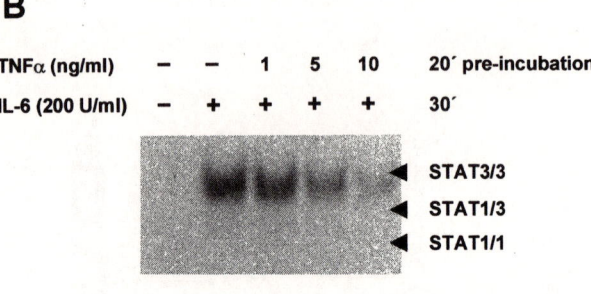

STAT3/3
STAT1/3
STAT1/1

C

| TNFα (10 ng/ml) | – | – | 20′ | 40′ | 20′ | pre-incubation |
| IL-6 (200 U/ml) | – | + | + | + | – | 15′ |

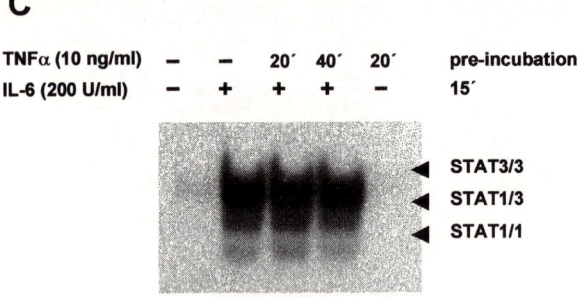

STAT3/3
STAT1/3
STAT1/1

Figure 15 TNF-α inhibits IL-6-induced STAT3 activation in macrophages but not in human hepatoma cells. Rat liver macrophages (**A**), RAW 264.7 mouse macrophages (**B**), and HepG2 cells (**C**) were pretreated with TNF-α at the concentrations indicated. At the different time-points IL-6 (200 U/ml) was added and incubation was continued as depicted. For the determination of STAT3 activation, cells were harvested and nuclear extracts were prepared; 5 μg of nuclear extracts were mixed with a ^{32}P-labelled oligonucleotide (mutated SIE probe of the c-fos promoter 5′-GAT CCG GGA GGG ATT TAC GGG AA ATG CTG-3′) and EMSAs were performed. The DNA–protein complexes formed were separated from the free probe by electrophoresis on a native 4.5% gel (lower panel)

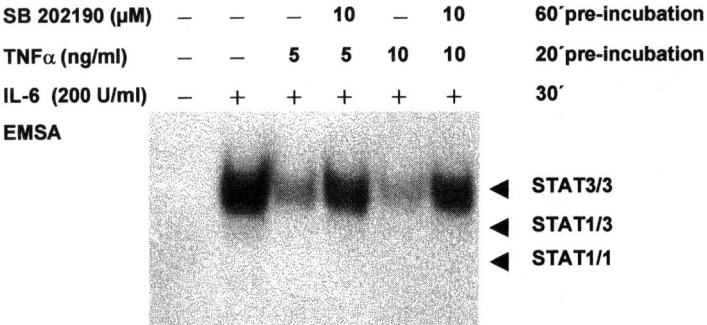

Figure 16 Inhibition of the p38-MAP-kinase restores the inhibitory effect of TNF-α on IL-6-induced STAT3 activation. Following a preincubation period of 40 min with SB 202190 at the concentrations indicated, RAW 264.7 cells were treated with TNF-α at the concentrations indicated, and incubation was continued for another 20 min. Then, cells were stimulated with IL-6 (200 U/ml) for a time period of 20 min. For the determination of STAT3 activation, cells were harvested and nuclear extracts were prepared. EMSAs were performed as described in the legend to Fig. 15

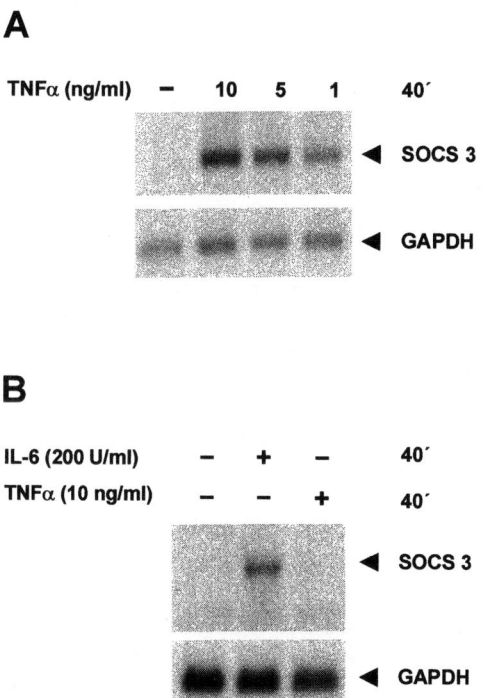

Figure 17 TNF-α induces SOCS3-mRNA in RAW 264.7 mouse macrophages but not in HepG2 cells. RAW 264.7 mouse macrophages (**A**) and HepG2 cells (**B**) were treated for 40 min with IL-6 (200 U/ml) or with TNF-α at the concentrations indicated. Cells were harvested for isolation of total RNA and subjected to Northern blot analyses for SOCS3 and GAPDH

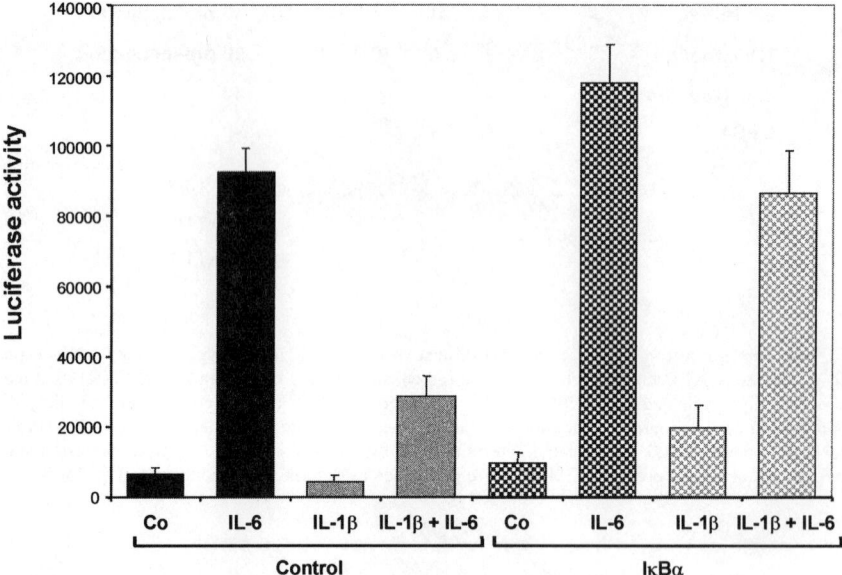

Figure 18 Overexpression of IκB-α restores the inhibitory effect of IL-1β on IL-6-induced α_2M promoter activity. HepG2 cells were co-transfected with the pGL3-Luc-α_2-macroglobulin (-215) reporter gene-construct, with the Lac-Z β-Gal construct and with IκB-α-cDNA. Cells were pretreated with IL-1β (100 U/ml) for 10 min as indicated, and then stimulated with IL-6 (100 U/ml) over 16 h. After lysis the luciferase activity was determined and normalized against β-galactosidase activity and protein content of the probe

rapidly induced by a number of cytokines such as IL-6 and IL-10[40]. SOCS proteins bind to the tyrosine-kinase domain of Janus kinases and thereby inhibit the tyrosine phosphorylation of the signal transducer gp130 and the STAT factors. We speculate that the inhibitory effect of TNF-α on the IL-6-induced STAT3 activation is due to SOCS3 induction.

Inhibition of IL-6-induced APP expression by IL-1β

A different mechanism was found to be responsible for the inhibition of IL-6-induced α_2M promoter activity by IL-1β using a reporter gene assay in HepG2 cells. Figure 18 shows that overexpression of IκBα, and in turn prevention of NF-κB activation, completely restores the inhibition of IL-6-induced α_2M promoter activity by IL-1β (Fig. 18). Since there exist overlapping regions within the binding sites of NF-κB and STAT3[41], the inhibitory effect of IL-1β on IL-6-induced α_2M promoter activity is very probably due to a competition between these two transcription factors.

Acknowledgements

The authors thank Dr Peter Freyer for his help with the artwork, and Silvia Cottin for the help with typing of this chapter. The experimental work performed in Aachen, and mentioned in this chapter, has been supported by grants from the Deutsche Forschungsgemeinschaft (Bonn) and the Fonds der Chemischen Industrie (Frankfurt).

References

1. Heinrich PC, Behrmann I, Müller-Newen G, Schaper F, Graeve L. IL-6-type cytokine signalling through the gp130/Jak/STAT pathway. Biochem J. 1998;334:297–314.

2. Guschin D, Rogers N, Briscoe J et al. A major role for the protein tyrosine kinase JAK1 in the JAK/STAT signal transduction pathway in reponse to interleukin-6. EMBO J. 1995;14:1421–9.

3. Rodig SJ, Meraz MA, White JM et al. Disruption of the Jak1 gene demonstrates obligatory and nonredundant roles of the Jaks in cytokine-induced biologic responses. Cell. 1998;93:373–83.

4. Heinrich PC, Behrmann I, Graeve L et al. The acute-phase response of the liver: molecular mechanism of IL-6 signalling from the plasma membrane to the nucleus. In: Hässinger D, Heinrich PC, editors. Signalling in the Liver. Proceedings of the International Falk Workshop (Part IV of the Liver Week, Freiburg 1997). Dordrecht: Kluwer; 1997:55–71.

5. Ballinger MD, Wells JA. Will any dimer do? Nature Struct Biol. 1998;5:938–40.

6. Yoshida K, Taga T, Saito M et al. Targeted disruption of gp130, a common signal transducer for the interleukin 6 family of cytokines, leads to myocardial and hematological disorders. Proc Natl Acad Sci USA. 1996;93:407–11.

7. Bravo J, Staunton D, Heath JK, Jones EY. Crystal structure of a cytokine-binding region of gp130. EMBO J. 1998;17:1665–74.

8. Kernebeck T, Pflanz S, Müller-Newen G et al. The signal transducer gp130: solution structure of the carboxy-terminal domain of the cytokine receptor homology region. Protein Sci. 1999;8:5–12.

9. Kurth I, Horsten U, Pflanz S et al. Activation of the signal transducer gp130 by both interleukin-6 and interleukin-11 requires two distinct binding epitopes. J Immunol. 1999;162:1480–7.

10. Gerhartz C, Heesel B, Sasse J et al. Differential activation of acute phase response factor/STAT3 and STAT1 via the cytoplasmic domain of the interleukin 6 signal transducer gp130 I. Definition of a novel phosphotyrosine motif mediating STAT1 activation. J Biol Chem. 1996;271:12991–8.

11. Shabo Y, Lotem J, Sachs L. Autoregulation of interleukin 6 and granulocyte-macrophage colony-stimulating factor in the differentiation of myeloid leukemic cells. Mol Cell Biol. 1989;9:4109–12.

12. Tomida M, Yamamoto-Yamaguchi Y, Hozumi M. Purification of a factor inducing differentiation of mouse myeloid leukemic M1 cells from conditioned medium of mouse fibroblast L929 cells. J Biol Chem. 1984;259:10978–82.

13. Rose TM, Bruce AG. Oncostatin M is a member of a cytokine family that includes leukemia-inhibitory factor, granulocyte colony-stimulating factor, and interleukin 6. Proc Natl Acad Sci USA. 1991;88:8641–5.

14. Kuropatwinski KK, De Imus C, Gearing D, Baumann H, Mosley B. Influence of subunit combinations on signaling by receptors for oncostatin M, leukemia inhibitory factor, and interleukin-6. J Biol Chem. 1997;272:15135–44.

15. Wu YY, Bradshaw RA. Induction of neurite outgrowth by interleukin-6 is accompanied by activation of Stat3 signaling pathway in a variant PC12 cell (E2) line. J Biol Chem. 1996;271:13023–32.

16. Estrov Z, Samal B, Lapushin R et al. Leukemia inhibitory factor binds to human breast cancer cells and stimulates their proliferation. J Interferon Cytokine Res. 1995;15:905–13.

17. Liu J, Spence MJ, Wallace PM, Forcier K, Hellstrom I, Vestal RE. Oncostatin M-specific receptor mediates inhibition of breast cancer cell growth and down-regulation of the c-myc proto-oncogene. Cell Growth Differ. 1997;8:667–76.

18. Behrmann I, Janzen C, Gerhartz C et al. A single STAT recruitment module in a chimeric cytokine receptor complex is sufficient for STAT activation. J Biol Chem. 1997;272:5269–74.

19. Gauldie J, Richards C, Harnish D, Lansdorp P, Baumann H. Interferon beta 2/B-cell stimulatory factor type 2 shares identity with monocyte-derived hepatocyte-stimulating factor and regulates the major acute phase protein response in liver cells. Proc Natl Acad Sci USA. 1987;84:7251–5.

20. Richards CD, Brown TJ, Shoyab M, Baumann H, Gauldie J. Recombinant oncostatin M stimulates the production of acute phase proteins in HepG2 cells and rat primary hepatocytes in vitro. J Immunol. 1992;148:1731–6.

21. Baumann H, Won KA, Jahreis GP. Human hepatocyte-stimulating factor-III and interleukin-6 are structurally and immunologically distinct but regulate the production of the same acute phase plasma proteins. J Biol Chem. 1989;264:8046–51.
22. Hermanns HM, Radtke S, Haan C et al. Contributions of leukemia inhibitory factor receptor and oncostatin M receptor to signal transduction in heterodimeric complexes with glycoprotein 130. J Immunol. 1999;163:6651–8.
23. Schaper F, Gendo C, Eck M et al. Activation of SHP2 via the IL-6 signal transducing receptor protein gp130 requires JAK1 and limits acute-phase protein expression. Biochem J. 1998;335: 557–65.
24. Stahl N, Farruggella TJ, Boulton TG, Zhong Z, Darnell JE Jr, Yancopoulos GD. Choice of STATs and other substrates specified by modular tyrosine-based motifs in cytokine receptors. Science. 1995;267:1349–53.
25. Starr R, Willson TA, Viney EM et al. A family of cytokine-inducible inhibitors of signalling. Nature. 1997;387:917–21.
26. Endo TA, Masuhara M, Yokouchi M et al. A new protein containing an SH2 domain that inhibits JAK kinases. Nature. 1997;387:921–4.
27. Naka T, Narazaki M, Hirata M et al. Structure and function of a new STAT-induced STAT inhibitor. Nature. 1997;387:924–9.
28. Nicholson SE, Willson TA, Farley A et al. Mutational analyses of the SOCS proteins suggest a dual domain requirement but distinct mechanisms for inhibition of LIF and IL-6 signal transduction. EMBO J. 1999;18:375–85.
29. Siewert E, Müller-Esterl W, Starr R, Heinrich PC, Schaper F. Different protein turnover of interleukin-6-type cytokine signalling components. Eur J Biochem. 1999;265:251–7.
30. Zohlnhöfer D, Graeve L, Rose-John S, Schooltink H, Dittrich E, Heinrich PC. The hepatic interleukin-6-receptor: down-regulation of the interleukin-6-binding subunit (gp80) by its ligand. FEBS Lett. 1992;306:219–22.
31. Dittrich E, Haft CR, Muys L, Heinrich PC, Graeve L. A di-leucine motif and an upstream serine in the interleukin-6 signal transducer gp130 mediate ligand-induced endocytosis and down-regulation of the IL-6 receptor. J Biol Chem. 1996;271:5487–94.
32. Thiel S, Behrmann I, Dittrich E et al. Internalization of the IL-6 signal transducer gp130 does not require activation of the JAK/STAT pathway. Biochem J. 1998;330:47–54.
33. Thiel S, Dahmen H, Martens A et al. Constitutive internalization and association with adaptor protein-2 of the interleukin-6 signal transducer gp130. FEBS Lett. 1998;441:231–4.
34. Thiel S, Behrmann I, Timmermann A et al. Identification of a Leu–Ile internalization motif within the cytoplasmic domain of the leukaemia inhibitory factor receptor. Biochem J. 1999;339: 15–19.
35. Bright JJ, Sriram S. TGF-beta inhibits IL-12-induced activation of Jak-STAT pathway in T lymphocytes. J Immunol. 1998;161:1772–7.
36. Sengupta TK, Schmitt EM, Ivashkiv LB. Inhibition of cytokines and Jak-STAT activation by distinct signaling pathways. Proc Natl Acad Sci USA. 1996;93:9499–504.
37. Bhat GJ, Abraham ST, Baker KM. Angiotensin II interferes with interleukin 6-induced Stat3 signaling by a pathway involving mitogen-activated protein kinase kinase 1. J Biol Chem. 1996;271:22447–52.
38. Sengupta TK, Talbot ES, Scherle PA, Ivashkiv LB. Rapid inhibition of interleukin-6 signaling and Stat3 activation mediated by mitogen-activated protein kinases. Proc Natl Acad Sci USA. 1998;95:11107–12.
39. van der Geer P, Hunter T, Lindberg RA. Receptor protein-tyrosine kinases and their signal transduction pathways. Annu Rev Cell Biol. 1994;10:251–337.
40. Ito S, Ansari P, Sakatsume M et al. Interleukin-10 inhibits expression of both interferon alpha- and interferon gamma-induced genes by suppressing tyrosine phosphorylation of STAT1. Blood. 1999;93:1456–63.
41. Zhang Z, Fuller GM. The competitive binding of STAT3 and NF-kappaB on an overlapping DNA binding site. Biochem Biophys Res Commun. 1997;237:90–4.

21
Cytokine gene transfer to the liver and regulation of the acute-phase response

C. D. RICHARDS, C. LANGDON, P. SIME and J. GAULDIE

INTRODUCTION

Many cytokines play multiple roles in the regulation of cell and tissue interaction. Different cytokine activities depend upon the target cell types, and action *in vivo* is governed by the distribution and concentration of cytokines throughout body fluids and organs. Effects on one organ may be similar or dissimilar to effects on other organs, depending on the amounts and types of responding cells, differences in signalling capacity between cell types from different organs, and interaction with other cytokines/mediators *in vivo*. The study of cytokine effects *in vivo* has been greatly facilitated by transgenic and gene knockout technology. In addition, local overexpression through other exogenous means such as viral gene expression vectors has also aided the characterization of cytokine function *in vivo*. We have used adenovirus vectors encoding several cytokines to transiently overexpress genes locally in order to study aspects of the inflammatory response.

Acute-phase responses to inflammation include fever, leucocytosis and the production of a heterogeneous group of proteins by the liver – the acute-phase proteins (APP)[1-5]. The induction of APP is thought to be a homeostatic response to inflammatory stimuli[5,6] and a number of these show anti-inflammatory properties[7] or inhibition of protease action at the inflammation sites. Cytokines that control liver hepatocyte response include the interleukin-6/leukaemia inhibitory factor (IL-6/LIF) family, which currently consists of IL-6, LIF, oncostatin M (OSM), IL-11, cardiotrophin-1 (CT-1) and ciliary neurotrophic factor (CNTF). These cytokines act at cell surface receptor complexes that include the signalling molecule gp130, and prominently activate the Jak/STAT pathway of signal transduction, as well as a variable AP-1 activation[8-10]. Hepatocytes possess these receptors and respond by the synthesis of several APP, termed type II APP such as haptoglobulin, fibrinogen and α_1-antichymotrypsin in humans, and haptoglobin, fibrinogen, α_1-cysteine protease inhibitor (α_1-CPI), and α_1-antichymotrypsin in rodents[4]. Regulation of genes of these proteins is dependent on the interaction of multiple transcription factors[4,5]. These act in *cis* or *trans* and generally act similarly across species of hepatocytes, although in some species specific differences do exist. The induction of hepatic APP synthesis by IL-6 is generally thought to contribute to anti-inflammatory properties of IL-6[11,12].

IL-1 and TNF have also been shown to directly stimulate a restricted set of APP (characterized as type I APP) and modulate the production of others. Thus, IL-1/TNF can stimulate α_1-acid glycoprotein (AGP), serum amyloid A protein, C-reactive protein and complement C3, and this stimulation can be synergistic in combination with IL-6. Both IL-1 and TNF are strong inducers of IL-6 expression in many cell types[13], and thus participate in generation of IL-6 from sites of inflammation. TGF-β, as well as other growth factors (IGF, HGF) have also been shown to modulate APP synthesis. TGF-β suppresses IL-1 stimulation but enhances IL-6 stimulation of type II APP genes[14,15]. Thus, the role of TGF-β compared to IL-6 is minor, but may significantly modify liver responses if expressed at significant levels.

Homeostasis of connective tissue (CT) components, that include CT cells and extracellular matrix (ECM), is largely controlled by growth factors and cytokines. These factors regulate cell activity, proliferation, and expression of ECM components as well as enzymes and their inhibitors that are needed for remodelling of CT. Remodelling is part of normal homeostasis (wound repair) as well as processes that catabolize CT or produce excess ECM (fibrosis). IL-1 and TNF are well established as acute inducers of tissue catabolism through stimulation of matrix metalloproteinases (MMPs), whereas TGF-β is well established as a strong stimulus of fibrotic (ECM deposition) through inhibition of MMP and enhancement of MMP inhibitors such as TIMP-1[16,17]. We have previously shown that adenovirus expressing active TGF-β_1 locally in lungs of rats and mice produced a dramatic fibrotic response accompanied by ECM deposition and expression of smooth muscle actin[18]. Of the IL-6 family of cytokines, OSM has strong activity regulating TIMP-1, IL-6 and other genes in CT cells[19–23]. The role of IL-6 cytokines in fibrosis *in vivo* is still not well established.

The purpose of this study was to examine the effects of systemic administration of adenovirus vectors that encode cytokines known to modulate liver responses on the basis of previous *in-vitro* work. Intravenous delivery of adenovirus vectors results in gene expression of inserted cytokines in the liver parenchyma and their overexpression for a period of 7–10 days. The response of the liver was determined by measuring APP and examining liver histology.

MATERIALS AND METHODS

Adenovirus type 5 (Ad) recombinant vectors (with E1 and E3 regions deleted) used in this study have been previously described elsewhere: Add170-3 (control vector with no inserted cytokine gene) and vector expressing murine IL-6 (AdmIL-6)[24,25]; vector expressing constitutively activated TGF-β_1 (AdTGF-β)[18]; vector expressing murine TNF-α (AdTNF)[26]; and vector expressing murine OSM[27]. Single doses of these vectors were administered to Sprague-Dawley rats

(200–225 g) through intravenous injections and effects were monitored for 28 days. Blood samples were taken from sequential tail bleeds at day 1 and 2, and then at sacrifice on days 3, 7, 14 and 28. Serum was decanted from clotted blood and stored at –20°C until analysis. Rocket electrophoresis was used as previously described[28] to assess levels of CPI and AGP. The B9 hybridoma proliferation assay was used to assess IL-6 levels in serum as previously described. Liver and lung tissue samples were fixed and stained (H&E) by standard procedures, and also immunostained for α smooth muscle actin as described[18].

RESULTS AND DISCUSSION

Adenovectors expressing TGF-β, mTNF-α, mIL-6 and mOSM were compared to the control virus Addl70-3 as to their ability to regulate liver responses. All vectors have been previously published as expressing biologically active cytokine, with effects demonstrated *in vitro* and *in vivo*. TNF, IL-6 and OSM vectors encode murine cytokines which we and others have shown can also regulate rat cell responses and interact with their respective rat receptors. The TGF-β virus encodes a mutated sequence of porcine TGF-β that is constitutively active, and regulates responses across all species tested.

The vectors were administered intravenously at 5×10^8 pfu/animal, and followed for 28 days. Vector expression of cytokine is typically for 3–7 days, and this study examined serum responses at days 1, 2, 3, 7, 14 and 28. Figure 1 shows the levels of α_1-CPI in serum, which has previously been established as a major APP in rats. Tail bleeds of untreated rats (control) showed a small (20%)

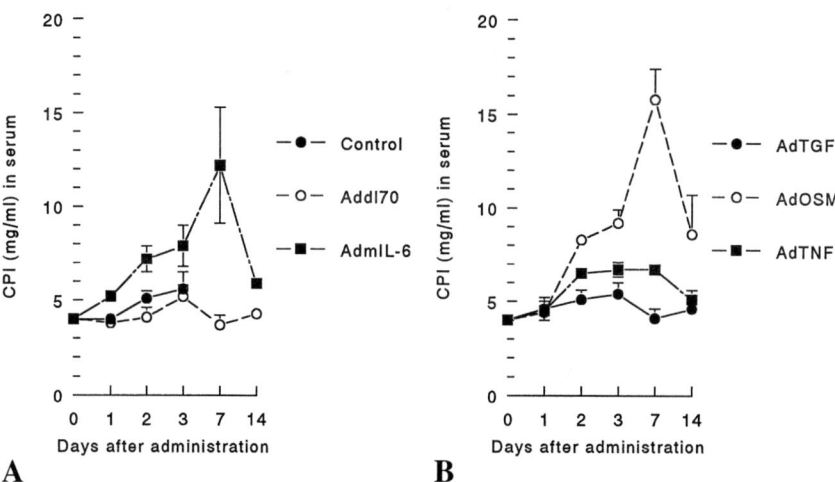

Figure 1 Serum levels of α-1-cysteine protease inhibitor (CPI) in rats treated with Ad5 vectors intravenously. Sprague-Dawley rats were treated with 5×10^8 pfu of: (**A**) Addl70, AdmIL-6 or left untreated (control); (**B**) AdTGF, AdmOSM or AdTNF. Serum levels of CPI were measured in the blood samples taken at the indicated times after treatment, using quantitative rocket electrophoresis. Each point is the mean and SD of $n = 3$ rats

increase (from 4 to 5 μg/ml) by day 3, which subsequently declined to day 0 levels. No significant difference from these levels was seen in rats treated with Add170 or with TGF-β, indicating a lack of effect of either of these cytokines on liver expression of α_1-CPI in this system (Fig. 1A). AdTNF-treated animals showed an increase of 40–45% evident on days 2, 3 and 7, which subsequently then decreased to control levels by day 14 (Fig. 1B). Rats treated with AdmIL-6 showed a larger increase evident at days 1, 2, 3, 7 and 14, with peak concentrations of 300% that of normal CPI levels at day 7. AdmOSM-treated rats (Fig. 1B) showed even higher levels of serum CPI again peaking at day 7 (15.5 μg/ml corresponding to approximately 400% of control levels). The effects of AdmOSM and AdmIL-6 are consistent with the documented direct effect of these cytokines on hepatocyte APP synthesis *in vitro*[22] and induction of serum levels of APP in mice *in vivo*[24,27].

Analysis of α_1-AGP levels showed that peak levels were seen at day 2 after treatment with AdTGF-β (approximately 200% of untreated or Add170-3), AdmIL-6 (approximately 560% of control), and AdmOSM (approximately 770% of control) (Fig. 2). These responses were thus similar in trend to those shown by CPI analysis, although earlier in peak responses. This probably reflects differences in the induction, expression and serum half-life of AGP versus CPI. TNF has been established as a strong inducer of type I APP such as α_1-AGP[4]. Levels of AGP were indeed highest in animals treated with AdTNF (approximately 950% of control) at day 2 and at day 3 (Fig. 2B) (approximately 860% of control). AdTNF showed a sustained induction of α_1-CPI at day 7 (Fig. 1) which may in part be mediated by the early induction of IL-6 in these animals. In contrast, both IL-6 and OSM have previously been established as

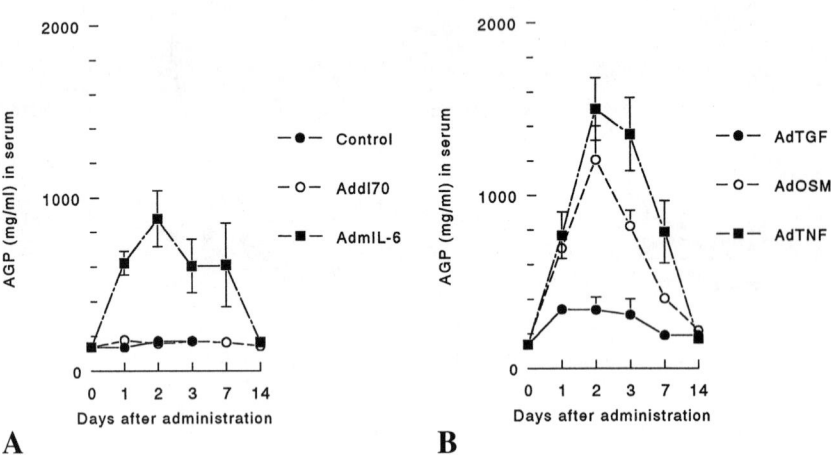

Figure 2 Serum levels of α-1-acid glycoprotein (AGP) in rats treated with Ad5 vectors intravenously. Sprague-Dawley rats were treated with 5×10^8 pfu of: (**A**) Add170, AdmIL-6 or left untreated (control); (**B**) AdTGF, AdmOSM or AdTNF. Serum levels of AGP were measured in the blood samples taken at the indicated times after treatment, using quantitative rocket electrophoresis. Each point is the mean and SD of $n = 3$ rats

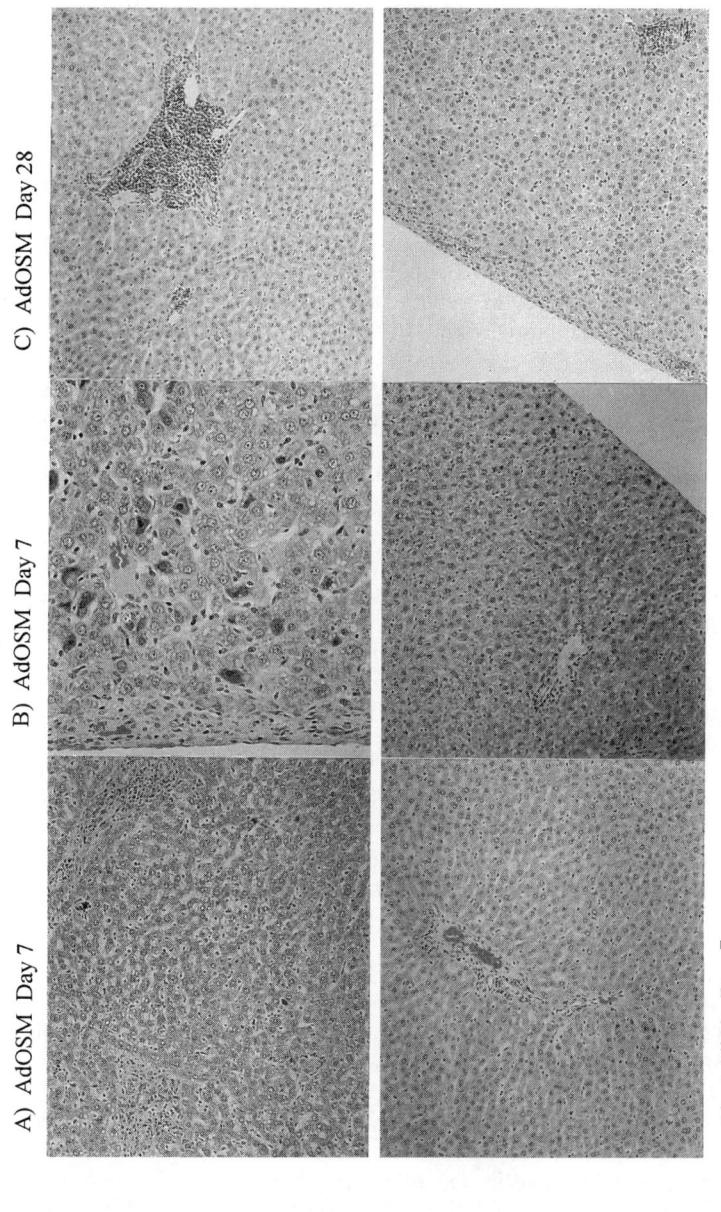

A) AdOSM Day 7

B) AdOSM Day 7

C) AdOSM Day 28

D) AddI70 Day 7

E) AdIL-6 Day 7

F) AdOSM Day 7

Figure 3 Liver histology of rats treated with AdmOSM. Sprague-Dawley rats were treated with 5×10^8 pfu AdmOSM or AdmIL-6 as described in the text. Animals were sacrificed at the indicated times and liver tissue samples were fixed, processed and stained by standard procedures. **A**: AdmOSM day 7, H&E stain 10× objective. **B**: AdOSM day 7, H&E stain 20× objective. **C**: AdOSM day 28, H&E stain, 10× objective. **D**: AddI70 day 7, H&E stain, 10× objective. **E**: AdIL-6 day 7, H&E stain, 10 × objective. **F**: AdOSM day 7, α-SM-actin immunostaining 10× objective

233

strong inducers of type II acute-phase reactants including α_1-CPI, and enhanced AGP levels but not to the same extent as TNF. This is consistent with the effects of TNF on type I APP and IL-6/LIF/OSM cytokines on type II APP.

Previous studies have shown that systemic administration of adenovirus vector expressing indicator genes results in infection of both liver and spleen[24,29]. Endothelial cells and hepatocytes are presumably a major target of systemic adenovirus infection, and expression of IL-6 or OSM in hepatic endothelium and parenchyma would provide high concentrations of local cytokine for direct effects on hepatocytes. OSM has previously been shown to regulate IL-6 expression by a number of different stromal cell types including endothelial cells[30]. To determine if indirect effects could be mediated through IL-6 in AdmOSM treatments, we assessed serum IL-6 levels in the serum of all animals using the B9 proliferation assay. Bioactive IL-6 levels were relatively low, with the exception of AdmIL-6-treated animals at day 3 (mean of 70 U/ml). Thus although CPI levels were higher with AdmOSM treatment (mean of 9 mg/ml CPI) at day 3, IL-6 levels were undetectable, suggesting IL-6 levels alone did not mediate OSM action on α_1-CPI levels.

We have previously shown that at high levels the AdTGF-β vector induces a dramatic fibrosis in lungs of rats or mice treated with intratracheal or intranasal administrations[18]. These effects were evident as early as day 3 after a single dose of vector and progressed over a period of 60 days to mortality from pulmonary fibrosis. To determine if histological evidence of inflammation or fibrosis was present in the lower level intravenous administrations used here, animals were sacrificed on days 3, 7, 14 and 28, and livers fixed and stained with H&E.

At the lower dose of vector used (5×10^8 pfu), we observed a number of histological changes over time in the liver, while lung tissue of the same individual rats did not show any evidence of alterations from normal untreated rats. No difference was observed in livers of rats treated with the control virus (Add 170-3) from untreated rats (Fig. 3D). The AdTGF-β treatment resulted in a mild, diffuse mononuclear cell infiltration in the liver parenchyma that was most evident at day 7, after which (day 14 and 28) the livers did not appear any different from control virus or untreated rats. Staining for α smooth muscle actin did not reveal any difference in the distribution or level of expression in these tissues. The AdTNF treatment also induced a diffuse mononuclear cell increase, most evident at day 7, that persisted until day 14, and after which the liver tissue was essentially normal in morphology.

The livers from animals treated with the AdmIL-6 and AdmOSM vectors were compared closely since the induction of liver APP responses (as measured by serum CPI) was similarly high. The AdmIL-6 vector, similar to vectors expressing TGF and TNF, caused some mononuclear cell infiltrate evident at day 7 (Fig. 3E), and liver tissue at day 14 was essentially normal in appearance. Interestingly, the AdmOSM vector induced several changes that were not evident in any of the other treatments. Mononuclear cell infiltration was seen as early as day 3, and was much more pronounced at day 7 (Fig. 3A and B), at which time there was increase in vacuolization of the hepatocyte cytoplasm, increase in darker staining (acidophilic) cells in H&E, and a marked increase in the number of mitotic figures. Thickening of the outer capsule (5–8 cell layer) was consistently evident (Fig. 3B) and staining for α smooth muscle actin

Table 1 TGF-β levels in rat liver tissue after intravenous delivery of AdTGF-β

Viral dose (pfu)	Active TGF-β (mean) (pg/g tissue)	Latent TGF-β (mean) (pg/g tissue)
5×10^8	78	2 666
1×10^9	244	6 480
5×10^9	370	13 638
7.5×10^9	2,283	66 778

Virus was delivered intravenously, and tissue taken at 72 h. TGF-β levels were measured by ELISA. In rats receiving control virus, at the highest dose, latent TGF-β measured 540 pg/g tissue (no active TGF-β was detected)

(SM-actin) showed increased detection around some portal triads and especially in the thickened layer of the capsule (Fig. 3F). By day 14 of AdmOSM treatment there was still some evidence of mononuclear infiltration that was more focused into aggregates, but capsule thickening and SM-actin presence generally appeared to be resolving. Day 28 of AdmOSM treatment showed aggregates of mononuclear cell accumulation (Fig. 3C); otherwise histology was normal.

In a separate series of studies in which increasing doses of the TGF-β vector were administered, liver tissue was removed and extracted at day 3. Levels of TGF-β were measured and showed (Table 1) that there was a dose relationship between the amount of virus delivered to the liver and the concentration of TGF in the tissue. At the higher dose used (7.5×10^9 pfu) there was over 2 ng/g of tissue of active TGF-β generated. This level of virus is the same as or higher than that used in our previous study of fibrogenesis in the lung[18]. In the case of lung, this caused a progressive and aggressive fibrogenic response resulting in complete and fatal fibrosis of the lung. There was marked induction of SM-actin containing myofibroblasts throughout the parenchyma and thickening of the pleura with extensive deposition of most connective tissue materials[18].

Contrary to these data in the lung, similar levels of TGF-β released in the liver lead to marked apoptosis of hepatocytes (Fig. 4A) and a transient, but resolving, appearance of SM-actin expressing cells within the stroma around the liver lobules (Fig. 4E). These changes never progressed to liver fibrosis and the changes were temporary with the liver returning to normal within the period of 14 to 21 days (Fig. 4F). When the liver capsule was examined there was a marked thickening and SM-actin expression (Fig. 4D), similar to that seen in the lung[18]. However, as with the other changes seen, this thickening resolved and returned to normal structure within the same 21-day period.

The fact that the same dose of vector and cytokine level gives a dramatic and progressive chronic fibrosis when expressed in the lung, but a resolving and mild indication of fibrogenesis when expressed in the liver, suggests that these two organs handle cytokine insults in a dramatically different manner. This indicates, overall, that the liver copes exceptionally well with transient physiological changes to cytokine levels as a result of inflammation. Further evidence of this resilience can be seen in the minimal changes observed after expression of the toxic cytokine TNF-α. In addition, these data indicate that insults by factors such as TGF-β, even at high levels, but which are short-lived, can lead to

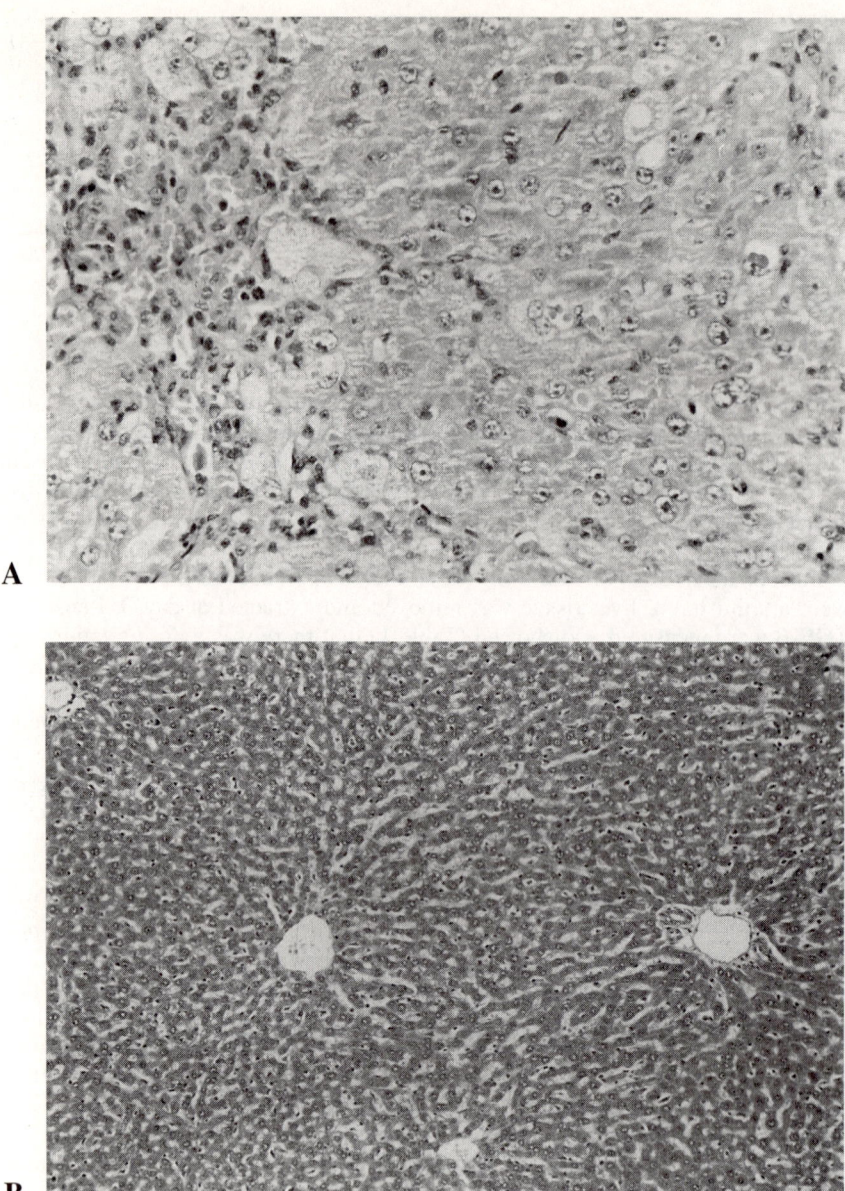

Figure 4 Liver histology of rats treated with high-dose AdTGFβ. Sprague-Dawley rats were treated with 7.5 × 10⁹ pfu of AdTGFβ or Addl-70 control vector as described. Animals were sacrificed at the indicated times and liver tissue samples were fixed, processed and stained by standard procedures. **A**: AdTGFβ day 3, H&E stain 10× objective. **B**: Addl-70 day 3, H&E stain 10× objective

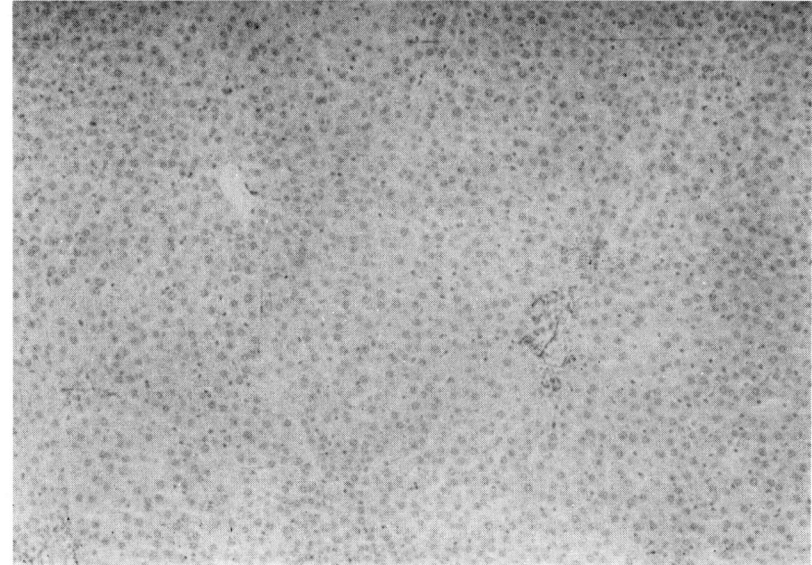

C

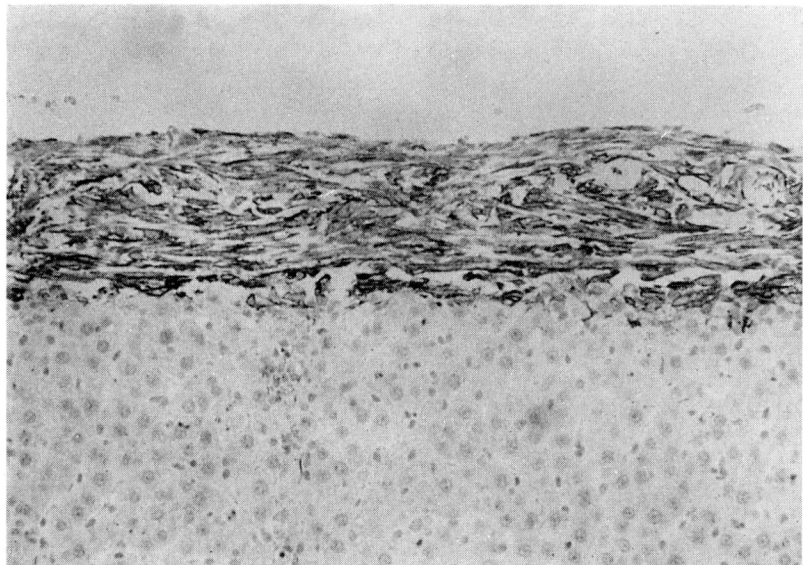

D

Figure 4 **C**: Addl-70 day 3, α-SM-actin immunostaining 10× objective. **D**: Capsule AdTGFβ day 3, α-SM-actin immunostaining 16× objective

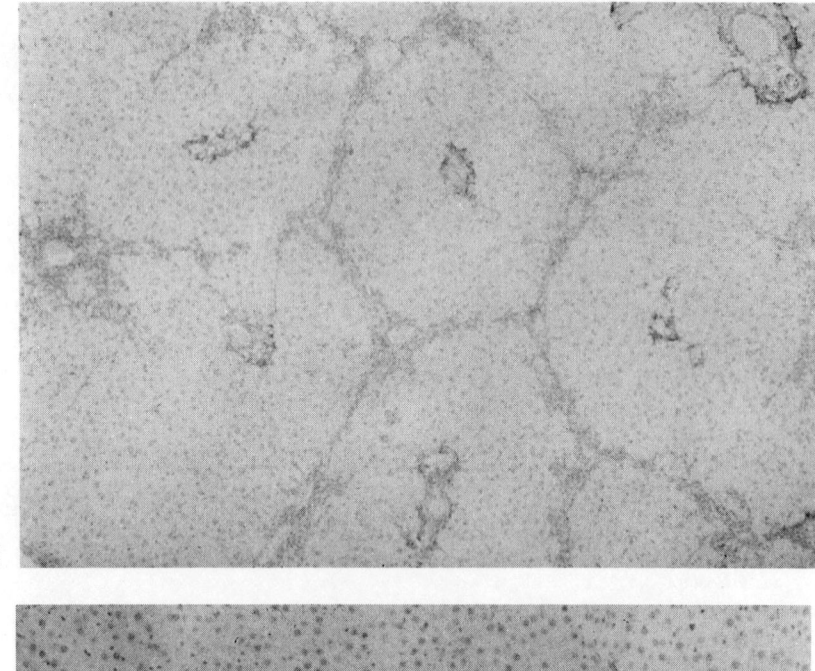

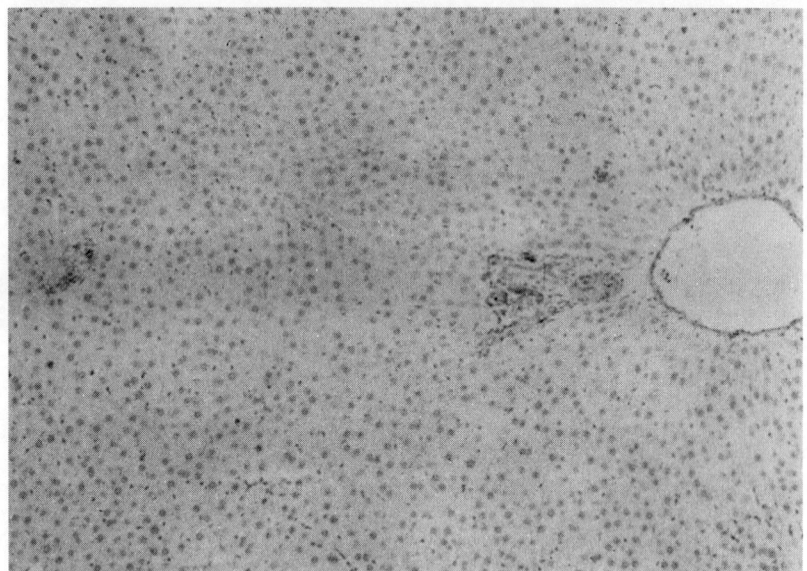

Figure 4 **E**: AdTGFβ day 3, α-SM-actin immunostaining 10× objective. **F**: AdTGFβ day 21, α-SM-actin immunostaining 10× objective

recovery of the liver. More chronic local release of these same factors is suggested to lead to progressive fibrosis, as seen in transgenic studies with the TGF-β gene being permanently driven to overexpression by the albumin promoter[31].

Acknowledgements

This research is supported by MRC Canada, Hamilton Health Sciences Corporation and St Joseph's Hospital. We thank J. A. Schroeder for excellent technical expertise, and S. DeSilvio for secretarial assistance.

References

1. Kushner, I, Mackiewicz A. Acute phase proteins as disease markers. Disease Markers. 1987;5:1.
2. Baumann H, Gauldie J. Regulation of hepatic acute phase plasma protein genes by hepatocyte stimulating factors and other mediators of inflammation. Mol Biol Med. 1990;7:147–59.
3. Heinrich PC, Castell JV, Andus T. Interleukin-6 and the acute phase protein. Biochem J. 1990;265:621–36.
4. Baumann H, Gauldie J. The acute phase response. Immunol Today. 1994;15:74–80.
5. Steel DM, Whitehead AS. The major acute phase reactants: C-reactive protein, serum amyloid P component and serum amyloid A protein. Immunol Today. 1994;15:81–8.
6. Koj A. Acute phase reactants – their synthesis, turnover and biological significance. Struct Funct Plasma Prot. 1974;1:73.
7. Tilg H, Vannier E, Vachino G, Dinarello CA, Mier JW. Antiinflammatory properties of hepatic acute phase proteins: preferential indiction of interleukin 1 (IL-1) receptor antagonist over IL-1 beta synthesis by human peripheral blood mononuclear cells. J Exp Med. 1993;178:1629–36.
8. Kishimoto T, Taga T, Akira S. Cytokine signal transduction. Cell. 1994;76:253–62.
9. Zhang X, Gu J, Lu Z et al. Ciliary neurotropic factor, interleukin 11, leukemia inhibitory factor, and oncostatin M are growth factors for human myeloma cell lines using the interleukin 6 signal transducer GP130. J Exp Med. 1994;177:1337–42.
10. Stahl N, Boulton TG, Farruggella T et al. Association and activation of Jak-Tyk kinases by CNTF-LIF-OSM-IL-6 beta receptor components. Science. 1994;263:92–5.
11. Tilg H, Trehu E, Atkins MB, Dinarello CA, Mier JW. Interleukin-6 (IL-6) as an anti-inflammatory cytokine: induction of circulating IL-1 receptor antagonist and soluble tumor necrosis factor receptor p55. Blood. 1994;83:113–18.
12. Xing Z, Gauldie J, Cox G et al. IL-6 is an antiinflammatory cytokine required for controlling local or systemic acute inflammatory responses. J Clin Invest. 1998;101:311–20.
13. Dinarello CA. Biological basis for interleukin-1 in disease. Blood. 1996;87:2095–147.
14. Mackiewicz A, Ganapathi MK, Shultz D et al. Transforming growth factor β_1 regulates production of acute-phase proteins. Proc Natl Acad Sci USA. 1990;87:1491–5.
15. Campos SP, Wang Y, Koj A, Baumann H. Divergent transforming growth factor-beta effects on IL-6 regulation of acute phase plasma proteins in rat hepatoma cells. J Immunol. 1993;151: 7128–37.
16. Matrisian LM. The matrix-degrading metalloproteinases. BioEssays. 1992;14:455–63.
17. Derynck R. TGF-beta-receptor-mediated signaling. TIBS. 1994;19:548–53.
18. Sime PJ, Xing Z, Graham FL, Csaky KG, Gauldie J. Adenovector-mediated gene transfer of active transforming growth factor-β1 induces prolonged severe fibrosis in rat lung. J Clinical Invest. 1997;100:768–76.
19. Richards CD, Shoyab M, Brown TJ, Gauldie J. Selective regulation of metalloproteinases inhibitor (TIMP-1) by oncostatin M in fibroblasts in culture. J Immunol. 1993;150:5596–603.
20. Richards CD, Agro A. Interaction between oncostatin M interleukin 1 and prostaglandin E_2 in induction of IL-6 expression in human fibroblasts. Cytokine. 1994;6:40–7.
21. Richards C, Langdon C, Botelho F, Brown TJ, Agro A. Oncostatin M inhibits IL-1-induced expression of IL-8 and granulocyte-macrophage colony-stimulating factor by synovial and lung fibroblasts. J Immunol. 1996;156:343–9.
22. Richards CD, Kerr C, Tanaka M et al. Regulation of tissue inhibitor of metalloproteinase-1 in fibroblasts and acute phase proteins in hepatocytes in vitro by mouse oncostatin M, cardiotrophin-1, and IL-6. J Immunol. 1997;159:2431–7.
23. Langdon CM, Leith J, Smith F, Richards CD. Oncostatin M stimulates monocyte chemoattractant protein-1- and interleukin-1-induced matrix metalloproteinase-1 production by human synovial fibroblasts in vitro. Arthritis Rheum. 1997;40:2139–46.
24. Braciak TA, Mittal SK, Graham FL, Richards CD, Gauldie J. Construction of recombinant human type 5 adenoviruses expressing rodent IL-6 genes. An approach to investigate in vivo cytokine function. J Immunol. 1993;151:5145–53.

25. Richards CD, Braciak T, Xing Z, Graham FL, Gauldie J. Adenovirus vectors for cytokine gene expression. Ann NY Acad Sci. 1995;762:282–93.
26. Sime PJ, Marr RA, Xing Z, Hewlett BR, Graham FL, Gauldie J. Transfer of tumor necrosis factor-alpha to rat lung induces severe pulmonary inflammation and patchy interstitial fibrogenesis with induction of transforming growth factor-beta 1 and myofibroblasts. Am J Pathol. 1998;153:825–32.
27. Kerr C, Langdon CM, Graham F, Gauldie J, Hara T, Richards CD. Adenovirus vector expressing mouse oncostatin M induces acute phase proteins and TIMP-1 expression in vivo in mice. J Interf Cyt Res. 1999;19:1195–205.
28. Richards CD, Brown TJ, Shoyab M, Baumann H, Gauldie J. Recombinant oncostatin-M stimulates the production of acute phase proteins in hepG2 cells and rat primary hepatocytes *in vitro*. J Immunol. 1992;148:1731–6.
29. Mittal SK, McDermott MR, Johnson DC, Prevec L, Graham FL. Monitoring foreign gene expression by a human adenovirus-based vector using the firefly luciferase gene as a reporter. Virus Res. 1993;28:67–90.
30. Brown TJ, Rowe JM, Liu J, Shoyab M. Regulation of interleukin-6 expression by oncostatin M. J Immunol. 1991;147:2175–80.
31. Sanderson N, Factor V, Nagy P *et al*. Hepatic expression of mature transforming growth factor $\beta1$ in transgenic mice results in multiple tissue lesions. Proc Natl Acad Sci USA. 1995;92: 2572–6.

22
The role of graft manipulation in the mechanism of primary non-function in liver transplantation: cytokines and transcription factors

R. G. THURMAN, P. SCHEMMER, C. A. BRADHAM,
T. G. LEHMANN, D. A. BRENNER, H. BUNZENDAHL,
B. U. BRADFORD, J. A. RALEIGH, G. E. ARTEEL,
R. F. STACHLEWITZ, H. CONNOR and R. MASON

INTRODUCTION

Graft manipulation

Primary non-function and dysfunction occur in 5–30% of liver transplantation cases, resulting either in the need for retransplantation or in the death of the recipient[1]. Since liver transplantation is the therapy of choice in an increasing number of liver diseases[2], and the organ pool is limited, there is an urgent need to understand the underlying mechanisms responsible for failure of transplanted livers. There are three crucial periods which can influence graft viability before rejection: harvest, cold storage and reperfusion. It has been demonstrated that reperfusion injury, rather than ischaemic cell damage developing during cold storage, predominates. This conclusion is based on the fact that after long cold storage in UW solution, reperfusion injury is minimized by Carolina Rinse solution[3]. Injury from ischaemic cold storage alone would have sufficient time to develop, but does not become apparent[3]. Several mechanisms, i.e. production of free radicals[4], disturbances of the microcirculation[5] and activation of the coagulation system[6], are probably involved in mechanisms of reperfusion injury. In addition, several cell types are involved, e.g. migration and activation of leucocytes[7] and damage to endothelial cells[8]. Further, Kupffer cells, the resident macrophages in the liver, are activated upon reperfusion[9], causing them to release toxic mediators such as superoxide radicals, tumour necrosis factor (TNF) and arachidonic acid derivatives[10–12].

Although TNF-α is implicated in reperfusion injury, the second messengers and signalling pathways activated during transplantation are unknown. The purpose of this study was to assess the activation of MAPKs and the transcription factor AP-1 in response to ischaemic cold storage and reperfusion following transplantation in the rat liver. The results demonstrate that JNK, but not ERK or p38, undergoes a potent, sustained induction upon reperfusion after transplantation. In addition, the DNA-binding activities of both AP-1 and NF-κB are elevated after reperfusion. The mRNAs for TNF-α and for *c-jun*, *junB*, and *c-fos* are induced in the transplanted liver. Finally, ceramide, but not diacylglycerol or sphingosine, is elevated in the transplanted liver. Ceramide is a second messenger generated by TNF-α, and an activator of JNK[13–15]. Since JNK activation preceded the elevations in ceramide and TNF-α mRNA, these results suggest that increased hepatic TNF-α and ceramide may perpetuate JNK induction, but are not the initiating signals of JNK activation during reperfusion injury in the transplanted liver.

The protective role of glycine

Glycine, a non-essential amino acid, is non-toxic, and has been shown to protect proximal tubules and hepatocytes[16] against hypoxia. Glycine also prevents nephrotoxicity caused by cyclosporin A[17]. Further, glycine added to a graft rinse solution reduced reperfusion injury and also improved initial graft function and survival after liver transplantation[16]. Moreover, glycine improved the hepatic microcirculation and reduced liver injury in a low-flow, reflow perfusion model[18]. A diet containing glycine improved survival of rats given endotoxin, most probably by inactivation of Kupffer cells, since TNF-α production was decreased[19]. Increases of intracellular calcium ($[Ca^{2+}]_i$) in Kupffer cells are essential for the release of prostanoids and inflammatory cytokines in response to stimuli such as endotoxin (LPS). Glycine prevents the increase of $[Ca^{2+}]_i$ by activating a glycine-gated chloride channel[20], which hyperpolarizes the cell membrane and makes Ca^{2+} influx via voltage-dependent Ca^{2+} channels more difficult. Thus, glycine blunted activation of Kupffer cells by LPS. This effect is important since activated Kupffer cells are involved in regulation of hepatic microcirculation, and several lines of evidence suggest that microcirculatory disturbances are a key factor in enhanced donor liver susceptibility to cold and warm ischaemia[21–23].

The purpose of this chapter is to review a new model of liver transplantation to evaluate the effect of manipulation during harvest, the effect of transplantation on cytokines and transcription factors, and to evaluate the protective effect of glycine and gene therapy.

METHODS

Liver transplantation

Orthotopic liver transplantation was performed in Sprague-Dawley rats. Donors and recipients were anaesthetized with methoxyfluorane. After explantation, livers were stored at 0–4°C for 24 h in UW solution. Grafts were rinsed with 10 ml of normal saline (18°C) and implanted by connecting the suprahepatic vena cava with a running 7/0 prolene suture, inserting cuffs into the corresponding vessels and anastomozing the bile duct and hepatic artery with an intra-luminal polyethylene splint. Transplantation required less than 40 min; during this time the portal vein was clamped for 12–15 min. After transplantation the recipients had free access to standard laboratory chow and tap water. Blood samples were collected from the inferior vena cava at sacrifice. Serum was obtained by centrifugation and stored at –80°C. AST and ALT activity were determined by standard enzymatic methods[24].

Western analysis

Nuclear extracts of liver (2.5 μg) was separated by electrophoresis on 10% acrylamide SDS gels, then transferred to Immobilon membranes (Millipore, Bedford, MA). Equal loading was confirmed by Ponceau S staining. JNK was detected using monoclonal anti-JNK-1 antibody (15701A, Pharmingen, San Diego, CA), and ERK was detected using polyclonal anti-ERK-1 antibody (K-23, Santa Cruz Biotechnology, Santa Cruz, CA). Antibody binding was detected using appropriate horseradish peroxidase-conjugated secondary antibodies (Santa Cruz Biotechnology, Santa Cruz, CA), and chemiluminescence (ECL kit, Amersham, Arlington Heights, IL).

Kinase assays

JNK kinase assays were performed as described elsewhere[25]. Briefly, 25 μg liver nuclear extract was incubated with recombinant GST-cJun substrate[26] con-jugated to glutathione-agarose beads (Pharmacia, Piscataway, NJ), extensively washed, then incubated in kinase reactions containing γ^{32}P-ATP as a phosphate donor. Substrate protein was resolved by gel electrophoresis, and phosphate incorporation was assessed by autoradiography and phosphorimager analysis (Molecular Dynamics, Sunnyvale, CA). ERK kinase assays were performed as described elsewhere[27]. Briefly, 25 μg liver nuclear extract was incubated with anti-ERK-2 antibody and protein A-conjugated sepharose beads (Pharmacia, Piscataway, NJ), extensively washed, then incubated in kinase reactions contain-ing γ^{32}P-ATP and recombinant substrate GST-ElkC[28] immobilized on glu-tathione-agarose beads. Similarly, p38 was immunoprecipitated with anti-p38 polyclonal antibody (the kind gift of R. Davis) and protein A-conjugated sepharose beads (Pharmacia, Piscataway, NJ), extensively washed, then incu-bated in kinase reactions containing γ^{32}P-ATP and recombinant substrate GST-ATF2 immobilized on glutathione-agarose beads (Pharmacia, Piscataway, NJ).

Electrophoretic mobility shift assays (EMSA)

Binding reactions were carried out for 20 min on ice, using 2.5 μg nuclear extract, 100 pg of ^{32}P-labelled DNA probes for the AP-1 consensus binding site, the NF-κB consensus binding site[29], or the HNF-1 binding site from the rat albumin promoter[30], with or without 20 ng unlabelled competitor probe[31]. Complexes were separated by electrophoresis on non-denaturing 5% acrylamide gels, and assessed by autoradiography and phosphorimager analysis (Molecular Dynamics, Sunnyvale, CA).

Liver nuclear extracts

Livers were collected after 24 h cold storage, 15 or 60 min after transplantation, or from untreated normal controls. After tissue samples were collected for RNA and lipid preparation, most of the liver was homogenized in homogenization buffer containing protease and phosphatase inhibitors. Nuclei were prepared using sucrose density gradient centrifugation, then lysed and extracts prepared as described elsewhere[32]. Protein was quantitated using the Bradford method (BioRad, Hercules, CA).

RNA preparation and Northern analysis

Total RNA was prepared from liver tissue samples as described elsewhere[33]; 25 μg RNA samples were separated by electrophoresis on 2.2 M formaldehyde, 1% agarose gels, then transferred to nylon membranes (MSI, Westboro, MA). cDNA probes for *c-jun*, *junB*, *c-fos*, and GAPDH were labelled using random priming (PrimeIt II, Stratagene, San Diego, CA). Membranes were hybridized and washed with a final stringency of 0.1X SSC, 0.1% SDS, then analysed by autoradiography and phosphorimager analysis (Molecular Dynamics, Sunnyvale, CA). Lipid extractions and diacylglycerol kinase assays to measure ceramide and diacylglycerol were performed as described elsewhere[34].

RT-PCR assay for TNF-α mRNA

One microgram of total liver RNA was reverse-transcribed using polyT oligo-nucleotide and MMLV reverse transcriptase (Perkin-Elmer/Applied Biosystems, Foster City, CA) in 25 μl. Rat β-actin was amplified using primers described elsewhere[35] in a 50 μl PCR reaction containing 1 mM MgCl$_2$, 50 mM Kcl, and 10 mM, Tris pH 8.3, using 1 μl of cDNA template. Rat TNF-α was amplified using primers TNF 5' (5'-CTG GCA GAG GAG GCT CTC CCC-3') and TNF3' (5'-CAG GTT CTC AGC GCT GAG C-3') in a 50 μl PCR reaction containing 1.5 mM MgCl$_2$, 25 mM KCl, 10 mM Tris, pH 9.2, 15% glycerol and 90 μg/ml BSA, using 5 μl cDNA template. PCR samples were analysed by agarose gel electrophoresis and ethidium bromide staining.

Adenoviruses

Ad5IκB, which expresses the IκB super-repressor, has been described elsewhere[36]. Ad5Luc was the kind gift of Dr Branko Stefanovic, and expresses luciferase driven by the CMV promoter. Adenoviruses were amplified in replication-permissive 293 cells and purified on CsCl gradients[37], then dialysed against 10 mM Tris pH 8.0, 100 mM NaCl, 1 mM MgCl$_2$, 3% glycerol for animal injections. Donor animals were infected by tail vein injection with the previously optimized dose of 10^{10} plaque-forming units (pfu) 24 h prior to liver explanation.

Recombinant adenovirus containing the transgene for either Zn/Cu-SOD (Ad-SOD1) or β-galactosidase (Ad-lacZ) was prepared as described elsewhere[38–40]. Briefly, the plasmid shuttle vectors pAd5-CMV-lacZ and pAd5-CMV-SOD1 were constructed by standard cloning protocols as described elsewhere[41]. The adenoviral shuttle plasmids were transfected into the permissive HEK 293 host cell line to generate recombinant Ad-lacZ and Ad-SOD1 adenoviruses. The virus isolates were plaque-purified and propagated in HEK 293 cells, isolated, concentrated, and titred by plaque assay to a stock titre of greater than 1×10^{11} pfu. Rats were injected intravenously with 1×10^9 pfu.

Histological procedures

Some rats were sacrificed 8 h after transplantation, and livers were fixed by perfusion with 4% paraformaldehyde in Krebs–Henseleit bicarbonate buffer (118 mM NaCl, 25 mM NaHCO$_3$, 1.2 mM KH$_2$PO$_4$, 1.2 mM MgSO$_4$, 4.7 mM KCl and 1.3 mM CaCl$_2$) at pH 7.6, embedded in paraffin, and processed for light microscopy (H&E staining). Liver damage was assessed by estimating the proportion of necrotic to non-necrotic areas as described elsewhere[5]. Briefly, five fields (400× magnification) were selected at random from at least four different sections per sample, and mean values were calculated. Eight hours after transplantation, and immediately after harvesting, liver samples were collected. Sections (6 μm) were cut on a rotary microtome and stained for ED1-positive Kupffer cells immunohistochemically using the DAKO Envision™ System and a primary anti-ED1 antibody (Biosource International, Camarillo, CA).

Determination of reduced, protein-bound pimonidazole by ELISA and immunohistochemistry

Pimonidazole is a 2-nitroimidazole which detects hypoxia in liver tissue[42]. Pimonidazole (120 mg/kg, 5 min before donor operation) was given intravenously and adducts were measured immediately following surgical harvest (25 min) in tissue homogenates with a competitive ELISA procedure described previously[43], modified for liver tissue[42] (Fig. 1). Protein levels in tissue homogenates were determined with the bicinchoninic acid (BCA) assay using a commercially available kit (Pierce Chemical Company, Rockford, IL). Paraffin blocks of formalin-fixed liver tissue were sectioned at 6 μm, and pimonidazole

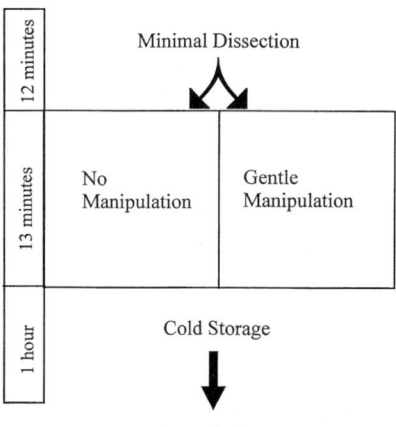

Figure 1   Model for gentle manipulation of the liver. The procedure is explained in the text

adducts were detected with a biotin–streptavidin–peroxidase indirect immuno-staining method using diaminobenzidine (DAB) as a chromogen[42]. After the immunostaining procedure, a counterstain of haematoxylin was applied. A Universal Imaging Corp. Image-1/AT image acquisition and analysis system (Chester, PA) incorporating an Axioskop 50 microscope (Carl Zeiss, Inc., Thornwood, NY) was used to capture the images[44].

RESULTS

Figure 1 depicts the method for gentle manipulation of livers during harvest[45]. Briefly, donor livers were harvested within 25 min prior to perfusion with cold UW solution. Minimal dissection was performed in a standardized fashion during the first 12 min, including freeing the organ from ligaments and cannula-tion of the bile duct. During the last 13 min, livers were either left alone or manipulated gently. Standardized gentle manipulation was carried out by touch-ing, retracting and moving the liver lobes *in situ* continuously. At 25 min, perfu-sion with 8 ml of cold Ringer's followed by 3 ml of cold UW solution was performed *in situ* via the portal vein. Cuffs were attached in the cold to the infra-hepatic vena cava and portal vein after explanation

Effects of gentle organ manipulation on liver injury, survival and hypoxia

In the non-manipulated group, survival was 100% after transplantation; how-ever, gentle manipulation decreased survival by 70%. In contrast, rats receiving manipulated livers from either $GdCl_3$- or glycine-pretreated donors survived as well as did non-manipulated controls (Fig. 2A). In all groups studied, tissue injury was undetectable prior to cold storage (Fig. 2B). In addition, non-manipulated grafts did not develop necrosis 8 h after transplantation; however, approximately 20% of the manipulated liver was necrotic at the same time. This damage was largely prevented by donor treatment before harvest with either $GdCl_3$ or glycine.

Pimonidazole, a 2-nitroimidazole hypoxia marker, binds to hypoxic liver cells *in vivo*[42]. As expected, pimonidazole binding predominates in pericentral regions where oxygen supply is naturally low. Gentle liver manipulation increased hypoxia about 2-fold in controls prior to cold storage ($p < 0.05$); however, after hepatic denervation or treatment with hexamethonium or intravenous glycine, pimonidazole binding was not different from controls (Fig. 3).

Cytokine and transcription factors are differently induced after liver transplantation

JNK, p38 and ERK are members of the MAPK family of signalling kinases. *In-vitro* kinase assays and immune-complex kinase assays were performed to assess the activities of JNK, p38 and ERK in the stored and transplanted rat liver. Hepatic p38 kinase activity was not altered by cold storage or by transplan-tation (Table 1). On the other hand, hepatic ERK was inhibited by ischaemic storage but was mildly activated at 15 min. At 60 min following transplantation,

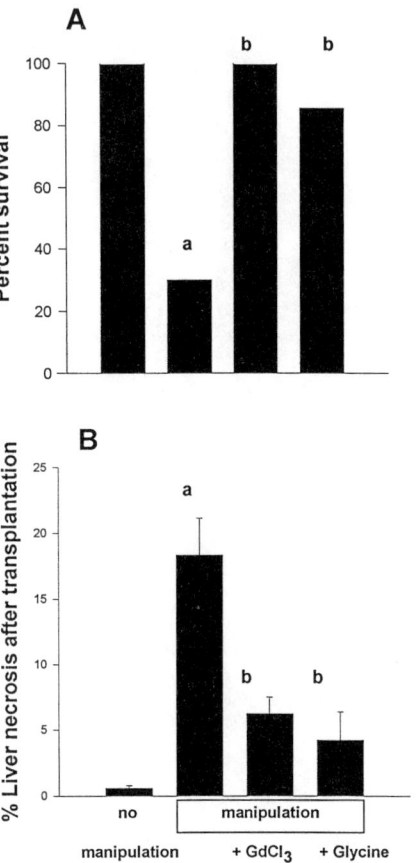

Figure 2   Effects of gentle organ manipulation on survival rates after liver transplantation. In panel **A**, donor livers were harvested within 25 min prior to perfusion with cold UW solution. After minimal dissection during the first 12 min livers were left alone or manipulated for the last 13 min as described in Materials and Methods. Some donor rats were pretreated with $GdCl_3$ or glycine. Liver grafts were stored in UW solution at 0–4°C for 1 h, and transplantation was performed using arterialization: (a) $p < 0.05$ compared to no manipulation; (b) compared to manipulation without pretreatment by Fisher exact test, $n = 5$–10. In panel **B**, liver grafts were removed from recipients 8 h after transplantation and liver damage was assessed by estimating the proportion of necrotic to non-necrotic areas in five fields selected at random from at least four different sections per sample. Subsequently, mean values were calculated. Some donors were treated with $GdCl_3$ or glycine before transplantation. Values are mean ± SEM ($p < 0.05$ by two-way ANOVA with Student–Newman–Keuls *post-hoc* test, $n = 4$–6 in each group): (a) $p < 0.05$ for comparison to no manipulation; (b) $p < 0.05$ compared to manipulation without pretreatment

ERK activity returned to control levels. Hepatic JNK was unaffected by cold storage, but was activated an average of 14-fold at 15 min and 27-fold at 60 min following transplantation. Thus, cold ischaemia did not activate any of the kinases (and inhibited ERK somewhat), while reperfusion associated with transplantation resulted in a relatively small, transient ERK activation, and a potent, sustained activation of JNK (Table 1).

247

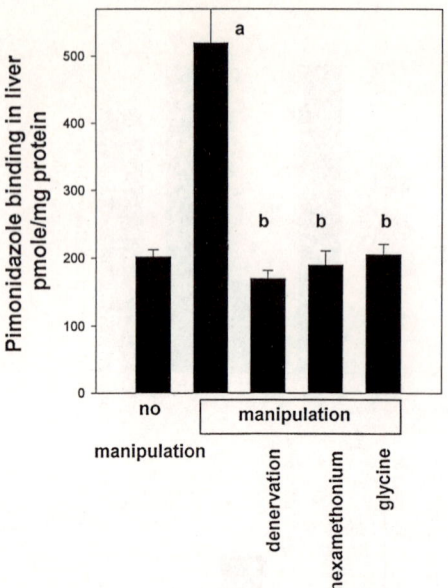

Figure 3 Gentle organ manipulation causes hypoxia after transplantation. Pimonidazole was given to donors prior to harvest as described in Materials and Methods, and pimonidazole binding was detected using a competitive ELISA. Some donors were pretreated with hexamethonium or glycine, or underwent hepatic denervation prior to manipulation. Results are means ± SEM; $n = 5$: (a) $p < 0.05$ for comparison to no manipulation; (b) $p < 0.05$ compared to manipulation

Cold ischaemic storage had no effect on NF-κB binding and elevated AP-1 binding slightly relative to the control. NF-κB binding was elevated an average of 2-fold at 15 min and 6-fold at 60 min. Further, AP-1 binding was unchanged at 15 min following transplantation, but was induced 5-fold at 60 min following transplantation. To determine whether the increase in AP-1 DNA binding activity corresponded with increased transcription, hepatic mRNA levels of the AP-1 components *c-jun*, *junB*, and *c-fos* were assessed. All three AP-1 components were induced 60 min following transplantation (Table 1).

Ceramides are produced by hydrolysis of sphingomyelin by sphingomyelinases[14], and have recently been shown to be important second messengers in response to TNF-α[13]. Accordingly, we measured total liver ceramide levels during cold storage and following transplantation. Following transplantation, ceramides were unchanged at 15 min and were elevated slightly at 60 min relative to the stored livers (Table 1). In contrast, the levels of diacylglycerol and sphingosine, other potential lipid second messengers, were unchanged by transplantation (data not shown).

To determine if TNF-α may contribute to the activation of AP-1 and NF-κB in the liver following transplantation, TNF-α mRNA levels were assessed by RT-PCR. TNF-α mRNA levels were induced at 60 min, but not at 15 min, following transplantation (Table 1).

Table 1 Effect of transplantation on activation of MAPKs, AP-1 and TNF (fold increase)

Minutes after transplant	JNK	ERK	P38	Ceramides	NF-κB	AP-1	cJun	junB	cfos	TNF α-mRNA
0	1	1	1	1	0	0	–	–	–	–
15	14	2.5	1	1	2	1	–	–	–	–
60	27	1	1	1.7	6	5	+	+	+	+

Numbers represent densitometric analysis which are based on fold increases. Parameters above were evaluated at 0, 15, and 50 min post-transplantation. Recombinant GST-cJun was incubated with 25 μg hepatic nuclear extracts from tissues collected at time points described above. JNK-mediated phosphorylation of GST-cJun was assessed by incorporation of γ-^{32}p-ATP, followed by SDS-PAGE, autoradiography, and phosphorimager analysis. AP-1 and NF-κB DNA binding activity was assessed using mobility shift assays. Nuclear extracts were incubated wiht 100 pg of labelled probe on ice for 20 min, followed by non-denaturing gel electrophoresis. Hepatic RNA was isolated and 20 μg RNA was subject to Northern analysis, to compare the mRNA levesl of c-jun, junB, and c-fos, as indicated. Filters were reprobed for GAPDH as a control for RNA integrity. Lipids were extracted from liver samples, and ceramides were determined. The mRnA levels for TNF-α and β-actin were assessed by RT-PCR. Data from ref. 69.

Role of NF-κB activation during transplantation

We next addressed the role of NF-κB activation during transplantation. NF-κB acts as a protective transcription factor in hepatocytes *in vitro* and following partial hepatectomy *in vivo*[39,41]. A mutant of IκB-α which is resistant to phosphorylation and degradation, and thus inhibits NF-κB activation, was used[36,46]. To assess the effect of blocking NF-κB activation in hepatocytes during transplantation, this IκB super-repressor was expressed in donor livers using adenoviral-mediated gene transfer. Donor animals were treated by tail vein injection 24 h prior to explantation with either the IκB adenovirus (Ad5IκB) or a control

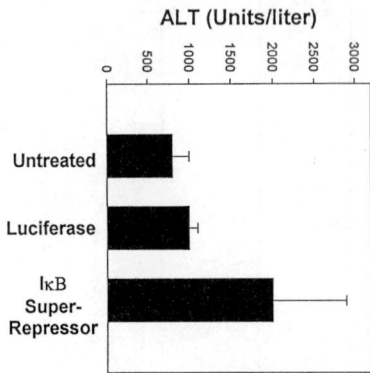

Figure 4 Expression of IκB super-repressor increases liver damage following liver transplantation. Serum ALT levels from recipients of untreated, luciferase- and IκB- super-repressor expressing allografts were determined after 3 h of transplantation. Results are presented as average ± SEM; *n* = 4 for each group

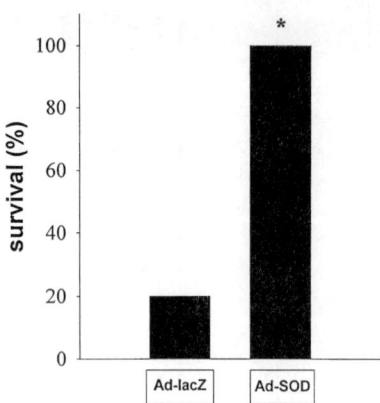

Figure 5 Effects of gene therapy with Ad-SOD1 on survival after liver transplantation. Donor rats were treated with Ad-SOD1 or Ad-lacZ intravenously 72 h prior to organ harvest. Organs were stored for 24 h in UW solution at 1–4°C and transplantation was performed using rearterialization. Survival was defined as animals alive for at least 7 days after transplantation. Values are mean ± SEM (*, $p < 0.001$ by two-way ANOVA with the Student–Newman–Keuls *post-hoc* test)

adenovirus expressing luciferase (Ad5Luc). Expression of the IκB super-repressor caused a greater increase in serum ALT levels at 3 h post-transplantation compared to either untreated transplants or luciferase-expressing transplants (Fig. 4). Moreover, NF-κB is activated by oxidants, and SOD decreases oxidants. In rats receiving Ad-lacZ-infected livers, survival was 20–25%. In contrast, all rats receiving an Ad-SOD1-infected organ survived (Fig. 5). There were no differences between recipients receiving Ad-lacZ-infected organs and controls, whereas differences compared to the Ad-SOD1-treated animals were significant.

DISCUSSION

Effect of manipulation

The organ transplantation procedure can be subdivided into three phases: harvest, cold storage and reperfusion. Previous studies on the mechanisms of graft injury leading to primary non-function and initial poor graft function focused on the cold storage[47–49] and reperfusion phases[50]. It has been concluded that most of the injury occurs as a result of reperfusion, since Carolina rinse solution used after cold storage minimized reperfusion injury after long-term immersion of the liver graft in cold UW solution where storage injury would have sufficient time to develop[3]. This study addressed injury resulting from gentle manipulation of the liver during harvest. When grafts were manipulated during harvest, survival decreased dramatically while serum AST and liver necrosis increased. This is important, since manipulation of the liver during harvest cannot be completely prevented in clinical liver transplantation. The working hypothesis to explain the observed effects of manipulation during harvest is as follows: manipulation causes disturbances in the microcirculation, creating hypoxia, followed by 'priming' or activation of Kupffer cells[9], which are known to play a role in reperfusion injury[51]. This causes aggravated reperfusion injury, which leads to poor initial graft function, early loss of the graft and death of the recipient.

Role of Kupffer cells

To test the hypothesis that Kupffer cells are involved in mechanisms of manipulation during harvest (see Fig. 1), donors were pretreated with GdCl$_3$, a rare-earth metal and selective Kupffer cell toxicant[52], or with glycine, a non-essential amino acid known to prevent Kupffer cell activation[19,20]. Interestingly, liver injury after transplantation due to graft manipulation during harvest was prevented by GdCl$_3$ and glycine, as shown by blunted increases in serum transaminases and necrosis (Fig. 2). Prevention of aggravated reperfusion injury under these conditions resulted in marked improvement in survival after transplantation. To test the working hypothesis that hepatic nerves are involved in mechanisms due to organ manipulation during harvest, livers were microsurgically denervated or ganglia were blocked before harvest. Indeed, these treatments prevented disturbances in microcirculation and hypoxia at harvest. Further, injury at reperfusion leading to impaired graft function and primary non-function after transplantation was prevented. This is consistent with the hypothesis that early disturbances of microcirculation and hypoxia are associated with hepatic innervation and translate into injury after reperfusion.

How can hepatic innervation be involved with injury developing at reperfusion? Laparatomy and mild abdominal exploration resulted in activation of nerves to the liver[53], and decreasing flow in both the hepatic artery and portal vein[54]. In perfused livers, stimulation of the hepatic nerves around the portal vein and the hepatic artery also enhanced glucose release[55–57], lowered portal flow[56,57], and decreased oxygen uptake due to disturbed hepatic microcirculation[56–58]. Hepatic parenchymal cells, Kupffer cells, endothelial cells and stellate cells receive efferent sympathetic innervation. In rats the parenchyma of the liver is poorly innervated at the periportal borders of the acinus[59]; however, signal conductance through cellular gap junctions occurs[60]. Direct stimulation of the mixed nerve bundle surrounding the hepatic artery produced a marked decrease of flow in both the hepatic artery and portal vein, disturbing the intrahepatic microcirculation. Indeed, in this study gentle *in-situ* organ manipulation disturbed hepatic microcirculation, which in turn caused hypoxia leading to production of oxidants (Fig. 3). In support of this hypothesis, Ad-SOD treatment prior to transplantation increases survival dramatically (Fig. 5).

Moreover, gentle manipulation of the liver during harvest activates the hepatic nerves which cause vasoconstriction in the liver reflected by impaired intrahepatic circulation, which in turn causes cellular hypoxia, followed by priming or activation of Kupffer cells[9,21–23,45]. This causes aggravated reperfusion injury, which leads to poor initial graft function, early loss of the graft, and death of the recipient. This is consistent with several lines of evidence which suggest that microcirculatory disturbances cause hypoxia with subsequent reperfusion injury[21–23].

Possible site of action of glycine

It is known that destruction of Kupffer cells, the major source of eicosanoids in the liver[61], reduces reperfusion injury[18]. Moreover, Kupffer cells release proteases and TNF-α upon activation[10]. A recent study has shown that glycine reduces TNF-α production and minimizes death induced by endotoxin, a known activator of Kupffer cells[19]. Indeed, TNF-α production after LPS increased significantly in Kupffer cells from manipulated livers; however, this effect was blunted when glycine was infused to the donor before manipulation ($p < 0.05$)[62]. Accordingly, it is proposed that glycine prevents activation of Kupffer cells at harvest, thereby minimizing reperfusion injury after transplantation. This effect is most probably related to actions on glycine-gated chloride channels of Kupffer cells or nerves.

Cytokines and transcription factors

Transplantation activated the transcription factor NF-κB (Table 1). In the transplanted liver, inhibiting NF-κB activation resulted in increased liver injury and the induction of hepatocyte apoptosis, demonstrating that NF-κB is protective to the liver following transplantation. Since NF-κB is also protective after partial hepatectomy[36], this suggests that NF-κB is a generally protective transcription factor to hepatocytes *in vitro* as well as *in vivo*. NF-κB activates expression of

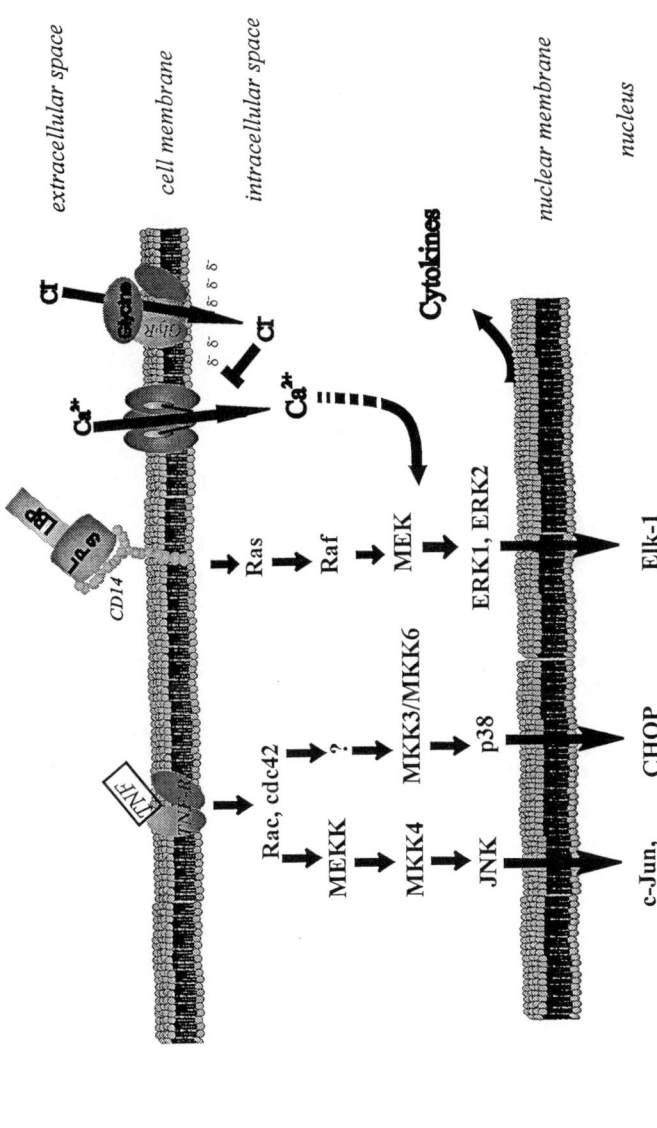

Figure 6 Diagram of proposed mechanism by which glycine prevents harvest-related injury. Gentle manipulation of the liver during harvest causes intrahepatic vasoconstriction, disturbances in microcirculation and hypoxia which is followed by 'priming' or activation of Kupffer cells. Activated Kupffer cells then release vasoactive substances, free radicals, cytokines and proteases which contribute to reperfusion injury developing upon transplantation, further impairing microcirculation. The production of some mediators released from Kupffer cells require an increase of intracellular calcium. When glycine is given a glycine-gated chloride channel (GlyR) in the membrane of Kupffer cells is activated, leading to chloride influx and to subsequent hyperpolarization of the membrane. This prevents activation of Kupffer cells, and the sequelae caused by manipulation. Cytokines such as TNF trigger the MAPK pathway leading to activation of JNK

genes which block caspase activation[63], possibly accounting for its protective effect. Many agents can inhibit NF-κB activation, including glucocorticoids, immunosuppressive agents, N-acetyl cysteine, superoxide dismutase and IκB super-repressor (Fig. 4). In SOD-treated livers subjected to ischaemia/reperfusion, NF-κB activity was partially inhibited, presumably by blocking the generation of oxidants which activate NF-κB[64]. Based on the results reported here, the effect of inhibiting NF-κB during ischaemia/reperfusion of liver transplants is hepatocyte apoptosis. Therapeutic strategies aimed at maintaining NF-κB activity while blocking oxidant production during the ischaemia/reperfusion of liver transplantation may be of clinical benefit. Indeed, gene therapy with SOD improved survival after transplantation dramatically[65] (Fig. 5).

Both NF-κB and AP-1 DNA binding activities are induced in the transplanted livers, which is consistent with increased TNF-α[66,67] (Table 1 and Fig. 6). The induction of AP-1 is further supported by induction of the mRNAs for the AP-1 components c-jun, junB, and c-fos after transplantation. JNK activity is increased before activation of AP-1 (Table 1). Reactive oxygen intermediates produced during reperfusion injury may arise in both hepatocytes and Kupffer cells, in addition to being induced by TNF-α, and may serve as second messengers for NF-κB activation[68]. Ceramide levels, but not sphingosine or diacylglycerol levels, were elevated after transplantation (Table 1). Ceramides are second messengers produced by the action of sphingomyelinase in response to TNF-α, and exogenous C2-ceramides activate JNK[14,15]. The relative timing of JNK activation and the increase in ceramides in the transplanted livers is inconsistent with ceramide acting as the initial activator of JNK, since JNK activation occurs earlier than the elevation of ceramides. However, increased ceramides may serve to prolong JNK induction or to modulate the outcome of the induced signal pathway. JNK activation also precedes the induction of TNF-α mRNA levels. Therefore, it is likely that increased hepatic TNF-α and ceramide levels perpetuate JNK induction, but are not the initiating signal (Table 1).

Conclusion and clinical implications

The data presented in this study are consistent with the hypothesis that gentle organ manipulation during harvest disturbs the hepatic microcirculation and causes hypoxia. This most probably plays a key role in mediating reperfusion injury via mechanisms involving Kupffer cells. If the effect of gentle manipulation is confirmed in humans, intravenous glycine, viral delivery of SOD, hepatic denervation and gene therapy before organ harvest, or the use of ganglionic blocking agents, could be used to lower the rate of primary graft nonfunction and dysfunction, increase survival, and lead to more efficient utilization of scarce organs.

Acknowledgements

This worth was supported in part by grants from NIH and by the Deutsche Forschungsgemeinschaft.

References

1. Ploeg RJ, D'Alessandro AM, Knechtle SJ *et al.* Risk factors for primary dysfunction after liver transplantation – a multivariate analysis. Transplantation. 1993;55:807–13.
2. Pichlmayr R, Ringe B, Lauchart W, Wonigeit K. Liver transplantation. Transplant Proc. 1987;19:103–12.
3. Gao W, Currin RT, Lemasters JJ, Connor HD, Mason RP, Thurman RG. Reperfusion rather than storage injury predominates following long-term (48 hrs) cold storage of grafts in UW solution: studies with Carolina Rinse in transplanted rat liver. Transplant Int. 1992;5:S329–35.
4. Marzi I, Zhong Z, Zimmermann FA, Lemasters JJ, Thurman RG. Xanthine and hypoxanthine accumulation during storage may contribute to reperfusion injury following liver transplantation in the rat. Transplant Proc. 1989;21:1319–20.
5. Thurman RG, Marzi I, Seitz G, Thies J, Lemasters JJ, Zimmermann FA. Hepatic reperfusion injury following orthotopic liver transplantation in the rat. Transplantation. 1988;46:502–6.
6. Gao W, Takei Y, Marzi I *et al.* Carolina Rinse solution: a new strategy to increase survival time after orthotopic liver transplantation in the rat. Transplantation. 1991;52:417–24.
7. Takei Y, Marzi I, Gao W, Gores GJ, Lemasters JJ, Thurman RG. Leukocyte adhesion and cell death following orthotopic liver transplantation in the rat. Transplantation. 1991;51:959–65.
8. Caldwell-Kenkel JC, Thurman RG, Lemasters JJ. Selective loss of nonparenchymal cell viability after cold ischemic storage of rat livers. Transplantation. 1988;45:834–7.
9. Lindert KA, Caldwell-Kenkel JC, Nukina S, Lemasters JJ, Thurman RG. Activation of Kupffer cells on reperfusion following hypoxia: particle phagocytosis in a low-flow, reflow model. Am J Physiol. 1992;262:G345–50.
10. Bouwens L. Structural and functional aspects of Kupffer cells. Revis Biol Cellular. 1988;16:69–94.
11. Cerra FB, West MA, Keller G, Mazuski J, Simmons RL. Hypermetabolism/organ failure: the role of the activated macrophage as a metabolic regulator. Prog Clin Biol Res. 1988;264:27–42.
12. Wardle EN. Kupffer cells and their function. Liver. 1987;7:63–75.
13. Dbaibo GS, Obeid LM, Hannun YA. Tumor necrosis factor-alpha (TNF-alpha) signal transduction through ceramide. Dissociation of growth inhibitory effects of TNF-alpha from activation of nuclear factor-kappa B. J Biol Chem. 1993;268:17762–6.
14. Hannun YA. The sphingomyelin cycle and the second messenger function of ceramide. J Biol Chem. 1994;269:3125–8.
15. Westwick JK, Bielawska AE, Dbaibo G, Hannun YA, Brenner DA. Ceramide activates the stress-activated protein kinases. J Biol Chem. 1995;270:22689–92.
16. Lemasters JJ, Thurman RG. Reperfusion injury after liver preservation for transplantation. Annu Rev Pharmacol Toxicol. 1997;37:327–38.
17. Thurman RG, Zhong Z, Frankenberg Mv, Stachlewitz RF, Bunzendahl H. Prevention of cyclosporin-induced nephrotoxicity with dietary glycine. Transplantation. 1997;63:1661–7.
18. Zhong Z, Jones S, Thurman RG. Glycine minimizes reperfusion injury in a low-flow, reflow liver perfusion model in the rat. Am J Physiol. 1996;270:G332–8.
19. Ikejima K, Iimuro Y, Forman DT, Thurman RG. A diet containing glycine improves survival in endotoxin shock in the rat. Am J Physiol. 1996;271:G97–103.
20. Ikejima K, Qu W, Stachlewitz RF, Thurman RG. Kupffer cells contain a glycine-gated chloride channel. Am J Physiol. 1997;272:G1581–6.
21. Teramoto K, Bowers JL, Kruskal JB, Clouse ME. Hepatic microcirculatory changes after reperfusion in fatty and normal liver transplantation in the rat. Transplantation. 1993;56:1076–82.
22. Hui A, Kawasaki S, Makuuchi M, Nakayama J, Ikegami T, Miyagawa J. Liver injury following normothermic ischemia in steatotic rat liver. Hepatology. 1994;20:1287–93.
23. Husberg BS, Genyk YS, Klintmalm GB. A new rat model for studies of the ischemic injury after transplantation of fatty livers: improvement after postoperative administration of prostaglandin. Transplantation. 1994;57:458.
24. Bergmeyer HU. Methods of Enzymatic Analysis, 1st edn. New York: Academic Press; 1988.
25. Westwick JK, Brenner DA. Methods for analyzing c-Jun kinase. Methods Enzymol. 1995;255:342–59.
26. Minden A, Lin A, Smeal T *et al.* c-Jun N-terminal phosphorylation correlates with activation of the JNK subgroup but not the ERK subgroup of mitogen-activated protein kinases. Mol Cell Biol. 1994;14:6683–8.

27. Lytton SD, Heland A, Zhang-Gouillon Z-Q *et al.* Autoantibodies against cytochromes P-4502E1 and P-4503A in alcoholics. Mol Pharmacol. 1999;55:223–33.
28. Marias R, Wynne J, Treisman R. The SRF accessory protein Elk-1 contains a growth factor-regulated transcriptional activation domain. Cell. 1993;73:381–93.
29. Baeuerle PA, Baltimore D. A 65 KD subunit of active NF-κB is required for inhibition of NF-κB by IκB. Genes Dev. 1989;3:1689–98.
30. Westwick JK, Weitzel C, Leffert HL, Brenner DA. Activation of Jun kinase is an early event in hepatic regeneration. J Clin Invest. 1995;95:803–10.
31. Hattori M, Tugores A, Westwick JK *et al.* Activation of activating protein 1 during hepatic acute phase response. Am J Physiol. 1993;264:G95–103.
32. Dignam JD, Lebovitz RM, Roeder RG. Accurate transcription by RNA polymerase II in a soluble extract from isolated mammalian cells. Nucleic Acids Res. 1983;11:1475–89.
33. Chirgwin JM, Przybyla AE, MacDonald RJ, Rutter WJ. Isolation of biologically active ribonucleic acid from sources enriched in ribonuclease. Biochemistry. 1979;18:5294–9.
34. Jayadev S, Liu B, Bielawska AE *et al.* Role for ceramide in cell cycle arrest. J Biol Chem. 1995;270:2047–52.
35. Kwon J, Chung IY, Benveniste EN. Cloning and sequence analysis of the rat tumor necrosis factor-encoding genes. Gene. 1993;132:227–36.
36. Brenner DA. Signal transduction during liver regeneration. J Gastroenterol Hepatol. 1998;13 (Suppl.):S93–5.
37. Graham FL, Prevec L. Methods for construction of adenovirus vectors. Mol Biotechnol. 1995;3:207–20.
38. Rigby PW. Cloning vectors derived from animal viruses. J Gen Virol. 1983;64:255–66.
39. Rosenfeld MA, Siegfried W, Yoshimura K *et al.* Adenovirus-mediated transfer of a recombinant alpha 1-antitrypsin gene to the lung epithelium *in vivo*. Science. 1991;252:431–4.
40. Rosenfeld MA, Siegfried W, Yoshimura K *et al.* Adenovirus-mediated transfer of a recombinant alpha 1-antitrypsin gene to the lung epithelium *in vivo*. Science. 1991;252:431–4.
41. Sambrook J, Fritsch EF, Maniatis T. Molecular Cloning: a Laboratory Manual, 2nd edn. Cold Spring Harbor, NY: Cold Spring Harbor Laboratory; 1989.
42. Arteel GE, Thurman RG, Yates JM, Raleigh JA. Evidence that hypoxia markers detect oxygen gradients in liver: pimonidazole and retrograde perfusion of rat liver. Br J Cancer. 1995;72:889–95.
43. Raleigh JA, La Dine JK, Cline JM, Thrall DE. An enzyme-linked immunosorbent assay for hypoxia marker binding in tumours. Br J Cancer. 1994;69:66–71.
44. Arteel GE, Iimuro Y, Yin M, Raleigh JA, Thurman RG. Chronic enteral ethanol treatment causes hypoxia in rat liver tissue *in vivo*. Hepatology. 1997;25:920–6.
45. Schemmer P, Schoonhoven R, Swenberg JA, Bunzendahl H, Thurman RG. Gentle *in situ* liver manipulation during organ harvest decreases survival after rat liver transplantation: role of Kupffer cells. Transplantation. 1998;65:1015–20.
46. Bradham CA, Qian T, Streetz K, Trautwein C, Brenner DA, Lemasters JJ. The mitochondrial permeability transition is required for tumor necrosis factor alpha-mediated apoptosis and cytochrome c release. Mol Cell Biol. 1998;18:6353–64.
47. Iu S, Harvey PRC, Makowka L, Pentrunka CN, Ilson RG, Strasberg SM. Markers of allograft viability in the rat. Transplantation. 1987;44:562–9.
48. Strasberg SM, Howard TK, Molmenti EP, Hertl M. Selecting the donor liver: risk factors for poor function after orthotopic liver transplantation. Hepatology. 1994;20:829–38.
49. Clavien PA, Harvey PRC, Strasberg SM. Preservation and perfusion injury in liver allografts. Transplantation. 1992;53:957–78.
50. Caldwell-Kenkel JC, Currin RT, Tanaka Y, Thurman RG, Lemasters JJ. Reperfusion injury to endothelial cells following cold ischemic storage of rat liver. Hepatology. 1989;10:292–9.
51. Bremer C, Bradford BU, Hunt KJ *et al.* Role of Kupffer cells in the pathogenesis of hepatic reperfusion injury. Am J Physiol. 1994;267:G630–6.
52. Hardonk MJ, Dijkhuis FWJ, Jonker AM. Selective depletion of Kupffer cells by gadolinium chloride attenuates both acute galactosamine-induced hepatitis and carbon tetrachloride toxicity in rats. In: Wisse E, Knook DL, Balabaud C, editors. Cells of the Hepatic Sinusoid. Leiden: Kupffer Cell Foundation; 1996:28–32.
53. Ji S, Beckh K, Jungermann K. Regulation of oxygen consumption and microcirculation by alpha-sympathetic nerves in the isolated perfused rat liver. FEBS Lett. 1984;167:117–22.

54. Lautt WW. Afferent and efferent neural roles in liver function. Prog Neurobiol. 1983;21:323–48.
55. Hartmann H, Beckh K, Jungermann K. Direct control of glycogen metabolism in the perfused rat liver by the sympathetic innervation. Eur J Biochem. 1982;123:521–6.
56. Beckh K, Hartmann H, Jungermann K. Modulation by insulin and glucagon of the activation of glycogenolysis by perivascular nerve stimulation in the perfused rat liver. FEBS Lett. 1982;146:69–72.
57. Beckh K, Balks HJ, Jungermann K. Activation of glycogenolysis and norepinephrine overflow in the perfused rat liver during repetitive perivascular nerve stimulation. FEBS Lett. 1982;149:261–5.
58. Seydoux J, Brunsmann MJ, Jeanrenaud B, Girardier L. Alpha-sympathetic control of glucose output of mouse liver perfused in situ. Am J Physiol. 1979;236:E323–7.
59. Forssmann WG, Ito S. Hepatocyte innervation in primates. J Cell Biol. 1977;74:299–313.
60. Metz W, Forssmann WG. Innervation of the liver in guinea pig and rat. Anat Embryol (Berl). 1980;160:239–52.
61. Decker K. The response of liver macrophages to inflammatory stimulation. Keio J Med. 1998;47:1–9.
62. Schemmer P, Bradford BU, Rose ML et al. Intravenous glycine improves survival in rat liver transplantation. Am J Physiol. 1999;276:G924–32.
63. Chu ZL, McKinsey TA, Liu L, Gentry JJ, Malim MH, Ballard DW. Suppression of tumor necrosis factor-induced cell death by inhibitor of apoptosis c-IAP2 is under NF-kappaB control. Proc Natl Acad Sci USA. 1997;94:10057–62.
64. Zwacka RM, Zhou W, Zhang Y et al. Redox gene therapy for ischemia/reperfusion injury of the liver reduces AP1 and NF-κB activation. Nature Med. 1999;4:698–704.
65. Lehmann TG, Wheeler MD, Schoonhoven R, Bunzendahl H, Samulski RJ, Thurman RG. Adenoviral gene delivery of Cu/Zn-superoxide dismutase minimizes liver injury and improves survival after liver transplantation in the rat. Hepatology. 1999 (In press).
66. Brenner DA, O'Hara M, Angel P, Chojkier M, Karin M. Prolonged activation of *jun* and collagenase genes by tumor necrosis factor-α. Nature (Lond). 1989;337:661–3.
67. Lowenthal JW, Ballard DW, Bogerd H, Bohnlein E, Greene WC. Tumor necrosis factor-alpha activation of the IL-2 receptor-alpha gene involves the induction of kappa B-specific DNA binding proteins. J Immunol. 1989;142:3121–8.
68. Schreck R, Rieber P, Baeuerle PA. Reactive oxygen intermediates as apparently widely used messengers in the activation of the NF-kB transcription factor and HIV-1. EMBO J. 1991;10:2247–58.
69. Bradham CA, Stachlewitz RF, Gao W et al. Reperfusion after liver transplantation in rats differentially activates the mitogen-activated protein kinases. Hepatology. 1997;25:1128–35.

23
Effect of lipopolysaccharides on hepatocellular transport processes

S. GRÜNE

INTRODUCTION

During sepsis the liver is one of the organs first affected[1]. Initially the organism reacts with a hyperdynamic circulation and hepatic centrilobular hypoxia[2,3], resulting in hepatocellular dysfunction[4-9].

Lipopolysaccharides (LPS) which are located on the outer membrane of Gram-negative bacteria, are thought to be one of the triggers of organ reaction to sepsis. Two effector molecules involved in the LPS response are the LPS binding protein (LBP) and CD14[10]. LBP appears to function as a catalytic transfer protein in delivering LPS to CD14[11]. CD14 is thought to be one of the important LPS recognition molecules. Membrane-bound CD14 (mCD14), which attaches to the cell surface, increases the sensitivity of macrophages to LPS[12,13]. A soluble form of CD14 (sCD14) is present in the plasma, and complexes of LPS and soluble CD14 sensitize CD14-negative cells, such as endothelial cells[14,15]. Another important LPS recognition molecule is the toll-like receptor protein (TLR). TLR has an extracellular domain and a cytoplasmic domain that is homologous to the interleukin-1 receptor. Six toll-like proteins are identified so far. CD14 seems to recruit LPS to the TLR proteins in order to activate the signalling cascade[16-18].

Bacteria and bacterial products enter the portal venous system. In the liver LPS induces a decrease in fenestration of the sinusoidal endothelial cells, accompanied by morphological evidence of enhanced endocytotic activity and cytoplasmic swelling[19]. This phenomenon can be observed from 3 h on, advancing up to 24 h. LPS is internalized and modified by Kupffer cells. Native LPS induces tumour necrosis factor (TNF-α) to a 5.7-fold higher level than the Kupffer cell modified LPS[20]. The uptake of LPS into the Kupffer cells occurs via a macropinocytic pathway[14], the uptake is unsaturable up to a concentration of 33 μg/ml[21,22]. LPS stimulation of Kupffer cells is not dependent on the uptake of LPS into the Kupffer cells. The stimulation results in a release of inflammatory mediators, including TNF-α, interleukin-1 (IL-1), interleukin-6, transforming growth factor-beta (TGF-β), nitric oxide, leukotrienes and prostanoids[23,24]. It is now thought that LPS is transported to the Golgi apparatus, and that this transport is necessary for at least some types of signal transduction by LPS[25]. Furthermore, LPS induces microtubule-dependent (IL-6 and TNF-α induction) and independent pathways (IL-1β and inducible nitric oxide synthetase) in Kupffer cells[26].

Hepatocytes express mCD14[15,27] and sCD14[28]. It is thought that sCD14 is somehow an acute-phase protein which is up-regulated by cytokines during endotoxaemia. Hepatocytes from LPS-treated animals express higher amounts of mCD14 and release more sCD14[15]. At low concentrations sCD14 can mediate the activation of mCD14-negative cells by LPS, but at high concentrations sCD14 can neutralize the effects of LPS[29].

The mechanism of LPS clearance in the liver has not yet been defined. It seems that LPS can be taken up by hepatocytes with or without prior contact to Kupffer cells. Hepatocytes have a higher capacity for taking up Kupffer cell-modified LPS than unmodified native LPS[20]. LPS is transported in vesicles through the hepatocytes and its biliary excretion is microtubule-dependent[30]. Fluorescein isothiocyanate labelled (FITC-) LPS was taken up by hepatocytes 5 min after injection into the portal vein and fluorescence was rapidly secreted into bile, peaking at 20 min[31].

It has not yet been elucidated whether LPS has a direct effect on the hepatocytes or whether effects are mediated through the Kupffer cells.

HEPATIC TRANSPORT PROCESSES DURING SEPSIS

Hepatocellular dysfunction due to LPS is characterized by a decrease in bilirubin transport[6], a decrease in bile salt uptake[23] and a decrease in the transport of organic anions such as indocyanine green[4,32] and sulphobromophthalein[5].

Transport in the liver is divided into (a) transport from the blood through the basolateral membrane of the hepatocyte, (b) transport through the hepatocyte, and (c) the excretion of the substances into the bile through the canalicular membrane.

Different transporting systems are expressed in the basolateral membrane (Fig. 1), which are affected during sepsis. The ATP-dependent multidrug resistance protein 1 (MRP1) transports bilirubin glucuronides[33], glutathione conjugates, LTC4 and bile acids[34,35] from the hepatocyte to the blood. It is up-regulated during sepsis[36].

Three different organic anion transporting polypeptides (OATPs) exist in the liver. OATP1 transports Na-independent bile acids, indocyanine green and bromosulphophthalein (BSP)[37]. OATP2 transports Na-independent bile acids, taurocholate, DHEAS, T4, BSP cardiac glycosides and pravastatin[38]. OATP3, which is only found at a low density in the liver[39], transports taurocholate, BSP, T3 and T4. OATP1 is down-regulated during sepsis[32,37].

LST1 is another transporter for organic anions, which is expressed exclusively in the liver[40] and transports eicosanoids (PGE$_2$), thromboxane B$_2$, leukotrienes C4 and E4). Thus far nothing is known about the effect of sepsis on this transporter. The Na$^+$-taurocholate cotransporting polypeptide (ntcp), which transports bile acids into hepatocytes[41], and the sodium–potassium ATPase which is necessary to maintain the membrane potential are also affected during sepsis[42,43].

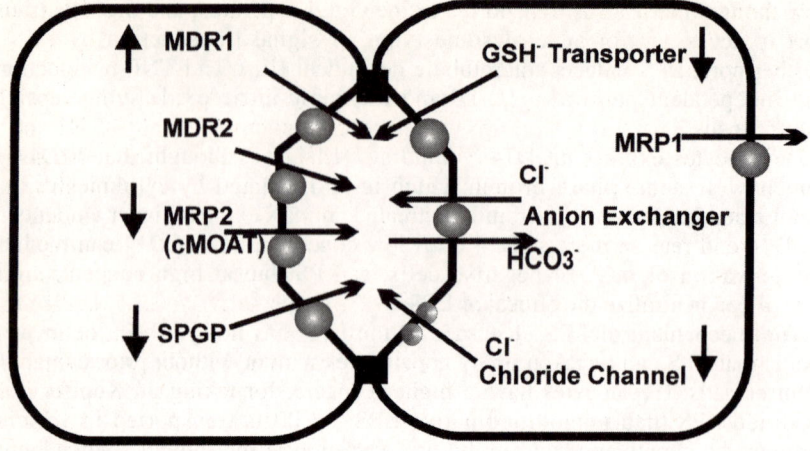

Figure 1 Effect of LPS on different canalicular transporters in the hepatocyte

On the canalicular side of the hepatocyte a group of transporters are necessary for detoxification (Fig. 2). The multidrug resistance protein 1 (MDR1) mediates biliary secretion of hydrophobic, cationic drugs[44,45]. Mdr2 plays a major role in the secretion of phospholipids in mice and rats[46], MDR3 secretes the phospholipids in humans[47].

MRP2 or cMOAT (canalicular multiorganic anion transporter) is responsible for the excretion of multivalent anionic conjugates such as indocyanine green from the hepatocyte into bile[48,49]. CMOAT is translocated in the early phase of

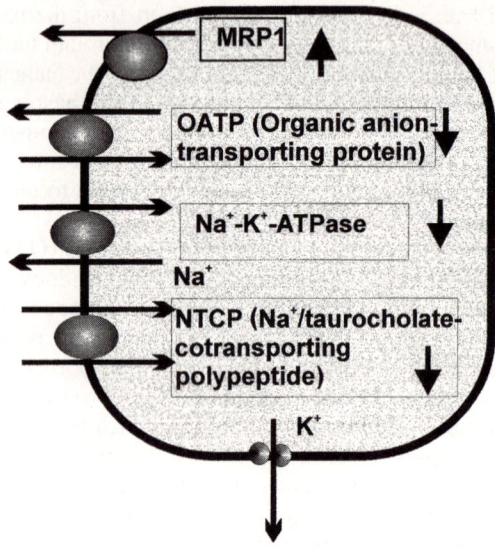

Figure 2 Effect of LPS on different transporters on the basolateral membrane in hepatocytes

LPS contact (less than 3 h) and down-regulated 5–12 h after the contact with LPS[7,48].

The transport capacity of the sister of P-glycoprotein (SPGP), which is a member of the ATP-binding cassette superfamily, is reduced during sepsis[50]. SPGP has slightly distinct transporting properties compared with MDR1 and is the ATP-dependent bile salt transporter on the canalicular membrane, also designated as bile salt exporting pump (BSEP) or BSEP/spgp[51,52]. Chloride channels change their conductance after LPS contact[53].

All the observed effects take place 2–18 h after exposing the liver to LPS. The aims of our study were to assess how early the uptake of an organic anion is affected by LPS administration in a perfused rat liver model, whether this effect is dose-dependent, and whether Kupffer cells play a role in the impairment of the organic anion uptake rate in our model. We chose indocyanine green as the organic anion for these studies because it is removed exclusively by the liver, it is secreted into bile in unmetabolized form, and it shares transport pathways with conjugated and unconjugated bilirubin. It is most probably taken up by OATP[54] and transported through the hepatocyte by vesicles[55]. It is assumed that the excretion is processed by the multidrug resistance-related protein 2 as one of the canalicular ICG transporters[56]. ICG itself causes a hyperpolarization of the hepatocytes by affecting the potassium conductance of the basolateral membrane[37].

MATERIALS AND METHODS

Materials

Indocyanine green (ICG) was obtained from Paesel and Lorei (Frankfurt, Germany); taurocholate (TC), lipopolysaccharides (Typ 0111:B6), gadolinium chloride ($GdCl_3$), 8-bromo-cyclic GMP (8-BrcGMP), collagen and collagenase were obtained from Sigma Chemicals; colloidal carbon was from Pelikan (No. 221135/Hannover, Germany). Male Wistar rats (180–280 g), obtained from Charles River Laboratories (Sulzbach, Germany), served as liver donors. All animals received care according to the criteria outlined in the 'Guide for the Care and Use of Laboratory Animals', according to the German law of animal protection.

Methods

Isolated perfused rat liver studies

Livers were surgically isolated and perfused *in situ* with a non-recirculating HCO_3^--containing balanced electrolyte solution, as previously described[57]. Each liver was perfused at a constant flow rate of 4 ml/min per gram liver weight. To evaluate the organ viability, hepatic O_2 uptake was determined from a continuous recording of O_2 tension in the perfusate with use of a Clark-type electrode placed in the perfusion inflow and outflow. Perfusate pH across the liver was continuously monitored using two in-line pH electrodes. The pressure in the perfusion system was monitored directly at inflow and outflow using a fluid pressure transducer, the output voltage signal was amplified by an analogue transducer manifold and sent to a computer. Compounds were infused by an external pump connected to the infusion cannula.

Experimental protocols were as follows: each liver was perfused for 130 min. After a 15 min equilibration period, ICG at different concentrations was infused for the entire perfusion period. From 25 min on, until the end of the perfusion, TC was infused at a concentration of 48.3 mg/kg per minute in order to achieve an ongoing bile flow. To determine the effect of LPS, LPS was infused in concentrations of 0.45, 0.9, and 1.44 mg/kg per minute from 40 to 70 min after the start of the experiment. Bile and perfusate outflow were collected every 5 min. The bile samples were collected in pre-weighed tubes and all samples were kept in the dark until photometric measurements. Every 30 min inflow perfusate was collected as a control. The samples were centrifuged for 10 min at 4000 rpm and 400 rpm respectively; 5 μl of the samples were taken and mixed with buffer which contained 2% albumin to stabilize the ICG. The ICG concentration was determined photometrically at 805 nm.

ICG uptake in primary cultured hepatocytes

Hepatocytes of $GdCl_3$-pretreated animals were isolated from rat liver using a previously described collagenase perfusion method[58]. Hepatocytes (less than 10% stainable by trypan blue) were used for each study. Four millilitres of freshly prepared hepatocytes were cultured for 1 h at 37C° in a buffer (pH 7.4) containing 20 mM Hepes, 140 mM NaCl, 5 mM KCl, 1 mM $MgSO_4$, 1 mM $CaCl_2$ and 0.8 mM KH_2PO_4, and the hepatocytes were allowed to attach to the collagen-coated Petri dishes. For every time-point two dishes were prepared with hepatocytes; two control dishes without hepatocytes were also prepared. Various concentrations of ICG were applied to the dishes to find the best ICG concentration for these experiments. Finally a concentration of 56 μg/ml cell suspension was used. In one group of experiments LPS was added at a concentration of 16 μg/ml cell suspension together with the ICG at the beginning of the experiment (time-point 0). As a control we treated primary cultured hepatocytes in another group of experiments with 8-BrcGMP (a cGMP-analogue which is able to enter the cell). 8-BrcGMP was added together with the ICG at the beginning of the experiment. At different time-points 400 μl of the supernatant of the different dishes were removed, prepared as described above, and the ICG concentration was determined photometrically at 805 nm. The uptake of ICG was followed for 2–4 h. All experiments described above were repeated in at least three different cell preparations.

Experiments with gadolinium chloride (GdCl$_3$)

To study the role of Kupffer cells in modulating the effect of LPS we treated a group of rats 24 h before the experiment with $GdCl_3$ at a dose of 1 mg/100 g body weight. To test the phagocytic capacity of Kupffer cells with and without $GdCl_3$, colloidal carbon (0.08 ml per 100 g body weight) was injected intravenously 30 min before sacrifice (24 h after a single injection of $GdCl_3$ as described earlier)[59]. The distribution of carbon in $GdCl_3$-treated livers and control livers was examined under a light microscope. The phagocytic activity in the gadolinium-treated group was decreased by 90% as compared to the untreated group.

Statistical analysis

Results are expressed as means ± SEM unless otherwise stated. Comparisons were made by repeated measures ANOVA or *t*-test as indicated.

RESULTS

In all experiments an ICG concentration of 57.8 mg/kg per minute was used. From 25 min after starting the ICG infusion to 130 min the uptake rate remained constant, resulting in a 63% (± 2%) uptake of the totally infused ICG. The different ICG dosages did not affect the perfusion pressure of the liver, the pH or the O_2 uptake (data not shown). During the observation period there was no significant change in pH and uptake rate of O_2, which was always above 2 μmol/g liver per minute.

ICG resulted in a decrease of bile flow over time, while the infusion of LPS (1.44 mg/kg per minute) did not result in an additional change in bile flow.

The clearance rate of ICG by the liver 40 min after LPS was added in a concentration of 1.44 mg/kg per minute (25 ± 8%) was significantly lower than in the control uptake experiments. At an LPS concentration of 0.9 mg/kg per minute the ICG extraction rate was 18% (± 6%) lower (not significant), and it decreased by 12.7% (± 7.4%) using an LPS concentration of 0.45 mg/kg per minute (not significant) (Fig. 3).

ICG concentrations in the bile were significantly lower if the livers were treated with LPS (Fig. 4).

In livers of animals which were pretreated with $GdCl_3$ at 24 h before the application of LPS, no decreased ICG uptake occurred (Fig. 5). No significant differences in pH, oxygen extraction or perfusion pressure were observed in the different treatment groups during the observation time.

Pretreatment with $GdCl_3$ and LPS resulted in a significant increase of the ICG excretion rate into the bile compared to other treatments. A significant reduction of ICG excretion into the bile was observed 15 min after the onset of LPS application. $GdCl_3$ alone did not result in any effect on ICG excretion or on bile flow.

The treatment of primary cultured hepatocytes with LPS (16 μg/ml supernatant), from $GdCl_3$-pretreated rats, did not change the uptake of ICG into the hepatocytes significantly (Fig. 6). In a control group treated with 8-BrcGMP we observed a significant increase (8 ± 3.6% SEM) of ICG-uptake as early as 30 min after application of 8-BrcGMP.

The viability of the hepatocytes was tested after 2 and 4 h. There was no change in viability after 2 h, 20% of the cells were stainable with trypan blue after 4 h, but there was no difference between the LPS-treated and untreated cells.

DISCUSSION

The administration of LPS resulted in a rapid (40 min) dose-dependent decrease of ICG uptake in the perfused rat liver. The effect of LPS on the hepatocytes occurred much earlier than previously described[60].

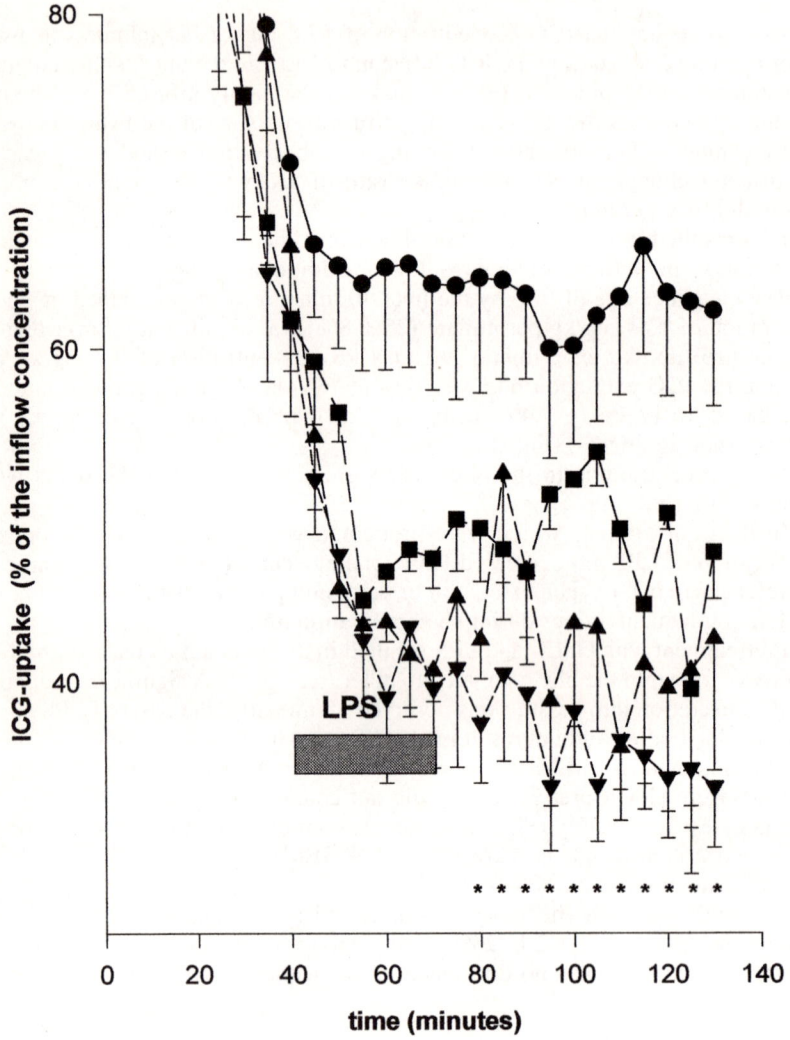

Figure 3 Effect of different concentrations of LPS on ICG uptake. The uptake of ICG into the liver is depicted as a percentage of the inflow concentration of ICG. Infusion with ICG started at 15 min (57.8 mg/kg per minute), infusion with taurocholate (TC) (48.3 mg/kg per minute) started at 25 min, administration of LPS in different concentrations (0.45, 0.9 and 1.44 mg/kg per minute) started at 40 min for 30 min. $n = 5$–6 for each treatment. *$p < 0.05$. Error bars represent SEM. (From ref. 32)

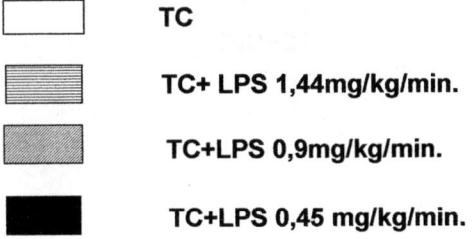

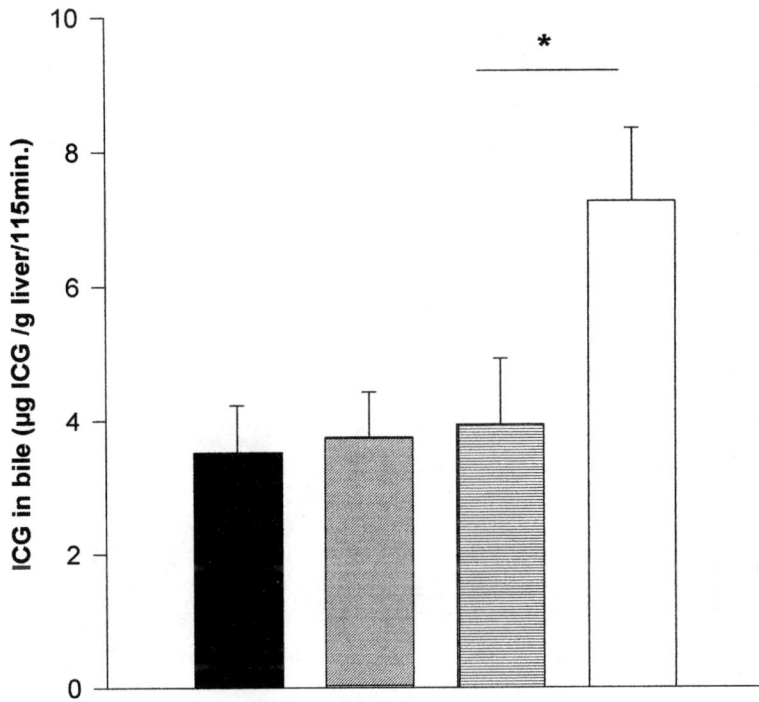

Figure 4 Effect of different concentrations of LPS on the excretion rate of ICG into bile. The excretion rate is depicted as excretion of ICG into the bile in μg/g liver over 115 min. Taurocholate (TC) was used at a concentration of 48.3 mg/kg per minute. The different concentrations of LPS were 0.45, 0.9 and 1.44 mg/kg per minute. $n = 5$–6 for every treatment. $*p < 0.05$. Error bars represent SEM. (From ref. 32)

We used concentrations of LPS between 0.45 and 1.44 mg/kg per minute. In the literature concentrations between 0.018 and 21.6 mg/kg per minute were used in liver perfusion systems and isolated hepatocytes[61–64]. The relatively high doses of LPS had to be administered since rat hepatocytes are less sensitive to LPS than, for example, human cells.

An increase in portal pressure with concomitant decrease of detoxification properties of the liver was observed in different studies[65–69]. Chronically

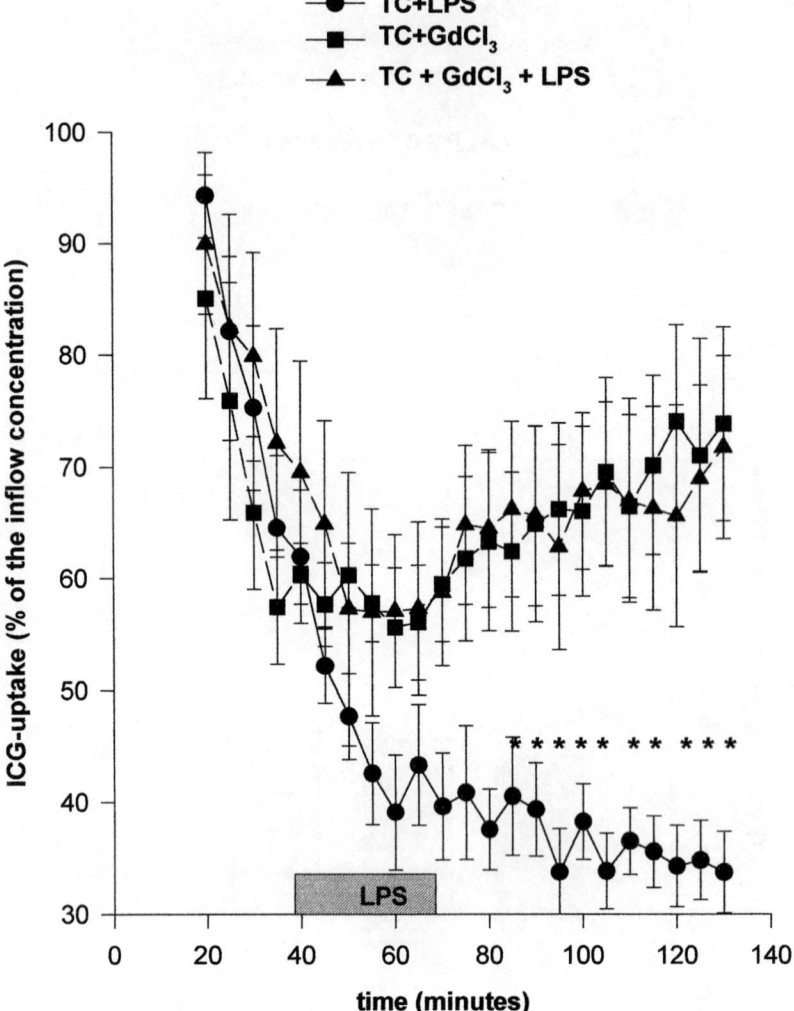

Figure 5 Effect of GdCl$_3$ on the uptake rate of ICG in the liver with and without LPS treatment. The effluent concentration of ICG is depicted as a percentage of the inflow concentration of ICG. Infusion with taurocholate (TC) (48.3 mg/kg per minute) started at 25 min, infusion with ICG (57.8 mg/kg per minute) started at 15 min, LPS (1.44 mg/kg per minute) started at 40 min (for 30 min). The animals were treated with GdCl$_3$ (10 mg/kg) 24 h before the experiment. $n = 5$ for every treatment. *$p < 0.05$. (From ref. 32)

intoxicated dogs (dimethylnitrosamine) showed a 50% increase of portal pressure[68]. Similar effects occurred in ethanol-treated animals[65]. The increase in portal pressure in these models is explained by a change of the normal architecture of the liver with, for example, increased periportal fibrosis. An acute increase in portal pressure and a significant impairment of hepatic uptake and secretory function could be observed in experiments using antiarrhythmic

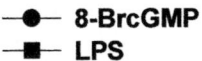

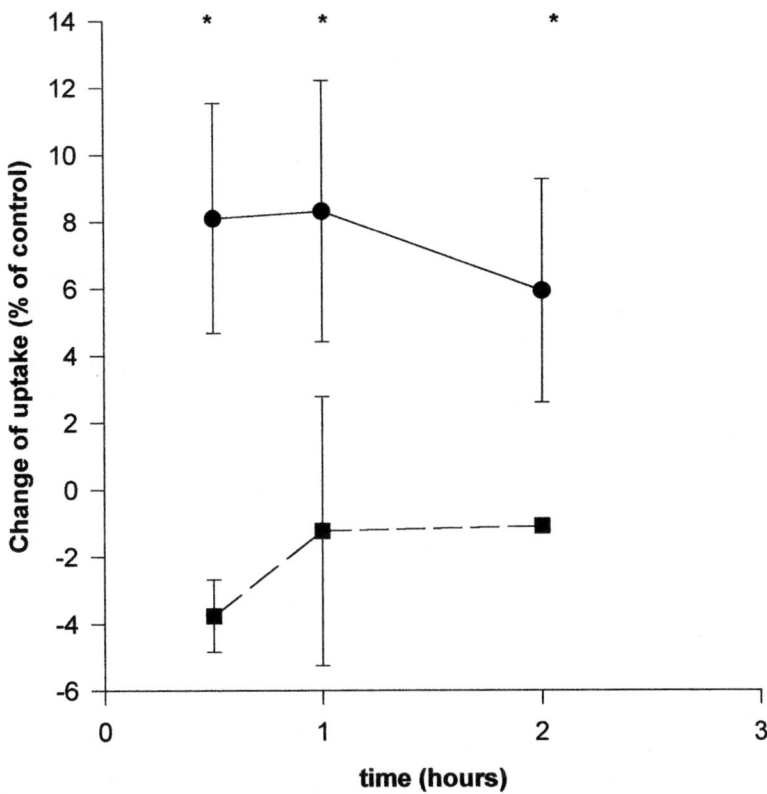

Figure 6 Effect of LPS and 8-BrcGMP on the ICG uptake in primary cultured hepatocytes. LPS (16 μg/ml supernatant) or 8-BrcGMP were added together with ICG (56 μg/ml supernatant) at the beginning of the experiment (time-point 0). The animals were pretreated with GdCl3 (10 mg/kg) for 24 h. The results are expressed as changes from the primary concentration in percentage. $n = 8$ for every treatment. *$p < 0.05$. Error bars represent SEM. (From ref. 32)

drugs[69]. Adenosine led to an acute increase of portal pressure[67]. The cause of the increase in portal pressure and the concomitant decrease of detoxification properties in these studies is thought to be due to impaired hepatic microcirculation[66]. In our experiments we monitored the portal pressure continuously. During our experimental procedure we did not observe a difference in portal pressure between the different treatment groups. Thus, in our experimental set-up an effect on liver microcirculation does not explain the rapid decrease in ICG uptake after LPS treatment.

Wang *et al.* could demonstrate that the application of TNF resulted in a significant reduction of the extraction rate of ICG after 1 h[70]. TNF is up-regulated 60–90 min, IL-1 3–4 h, and IL-6 4–8 h after application of endo-toxin[71]. The observed effect on the hepatocytes therefore has to be a direct effect of LPS on the hepatocytes or a Kupffer cell effect which is mediated through transmitters other than TNF or the mentioned cytokines. It was also shown that endotoxin in combination with different cytokines stimulated cGMP production by the hepatocyte[61]. Blocking Kupffer cells using $GdCl_3$, in our liver perfusion model, normalized the uptake rate of ICG into the hepatocytes, indicating a Kupffer cell-dependent mechanism for this LPS-induced hepatocellular dysfunc-tion. In addition, in primary cultured hepatocytes there was no direct and rapid effect of LPS on the ICG uptake rate into hepatocytes, and the application of 8-BrcGMP resulted in a significant increase in ICG uptake into primary cultured hepatocytes within the first 0.5 h. 8-BRcGMP is a cGMP-analogue which is able to enter the cell. CGMP itself is an intracellular second messenger which is upregulated, for example, by nitric oxide and atrial natriuretic peptide in hepato-cytes. Bilzer et al.[72] demonstrated that cGMP has a protective effect on hepato-cytes in oxidative stress. While cGMP has no effect on the excretion rate of organic anions[73], our data show an increased uptake of the organic anion ICG.

Endotoxin-induced cytokines seem to be responsible for a reduction in ICG uptake observed as early as 2 h after LPS contact with the liver. Different trans-mitters seem to be responsible for this rapid effect. As well as the cytokines, the production of other mediators such as thromboxane, different prostaglandins, prostacyclin and leukotrienes is up-regulated in Kupffer cells[74,75]. Up-regulation of these mediators depends on the dose of LPS[75].

Our results show different effects of LPS on the uptake of ICG and on its excretion into bile. The latter effect was not dose-dependent. Even with the smallest dose of LPS used (0.45 mg/kg per minute) a decrease in biliary excre-tion was observed starting 15 min after LPS administration. Utili et al.[63], using 20 μg/ml perfusate, found an almost instant decrease of bile salt-independent bile flow. They also found a reduction of the secretion of sulphobromoph-thalein into the bile by 36%. In our system it is not possible to assess the decreasing effect of LPS on bile flow because ICG itself leads to a bile flow reduction[76]. The reduction of ICG excretion after LPS administration was bile flow-independent.

Bilirubin, ICG and sulphobromophthalein seem to be taken up into the hepa-tocyte by the organic anion-transporting polypeptide (oatp)[54], whereas the excre-tory route of ICG into bile is so far not known. Work from Sathirakul et al.[56] and Takikawa et al.[77] suggests that there is a predominant transport system for BSP and DBSP which also transports cefodizime and LTC_4, and a distinct transport system for ICG which is thought to be MRP2.

$GdCl_3$ treatment does not abolish all effects of Kupffer cells. Phagocytic prop-erties are down-regulated to 90%. The PGE_2 concentration is still 35% higher than in unstimulated (not LPS-stimulated) livers[78]. The release of NO is signifi-cantly decreased[79] if Kupffer cells are treated with $GdCl_3$.

In conclusion, we demonstrated a rapid dose-dependent endotoxin-induced reduction in ICG transport at both the sinusoidal (40 min) and canalicular (15 min) membrane. This effect is likely to be a Kupffer cell-mediated effect since LPS is not able to induce this hepatocellular dysfunction in primary cul-tured hepatocytes, and $GdCl_3$ treatment abolishes the LPS effect. Cytokines are unlikely to function as mediators because the effects are too fast to be caused by an up-regulation of cytokines. Further studies are necessary to determine whether prostanoids, nitric oxide or other second messengers might be responsible for the observed rapid LPS effect.

References

1. Wang P, Zhou M, Rana MW, Ba ZF, Chaudry IH. Differential alterations in microvascular perfusion in various organs during early and late sepsis. Am J Physiol. 1992;263:G38–43.
2. Dahn MS, Wilson RF. Hepatic parenchymal oxygen tension following injury and sepsis. Arch Surg. 1990;125:441–3.
3. Harken AH, Lillo RS, Hufnagel HV. Direct influence of endotoxin on cellular respiration. Surg Gynecol Obstet. 1978;140:858–60.
4. Wang P, Zheng F, Ba, Chaudry IH. Hepatic extraction of indocyanine green is depressed early in sepsis despite increased hepatic blood flow and cardiac output. Arch Surg. 1991;126:219–24.
5. Bolder U, Ton-Nu H-T, Schteingart CD, Frick E, Hofmann AF. Hepatocyte transport of bile acids and organic anions in endotoxemic rats: impaired uptake and secretion. Gastroenterology. 1997;112:214–25.
6. Roelofsen H, Veere CNVD, Ottenhoff R, Schoemaker B, Jansen PLM, Oude-Elferink RPJ. Decreased bilirubin transport in the perfused liver of endotoxemic rats. Gastroenterology. 1994;107:1075–84.
7. Roelofsen H, Schoemaker B, Bakker C, Ottenhoff R, Jansen PLM, Oude-Elferink RPJ. Impaired hepatocanicular organic anion transport in endotoxemic rats. Am J Physiol. 1995;269:G427–34.
8. Grüne S, Michl M, Schölmerich J, Holstege A. Uptake of indocyanine green (ICG) into the liver is rapidly decreased by lipopolysaccharide (LPS). Gastroenterology. 1997;112:A1275.
9. Grüne S, Michl M, Schinharl D et al. Depression of Kupffer cell function abolishes the rapid effect of LPS on the indocyanine green uptake-rate in the rat liver. Gastroenterology. 1998;113:A7.
10. Gegner JA, Ulevitch RJ, Tobias PS. Lipopolysaccharide (LPS) signal transduction and clearance. Dual roles for LPS binding protein and membrane CD14. J Biol Chem. 1995;270:5320–5.
11. Tapping RI, Tobias PS. Cellular binding of soluble CD14 requires lipopolysaccharide (LPS) and LPS-binding protein. J Biol Chem. 1997;272:23157–64.
12. Enomoto N, Ikejima K, Bradford B et al. Alcohol causes both tolerance and sensitization of rat Kupffer cells via mechanisms dependent on endotoxin. Gastroenterology. 1998;115:443–51.
13. Lukkari TA, Jarvelainen HA, Oinonen T, Kettunen E, Lindros KO. Short-term ethanol exposure increases the expression of Kupffer cell CD14 receptor and lipopolysaccharide binding protein in rat liver. Alcohol Alcoholism 1999;34:311–19.
14. Poussin C, Foti M, Carpentier JL, Pugin J. CD14-dependent endotoxin internalization via a macropinocytic pathway. J Biol Chem. 1998;273:20285–91.
15. Liu S, Khemlani LS, Shapiro RA et al. Expression of CD14 by hepatocytes: upregulation by cytokines during endotoxemia. Infect Immun. 1998;66:5089–98.
16. Chow JC, Young DW, Golenbock DT, Christ WJ, Gusovsky F. Toll-like receptor-4 mediates lipopolysaccharide-induced signal transduction. J Biol Chem. 1999;274:10689–92.
17. Cario E, Rosenberg IM, Brandwein SL, Beck PL, Reinecker HC, Podolsky DK. Lipopolysaccharide activates distinct signaling pathways in intestinal epithelial cell lines expressing toll-like receptors. J Immunol. 2000;164:966–72.
18. Modlin RL, Brightbill HD, Godowski PJ. The toll of innate immunity on microbial pathogens. N Engl J Med. 1999;340:1834–5.
19. Sarphie TG, Deaciuc IV. Liver sinusoid during chronic alcohol consumption in the rat: an electron microscopic study. Alocohol Clin Exp Res. 1995;19:291–8.
20. Treon SP, Thomas P. Lipoloysaccharide (LPS) processing by Kupffer cells releases a modified LPS with increased hepatocyte binding and decreased tumor necrosis factor-alpha stimulatory capacity. Proc Soc Exp Biol Med. 1993;202:153–8.
21. Fox ES, Thomas P. Uptake and modification of [124]I-lipopolysaccharide by isolated rat Kupffer cells. Hepatology. 1988;8:1550–6.
22. Fox ES, Thomas P. Comparative studies of endotoxin uptake by isolated rat Kupffer and peritoneal cells. Infect Immun. 1987;55:2962–6.

23. Whiting JF, Green RM, Rosenbluth AB, Gollan JL. Tumor necrosis factor-alpha decreases hepatocyte bile salt uptake and mediates endotoxin-induced choleostasis. Hepatology. 1995;22: 1273–8.
24. Luster MI, Germolec DR. Endotoxin-induced cytokine gene expression and excretion in the liver. Hepatology. 1994;19:480–8.
25. Thieblemont N, Wright SD. Transport of bacterial lipopolysaccharide to the Golgi apparatus. J Exp Med. 1999;190:523–34.
26. Rao P, Falk LA. Colchicine down-regulates lipolysaccharide-induced granulocyte-macrophage colony-stimulating factor production in murine macrophages. J Immunol. 1997;159:3531–9.
27. Fearns C, Kravchenko VV, Ulevitch RJ, Loskutoff DJ. Murine CD14 gene expression in vivo: extramyeloid synthesis and regulation by lipopolysaccharide. J Exp Med. 1995;181:857–66.
28. Su GL, Dorko K, Strom SC, Nussler AK, Wang SC. CD14 expression and production by human hepatocytes. J Hepatol. 1999;31:435–42.
29. Haziot A, Rong GW, Lin XY, Silver J, Goyert SM. Recombinant soluble CD14 prevents mortality in mice treated with endotoxin (lipopolysaccharide). J Immunol. 1995;154:6529–32.
30. Hori Y, Takeyama Y. Impaired transport of lipopolysaccharide across the hepatocytes in rats with cerulein-induced experimental pancreatitis. Pancreas. 1998;16:148–53.
31. Mimura Y, Sakisaka S, Harada M, Sata M, Tanikawa K. Role of hepatocytes in direct clearance of lipopolysaccharide in rats. Gastroenterology. 1995;109:1969–76.
32. Grüne S, Michl M, Schinharl D et al. Rapid effects of lipopolysaccharides on the indocyanine green-clearance of the rat liver. Eur J Gastroenterol Hepatol. (In press).
33. Jedlitschky G, Leier I, Buchholz U, Hummel-Eisenbeiss J, Burchell B, Keppler D. ATP-dependent transport of bilirubin glucuronides by the multidrug resistance protein MRP1 and its hepatocyte canalicular isoform MRP2. Biochem J. 1997;327:305–10.
34. Hirohashi T, Suzuki H, Sugiyama Y. Characterization of the transport properties of cloned rat multidrug resistance-associated protein 3 (MRP3). J Biol Chem. 1999;274:15181–5.
35. Bakos E, Evers R, Szakacs G et al. Functional multidrug resistance protein (MRP1) lacking the N-terminal transmembrane domain. J Biol Chem. 1998;273:32167–75.
36. Vos TA, Hooiveld GJ, Koning H et al. Up-regulation of the multidrug resistance genes, Mrp1 and Mdr1b, and down-regulation of the organic anion transporter, Mrp2, and the bile salt transporter, Spgp, in endotoxemic rat liver. Hepatology. 1998;28:1637–44.
37. Lund M, Kang L, Tygstrup N, Wolkoff AW, Ott P. Effect of LPS on transport of indocyanine green and alanine uptake in perfused rat liver. Am J Physiol. 1999;277:G91–100.
38. Hsiang B, Zhu Y, Wang Z et al. A novel human hepatic organic anion transporting polypeptide (OATP2). Identification of a liver-specific human organic anion transporting polypeptide and identification of rat and human hydroxymethylglutaryl-CoA reductase inhibitor transporters. J Biol Chem. 1999;274:37161–8.
39. Abe T, Kakyo M, Sakagami H et al. Molecular characterization and tissue distribution of a new organic anion transporter subtype (oatp3) that transports thyroid hormones and taurocholate and comparison with oatp2. J Biol Chem. 1998;273:22395–401.
40. Abe T, Kakyo M, Tokui T et al. Identification of a novel gene family encoding human liver-specific organic anion transporter LST-1. J Biol Chem. 1999;274:17159–63.
41. Stieger B, Hagenbuch B, Landmann L, Hochli M, Schroeder A, Meier PJ. In situ localization of the hepatocytic Na+/taurocholate cotransporting polypeptide in rat liver. Gastroenterology. 1994;107:1781–7.
42. Green RM, Beier D, Gollan JL. Regulation of hepatocyte bile salt transporters by endotoxin and inflammatory cytokines in rodents. Gastroenterology. 1996;111:193–8.
43. Moseley RH, Wang W, Takeda H et al. Effect of endotoxin on bile acid transport in rat liver: a potential model for sepsis-associated cholestasis. Am J Physiol. 1996;271:G137–46.
44. Szabo K, Welker E, Bakos et al. Drug-stimulated nucleotide trapping in the human multidrug transporter MDR1. Cooperation of the nucleotide binding domains. J Biol Chem. 1998;273: 10132–8.
45. Müller M, Mayer R, Hero U, Keppler D. ATP-dependent transport of amphiphilic cations across the hepatocyte canalicular membrane mediated by mdr 1 P-glycoprotein. FEBS Lett. 1994;343:168–72.
46. Oude-Elferink RPJ, Tytgat GN, Groen AK. Hepatic canalicular membrane 1: the role of mdr2 P-glycoprotein in hepatobiliary lipid transport. FASEB J. 1997;11:19–28.
47. Kamisako T, Gabazza EC, Ishihara T, Adachi Y. Molecular aspects of organic compound transport across the plasma membrane of hepatocytes. J Gastroenterol Hepatol. 1999;14:405–12.

48. Kubitz R, Wettstein M, Warskulat U, Häussinger D. Regulation of the multidrug resistance protein 2 in the rat liver by lipopolysaccharide and dexamethasone. Gastroenterology. 1999;116:401–10.
49. Keppler D, König J. Hepatic canalicular membrane 5: expression and localization of the conjugate export pump encoded by the MRP2 (cMRP/cMOAT) gene in liver. FASEB J. 1997;11: 509–16.
50. Green RM, Hoda F, Ward KL. Molecular cloning and characterization of the murine bile salt export pump. Gene. 2000;241:117–23.
51. Lecureur V, Sun D, Hargrove P et al. Cloning and expression of murine sister of P-glycoprotein reveals a more discriminating transporter than MDR1/P-glycoprotein. Mol Pharmacol. 2000;57:24–35.
52. Gerloff T, Stieger B, Hagenbuch B et al. The sister of P-glycoprotein represents the canalicular bile salt export pump of mammalian liver. J Biol Chem. 1998;273:10046–50.
53. Xue-Jun Meng, Carruth MW, Weinman SA. Leukotriene D4 activates a chloride conductance in hepatocytes from lipopolysaccharide-treated rats. J Clin Invest. 1997;99:1–8.
54. Kullak-Ublick G-A, Hagenbuch B, Stieger B, Wolkoff AW, Meier PJ. Functional characterisation of the basolateral rat liver organic anion transporting polypeptide. Hepatology. 1994;20:411–16.
55. Takikawa H, Sano N, Akimoto K, Ogasawara T, Yamanaka M. Effects of colchicine and phenothiazine on biliary excretion of organic anions in rats. J Gastroenterol Hepatol. 1998;13: 427–32.
56. Sathirakul K, Suzuki H, Yasuda K et al. Kinetic analysis of hepatobiliary transport of organic anions in Eisai hyperbilirubinemic mutant rats. J Pharmacol Exp Ther. 1993;265:1301–12.
57. Myers NC, Grüne S, Jameson HL, Anwer MS. CGMP stimulates bile acid-independent bile formation and biliary bicarbonate excretion. Am J Physiol. 1996;270:G418–24.
58. Grüne S, Engelking LR, Anwer MS. Role of intracellular calcium and protein kinases in the activation of hepatic Na+/taurocholate cotransport by cyclic AMP. J Biol Chem. 1993;268: 17734–41.
59. Hardonk JM, Dijkhuis FWJ, Hustaert CE, Koudstaal J. Heterogeneity of rat liver and spleen macrophages in gadolinium chloride-induced elimination and repopulation. J Leukocyte Biol. 1992;52:296–302.
60. Wang P, Chaudry IH. Mechanism of hepatocellular dysfunction during hyperdynamic sepsis. Am J Physiol. 1996;270:R927–38.
61. Geller DA, Nussler AK, Silvio MD et al. Cytokines, endotoxin, and glucocorticoids regulate the expression of inducible nitric oxide synthase in hepatocytes. Proc Natl Acad Sci USA. 1993;90:522–6.
62. Kurose I, Shinzo K, Ishii H et al. Nitric oxide mediates lipopolysaccharide-induced alteration of mitochondrial function in cultured hepatocytes and isolated perfused liver. Hepatology. 1993;18:380–8.
63. Utili R, Abernathy CO, Zimmerman HJ. Inhibition of Na+, K+-adenosinetriphosphatase by endotoxin: a possible mechanism for endotoxin-induced cholestasis. J Infect Dis. 1977;136:583–7.
64. Kmiec Z, Hughes RD, Moore KP et al. Effect of supernatants from Kupffer cells stimulated with galactosamine and endotoxin on the function of isolated rat hepatocytes. Hepatogastroenterology. 1993;40:259–61.
65. Cruz MA, Bravo I, Rojas S, Gallardo V. Effects of ethanol ingestion on amino acid uptake in the dog liver in vivo. Pharmacology. 1985;30:12–19.
66. Akerboom T, Lenzen R, Schneider I, Sies H. Cholestasis and changes in the microcirculation of perfused rat liver caused by the calcium ionophore A23187 and type I antiarrhythmic drugs. Biochem Pharmacol. 1987;36:3037–42.
67. Nukina S, Fusaoka T, Thurman RG. Glycogenolytic effect of adenosine involves ATP from hepatocytes and eicosanoids from Kupffer cells. Am J Physiol. 1994;266:G99–105.
68. Kawasaki S, Umekita N, Beppu T et al. Hepatic transport of indocyanine green in dogs chronically intoxicated with dimethylnitrosamine. Toxicol Appl Pharmacol. 1984;75:309–17.
69. Lenzen R, Stremmel W, Strohmeyer G. Antiarrythmic drugs impair hepatic uptake and secretory function by different mechanisms in the isolated perfused rat liver. Biochim Biophys Acta. 1991;1074:406–12.
70. Wang P, Ayala F, Ba ZF, Zhou M, Perrin MM, Chaudry IH: Tumor necrosis factor-alpha produces hepatocellular dysfunction despite normal cardiac output and hepatic microcirculation. Am J Physiol. 1993;265:G126–32.

71. Neugebauer EA, Holaday JW, II. Physicochemical characteristics of endotoxins. In: Neugebauer EA, Holaday JW, editors. Handbook of Mediators in Septic Shock. Ann Arbor: CRC Press; 1993:4–17.
72. Bilzer M, Jaeschke H, Vollmar AM, Paumgartner G, Gerbes AL. Prevention of Kupffer cell-induced oxidant injury in rat liver by atrial natriuretic peptide. Am J Physiol. 1999;276: G1137–44.
73. St-Pierre M, Dufour J-FJ, Arias IM. Stimulation of bile acid independent bile flow with bromo-cyclic guanosine monophosphate. Hepatology. 1996;24:1487–91.
74. Kim Y-I, Kai T, Ktiano S et al. Hepatoprotection by a PGI2 analogue in complete warm ischemia of the pig liver. Transplantation. 1994;58:875–9.
75. Brouwer A, Barelds RJ, Leeuw AMD et al. Isolation and culture of Kupffer cells from human liver, ultrastructure, endocytosis and prostaglandin synthesis. J Hepatol. 1988;6:36–49.
76. Horak W, Grabner G, Paumgartner G. Inhibition of bile salt-independent bile formation by indo-cyanine green. Gastroenterology. 1973;64:1005–12.
77. Takikawa H, Nshikawa K, Sano N, Yamanaka M, Hrie T. Mechanisms of biliary excretion of lithocholate-3-sulfate in Eisai hyperbilirubinemic rats (EHBR). Dig Dis Sci. 1995;40:1792–7.
78. Roland CR, Nazruddin B, Nakafusa Y, Mohanakumar T, Flye MW. Prevention of endotoxin-induced mortality is associated with blockade of both PGE2 synthesis and calcium flux in Kupffer cells. Gastroenterology. 1998;213:A264.
79. Roland CR, Naziruddin B, Mohanakumar T, Flye MW. Gadolinium chloride inhibits Kupffer cell nitric oxide synthase (iNOS) induction. J Leukocyte Biol. 1996;60:487–92.

24
Hepatic actions of endothelin-1

A. MALLAT and S. LOTERSZTAJN

INTRODUCTION

Identified by Yanagisawa and co-workers a little more than a decade ago as the most potent vasoconstrictor yet described, endothelin-1 (ET-1) is the topic of an extensive litterature describing a wide variety of ubiquitous vascular and non-vascular effects and their involvement in physiological and pathological processes[1-4]. In recent years the availability of transgenic models, and of an increasing number of ET receptor agonists and antagonists, has confirmed the crucial role of the peptide in diverse pathophysiological cardiovascular or renal conditions, such as chronic heart failure, hypertension, stroke or renal failure[5,6]. At the same time, evidence for crucial vascular and non-vascular functions of ET-1 in the liver has emerged. The peptide was shown to affect processes as diverse as glycogenolysis, bile secretion, intrahepatic resistance or stellate cell function. Moreover, overactivity of the ET system is now increasingly implicated in the pathogenesis of portal hypertension, hepatic ischaemia–reperfusion injury and in liver fibrogenesis[2,7]. This chapter will summarize current knowledge on hepatic actions of ET-1 in health and disease, following a brief overview of the biology of ET-1 and its receptors.

ET-1: GENERAL OVERVIEW

Synthesis

ET-1 belongs to a family of three homologous 21 amino-acid peptides (ET-1, ET-2 and ET-3) which are encoded by distinct genes[3,4]. Expression of ET-1 is modulated by diverse stimuli at the gene level: main inducers include cytokines, growth factors, hypoxia and mechanical fluid shear stress, while vasodilators such as nitric oxide or natriuretic peptides down-regulate expression of pre-proET-1 mRNA. The endothelin synthesis pathway has largely been elucidated in recent years. Peptides arise through maturation of an inactive precursor by sequential proteolytic steps: preproendothelin is initially processed at dibasic sites into a 39 amino-acid peptide, big-ET, by an as-yet-unidentified furin-like protease; mature peptides are further generated from big-ET by a membrane-bound metalloproteinase, ET-converting enzyme-1 (ECE-1) which has primarily been identified in endothelial cells[8]. Alternatively spliced isoforms of ECE-1 have been reported: ECE-1α is predominantly expressed in microsomal fractions and converts endogenously produced big-ET, while ECE-1β predominantly behaves as an ectoenzyme expressed at the cell surface and involved in the cleavage of extracellular big-ET[9].

Endothelin receptors and transduction pathways

Physiological effects of endothelins are mediated by two related G protein-coupled receptors: the selective ETA receptor shows much greater affinity for ET-1 than for ET-2 and ET-3, while the non-selective ETB subtype binds all three isopeptides with similar affinity[10]. A third receptor, ETC, cloned in *Xenopus laevis*, has no mammalian counterpart yet identified. Availability of specific agonists or antagonists of ETA and ETB receptors allows discrimination of their functions[6]. ETA and ETB receptors show intricate vasoregulatory effects. Hence, contraction of vascular smooth muscle cells is predominantly mediated by ETA, but constricting effects of ETB have also been demonstrated in selected territories. Constrictor tone is, however, modulated by ETB receptors on endothelial cells, owing to secretion of relaxing nitric oxide[11]. These dual effects account for the biphasic pressor response to an infusion of ET-1[12].

Binding of ET-1 to its receptors is unique, in that it is very prolonged[10]. Processes that govern termination of ET signalling are progressively unravelled. ETB receptors are rapidly inactivated by phosphorylation, while termination of ETA-mediated signalling is slower and depends upon internalization[9]. In keeping with the diversity of their functions, ET receptors activate various effectors, promoting regulation of cytosolic calcium, increases or decreases in cyclic AMP, stimulation of prostaglandin synthesis or activation of tyrosine kinases[2]. These diverse mediators show cell or tissue specificity.

Ubiquitous distribution of ET-1 and its receptors

ET-1 and ET receptors are widely distributed. Tissues that produce the peptide express ET binding sites, suggesting a predominant autocrine/paracrine mode of action. This assumption is further supported by the fact that plasma concentrations of ET are low in the picomolar range, far below the nanomolar pharmacological threshold. In addition, rapid clearance by the lungs and the liver results in a very short half-life of the peptide (1 min)[13,14].

The ET-1 system in the normal liver

The liver appears as a central target of ET-1, with both hepatic production of the peptide and wide distribution of its receptors in the various liver cell types (Fig. 1). As shown by immunocytochemistry and *in-situ* hybridization, ET-1 is physiologically produced at low levels by non-parenchymal cells, predominantly in sinusoidal cells[15,16]. As in other organs, expression of the protein is regulated at the gene level by cytokines, through autocrine/paracrine interactions. Hence, systemic administration of endotoxin promotes the release of TGF-β by Kupffer cells, leading to increased secretion of ET-1 by endothelial cells[17,18]. Binding

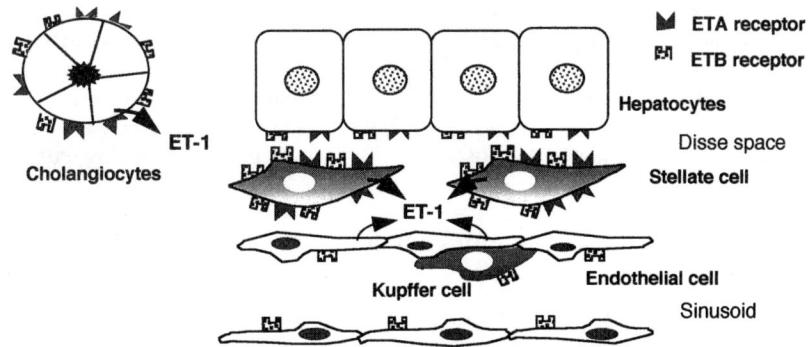

Figure 1 Sources of endothelin-1 in the normal liver and distribution of its receptors

sites for ET-1 appear most numerous on stellate cells, as indicated by *in-vivo* and culture studies, but significant numbers are also expressed by hepatocytes, cholangiocytes, endothelial cells and Kupffer cells[15,19–21]. Figure 1 shows that both ETA and ETB receptors are found on hepatocytes, stellate cells and cholangiocytes, while endothelial cells and Kupffer cells selectively harbour ETB receptors[15,19–21].

MULTIPLE EFFECTS OF ET-1 IN THE HEALTHY LIVER (Fig. 2)

Regulation of glycogenolysis

ET-1 promotes long-lasting activation of glycogenolysis, as shown in hepatocyte cultures and in the isolated perfused liver[21–23]. This metabolic effect is mediated

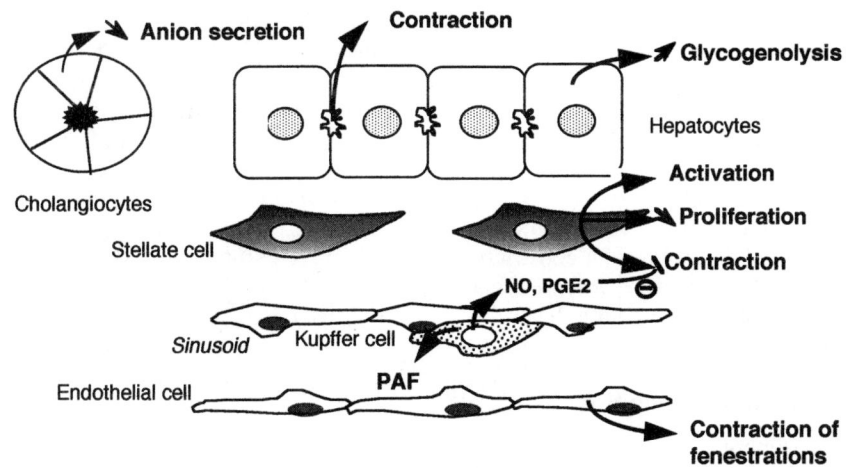

Figure 2 Hepatic actions of ET-1 at the cell level

by ETB receptors and the sequence of molecular events has been elucidated for the most part[21,23]. Stimulation of ETB receptors promotes activation of two distinct heterotrimeric G proteins, resulting in an increase in free cytosolic calcium: a Gq-mediated pathway promotes activation of phospholipase C, leading to IP3-induced calcium release into the cytosol, while a Gs-mediated pathway results in inhibition of the plasma membrane calcium pump, thereby blocking extrusion of calcium from the cell.

Regulation of hepatic haemodynamics

Shortly after its discovery, ET-1 was shown to elicit marked vasoconstriction in the portal territory. Intraportal or systemic infusion of exogenous ET-1 promotes a potent and sustained increase in intrahepatic resistance and portal pressure[22,24,25]. This constricting effect also occurs following endogenous hepatic production of ET-1[26]. Targets of ET-1 in the hepatic vasculature have been investigated by means of intravital microscopy, which enables one to delineate changes in haemodynamics of the liver microcirculation at the sinusoidal level. It was shown that ET-1 affects portal haemodynamics by constricting both portal venules and sinusoids[25,27].

That sinusoids may regulate their calibre raised the question as to the identity of the cell responsible for constriction. The hypothesis of a major role of stellate cells soon emerged. These cells display a star-like morphology, encircling sinusoids, and are therefore in an ideal position to regulate sinusoidal blood flow[28]. Numerous studies have shown that stellate cells display prolonged reversible constriction in response to ET-1[15,29,30]. This effect shows some degree of inter-species difference, being mediated by ETA and ETB receptors in human and rat cells, respectively[16,31]. Importantly, in culture studies, contractile properties of stellate cells are restricted to their myofibroblastic activated phenotype, while cultures of vitamin-A rich stellate cells isolated from normal livers do not show show any evidence of contraction[32]. These observations are nevertheless challenged by *in-vivo* videomicroscopy, which provides indirect evidence for contraction of quiescent stellate cells in the normal liver by demonstrating that sites of constriction or dilation of sinusoids colocalize with the body of stellate cells[27,33].

The respective roles of ETA and ETB receptors, and their site of action, may vary according to species or to experimental conditions, but most studies conclude that both subtypes contribute to contraction of vascular smooth muscle cells located in portal venules[27,34–36]. Receptors involved in the regulation of microcirculation at the sinusoidal level are a matter of controversy. One study suggested that sinusoidal constriction depends on ETA stimulation, while ETB-mediated effects were observed in a separate work[27,35].

Altogether these data indicate that ET-1 is a physiological regulator of portal and sinusoidal resistance.

Regulation of bile flow

Experimental studies have shown that ET-1 may diversely affect bile flow. Infusion of low concentrations of ET-1 in the isolated perfused liver promotes bile acid-dependent bile flow[37]. This choleretic effect is probably of dual origin, resulting from an increase in hepatocyte vesicular transport and secretion of bile acids, and from an enhancement of contraction of bile canaliculi[37,38]. Conversely, high concentrations of the peptide reduce bile flow. Cholestatic effects are in part consecutive to impairment of liver blood flow[37,39]; in addition, ET-1 also directly reduces ductal bile secretion, which accounts for 10–40% of the total bile volume in the normal liver, but shows large increases during cholestatic diseases. ET-1 lowers secretin-induced choleresis and secretin-stimulated bicarbonate secretion originating from cholangiocytes and gallbladder epithelial cells[40,41]. Altogether, these results suggest that ET-1 might be involved in the pathogenesis of cholestasis during chronic liver diseases.

Effects of ET-1 on Kupffer cells and sinusoidal endothelial cells

While ET-1 promotes constriction of stellate cells, the peptide simultaneously stimulates production of vasodilatory mediators by neighbouring Kupffer cells. Stimulation of ETB receptors induces expression of inducible nitric oxide and the subsequent release of nitric oxide, as well as secretion of prostaglandin E_2, two compounds that relax stellate cells[42,43].

Whether ET-1 also induces production of vasodilating nitric oxide by sinusoidal endothelial cells in a similar manner to what is found in other vascular beds has not yet been demonstrated. However, this hypothesis is supported by the finding that infusion of an ETB agonist in the portal vein simultaneously promotes vasoconstriction and the release of vasodilating nitric oxide[36]. Finally, ETB receptors located on sinusoidal cells elicit contraction of endothelial fenestrations, resulting in impaired exchanges between sinusoidal capillaries and hepatocytes[44,45].

ET-1 AND LIVER INJURY

Hepatic ischaemia–reperfusion injury

Reperfusion injury is a serious consequence of hepatic ischaemia, occurring during liver resection or organ preservation before transplantation. Microcirculatory impairment is central to the development of this process and has recently been linked to ET-1. It was shown that the peptide is overproduced in the vascular spaces during harvesting and cold preservation of the liver[46]. In addition, experimental ischaemia induced by portal clamping is associated with a rapid increase of ET-1 in the liver, and in the hepatic and portal venous blood[47,48]. Overproduction of ET-1 is temporally related to an increase in portal pressure and to alterations of the liver microcirculation[47,48]. Finally, reperfusion injury may be circumvented by the administration of neutralizing ET antibodies or of non-selective ETA/ETB antagonists during the ischaemic phase[48–50]. These observations suggest that ET receptor antagonists might offer new therapeutic avenues for the prevention of hepatic ischaemia–reperfusion injury. In line with these observations, recent studies suggest that this pharmacological approach may also be of value for the prevention of hepatic allograft dysfunction following transplantation from non-heart-beating donors[51].

ET-1 and chronic liver diseases

Up-regulation of the endothelin system

Several studies have pointed out major changes in the pattern of expression of ET-1 and its receptors during chronic liver diseases. Plasma concentrations of ET-1 increase by 2–5-fold in patients with cirrhosis, and show a fairly good correlation with the severity of the disease[52–54]. More importantly, hepatic synthesis of ET-1 is highly up-regulated. Surgical samples of cirrhosis show marked overexpression of ET-1, predominantly originating from myofibroblastic stellate cells, but also from endothelial cells and cholangiocytes[16]. Similar findings arise from an experimental model of fibrogenesis induced by tetrachloride intoxication[55,56]. In keeping with these observations, endothelial and/or stellate cells display enhanced ET-1 synthesis in response to PDGF and TGF-β, two factors highly expressed in the diseased liver[16,17].

Chronic liver disease is also accompanied by a marked up-regulation of ET receptors, as evidenced in homogenates of human cirrhotic surgical samples and in myofibroblastic stellate cells isolated from rats with experimental liver fibrosis[56,57]. Interestingly, ETB receptors appear to be preferentially up-regulated in myofibroblastic stellate cells. This shift of expression in ET receptors could originate from paracrine effects of fibrogenic cytokines and oxygen radicals expressed in the diseased liver. It was shown that PDGF, thrombin and superoxides selectively up-regulate ETB receptors in human myofibroblastic stellate cells in culture[58,59].

Finally, it has recently been suggested that myofibroblastic activation of stellate cells during liver injury is associated with an increased sensitivity of ETA receptors to low picomolar concentrations of the peptide[60]. Molecular mechanisms underlying sensitization of stellate cells to the peptide are presently unknown.

Altogether, these observations have set the stage for investigations aiming at elucidating the role of ET-1 in the pathogenesis of chronic liver diseases.

Pathophysiology of portal hypertension

A number of studies have investigated whether ET-1 is part of the processes leading to elevation of intrahepatic resistance and development of portal hypertension associated with chronic liver diseases, and several observations support this hypothesis. In carbon tetrachloride-induced experimental cirrhosis, stellate cells show a progressive increase in contractility in response to ET-1, that correlates with their degree of myofibroblastic activation[61]. In that same model, sarafotoxin S6C, a selective ETB agonist, induces greater elevation of portal pressure in cirrhotic animals, as compared to controls[61]. In keeping with these observations, portal rings isolated from rats with bile duct ligation show increased response to ET-1[62]. In aggregate, these results strongly suggest that the peptide is involved in the increase in intrahepatic resistance that contributes to the generation of portal hypertension. More conclusive evidence stems from the effects of ET antagonists in experimental models. In portal hypertension induced by carbon tetrachloride or bile duct ligation, portal infusion of a selective ETA receptor antagonist, or of a mixed ETA/ETB antagonist, lowers the high portal pressure of these animals[61,62]. In addition, three studies recently reported that acute administration of a non-selective ETA/ETB antagonist decreases portal pressure *in vivo* in these same models, an effect that was attributed to a decrease in hepatic portocollateral resistance[45,63,64].

Pathophysiology of liver fibrogenesis

Considering the crucial role of stellate cells in the development of liver fibrosis[28], and the abundance of ET receptors on these cells, several studies have investigated the role of ET-1 in the pathophysiology of cirrhosis. Various effects of ET-1 were observed, depending on the stage of activation of stellate cells. In quiescent vitamin-A-rich rat stellate cells, ET-1 promotes myofibroblastic transdifferentiation[65]. In addition, cells at early stages of culture show a weak mitogenic response to ETA receptor stimulation[16]. However, opposite trends are found in fully activated myofibroblastic stellate cells. We found that ET-1 is a potent growth inhibitor for these cells, via ETB receptors[20]. We investigated the transduction pathway involved in the antiproliferative effect of ET-1 and found that endogenous production of growth-inhibitory prostaglandins (PGI_2) and PGE_2 is central to this process[20,66,67] (Fig. 3); indeed, stimulation of ETB receptors activates within minutes the production of PGI_2 and PGE_2 by endogenous type 2 cyclooxygenase (COX-2). Released prostaglandins in turn promote

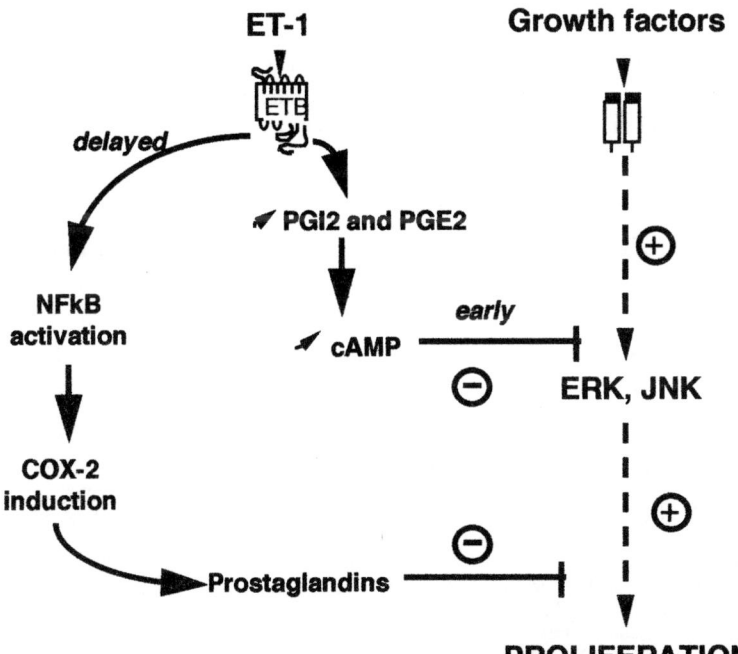

Figure 3 Inhibition of proliferation of myofibroblastic stellate cells by endothelin-1: molecular mechanisms

autocrine synthesis of cyclic AMP, which inhibits early steps of the mitogenic cascade elicited by growth factors by decreasing activation of two members of the MAP kinase family, ERK (extracellular-regulated kinase) and JNK (c-Jun kinase). In addition, stimulation of ETB receptors also promotes growth inhibition by a delayed mechanism. This involves activation of the nuclear transcription facor NF-κB, leading to induction of the expression of COX-2 and late synthesis of growth-inhibitory prostaglandins which interfere with cell proliferation by an as-yet-undefined mechanism. Interestingly, this prostaglandin/cyclic AMP pathway selectively up-regulates expression of ETB receptors by hepatic myofibroblasts, thereby amplifying the growth-inhibitory response to ET-1[66]. Altogether, these results indicate that ET-1 may have a dual role during liver fibrogenesis. At early stages of liver injury the peptide displays profibrogenic properties by accelerating myofibroblastic activation. In contrast, at later stages, ET-1 limits fibrogenesis by inhibiting accumulation of myofibroblasts, following stimulation of up-regulated ETB receptors. In this regard we recently found that fibrogenic growth factors such as PDGF or thrombin up-regulate ETB receptors, amplifying the growth-inhibitory response to ET-1[58]. This negative feedback therefore limits accumulation of myofibroblasts elicited by these growth factors.

In line with the dual effects of ET-1 in stellate cell cultures, endothelin antagonism in experimental fibrosis has yielded conflicting results. Administration of a non-selective ETA/ETB antagonist, bosentan, decreased liver fibrosis following chronic intoxication by tetrachloride in one study[65]. However, in that same experimental model a separate study found that a second-generation non-selective ET receptor antagonist aggravated the development of liver fibrosis, in keeping with antifibrogenic properties of ETB receptors[68]. Future studies should therefore particularly investigate the effects of selective ETA or ETB antagonists in experimental models of liver fibrosis in order to elucidate these discrepancies.

References

1. Goldie RG. Endothelins in health and disease: an overview. Clin Exp Pharmacol Physiol. 1999;26:145–8.
2. Mallat A, Lotersztajn S. Multiple hepatic functions of endothelin-1: physiopathological relevance. J Hepatol. 1996;25:405–13.
3. Masaki T, Yanagisawa M, Goto K. Physiology and pharmacology of endothelins. Med Res Rev. 1992;12:391–421.
4. Miyauchi T, Masaki T. Pathophysiology of endothelin in the cardiovascular system. Annu Rev Physiol. 1999;61:391–415.
5. Benigni A, Remuzzi G. Endothelin antagonists. Lancet. 1999;353:133–8.
6. Douglas SA. Clinical development of endothelin receptor antagonists. Trends Pharmacol Sci. 1997;18:408–12.
7. Mallat A. Hepatic stellate cells and intrahepatic modulation of portal pressure. Digestion. 1998;59:416–19.
8. Turner AJ, Barnes K, Schweizer A, Valdenaire O. Isoforms of endothelin-converting enzyme: why and where? Trends Pharmacol Sci. 1998;19:483–6.
9. Webb DJ, Monge JC, Rabelink TJ, Yanagisawa M. Endothelin: new discoveries and rapid progress in the clinic. Trends Pharmacol Sci. 1998;19:5–8.
10. Pollock DM. Endothelin receptor subtypes and tissue distribution. In: Highsmith RM, Highsmiths RM, editor. Endothelin: Molecular Biology, Physiology, and Pathology. Totowa: 1998:1–29.
11. Douglas SA, Meek TD, Ohlstein EH. Novel receptor antagonists welcome a new era in endothelin biology. Trends Biochem Sci. 1994;15:313–16.

12. Yanagisawa M, Kurihara H, Kimura S *et al.* A novel potent vasoconstrictor peptide produced by vascular endothelial cells [See comments]. Nature. 1988;332:411–15.

13. Fukuroda T, Fujikawa T, Ozaki S, Ishikawa K, Yano M, Nishikibe M. Clearance of circulating endothelin-1 by ETB receptors in rats. Biochem Biophys Res Commun. 1994;199:1461–5.

14. Anggard E, Galton S, Rae G *et al.* The fate of radioiodinated endothelin-1 and endothelin-3 in the rat. J Cardiovascul Pharmacol. 1989;13:S46–S49.

15. Housset C, Rockey DC, Bissell DM. Endothelin receptors in rat liver: lipocytes as a contractile target for endothelin 1. Proc Natl Acad Sci USA. 1993;90:9266–70.

16. Pinzani M, Milani S, De Franco R *et al.* Endothelin-1 is overexpressed in cirrhotic liver and exerts multiple effects on activated hepatic stellate cells. Front Endocrinol. 1995;15:77–9.

17. Eakes AT, Olson MS. Regulation of endothelin synthesis in hepatic endothelial cells. Am J Physiol. 1998;274:G1068–76.

18. Rieder H, Ramadori G, Meyer Z, Meyer zum Büschenfelde KH. Sinusoidal endothelial liver cells *in vitro* release endothelin – augmentation by transforming growth factor b and Kupffer cell-conditioned media. Klin Wochenschr. 1991;69:387–91.

19. Gondo K, Ueno T, Sakamoto M, Sakisaka S, Sata M, Tanikawa K. The endothelin-1 binding site in rat liver tissue: light- and electron-microscopic autoradiographic studies. Gastroenterology. 1993;104:1745–9.

20. Mallat A, Fouassier L, Preaux AM *et al.* Growth inhibitory properties of endothelin-1 in human hepatic myofibroblastic Ito cells. An endothelin B receptor-mediated pathway. J Clin Invest. 1995;96:42–9.

21. Jouneaux C, Mallat A, Serradeil-Le Gal C, Goldsmith P, Hanoune J, Lotersztajn S. Coupling of endothelin B receptors to the calcium pump and phospholipase C via Gs and Gq in rat liver. J Biol Chem. 1994;269:1845–51.

22. Gandhi CR, Stephenson K, Olson MS. Endothelin, a potent peptide agonist in the liver. J Biol Chem. 1990;265:17432–5.

23. Serradeil-Le Gal C, Jouneaux C, Sanchez-Bueno A *et al.* Endothelin action in rat liver. Receptors, free Ca^{2+} oscillations, and activation of glycogenolysis. J Clin Invest. 1991;87:133–8.

24. Tran-Thi TA, Kawada N, Decker K. Regulation of endothelin-1 action on the perfused rat liver. Febs Lett. 1993;318:353–7.

25. Zhang JX, Pegoli WJ, Clemens MG. Endothelin-1 induces direct constriction of hepatic sinusoids. Am J Physiol. 1994;266:G624–32.

26. Oshita M, Takei Y, Kawano S *et al.* Roles of endothelin-1 and nitric oxide in the mechanism for ethanol-induced vasoconstriction in rat liver. J Clin Invest. 1993;91:1337–42.

27. Zhang JX, Bauer M, Clemens MG. Vessel- and target cell-specific actions of endothelin-1 and endothelin-3 in rat liver. Am J Physiol. 1995;269:G269–77.

28. Friedman SL. The cellular basis of hepatic fibrosis. N Engl J Med. 1993;328:1828–35.

29. Pinzani M, Failli P, Ruocco C *et al.* Fat-storing cells as liver-specific pericytes. Spatial dynamics of agonists-stimulated calcium transients. J Clin Invest. 1992;90:642–6.

30. Kawada N, Tran-Thi TA, Klein H, Decker K. The contraction of hepatic stellate (Ito) cells stimulated with vasoactive substances. Possible involvement of endothelin 1 and nitric oxide in the regulation of the sinusoidal tonus. Eur J Biochem. 1993;213:815–23.

31. Rockey DC. Characterization of endothelin receptors mediating rat hepatic stellate cell contraction. Biochem Biophys Res Commun. 1995;207:725–31.

32. Rockey DC, Housset CN, Friedman SL. Activation-dependent contractility of rat hepatic lipocytes in culture and *in vivo*. J Clin Invest. 1993;92:1795–804.

33. Suematsu M, Goda N, Sano T *et al.* Carbon monoxide: an endogenous modulator of sinusoidal tone in the perfused rat liver [See comments]. J Clin Invest. 1995;96:2431–7.

34. Wang HG, Shibamoto T, Miyahara T. Endothelin-1 selectively contracts portal vein through both ETA and ETB receptors in isolated rabbit liver. Am J Physiol. 1997;273:G1036–43.

35. Ito Y, Katori M, Majima M, Kakita A. Constriction of mouse hepatic venules and sinusoids by endothelins through ETB receptor subtype. Int J Microcirc Clin Exp. 1996;16:250–8.

36. Higuchi H, Satoh T. Endothelin-1 induces vasoconstriction and nitric oxide release via endothelin ET(B) receptors in isolated perfused rat liver. Eur J Pharmacol. 1997;328:175–82.

37. Tanaka A, Katagiri K, Hoshino M, Hayakawa T, Tsukada K, Takeuchi T. Endothelin-1 stimulates bile acid secretion and vesicular transport in the isolated perfused rat liver. Am J Physiol. 1994;266:G324–9.

38. Kamimura Y, Sawada N, Aoki M, Mori M. Endothelin-1 induces contraction of bile canaliculi in isolated rat hepatocytes. Biochem Biophys Res Commun. 1993;191:817–22.

39. Isales CM, Nathanson MH, Bruck R. Endothelin-1 induces cholestasis which is mediated by an increase in portal pressure. Biochem Biophys Res Commun. 1993;191:1244–51.
40. Fouassier L, Chinet T, Robert B et al. Endothelin-1 is synthesized and inhibits cyclic adenosine monophosphate-dependent anion secretion by an autocrine/paracrine mechanism in gallbladder epithelial cells. J Clin Invest. 1998;101:2881–8.
41. Caligiuri A, Glaser S, Rodgers RE et al. Endothelin-1 inhibits secretin-stimulated ductal secretion by interacting with ETA receptors on large cholangiocytes. Am J Physiol. 1998;275:G835–46.
42. Stephenson K, Gupta A, Mustafa SB, Halff GA. Endothelin-stimulated nitric oxide production in the isolated Kupffer cell. J Surg Res. 1997;73:149–54.
43. Gandhi CR, Stephenson K, Olson MS. A comparative study of endothelin- and platelet-activating-factor-mediated signal transduction and prostaglandin synthesis in rat Kupffer cells. Biochem J. 1992;281:485–92.
44. Oda M, Kamegay Y, Yokomori H, Han JY, Akiba Y, Nakamura M. Roles of plasma membrane Ca ATPase in the relaxation and contraction of hepatic sinusoidal endothelial fenestrae. Effects of prostaglandin E1 and endothelin 1. In: Wisse E, Knook DL, Balabaud C, editors. Cells of the Hepatic Sinusoid. Leiden: 1997:313–17.
45. Reichen J, Gerbes AL, Steiner MJ, Sagesser H, Clozel M. The effect of endothelin and its antagonist Bosentan on hemodynamics and microvascular exchange in cirrhotic rat liver. J Hepatol. 1998;28:1020–30.
46. Stansby G, Fuller B, Jeremy J, Cheetham K, Rolles K. Endothelin release – a facet of reperfusion injury in clinical liver transplantation. Transplantation. 1992;56:239–40.
47. Kawamura E, Yamanaka N, Okamoto E, Tomoda F, Furukawa K. Response of plasma and tissue endothelin-1 to liver ischemia and its implication in ischemia–reperfusion injury. Hepatology. 1995;21:1138–43.
48. Goto M, Takei Y, Kawano S et al. Endothelin-1 is involved in the pathogenesis of ischemia/reperfusion liver injury by hepatic microcirculatory disturbances. Hepatology. 1994;19:675–81.
49. Dhar DK, Yamanoi A, Ohmori H et al. Modulation of endothelin and nitric oxide: a rational approach to improve canine hepatic microcirculation. Hepatology. 1998;28:782–8.
50. Pannen BH, Al-Adili F, Bauer M, Clemens MG, Geiger KK. Role of endothelins and nitric oxide in hepatic reperfusion injury in the rat. Hepatology. 1998;27:755–64.
51. Fukunaga K, Takada Y, Mei G et al. An endothelin receptor antagonist ameliorates injuries of sinusoid lining cells in porcine liver transplantation [published erratum appears in Am J Surg. 1999;178:436]. Am J Surg. 1999;178:64–8.
52. Asbert M, Ginès A, Ginès P et al. Ciculating levels of endothelin in cirrhosis. Gastroenterology. 1993;104:1485–91.
53. Moore K, Wendon J, Frazer M, Karani J, Williams R, Badr K. Plasma endothelin immunoreactivity in liver disease and the hepatorenal syndrome. N Engl J Med. 1992;327:1774–8.
54. Uchihara M, Izumio N, Sato C, Marumo F. Clinical significance of elevated plasma endothelin concentration in patients with cirrhosis. Hepatology. 1992;16:95–9.
55. Rockey DC, Fouassier L, Chung JJ et al. Cellular localization of endothelin-1 and increased production in liver injury in the rat: potential for autocrine and paracrine effects on stellate cells. Hepatology. 1998;27:472–80.
56. Gandhi CR, Nemoto EM, Watkins SC, Subbotin WM. An endothelin receptor antagonist TAK-004 ameliorates carbon tetrachloride-induced acute liver injury and portal hypertension in rats. Liver. 1998;18:39–48.
57. Leivas A, Jimenez W, Bruix J et al. Gene expression of endothelin-1 and ET(A) and ET(B) receptors in human cirrhosis: relationship with hepatic hemodynamics. J Vasc Res. 1998;35:186–93.
58. Mallat A, Gallois C, Tao J et al. Platelet-derived growth factor-BB and thrombin generate positive and negative signals for human hepatic stellate cell proliferation. Role of a prostaglandin/cyclic AMP pathway and cross-talk with endothelin receptors. J Biol Chem. 1998;273:27300–5.
59. Gabriel A, Kuddus RH, Rao AS, Watkins WD, Gandhi CR. Superoxide-induced changes in endothelin (ET) receptors in hepatic stellate cells. J Hepatol. 1998;29:614–27.
60. Reinehr RM, Kubitz R, Peters-Regehr T, Bode JG, Haussinger D. Activation of rat hepatic stellate cells in culture is associated with increased sensitivity to endothelin 1. Hepatology. 1998;28:1566–77.

61. Rockey DC, Weisiger RA. Endothelin induced contractility of stellate cells from normal and cirrhotic rat liver: implications for regulation of portal pressure and resistance. Hepatology. 1996;24:233–40.
62. Kamath PS, Tyce GM, Miller VM, Edwards BS, Rorie DK. Endothelin-1 modulates intrahepatic resistance in a rat model of noncirrhotic portal hypertension. Hepatology. 1999;30:401–7.
63. Kojima H, Yamao, J, Tsujimoto T, Uemura M, Takaya A, Fukui H. Mixed endothelin receptor antagonist, SB209670, decreases portal pressure in biliary cirrhotic rats *in vivo* by reducing portal venous system resistance. J Hepatol. 2000;32:43–50.
64. Sogni P, Moreau R, Gomola A *et al.* Beneficial hemodynamic effects of bosentan, a mixed ET(A) and ET(B) receptor antagonist, in portal hypertensive rats. Hepatology. 1998;28:655–9.
65. Rockey DC, Chung JJ. Endothelin antagonism in experimental hepatic fibrosis. Implications for endothelin in the pathogenesis of wound healing. J Clin Invest. 1996;98:1381–8.
66. Mallat A, Preaux AM, Serradeil-Le Gal C *et al.* Growth inhibitory properties of endothelin-1 in activated human hepatic stellate cells: a cyclic adenosine monophosphate-mediated pathway. Inhibition of both extracellular signal-regulated kinase and c-Jun kinase and upregulation of endothelin B receptors. J Clin Invest. 1996;98:2771–8.
67. Gallois C, Habib A, Tao J *et al.* Role of NF-kappaB in the antiproliferative effect of endothelin-1 and tumor necrosis factor-alpha in human hepatic stellate cells. Involvement of cyclooxygenase-2. J Biol Chem. 1998;273:23183–90.
68. Poo JL, Jimenez W, Maria Munoz R *et al.* Chronic blockade of endothelin receptors in cirrhotic rats: hepatic and hemodynamic effects. Gastroenterology. 1999;116:161–7.

25
Mechanisms of bile acid-induced cell death

M. E. GUICCIARDI, W. A. FAUBION, S. F. BRONK,
P. J. ROBERTS and G. J. GORES

INTRODUCTION

Cholestasis is a common feature of many human liver diseases. Although the initial insult in these disorders is usually directed to the bile ducts, the progression of the disease is promoted by direct damage to the hepatocytes[1]. During cholestasis the impairment of bile flow leads to retention of hydrophobic and potentially toxic bile salts within the hepatocytes, which cause hepatocellular injury[2,3]. We previously demonstrated that cholestatic liver injury results, at least in part, from the induction of hepatocyte apoptosis by toxic bile salts[4,5]. Thus, further insight into the mechanisms of bile salt-induced apoptosis is of clinical and scientific relevance as this information may lead to new strategies for the treatment of these liver diseases.

Activation of death receptors is a common mechanism for the induction of apoptosis[6,7]. Death receptors are members of the tumour necrosis factor/nerve growth factor superfamily of membrane receptors, characterized by a sequence of 60–80 amino acids within the cytoplasmic tail called the death domain, which enables the receptor to engage the apoptotic signal[8,9]. Death receptors include Fas/CD95, tumour necrosis factor receptor-1 (TNF-R1), death receptor 3 (DR3), and tumour necrosis factor-related apoptosis-inducing ligand (TRAIL) receptors 1 and 2. Fas is one of the best-characterized death receptors. Fas is highly expressed in the liver and its key role in liver pathophysiology and homeostasis has been amply documented[10,11]. Activation of this death receptor *in vivo* by injection of an agonistic antibody in mice is associated with fulminant hepatic liver failure and death of the animal[12]. Stimulation of the Fas receptor usually occurs by engagement of the natural ligand FasL or agonistic anti-Fas antibodies. This binding results in oligomerization of the receptor and recruitment of the adapter molecule Fas-associated protein with death domain (FADD), which in turn binds to and activates the proximal protease caspase 8, forming the so-called death inducing signalling complex (DISC)[13]. Caspase 8 can then induce apoptosis by initiating a direct caspase cascade by cleaving caspase 3 and other distal effector proteases, which play a crucial role in mediating the intracellular events culminating in the morphological changes of apoptosis[14,15]. Activation of Fas can also trigger apoptosis through a mitochondrial-dependent pathway[16]. In this model, mitochondrial dysfunction occurs following the formation of the DISC, resulting in the release of cytochrome-c, a protein normally residing in the mitochondrial intermembrane space. The released cytochrome-c then binds to the cytosolic apoptosis activating factor-1 (Apaf-1) and procaspase 9, leading to activation of caspase 9. Activated caspase 9 directly cleaves procaspase 3 to active caspase 3[17], which in turn processes and activates other downstream caspases. The link between the activation of caspase 8 occurring at the DISC and the mitochondrial damage is still to be fully elucidated, but recent studies indicated that Bid, a novel pro-apoptotic member of the Bcl-2 family, might be a possible candidate for this role[18,19].

Based on these observations the overall objective of this study was to further elucidate the molecular mechanisms of bile salt-induced apoptosis by investigating if Fas is required for bile salt-mediated apoptosis.

EXPERIMENTAL PROCEDURES

Culture of McNtcp.24 cells and mouse hepatocytes

For the present study we used the rat hepatoma McNtcp.24 cell line and cultures of primary mouse hepatocytes. McNtcp.24 cells are derived from the McArdle-RH7777 rat hepatoma cell line after stable transfection with the sodium-dependent taurocholate cotransporting polypeptide (Ntcp), and transport bile salts into and out of the cells at a rate virtually identical to primary hepatocytes[20]. Fas-defective (*lpr*), FasL-defective (*gld*), tumour necrosis factor receptor-1 (TNF-R1) knockout, and wild-type male mice (MRLMPJ +/+) were obtained from Jackson Laboratories (Bar Harbor, Maine). Bile salt-mediated apoptosis of hepatocytes was assessed in serum- and insulin-free media.

Quantification of apoptosis

Apoptosis was quantitated as previously described by assessing the nuclear changes of apoptosis using the nuclear binding dye 4′,6′-diamidino-2-phenylindole dihydrochloride (DAPI) and fluorescence microscopy[22].

Caspase 8 activation

Immunoblot analysis for caspase 8 was performed using whole-cell lysates as described by Martins *et al.*[23]. A rabbit anti-caspase 8 (generous gift from Dr Anu Srinivasan, IDUN, San Diego, CA) was used as primary antibody. Horseradish peroxidase-conjugated goat anti-rabbit IgG (Santa Cruz Biochemicals, Santa Cruz, CA) was used as secondary antibody. The blot was visualized using chemiluminescent substrate (ECL; Amersham, Arlington Heights, IL).

Caspase 8 activity was also measured in cytosolic extracts using the fluorogenic substrate IETD-AFC, as we previously described in detail[24].

RESULTS AND DISCUSSION

We previously demonstrated that the toxic bile salt glycochenodeoxycholate (GCDC), whose serum concentration is significantly increased during cholestasis, induces hepatocyte apoptosis *in vitro* when used at concentration > 50 μmol/L[4]. However, we found that, in order to cause apoptosis, GCDC must be efficiently transported into the cells. Indeed, a 2 h treatment with GDCD induced dose-dependent apoptosis in McNtcp.24 cells, which efficiently transport bile salts, but no apoptosis was observed in the parental cell line which lacks the bile salt transporter (Fig. 1). This observation suggests that GCDC-mediated apoptosis is triggered by intracellular events that occur when the intracellular concentration of GCDC is increased.

To test the hypothesis the death receptors are involved in bile salt-mediated apoptosis, we treated hepatocytes obtained from mice with deficient death receptors with GCDC (Fig. 2). Mouse hepatocytes from the Fas-deficient *lpr* mice were insensitive to GCDC cytotoxicity, suggesting that GCDC kills by a Fas-dependent mechanism. In contrast, FasL-deficient *gld* mouse hepatocytes underwent apoptosis during treatment with toxic bile salts. To determine if other death receptors might be involved in bile salt-induced apoptosis, we used mouse hepatocytes from TNF-R1 knockout mice. Hepatocytes from TNF-R1 knockout mice were as sensitive as the wild-type to GCDC, suggesting that TNF-R1 is not

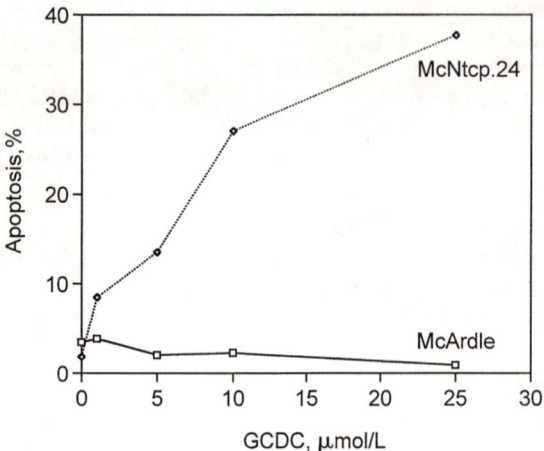

Figure 1 Bile salts-induced apoptosis requires the bile salt transporter. McNtcp.24 cells, stably transfected with the sodium-dependent taurocholate cotransporting polypeptide (Ntcp), and the parental McArdle-RH7777 rat hepatoma cell line, which lacks the bile salt transporter, were treated with increasing concentrations of GCDC for 2 h. Apoptosis was quantitated morphologically using DAPI staining and fluorescence microscopy. Cells were considered apoptotic based on the classic features of apoptosis (chromatin condensation, nuclear fragmentation)

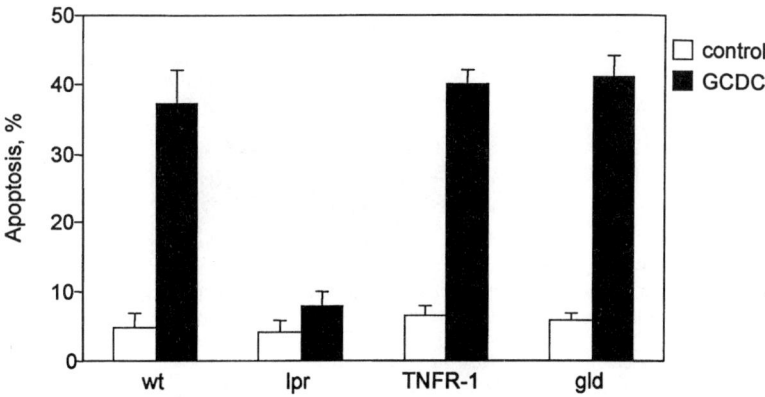

Figure 2 GCDC-induced hepatocyte apoptosis is mediated by a Fas-dependent, FasL- and TNFR-1-independent mechanism. Hepatocytes were isolated from Fasdeficient (*lpr*), FasL-deficient (*gld*), TNFR-1-knockout, and wild-type mice and cultured in media for 24 h. Cells were then incubated in the presence or in the absence (control) of 50 μmol/L GCDC for 4 h. Apoptosis was quantitated morphologically. Data are expressed as mean ± SED

involved in bile salt-mediated apoptosis. These data suggest that GCDC induces apoptosis by a Fas receptor-dependent, FasL-independent mechanism. Further studies are needed to investigate the possible role of other death receptors (i.e. TRAIL).

We next determined whether treatment with GCDC could induce oligomerization of Fas receptor. Fas is normally present on the plasma membrane in a monomeric form; stimulation of Fas results in aggregation to form trimers, which efficiently recruit FADD and caspase 8, promoting activation of caspase 8 and inducing a caspase cascade. By performing immunoprecipitation in the presence of limiting amount of anti-Fas antibody, we were able to detect Fas only in McNtcp.24 cells stimulated with 50 μmol/L GCDC, whereas no Fas was precipitated from untreated cells (data not shown). Since, under such conditions, oligomerized Fas is precipitated more efficiently than the monomeric receptor, we concluded that GCDC induces oligomerization of Fas. On the other hand, when we performed immunoprecipitation in the presence of excess amounts of anti-Fas antibody, which allows the precipitation of all the Fas expressed in the cells, we found that the amount of Fas protein was the same before and after GCDC treatment, demonstrating that GCDC does not induce overexpression of Fas receptor.

Because Fas-dependent apoptosis is associated with processing of procaspase 8 to active caspase 8 in the DISC, we finally tested whether GCDC could induce activation of caspase 8. Immunoblot analysis of caspase 8 on cell lysate from McNtcp.24 cells showed a 40% reduction of the 55–53 kDa fragment, corresponding to the zymogen form of the enzyme, upon 2 h treatment with GCDC, consistent with the processing of the proenzyme into the active fragments of 18–20 κDa and 10 κDa, respectively (Fig. 3). Moreover, cytosolic activity of caspase 8, measured as hydrolytic activity of the fluorogenic substrate IETD-AFC, increased four-fold within 2 h of treatment with GCDC (Fig. 4).

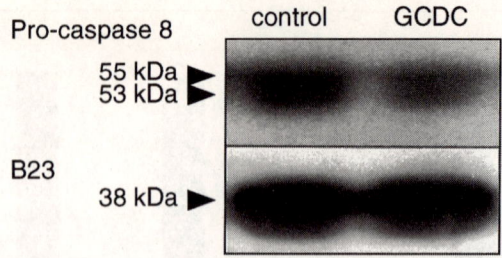

Figure 3 Caspase 8 is processed upon treatment with GCDC. McNtcp.24 cells were incubated in the presence or in the absence (control) of 50 μmol/L GCDC for 2 h. Immunoblot analysis for caspase 8 was performed using whole-cell lysates. The reduction of the 55–53 kDa fragment in GCDC-treated cells confirms the processing of the proenzyme into the active forms. Immunoblot analysis for the protein B23 was performed as protein loading control

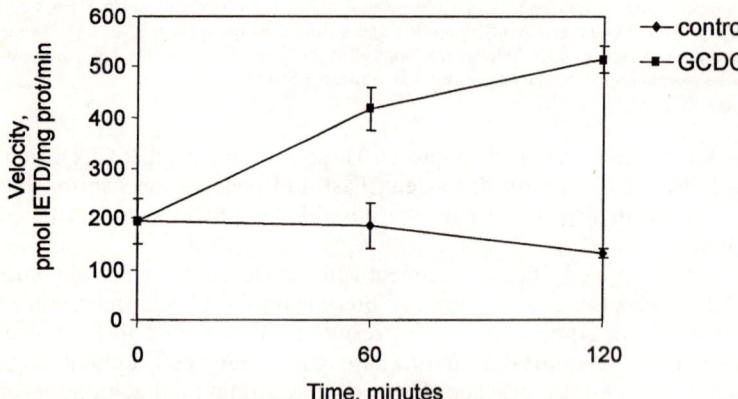

Figure 4 Caspase 8 activity increases in hepatocytes upon treatment with GCDC. McNtcp.24 cells were incubated in the presence or in the absence (control) of 50 μmol/L GCDC. At the indicated time points, caspase 8 activity was measured fluorometrically in the cytosolic extracts, using the fluorogenic substrate IETD-AMC. Data are indicated as mean ± SEM

Altogether, these data demonstrate that caspase 8 is activated during GCDC-induced apoptosis.

CONCLUSION

In summary, the present study demonstrates that: (a) GCDC causes apoptosis only in cells that efficiently transport bile salts; (b) GCDC induces apoptosis in a Fas-dependent, but FasL-independent manner; and (c) GCDC-mediated apoptosis signals through the Fas pathway, promoting Fas oligomerization and caspase 8 activation. Nevertheless, the mechanism by which toxic bile salts activate the Fas system is still unclear. Providing further insight into this mechanism, as well as identifying other molecules involved in the transduction of the apoptotic signal induced by bile salts, might be of great importance for developing new therapeutic approaches for cholestatic liver diseases.

References

1. Schmucker DL, Otha M, Kanai S, Sato Y, Kitani K. Hepatic injury induced by bile salts: correlation between biochemical and morphological events. Hepatology. 1990;12:1216–21.
2. Greim H, Trulzsch D, Roboz J *et al.* Mechanism of cholestasis: 5. Bile acids in normal rat liver and in those after bile duct ligation. Gastroenterology. 1972;63:837–45.
3. Greim H, Trulzsch D, Czygan P *et al.* Mechanism of cholestasis: 6. Bile acids in human livers with or without biliary obstruction. Gastroenterology. 1972;63:846–50.
4. Patel T, Bronk SF, Gores GJ. Increases of intracellular magnesium promote glycochenodeoxycholate-induced apoptosis in rat hepatocytes. J Clin Invest. 1994;94:2183–92.
5. Kwo P, Patel T, Bronk SF, Gores GJ. Nuclear serine protease activity contributes to bile acid-induced apoptosis in hepatocytes. Am J Physiol. 1995;268:G613–21.
6. Nagata S. Apoptosis by death factor. Cell. 1997;88:355–65.
7. Ashkenazi A, Dixit VM. Death receptors: signaling and modulation. Science. 1998;28:1305–8.
8. Smith CA, Farrah T, Goodwin RG. The TNF receptor superfamily of cellular and viral proteins: activation, costimulation, and death. Cell. 1994;76:959–62.
9. Tartaglia LA, Ayres TM, Wong GHW, Goeddel DV. A novel domain within the 55 kd TNF receptor signals cell death. Cell. 1993;74:845–53.
10. Faubion WA, Gores GJ. Death receptors in liver biology and pathobiology. Hepatology. 1999;29:1–4.
11. Galle PR, Hofmann WJ, Walczak H *et al.* Involvement of the CD95 (APO-1/Fas) receptor and ligand in liver damage. J Exp Med. 1995;182:1223–30.
12. Ogasawara J, Watanabe-Fukunaga R, Adachi M *et al.* Lethal effect of the anti-Fas antibody in mice. Nature. 1993;364:806–9.
13. Chinnaiyan AM, Tepper CG, Sedlin MF *et al.* FADD/MORT1 is a common mediator of CD95 (Fas/APO-1) and tumor necrosis factor receptor-induced apoptosis. J Biol Chem. 1996;271:4961–5.
14. Muzio M, Chinnaiyan AM, Kischkel FC *et al.* FLICE, a novel FADD-homologous ICE/CED-3-like protease, is recruited to the CD95 (Fas/APO-1) death-inducing signaling complex. Cell. 1996;85:817–27.
15. Salvesen GS, Dixit VM. Caspases: intracellular signaling by proteolysis. Cell. 1997;91:443–6.
16. Scaffidi C, Fulda S, Srinivasan A *et al.* Two CD95 (APO-1/Fas) signaling pathways. EMBO J. 1998;17:1675–87.
17. Li P, Nijhawan D, Budihardjo I *et al.* Cytochrome c and d-ATP-dependent formation of Apaf-1/caspase 9 complex initiates an apoptotic protease cascade. Cell. 1997;91:479–89.
18. Luo X, Budihardjo I, Zou H, Slaughter C, Wang X. Bid, a Bcl-2 interacting protein, mediates cytochrome c release from mitochondria in response to activation of cell surface death receptors. Cell. 1998;94:481–90.
19. Li H, Zhu H, Xu CJ, Yuan J. Cleavage of BID by caspase 8 mediates the mitochondrial damage in the Fas pathway of apoptosis. Cell. 1998;94:491–501.
20. Torchia EC, Shapiro RJ, Agellon LB. Reconstitution of bile acid transport in the rat hepatoma McArdle RH-7777 cell line. Hepatology. 1996;24:206–11.
21. Spivey JR, Bronk SF, Gores GJ. Glycochenodeoxycholate-induced lethal hepatocellular injury in rat hepatocytes. Role of ATP depletion and cytosolic free calcium. J Clin Invest. 1993;92:17–24.
22. Que FG, Gores GJ, LaRusso NF. Development and initial application of an *in vitro* model of apoptosis in rodent cholangiocytes. Am J Physiol. 1997;272:G106–15.
23. Martins LM, Kottke T, Mesner PW *et al.* Activation of multiple interleukin-1beta converting enzyme homologous in cytosol and nuclei of HL-60 cells during etoposide-induced apoptosis. J Biol Chem. 1997;272:7421–30.
24. Faubion WA, Guicciardi ME, Miyoshi H *et al.* Toxic bile salts induce rodent hepatocyte apoptosis via direct activation of Fas. J Clin Invest. 1999;103:137–45.

26
Death receptor-mediated programmed cell death in the liver

P. R. GALLE, S. KANZLER and S. STRAND

INTRODUCTION

During the past 30 years it has been increasingly recognized that programmed cell death, apoptosis, is an integral part of life. Apoptosis plays a role during development and organ shaping and is involved in many physiological processes. In addition, today it is clear that apoptosis is involved in the pathogenesis of many diseases; in fact there is hardly any disease in which apoptosis, either too much or too little, does not play a role.

DEATH-RELATED RECEPTORS

Among the different ways to die, apoptosis by activation of death factors expressed on the cell surface has gained much attention. Death factors are members of the tumour necrosis factors/nerve growth factors superfamily of receptors. In the liver the death receptors CD95, TNF-R1, TNF-R2, TGF-β receptor and TRAIL R2, TRAIL R3, TRAIL R4 have been detected. These death receptors share certain similarities such as two to five copies of cysteine-rich extracellular repeats and an intracellular death domain which is important for transduction of the apoptotic signal.

Fas receptor/Fas ligand

Fas (CD95/APO-1) is a type l-membrane protein[1,2]. Fas and TNF-R1 are both death receptors that belong to the tumour necrosis factor (TNF)/nerve growth factor (NGF) receptor superfamily, which also includes TNF-R2 (p75), the receptor for lymphotoxin-β, the NGF receptor, CD40, CD27 and CD30[3]. This family is still growing, and new members have recently been identified[4–6]. Fas is highly expressed in activated mature lymphocytes, or lymphocytes transformed with human T-cell leukaemia virus (HTLV-1), human immunodeficiency virus (HIV), or Epstein–Barr virus (EBV). Additionally, many non-lymphoid tissues such as the liver are Fas-positive[7,8]. Binding of Fas by its ligand (CD95L, FasL) or by anti-Fas antibodies results in receptor crosslinking and apoptosis of Fas-positive cells. FasL is a 40 kDa type II transmembrane protein that mediates apoptosis in sensitive target cells[9]. FasL can be protolytically cleaved from the membrane by a metalloproteinase and occurs in a soluble form. Thus, FasL may act as a cytotoxic effector at a distant site from the producer cell. The Fas-mediated intracellular pathway has recently been partially elucidated. Ligation of Fas results in receptor oligomerization, leading to recruitment of the adaptor protein, FADD (Fas-associated protein with death domain) to the death domain of Fas. This complex leads to the recruitment of FLICE (caspase 8) and the activation of further downstream caspases or the mitochondrial pathway, eventually resulting in apoptosis[10,11]. Very recently it has been shown that the bid protein – a member of the proapoptotic bcl-2 family – is a critical substrate for signalling by death receptor agonists, since injection of antibodies against Fas did not lead to massive apoptosis in bid-deficient mice as observed in control animals.

Furthermore, it was shown that mitochondrial dysfunction, as well as effector caspase activity, was reduced in these animals[12].

The fact that FasL is primarily expressed by activated T cells in order to maintain peripheral T and B cell homeostasis suggested that this signalling pathway would have an important role in immune-mediated liver injury, such as autoimmune hepatitis. In addition, several studies have given evidence that Fas signalling may also be functional in a variety of injuries, including toxic damage (see below). Hepatocytes constitutively express Fas and may up-regulate expression of this receptor in a variety of liver diseases, such as viral hepatitis or alcohol-induced liver disease[7,13,14]. Intraperitoneal injection of agonistic anti-Fas antibodies leads to massive hepatocyte apoptosis with subsequent fulminant liver failure[8]. In chronic hepatitis C virus infection it has been shown by immunohistochemical studies that staining for Fas was mainly found in hepatocytes in areas of 'piecemeal necrosis' and lymphocytic infiltrates[13]. Since FasL is constitutively expressed on cytotoxic lymphocytes it is conceivable that T-cell-mediated immune response leading to apoptosis is transduced by the Fas pathway in viral as well as in autoimmune liver disease. Additionally, Fas-mediated apoptosis of target cholangiocytes may also occur via cytotoxic lymphocytes in liver allograft rejection and in primary biliary cirrhosis.

Under pathophysiological conditions hepatocytes may also express Fas ligand, raising the possibility that a Fas ligand-positive hepatocyte may induce apoptosis in a Fas-positive neighbour, an example of fratricide[7].

TNF/TNF-receptor/TRAIL

Tumour necrosis factor (TNF) is a pleiotropic cytokine primarily produced by macrophages, but in smaller amounts also by several other cell types. In the liver TNF is primarily produced by cholangiocytes and Kupffer cells. TNF exerts a wide spectrum of cellular responses, including fever, shock, tissue injury, tumour necrosis, anorexia, induction of other cytokines and immunoregulatory molecules, cell proliferation, differentiation and apoptosis[15]. TNF interacts with two receptors, TNF-R1 (p55) and TNF-R2 (p75), which are encountered in most cell types[16]. The intracellular domain of TNF-R1 has a death domain, whereas that of TNF-R2 does not[17]. It seems that TNF-R2 is a poor inducer of apoptosis and rather exerts antiapoptotic action via the transcription factor nuclear factor κB (NF-κB). Apoptosis induced by TNF-R1 ligation, like Fas stimulation, requires receptor oligomerization and can use the FADD/caspase pathway via the adaptor protein TRADD (TNF receptor-associated protein with death domain; for review see ref. 18). TNF-R1 is highly expressed in hepatocytes and Kupffer cells. Its expression in cholangiocytes, endothelial and stellate cells remains to be determined. Normal hepatocytes are resistant to TNF toxicity, but can be sensitized to TNF cytotoxicity by inhibition of RNA synthesis[19], or by repression of activation of NF-κB[20]. TNF causes liver injury by inducing hepatocyte apoptosis under different pathological conditions such as LPS-induced Kupffer cell activation, ischaemia–reperfusion injury, and the cytokine syndrome associated with septic shock. TNF serum levels are increased in patients with alcoholic hepatitis, and TNF levels correlate inversely with patient survival. It was shown that antibodies to TNF attenuate hepatic necrosis and inflammation caused by chronic exposure to alcohol in the rat[21]. In addition, TNF serum levels are clearly elevated in patients with fulminant hepatitis[22]. Both hepatitis B and C virus infection induce TNF expression in human liver and human hepatoma cell lines[23]. TNF also plays a critical role in liver injury induced by concavalin A, a model relevant to inflammatory liver injury[24].

TRAIL (TNF-related apoptosis-inducing ligand), also called Apo2 ligand, is a further member of the TNF superfamily[25,26]. It is a type II membrane protein and transcripts have been detected in a variety of human tissues. Four closely related receptors bind TRAIL: death receptor 3 (DR3), DR4 and DR5, which contain cytoplasmic death domains and signal apoptosis, and a non-signalling decoy receptor (DcR) that lacks a cytoplasmic tail and inhibits TRAIL function. TRAIL has been shown to induce apoptosis in various cell lines of diverse origin.

TGF-β_1/TGF-receptor

Transforming growth factor-β_1 (TGF-β_1) is the prototype and best characterized of three TGF-β isoforms (TGF-β_1, TGF-β_2 TGF-β_3) encountered in mammalian species. It is a highly conserved molecule with one of the most versatile signalling functions regulating cell growth, differentiation, migration, expression of extracellular matrix and death (for review see ref. 27). In its biologically active form TGF-β_1 consists of a 25 kDa homodimer linked by disulphide bonds. TGF-β_1 is secreted in a biologically inactive form as a complex consisting of two units of the large precursor segment of TGF-β_1 propeptide linked to the mature TGF-β_1 dimer. Conversion of the latent complex to the mature, biologically active form is achieved *in vitro* by acid, alkali, heat or proteases. *In-vivo* mechanisms of TGF-β_1 activation are not fully understood, but seem to involve proteases. TGF-β_1 conveys signals via two serine/threonine kinase receptors, type I and type II, both of which are necessary for signal transduction and are found ubiquitously[28]. The type II TGF-β-receptor determines ligand specificity and is able to interact with different type I receptor isoforms. Activation of the kinase domain of the type I receptor leads to signal transduction to downstream effectors. Increased hepatic levels of TGF-β_1 can be found in a variety of acute and chronic liver diseases such as viral or autoimmune hepatitis or experimentally after CCl_4 administration, bile duct ligation or schistosomiasis infection[29,30].

There is now a large body of evidence that TGF-β_1 and activin A, another member of the TGF-β superfamily, induce hepatocellular apoptosis *in vitro* and *in vivo*[31]. An important mechanism for TGF-β-induced apoptosis might be induction of proapoptotic genes such as *p53* and *bax*, as has been shown for liver epithelial cells[32]. On the other hand, Saile and co-workers have recently shown that TGF-β and/or TNF may inhibit apoptosis in activated hepatic stellate cells *in vitro*[33]. These results indicate that the mechanism of TGF-β_1-induced apoptosis may differ depending on cell type and state of activation.

SUMMARY

Cell death has been recognized as a tightly controlled mechanism which is of similar importance to proliferation. The relevance of death receptors in liver disease suggests them as future targets for therapeutic intervention.

References

1. Itoh N, Yonehara S, Ishii A *et al.* The polypeptide encoded by the cDNA for human cell surface antigen Fas can mediate apoptosis. Cell. 1991;66:233–43.
2. Oehm A, Behrmann I, Falk W *et al.* Purification and molecular cloning of the APO-1 cell surface antigen, a member of the tumor necrosis factor/nerve growth factor receptor superfamily. Sequence identity with the Fas antigen. J Biol Chem. 1992;267:10709–15.
3. Nagata S, Golstein P. The Fas death factor. Science. 1995;267:1449–56.
4. Chinnaiyan AM, O'Rourke K, Yu GL *et al.* Signal transduction by DR3, a death domain-containing receptor related to TNFR-1 and CD95. Science. 1996;274:990–2.
5. Brojatsch J, Naughton J, Rolls MM, Zingler K, Young JA. CAR1, a TNFR-related protein, is a cellular receptor for cytopathic avian leukosis–sarcoma viruses and mediates apoptosis. Cell. 1996;87:845–55.
6. Montgomery RI, Warner MS, Lum BJ, Spear PG. Herpes simplex virus-1 entry into cells mediated by a novel member of the TNF/NGF receptor family. Cell. 1996;87:427–36.
7. Galle PR, Hofman WJ, Walczak H *et al.* Involvement of the CD95 (APO-1/Fas) receptor and ligand in liver damage. J Exp Med. 1995;182:1223–30.
8. Ogasawara J, Watanabe-Fukunaga R, Adachi M *et al.* Lethal effect of the anti-Fas antibody in mice. Nature. 1993;364:806–9.
9. Suda T, Takahashi T, Golstein P, Nagata S. Molecular cloning and expression of the Fas ligand, a novel member of the tumor necrosis factor family. Cell. 1993;75:1169–78.
10. Medema JP, Scaffidi C, Kischkel FC *et al.* FLICE is activated by association with the CD95 death-inducing signaling complex (DISC). EMBO J. 1997;16:2794–804.
11. Muzio M, Chinnaiyan AM, Kischkel FC *et al.* FLICE, a novel FADD-homologous ICE-CED-3-like protease, is recruited to the CD95 (Fas/APO-1) death-inducing signaling complex. Cell. 1996;85:817–27.
12. Yin XM, Wang K, Gross A *et al.* Bid-deficient mice are resistant to Fas-induced hepatocellular apoptosis. Nature. 1999;400:886–91.
13. Hiramatsu N, Hayashi N, Katayama K *et al.* Immunohistochemical detection of Fas antigen in liver tissue of patients with chronic hepatitis C. Hepatology. 1994;19:1354–9.
14. Galle PR, Krammer PH. CD95-induced apoptosis in human liver disease. Semin Liver Dis. 1998;18:141–51.
15. Baker SJ, Reddy EP. Modulation of life and death by the TNF receptor superfamily. Oncogene. 1998;17:3261–70.
16. Tartaglia LA, Goeddel DV. Two TNF receptors. Immunol Today. 1992;13:151–3.
17. Tartaglia LA, Rothe M, Hu YF, Goeddel DV. Tumor necrosis factor's cytotoxic activity is signaled by the p55 TNF receptor. Cell. 1993;73:213–6.
18. Faubion WA, Gores GJ. Death receptors in liver biology and pathobiology. Hepatology. 1999;29:1–4.

19. Leist M, Gantner F, Bohlinger I, Germann PG, Tiegs G, Wendel A. Murine hepatocyte apoptosis induced *in vitro* and *in vivo* by TNF-α requires transcriptional arrest. Immunology. 1994;153:1778–88.
20. Xu Y, Bialik S, Jones BE *et al.* NF-kappaB inactivation converts a hepatocyte cell line TNF-alpha response from proliferation to apoptosis. Am J Physiol. 1998;275:C1058–66.
21. Iimuro Y, Gallucci RM, Luster MI, Kono H, Thurman RG. Antibodies to tumor necrosis factor alfa attenuate hepatic necrosis and inflammation caused by chronic exposure to ethanol in the rat. Hepatology. 1997;26:1530–7.
22. Muto Y, Nouri-Aria KT, Meager A, Alexander GJ, Eddleston AL, Williams R. Enhanced tumour necrosis factor and interleukin-1 in fulminant hepatic failure. Lancet. 1988;2:72–4.
23 Gonzalez-Amaro R, Garcia-Monzon C, Garcia-Buey L *et al.* Induction of tumor necrosis factor alpha production by human hepatocytes in chronic viral hepatitis. J Exp Med. 1994;179:841–8.
24. Tagawa Y, Sekikawa K, Iwakura Y. Suppression of concanavalin A-induced hepatitis in IFN-gamma (–/–) mice, but not in TNF-alpha (–/–) mice: role for IFN-gamma in activating apoptosis of hepatocytes. J Immunol. 1997;159:1418–28.
25. Wiley SR, Schooley K, Smolak PJ *et al.* Identification and characterization of a new member of the TNF family that induces apoptosis. Immunity. 1995;3:673–82.
26. Pitti RM, Marsters SA, Ruppert S, Donahue CJ, Moore A, Ashkenazi A. Induction of apoptosis by Apo-2 ligand, a new member of the tumor necrosis factor cytokine family. J Biol Chem. 1996;271:12687–90.
27. Roberts AB, Sporn MB. Physiological actions and clinical applications of transforming growth factor-beta (TGF-beta). Growth Factors. 1993;8:1–9.
28. Derynck R. TGF-beta-receptor-mediated signaling. Trends Biochem Sci. 1994;19:548–53.
29. Bayer EM, Herr W, Kanzler S *et al.* Transforming growth factor-beta 1 in autoimmune hepatitis: correlation of liver tissue expression and serum levels with disease activity. Hepatology. 1998;28:803–11.
30. Castilla A, Prieto J, Fausto N. Transforming growth factors beta 1 and alpha in chronic liver disease. Effects of interferon alfa therapy. N Engl J Med. 1991;324:933–40.
31. Oberhammer FA, Pavelka M, Sharma S *et al.* Induction of apoptosis in cultured hepatocytes and in regressing liver by transforming growth factor beta 1. Proc Natl Acad Sci USA. 1992;89:5408–12.
32. Teramoto T, Kiss A, Thorgeirsson SS. Induction of p53 and Bax during TGF-beta 1 initiated apoptosis in rat liver epithelial cells. Biochem Biophys Res Commun. 1998;251:56–60.
33. Saile B, Matthes N, Knittel T, Ramadori G. Transforming growth factor beta and tumor necrosis factor alpha inhibit both apoptosis and proliferation of activated rat hepatic stellate cells. Hepatology. 1999;30:196–202.

27
Induction of liver apoptosis by toxins

P. BRISSOT, N. RAKBA, P. LOYER, C. PIGEON, B. TURLIN,
O. LORÉAL, C. GUGUEN-GUILLOUZO and G. LESCOAT

INTRODUCTION

Apoptosis, also termed programmed cell death, is a highly conserved process for deleting old, damaged cells, or deleterious cells. Its rate is coupled with the rate of mitosis, which contributes to cell homeostasis (balance proliferation/apoptosis). Apoptosis is morphologically defined by nuclear (DNA) and cell fragmentation with the formation of membrane-bound fragments containing viable organelles referred to as apoptotic bodies. Apoptotic bodies are phagocytosed by neighbouring cells or professional macrophages. Typically, the maintained integrity of the subcellular fragments avoids the release of potentially toxic intracellular constituents, accounting for the absence of an inflammatory response. In contrast and schematically, lethal cell injury by necrosis is characterized by cell swelling, loss of membrane integrity, cytolysis and subsequent inflammation[1-4].

In the normal liver it is estimated that only < 0.1–0.5% of hepatocytes are identified as apoptotic cells. This small number is probably due to the fact that apoptosis is a rapid process (over 2–4 h) followed by immediate phagocytosis of apoptotic cells. Therefore, an apparently small rate of apoptosis can correspond with important effects on the whole liver: a rate of 3% hepatocyte apoptosis in the absence of regeneration would result in a 25% reduction in liver mass over 2–3 days[5].

In the diseased liver, dysregulation of apoptosis has been implicated in various conditions[6,7]:

1. Ischaemia/reperfusion injury of the liver. Ischaemia and reperfusion release mediators such as TNF-α, which is known to produce apoptosis. They also release free radicals which cause apoptosis of sinusoidal endothelial cells.
2. Viral hepatitis. Councilman bodies (also called acidophilic bodies), a characteristic feature of viral hepatitis, are compatible with apoptotic bodies. A higher number of apoptotic hepatocytes, as compared to healthy subjects,

has been found, and there is evidence that immune (cytotoxic T lymphocytes)-mediated pathways of apoptosis are activated[8].

3.   Diseases of the bile ducts. Chronic non-suppurative destructive cholangitis (primary biliary cirrhosis) has been associated with a high rate of apoptosis[9]. Patel *et al.*[10] reported that toxic bile salts directly induced apoptosis in hepatocytes.

4.   Hepatocarcinogenesis. An increased rate of apoptosis has been reported[11], and might contribute to slow down tumour growth.

This chapter deals with apoptosis induced by hepatotoxins, and will consider successively the following agents: alcohol, iron, copper and endotoxins.

ALCOHOL AND APOPTOSIS[12]

Cell death in alcoholic liver disease (ALD) has generally been attributed to necrosis, especially through acetaldehyde production, mitochondrial dysfunction, and neutrophil infiltration with subsequent oxidative stress. However, apoptosis also plays a crucial role in alcohol-induced liver injury.

Increased apoptosis due to alcohol has been documented in human, animal and *in-vitro* studies:

1.   In human alcoholic liver disease, using the expression of a phenotypic marker of apoptosis (the Lewis antigen) and the TUNEL assay, Kawahara *et al.*[13] showed that these markers were expressed in hepatocytes containing Mallory bodies, a characteristic pathological feature of alcoholic hepatitis. Zhao *et al.*[14] reported enhanced apoptosis in ALD, especially in areas of severe (fibrotic) injury.

2.   In alcohol-fed rats, Benedetti *et al.*[15] reported that hepatocyte apoptosis was localized up to the fifth perivenular row (instead of the first two rows in normal animals). Using the intragastric feeding rat model, Yacoub *et al.*[16] showed that the highest number of apoptotic cells were seen in the group of rats exhibiting liver injury. Mice chronically exposed to ethanol vapour by inhalation exhibited an increase in hepatocytic apoptosis which was reversible after stopping exposure[17].

3.   *In vitro*, Wu and Cederbaum[18,19] showed apoptosis in HepG2 cell lines expressing human cytochrome P-4502E1. In hepatocytes isolated from Wistar rats, and cultured in the presence of alcohol, the amount of fragmented DNA and the number of apoptotic hepatocytes were increased by ethanol[20].

Several mechanisms can be involved:

1.   *The 'death receptor' pathway.* Among various cell surface cytokine receptors belonging to the TNF/NGF-receptor superfamily (TNF = tumor necrosis factor; NGF = nerve growth factor), CD95 (Fas/Apo-1) and TNF receptor 1 (TNF-R1) are particularly implicated in apoptosis triggering[21]. *Concerning the CD95 system*, increased levels of soluble Fas ligand, in correlation with the severity of alcoholic hepatitis, have been reported[22]. In liver tissue from 13 patients with alcoholic cirrhosis, although CD95 receptor expression was not

found to be up-regulated (in contrast with chronic HBV hepatitis and acute liver failure), high CD95 ligand mRNA expression was found in hepatocytes[23]. The liver being CD95-receptor positive, the presence of CD95 ligand mRNA and receptor in the same cell has led to the hypothesis by Galle and Krammer[21] that hepatocytes could be not only target but also effector cells. Membrane-bound CD95 ligand could interact with the CD95 receptor of a neighbouring hepatocyte, therefore acting as a 'fratricide'. Alternatively, CD95-mediated apoptosis could occur in an autocrine or paracrine fashion due to the release of a soluble ligand. *Concerning the TNF-R1 system,* increased plasma TNF-α activity has been documented in alcoholic liver disease[24-26]. The concentrations of hepatocyte TNF receptors 1 (and 2) are increased during chronic ethanol administration to rats[27], and, in patients with alcoholic hepatitis, strong cytoplasmic staining for both receptors has been reported using immunoperoxidase techniques[28]. Therefore, signalling through CD95 and TNF-α is likely to represent important pathways for apoptosis in alcoholic liver disease.

2. *The role of oxidative stress.* This is suggested by data indicating the role of cytochrome P4502E1 (CYP2E1). Using stable HepG2 cell lines which express this cytochrome, Wu and Cederbaum[19] demonstrated that ethanol-induced apoptosis was dependent on CYP2E1 since: (a) DNA fragmentation, caspase 1 and 3 activation and apoptotic morphological changes were not found in HepG2 cells that do not express this cytochrome; (b) apoptosis was decreased or prevented by 4-methylpyrazole, an effective inhibitor of ethanol oxidation by CYP2E1; (c) it was prevented by trolox, an anti-oxidative agent. Therefore, the sequential events leading to apoptosis could be ethanol oxidation by CYP2E1, production of a pro-oxidative state and activation of caspases which play a key role in the proteolytic cascade leading to the final events of apoptosis.

3. *The transforming growth factor (TGF)-beta$_1$ system.* It has been shown by Oberhammer *et al.*[29] that the fibrogenic cytokine TGF-β_1, secreted by Kupffer and stellate cells in alcoholic liver disease, induced apoptosis in cultured hepatocytes.

IRON AND APOPTOSIS

Iron excess is known to produce (or contribute to) liver cell damage, in three main ways as illustrated especially by the liver picture of genetic haemochromatosis. First, it can generate liver cell death as shown by slight biochemical cytolysis (i.e. hypertransaminasaemia) and pathologically by the feature described as 'sideronecrosis'. Secondly, there is constitution of fibrosis and cirrhosis. Thirdly, hepatocellular carcinoma may develop[30,31]. The main mechanism advocated for these deleterious effects is iron-related lipid peroxidation producing initial alterations of cellular membranes and organelles such as mitochondria, microsomes and lysosomes[32-34]. Additional mechanisms of iron toxicity can be proposed: (a) TGF-β_1 has been found by Houglum *et al.*[35] to co-localize with iron and MDA protein adducts in the liver of untreated haemochromatosis patients, with normalization after iron removal. (b) The role of iron *per se* (i.e. independently of cirrhosis) in the carcinogenetic process is suggested by the rare but possible development of hepatocellular carcinoma in cirrhosis-free haemochromatosis patients[36]. Moreover, hepatocellular carcinoma patients with neither haemochromatosis nor cirrhosis present with an increase in liver iron content in non-tumoral areas[37]. Experimentally, our group showed, in rat hepatocytes stimulated by EGF/pyruvate, that iron induced DNA synthesis, and that this induction was likely to be related both to cell proliferation and DNA repair of iron-induced DNA damage[38].

When considering these various mechanisms of hepatic iron toxicity, apoptosis might be involved in each of them: oxidative stress[39], as well as TGF-β_1, are putative apoptosis inducers, and apoptosis may also occur as a compensatory mechanism to the proliferative effect of iron. However, despite these theoretical mechanistic considerations, one must admit that evidence for liver iron-induced apoptosis has not been widely reported:

1. Experimentally, it has been shown in the Long-Evans Cinnamon rat model, in which an iron-regular diet is followed by fulminant hepatitis and liver cancer with numerous apoptotic bodies, that iron deprivation prevented these hepatic complications together with marked inhibition of apoptosis[40].
2. In humans, Zao *et al.*[41] studied three situations of iron overload: genetic hemochromatosis (34 cases, among whom 17 were in the cirrhotic stage), mild to moderate iron overload not related to homozygous hemochromatosis (24 cases), and transfusional iron overload (five cases). Apoptosis was assessed by use of DNA nick-end labelling (TUNEL). The results indicated that: (a) an increased apoptotic rate of hepatocytes occurs in chronic hepatic iron overload; (b) the increase was greater in haemochromatosis; (c) the location of apoptosis was, in haemochromatosis, pericentral (perivenular), in contrast to the two other groups of hepatic iron overload. Globally, these data suggest that iron overload can be an apoptotic inducer.

Some data report the pro-apoptotic effect of *iron deprivation* produced by iron chelators. Although apparently inconsistent with the above-mentioned results concerning iron-induced apoptosis, it should be kept in mind that iron deprivation applied to proliferative cells (i.e. as potential anticancer agent) is a different situation from applying a chelator in order to eliminate cellular iron overload (i.e. as a therapeutic tool for iron excess). Desferrioxamine (DFO) has been shown to produce apoptosis in some non-hepatic proliferative cell lines but, as stressed by Richardson[42], DFO did not result in apoptosis in all cell lines, and apoptosis was only observed, after a 24-h incubation, at concentrations of 0.5–2.5 mM, which are well above therapeutically obtainable levels (8–20 μM). Similar data were observed in our group[43] using DFO in the human hepatoblastoma cell line HepG2. However, when a new synthetic iron chelator (O-Trensox) was applied to this cellular model, we obtained a strong inhibition of proliferation, cell cycle arrest mainly in G1 phase and apoptosis, demonstrated by Hoechst staining, at a concentration of 20 μM after 48 h of exposure. Whether this apoptotic effect was the result of iron deprivation *per se*, or involved other metal chelating properties, remains to be determined.

COPPER AND APOPTOSIS

Hepatic copper overload is responsible for progressive liver injury and eventual cirrhosis in Wilson's disease and Indian childhood cirrhosis. Like iron, copper catalyses the formation of oxyradicals with subsequent lipid peroxidation which damages membranes and intrahepatocytic organelles (lysosomes, mitochondria) and even DNA[33,34,44,45].

The apoptotic effect of copper onto the liver has been documented both *in vivo* and *in vitro*. During chronic copper poisoning in sheep, apoptosis was observed in all zones of the hepatic lobule[46]. However, the major contribution in this field was provided by Strand *et al.*[47]. Studying four patients with fulminant hepatic failure due to Wilson's disease, hepatic apoptosis and expression of CD95L and CD95L mRNA were detected. Using HepG2 cells exposed to copper, they demonstrated hepatocytic apoptosis by confocal laser scan analysis after TUNEL staining, and FACS analysis after propidium iodide staining. Apoptosis could be reduced by a neutralizing anti-CD95L antibody (NOK-1). The antioxidant and glutathione precursor *N*-acetylcysteine resulted in reduced CD95L mRNA. On the whole, these data indicate that copper induces hepatic apoptosis via the CD95 (APO1-Fas) system, and suggest that the initiating event is represented by copper-induced oxidative stress.

APOPTOSIS AND ENDOTOXIN

Endotoxin, which corresponds to the bacterial cell wall component lipo-polysaccharide (LPS), causes sequestration of neutrophils within the hepatic sinusoids without significant liver injury[48]. Using both *in-vivo* (rats) and *in-vitro* (rat hepatocyte and/or Kupffer cell cultures) models, Hamada *et al.*[49] showed that activation of Kupffer cells, TNF-α and caspases downstream of TNF-R1 were involved in hepatocyte apoptosis induced by LPS.

When combined with galactosamine (GalN), which selectively depletes hepatic uridine nucleotides leading to transcriptional block, acute hepatic failure occurs. Leist *et al.*[50] demonstrated that TNF-α-induced hepatocyte apoptosis preceded liver failure in this experimental murine shock. Neutrophil trans-migration was identified, in this model, as a critical step in the development of massive hepatocellular necrosis[48]. Activation of caspase 3 (CPP32)-like proteases was shown to be critical for the development of TNF-α-induced parenchymal cell apoptosis[51]. Recently, Lawson *et al.*[52] showed that pretreat-ment with uridine of GalN/endotoxin mice markedly reduced apoptosis and neutrophil transmigration, and prevented hepatocyte necrosis and transaminase release. These data led to the conclusion that excessive apoptosis represents an important signal for transmigration of primed neutrophils sequestered in sinu-soids during endotoxaemia *in vivo*. Maher and Gores, in a recent editorial[53], propose the following synthetic scheme of events in endotoxin/galactosamine induced liver injury: endotoxin-induced TNF-α which in turn leads to neutrophil sequestration in the hepatic sinusoids, galactosamine sensitizes hepatocytes to TNF-mediated apoptosis, and this signals sequestered neutrophils to invade the parenchymal cells and cause hepatocyte necrosis.

These data on the relationship between endotoxin, apoptosis and necrosis may have important clinical relevance. It is well known that plasma endotoxin levels are increased in cirrhosis[54], in relation to the severity of liver dysfunction[55,56]. Especially, endotoxin is frequently increased in the blood of alcoholics[57], and in some animal models of alcoholic liver disease[58].

SUMMARY

In conclusion, induction of apoptosis by toxins is involved in the pathogenesis of a variety of hepatic complications. This new comprehensive approach to liver diseases now paves the road for novel therapeutic strategies in liver conditions involving uncontrolled apoptosis.

Acknowledgements

This work was supported in part by EEC Biomed 2, Association Fer et Foie, and Association pour la Recherche sur le Cancer (Grant 5617).

References

1. Rosser BG, Gores GJ. Liver cell necrosis: cellular mechanisms and clinical implications. Gastroenterology. 1995;108:252–75.
2. Galle PR. Apoptosis in liver disease. J Hepatol. 1997;27:405–12.
3. Feldmann G. Liver apoptosis. J Hepatol. 1997;26(Suppl. 2):1–11.
4. Berk PD, Gores GJ. Apoptosis as a mechanism of liver disease. Semin Liver Dis. 1998;2:103–90.
5. Bursch W, Paffe S, Putz B, Barthel G, Schulte-Hermann R. Determination of the length of the histological stages of apoptosis in normal liver and in altered hepatic foci of rats. Carcinogenesis. 1990;11:847–53.
6. Patel T, Roberts LR, Jones BA, Gores GJ. Dysregulation of apoptosis as a mechanism of liver disease. Semin Liver Dis. 1998;2:105–14.
7. Miyoshi H, Gores GJ. Apoptosis of the liver: relevance for the hepatobiliary–pancreatic surgeon. J Hepatobiliary Pancreat Surg. 1998;5:409–15.
8. Lau JYN, Xie X, Lai MMC, Wu PC. Apoptosis and viral hepatitis. Semin Liver Dis. 1998;18:169–76.
9. Kuroki T, Kawakita N, Nakatani K, Hisa T, Kitada T, Sakaguchi H. Expression of antigens related to apoptosis and cell proliferation in chronic non suppurative destructive cholangitis in primary biliary cirrhosis. Virchows Arch. 1996;429:119–29.
10. Patel T, Bronk SF, Gores GJ. Increase of intracellular magnesium promotes glycodeoxycholate-induced apoptosis in rat hepatocytes. J Clin Invest. 1994;94:2183–92.
11. Bursch W, Grasl-Kraupp B, Ellinger A et al. Active cell death: role in hepatocarcinogenesis and subtypes. Biochem Cell Biol. 1994;72:669–75.
12. Nanji AA. Apoptosis and alcoholic liver disease. Semin Liver Dis. 1998;18:187–90.
13. Kawahara H, Matsuda Y, Takase S. Is apoptosis involved in alcoholic hepatitis? Alcohol. 1994;29(Suppl. 1):113–18.
14. Zhao M, Laissue J, Zimmermann A. TUNEL-positive hepatocytes in alcoholic liver disease. A retrospective biopsy study using DNA nick end-labelling. Virchows Arch. 1997;431:337–44.
15. Benedetti A, Jezequel AM, Orlandi F. A quantitative evaluation of apoptotic bodies in rat liver. Liver. 1988;8:172–7.
16. Yacoub LK, Fogt F, Griniuviene B, Nanji AA. Apoptosis and Bcl-2 protein expression in experimental alcoholic liver disease in the rat. Alcohol Clin Exp Res. 1995;19:854–9.
17. Goldin RD, Hunt NC, Clark J, Wickramasinghe SN. Apoptotic bodies in a murine model of alcoholic liver disease: reversibility of ethanol-induced changes. J Pathol. 1993;171:73–6.
18. Wu D, Cederbaum AI. Ethanol cytotoxicity to a transfected HepG2 cell line expressing human cytochrome P-4502E1. J Biol Chem. 1996;271:23914–19.

19. Wu D, Cederbaum AI. Ethanol-induced apoptosis to stable HepG2 cell lines expressing human cytochrome P-4502E1. Alcohol Clin Exp Res. 1999;23:67–76.
20. Kurose I, Higuchi H, Miura S *et al.* Oxidative stress-mediated apoptosis of hepatocytes exposed to acute ethanol intoxication. Hepatology. 1997;25:368–78.
21. Galle PG, Krammer PH. CD95-induced apoptosis in human liver disease. Semin Liver Dis. 1998;18:141–51.
22. Taieb J, Mathurin P, Poynard T, Gougero-Pocidalo MA, Chollet-Martin S. Raised plasma soluble Fas and Fas-ligand in alcoholic liver disease. Lancet. 1998;351:1930–1.
23. Galle PR, Hofmann WJ, Walczak H *et al.* Involvement of the CD95 (APO-1/Fas) receptor and ligandin liver damage. J Exp Med. 1995;182:1223–30.
24. McClain C, Hill D, Schmidt J, Diehl AM. Cytokines and alcoholic liver disease. Semin Liver Dis. 1993;13:170–82.
25. Khoruts A, Stahnke L, McClain C, Logan G, Allen JI. Circulating tumor necrosis factor, interleukin-1 and interleukin-6 concentrations in chronic alcoholic patients. Hepatology. 1991;13:267–76.
26. Felver ME, Mezey E, McGuire M *et al.* Plasma tumor necrosis factor alpha predicts decreased long-term survival in severe alcoholic hepatitis. Alcohol Clin Exp Res. 1990;14:255–9.
27. Deaciuc IV, D'Souza NB, Spitzer JJ. Tumor necrosis factor-alpha cell-surface receptors of liver parenchymal and nonparenchymal cells during acute and chronic alcohol administration to rats. Alcohol Clin Exp Res. 1995;19:332–8.
28. Spengler U, Zachoval R, Gallati H *et al.* Serum levels and *in situ* expression of TNF-alpha and TNF-alpha binding proteins in inflammatory liver diseases. Cytokine. 1996;8:864–72.
29. Oberhammer FA, Pavelka M, Sharma S *et al.* Induction of apoptosis in cultures hepatocytes and in regressing liver by transforming growth factor beta 1. Proc Natl Acad Sci USA. 1992;89:5408–12.
30. Deugnier YM, Loréal O, Turlin B *et al.* Liver pathology in genetic hemochromatosis: a review of 135 homozygous cases and their bioclinical correlations. Gastroenterology. 1992;102:2050–9.
31. Brissot P, Deugnier Y. Genetic hemochromatosis. In: McIntyre N, Benhamou JP, Bircher J, Rizzetto M, Rodes J, editors. Oxford Textbook of Clinical Hepatology. Oxford: Oxford University Press; 1999:1379–91.
32. Bacon BR, Britton RS. The pathology of hepatic iron overload: a free radical-mediated process? Hepatology. 1990;211:127–30.
33. Brissot P, Loréal O, Hubert N *et al.* Chronic metal overload and hepatic damage. In: Clément B, Guillouzo A, editors. Cellular and Molecular Aspects of Cirrhosis. Colloque INSERM/John Libbey Eurotext; 1992, Vol. 216:13–23.
34. Britton RS. Metal-induced hepatotoxicity. Semin Liver Dis. 1996;16:3–12.
35. Houglum K, Ramm GA, Crawford DHG, Witzum JL, Powell LW, Chojkier M. Excess iron induces hepatic oxidative stress and transforming growth factor beta1 in genetic hemochromatosis. Hepatology. 1997;26:605–10.
36. Deugnier YM, Guyader D, Crantock L *et al.* Primary liver cancer in genetic hemochromatosis: a clinical, pathological, and pathogenetic study of 54 cases. Gastroenterology. 1993;104:228–34.
37. Turlin B, Juguet F, Moirand R *et al.* Increased liver iron stores in patients with hepatocellular carcinoma developed in a noncirrhotic liver. Hepatology. 1995;22:446–50.
38. Chenoufi N, Loréal O, Drénou B *et al.* Iron may induce both DNA synthesis and repair in rat hepatocytes stimulated by EGF/pyruvate. J Hepatol. 1997;26:650–8.
39. Buttke TM, Sandstrom PA. Oxidative stress as a mediator of apoptosis. Immunol Today. 1994;15:7–10.
40. Kato J, Kobune M, Kohgo Y *et al.* Hepatic iron deprivation prevents spontaneous development of fulminant hepatitis and liver cancer in Long–Evans Cinnamon rats. J Clin Invest. 1996;98:923–9.
41. Zhao M, Laissue JA, Zimmermann A. Hepatocyte apoptosis in hepatic iron overload diseases. Histol Histopathol. 1997;12:367–74.
42. Richardson DR. Potential of iron chelators as effective antiproliferative agents. Can J Physiol Pharmacol. 1997;75:1164–80.
43. Rakba N, Loyer P, Delcros JG *et al.* Comparison of antiproliferative and apoptotic effects of O-Trensox, a new synthetic iron chelator, and desferrioxamine in the human hepatoblastoma cell line HepG2. AASLD, Dallas, November 1999 A (in press).

44. Sokol RJ, Twedt D, McKim JM *et al.* Oxidant injury to hepatic mitochondria in patients with Wilson's disease and Bedlington terriers with copper toxicosis. Gastroenterology. 1994;107:1788–98.

45. Li Y, Togashi Y, Sato S *et al.* Spontaneous hepatic copper accumulation in Long–Evans Cinnamon rats with hereditary hepatitis. A model of Wilson's disease. J Clin Invest. 1991;87:1858–61.

46. King TP, Bremmer I. Autophagy and apoptosis in liver during the prehaemolytic phase of chronic copper poisoning in sheep. J Comp Pathol. 1979;89:515–30.

47. Strand S, Hofmann WJ, Grambihler A *et al.* Hepatic failure and liver cell damage in acute Wilson's disease involve CD95 (APO-1/Fas) mediated apoptosis. Nature Med. 1998;4:588–93.

48. Chosay JG, Essani NA, Dunn CJ, Jaeschke H. Neutrophil margination and extravasation in sinusoids and venules of liver during endotoxin-induced injury. Am J Physiol. 1997;272:G1195–200.

49. Hamada E, Nishida T, Uchiyama Y *et al.* Activation of Kupffer cells and caspase-3 involved in rat hepatocyte apoptosis induced by endotoxin. J Hepatol. 1999;30:807–18.

50. Leist M, Gantner F, Bohlinger I, Tiegs G, Germann PG, Wendel A. Tumor necrosis factor-induced hepatocyte apoptosis precedes liver failure in experimental murine shock models. Am J Pathol. 1995;146:1220–34.

51. Jaeschke H, Fisher MA, Lawson JA, Simmons CA, Farhood A, Jones DA. Activation of caspase 3 (CPP32)-like proteases is essential for THF-alpha-induced hepatic parenchymal cell apoptosis and neutrophil-mediated necrosis in a murine endotoxin shock model. J Immunol. 1998;160: 3480–6.

52. Lawson JA, Fisher MA, Simmons CA, Farhood A, Jaeschke H. Parenchymal cell apoptosis as a signal for sinusoidal sequestration and transendothelial migration of neutrophils in murine models of endotoxin and Fas-antibody-induced liver injury. Hepatology. 1998;28:761–7.

53. Maher JJ, Gores GJ. Apoptosis: silent killer or neutral bomb? Hepatology. 1998;28:865–7.

54. Lumsden AB, Henderson JM, Kutner MH. Endotoxin levels measured by a chromogenic assay in portal, hepatic and peripheral venous blood in patients with cirrhosis. Hepatology. 1988;8:232–6.

55. Lin R, Lee F, Lee S *et al.* Endotoxemia in patients with chronic liver diseases: relationship to severity of liver diseases, presence of oesophageal varices, and hyperdynamic circulation. J Hepatol. 1995;22:165–72.

56. Ferro D, Quintarelli C, Lattuada A *et al.* High plasma levels of von Willebrand factor as a marker of endothelial perturbation in cirrhosis: relationship to endotoxinemia. Hepatology. 1996;23:1377–83.

57. Bode C, Kugler V, Bode JC. Endotoxemia in patients with alcoholic and non-alcoholic cirrhosis and in subjects with no evidence of chronic liver disease following acute alcohol excess. J Hepatol. 1987;4:8–14.

58. Nanji AA, Khettry U, Sadrzadeh SMH, Yamanaka T. Severity of liver injury in experimental alcoholic liver disease. Am J Pathol. 1993;142:367–73.

28
Apoptosis induced by tumour necrosis factor α in human hepatoma cell lines

S. ROUSSET, A. BRINGUIER, B. LARDEUX and G. FELDMANN

INTRODUCTION

Tumour necrosis factor alpha (TNF-α), a cytokine characterized 25 years ago[1], is produced by macrophages and in the liver by Kupffer cells. It exerts several pleiotropic functions on hepatocytes[2], one of which, cell proliferation, has recently been analysed in detail[3]. TNF-α is also known to induce cytotoxicity, at least in several tumoral cell lines[4]. The nature of cell death, necrosis or apoptosis, due to TNF-α is still debated. However, recent results have demonstrated that the cytokine was capable of inducing apoptosis in murine hepatocytes either *in vivo*[5] or *in vitro*[6], but when special conditions were used, i.e. when transcriptional inhibitors such as actinomycin D, galactosamine or α-amanitin were added to TNF-α[5,6]. In another respect we now know many details on TNF-α signalling pathways, explaining why the same cytokine could exert cell proliferation or apoptosis. Before briefly reviewing these pathways it must be recalled that TNF-α belongs to the TNF superfamily, a large family of peptides which also contains the Fas ligand responsible for apoptotic cell death when it binds to the Fas/Apo-1 receptor[7]. When TNF-α binds to TNF-R1, its main cell receptor, it triggers a trimerization of the receptor and a cascade of cellular protein interactions ending either in cell survival or in cell death. The intracellular domain of TNF-R1 asssociates with TRADD (TNF-R1-associating-death-domain), an adaptor protein which recruits various signalling molecules that have both death-promoting and death-preventing effects. Death promotion is caused by recruitment of FADD (Fas-associating-death-domain) by TRADD[8]. This causes the same pro-apoptotic effects observed after the recruitment of FADD by Fas[9]. Briefly FADD recruits procaspase 8, which autoactivates into the active caspase 8. The latter activates other caspases and also causes the cleavage of BID[10], a pro-apoptotic member of the Bcl-2 family[11]. Translocation of truncated BID to mitochondria causes the release of cytochrome-c[10] and AIF (apoptosis-inducing factor)[12] in the cytosol. In the presence of dATP and APAF1 (apoptosis-protease-activating factor 1) cytochrome-c activates caspase 9[13] and then the caspase cascade, in particular caspases 3 and 7. Proteolysis and DNA fragmentation occur secondary to the conjugate actions of caspases and AIF and lead to apoptosis. Regulation of TNF-α-pro-apoptotic action could depend, at least in part, on the action of the other members of the Bcl-2 family[9]. In addition to recruiting the pro-apoptotic FADD adaptor protein, TRADD also recruits RIP (receptor-interacting protein) and TRAF2 (TNF-receptor-associated factor 2)[9]. These two polypeptides mainly signal for anti-apoptotic effects. First TRAF2 activates the Jun-NH$_2$-terminal kinase (JNK)/AP1 system which plays a role probably important in hepatocyte proliferation[14]. Second, TRAF2 and RIP cause the proteosomal degradation of IκB, an inhibitor of NF-κB that normally maintains NF-κB in an inactive cytosolic complex[15]. The resulting translocation of NF-κB into the nucleus may induce cell survival[16]. The role of NF-κB in TNF-α-induced apoptosis has been illustrated by Beg and Baltimore[17], who reported that TNF-α knockout mice exhibited liver apoptosis, and by Bellas et al.[18], who showed that inhibition of IκB degradation prevented nuclear translocation of NF-κB and also induced a massive apoptosis in murine hepatocytes.

These last results confirm that it is possible to promote the TNF-α pro-apoptotic effects at the expense of cell proliferation, at least in normal hepatocytes. Two means are available: one unspecific, which is based on the use of transcriptional inhibitors preventing the transcription of anti-apoptotic genes such as those of NF-κB or AP1; and a more specific one which acts on the cytosolic NF-κB/IκB complex. However the situation is more complicated in hepatoma cell lines since these cells proliferate spontaneously and are not very susceptible to apoptotic agents, perhaps because they express, as we observed for many of them (personal results), a large amount of anti-apoptotic proteins. At least to our knowledge, only one hepatoma cell line, HepG2, has been investigated to test the TNF-α-pro-apoptotic effects, and apoptosis was observed only when transcriptional inhibitors were used[6]. So the aim of this work was to study the behaviour of several human hepatoma cell lines when submitted to TNF-α either alone or associated with actinomycin D. In addition the behaviour of some anti-apoptotic proteins, such as Bcl-2[11] and HSP70[19], was also investigated. We plan to inhibit these two proteins using an antisense strategy to sensitize the tumoral cells to the apoptotic effect of TNF-α alone.

MATERIAL AND METHODS

Material

Five human hepatoma cell lines – HepG2, Hep3B, SKHep1, Chang Liver, and IHH (immortalized human hepatocytes), with the first four provided by ATCC (Rockville, MD, USA) and IHH provided by Moshage (Groningen, the Netherlands)[20] – were cultured in MEM Eagle medium (Life Technologies, Grand Rapids, NY, USA) supplemented with 10% fetal calf serum and antibiotics under a 95% O_2, 5% CO_2 atmosphere. When the cells were at semiconfluency, TNF-α (R&D Systems, Abingdon, UK), at a concentration of 50 or

200 IU/ml, was added to the culture medium. In some experiments actinomycin D (Sigma, St Louis, MO, USA) at a concentration of 0.8 mM, was added 30 min before TNF-α. In all cases the effects were observed after 24 or 48 h.

Methods

Several different methods were used in the five cell lines to investigate: (1) the effects of TNF-α on cell proliferation, necrosis and apoptosis; (2) some of the proteins acting in TNF-α signalling pathways; and (3) the presence of anti-apoptotic proteins Bcl-2 and HSP70.

Effects of TNF-α on cell proliferation, necrosis and apoptosis

Cell proliferation was measured by radioactive thymidine incorporation in counts/min (cpm), and the number of cells was estimated studying the specific optical density (OD) after crystal violet staining. The ratio of cpm/OD gave the cell proliferation induced by TNF-α.

For necrosis, measurements of lactate dehydrogenase (LDH) activity in the supernatants of cell cultures were made by using the LDH kit test from Merck Diagnostics (Paris, France) according to the manufacturer's instructions. Apoptosis was studied using three different techniques:

1. Staining of the cells by DAPI to study chromatin condensation and/or nuclear fragmentation.
2. DNA electrophoresis to study the formation of oligonucleosomes and nucleosomes.
3. Behaviour of poly-(ADP)-ribose-polymerase (PARP), an enzyme cleaved by caspase 3 during apoptosis[21], by immunoblotting of nuclear extracts with specific monoclonal anti-PARP antibody (Pharmingen, San Diego, CA, USA). The bands obtained were semi-quantified by software Candela (Microvision, Les Ulys, France).

Proteins acting in the TNF-α signalling pathway

TNF-R1, the main receptor of TNF-α, was studied in all cell lines by immunoblotting with specific anti-TNF-R1 monoclonal antibodies (R&D Systems). The presence of TRADD and FADD, and their behaviour with TNF-α and/or actinomycin D, was analysed in two cell lines only (HepG2 and IHH) by immunoblotting with specific anti-TRADD or anti-FADD monoclonal antibodies (Immunotech, Marseilles, France).

Presence of anti-apoptotic proteins Bcl-2 and HSP70 and quantification of HSP70 mRNA

The two proteins Bcl-2 and HSP70 were studied by immunoblotting in all the cell lines with specific monoclonal anti-Bcl-2 (Santa Cruz Biotechnology, Santa Cruz, CA, USA) or anti-HSP70 (Pharmingen) antibodies. In addition the amount of HSP70 mRNA was measured by ribonuclease protection assay (RPA) according to the method already described in the laboratory[22]. Briefly, molecular hybridization of Hep3B, SKHep1 and normal liver lysates was made with specific HSP70 riboprobe (cRNA) obtained after RT-PCR with specific primers of HSP70 from total RNA coming from Hep3B, SKHep1 or hepatocytes. The amount of HSP70 mRNA was related to the amount of a reference gene, GAPDH mRNA.

RESULTS

Effects of TNF-α

Cell proliferation

After 24 h (Fig. 1), only the SKHep1 cells were proliferating after TNF-α addition, particularly with a dose of 50 IU/ml. After 48 h, HepG2 cells proliferated with TNF-α in a dose-dependent manner, while Chang Liver was particularly sensitive to 50 IU/ml of TNF-α (data not shown).

Necrosis

After 24 or 48 h no increase in LDH activity was observed in supernatants of cells submitted to TNF-α alone, whatever the dose used. When actinomycin D (actD) was added before TNF-α, cytolysis was observed in the five cell lines, but this effect was not increased when TNF-α was added, whatever the dose.

Apoptosis

Apoptosis was investigated first by DAPI staining. For IHH and HepG2 cell lines no apoptotic figures were observed with TNF-α alone, whatever the dose, or after pretreatment with actD. Similar results were obtained for Hep3B,

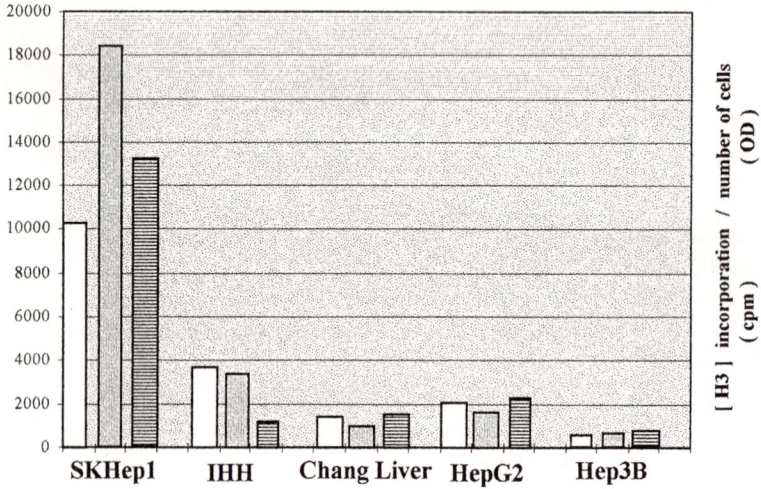

Figure 1 Measure of cell proliferation of SKHep1, IHH, Chang Liver, HepG2 and Hep3B cell lines after 24 h of treatment with TNF-α □, control; ▨ , 50 IU/ml TNF-α; ▥ , 200 IU/ml TNF-α. Only SKHep1 cells proliferate with TNF-α, especially with a dose of 50 IU/ml

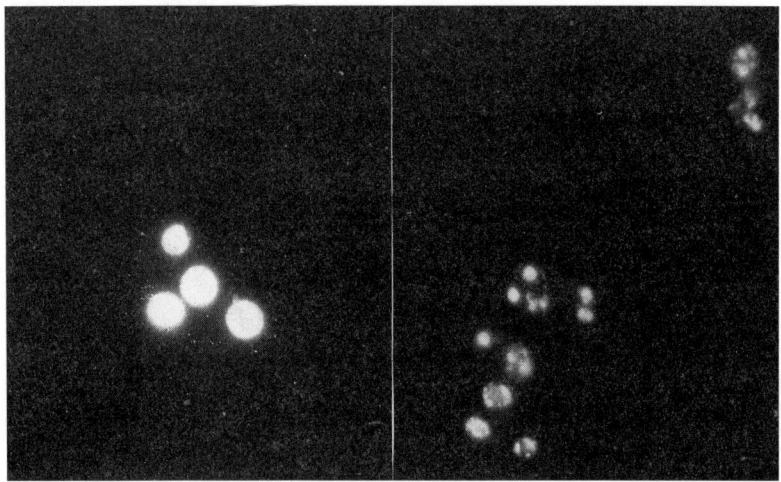

Figure 2 DAPI staining on Chang Liver cells after 24 h. **A**: control; **B**: after pretreatment with actD (0.8 μM) and TNF-α (50 IU/ml). Apoptotic figures (chromatin condensation and nuclear fragmentation) are observed in (**B**) while nuclei are normal in (**A**). (×250)

SKHep1 and Chang Liver with TNF-α alone, while after pretreatment with actD, apoptotic figures (chromatin condensation and/or nucleus fragmentation) were observed with the two doses of TNF-α in the three cell lines (Fig. 2).

Apoptosis was then studied by DNA electrophoresis to investigate the formation of oligonucleosomes and nucleosomes, after 12 or 24 h of treatment with actD and TNF-α. Figure 3 presents the results obtained with the SKHep1 cell line. After 12 h, DNA fragmentation was observed with actD, but this fragmentation was not increased with TNF-α. After 24 h, DNA fragmentation obtained with actD was increased with TNF-α, especially with a dose of 50 IU/ml.

Apoptosis was also investigated by immunoblotting of PARP. After 12 h (Fig. 4), no PARP cleavage was observed for Chang Liver and Hep3B cells in the samples when actD was absent, while when actD was added, a PARP cleavage was observed. This cleavage was increased 1.3 times for Chang Liver cells with TNF-α, whatever the dose; 1.2 times with 50 IU/ml TNF-α and 2.8 times with 200 IU/ml TNF-α for Hep3B cells. For SKHep1 cells the cleavage of PARP was similar in the samples treated with actD, with or without TNF-α. For IHH no cleavage was observed, and for HepG2 no significant cleavage was recorded, whatever the conditions used. After 24 h the cleavage of PARP was similar in the samples treated with actD with or without TNF-α in Chang Liver cells, while the cleavage observed with actD was increased 3.5 times with 50 IU/ml TNF-α in SKHep1 cells; for Hep3B, HepG2 and IHH, no significant cleavage was observed (data not shown).

Proteins acting in the TNF-α signalling pathway

A band corresponding to the apparent molecular weight of TNF-R1 (55 kDa) was observed by immunoblotting in each hepatoma cell line (Fig. 5). TRADD

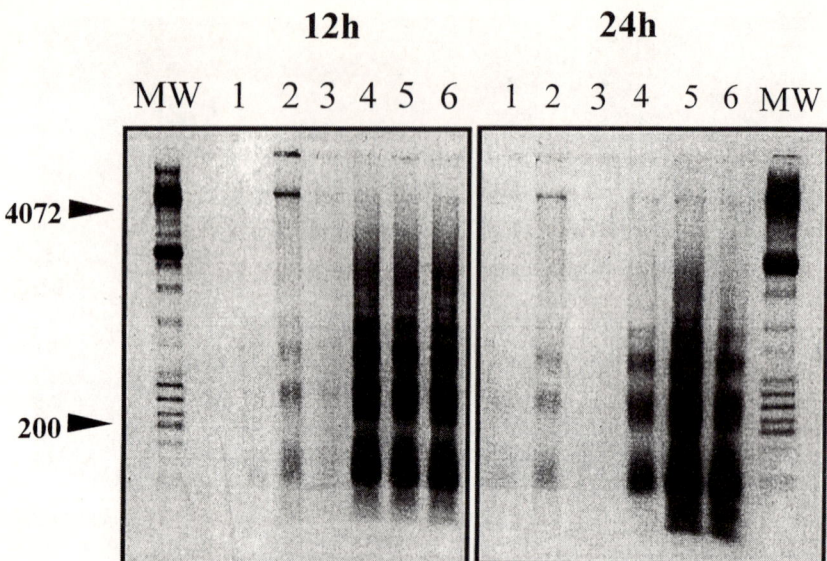

Figure 3 DNA gel electrophoresis, of SKHep1 cells after 12 or 24 h of treatment. Lines 1: control; 2: TNF-α (50 IU/ml); 3: TNF-α (200 IU/ml); 4: actD (0.8 μM); 5: actD (0.8 μM) + TNF-α (50 IU/ml); 6: actD (0.8 μM) + TNF-α (200 IU/ml). (MW = molecular weight). DNA fragmentation observed at 24 h with actD is increased with TNF-α

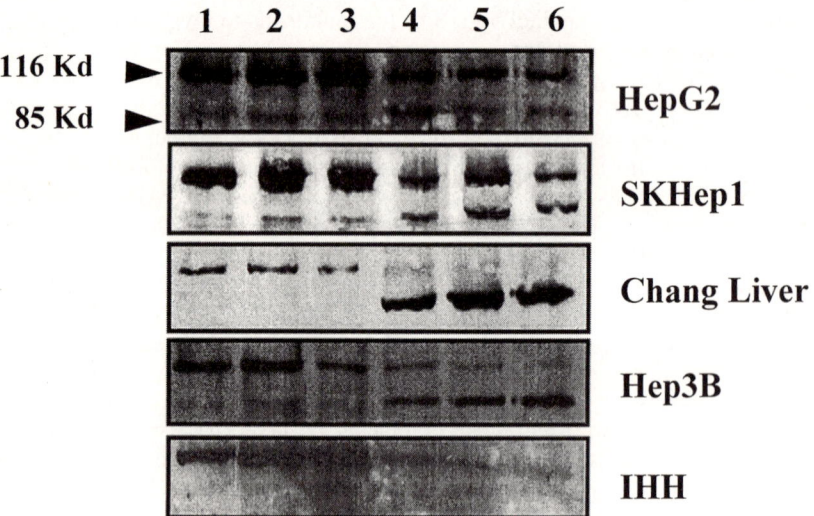

Figure 4 PARP immunoblotting on HepG2, SKHep1, Chang Liver, Hep3B and IHH cell lines after 12 h of treatment. Lines 1: control; 2: TNF-α (50 IU/ml); 3: TNF-α (200 IU/ml); 4: actD (0.8 μM); 5: actD (0.8 μM) + TNF-α (50 IU/ml); 6: actD (0.8 μM) + TNF-α (200 IU/ml). No PARP cleavage was observed for Chang Liver or Hep3B cells in the samples when actD was absent, but when actD was added a PARP cleavage was observed and this cleavage was increased with TNF-α. For SKHep1 cells the cleavage of PARP was similar in the samples treated with actD, with or without TNF-α. For IHH and HepG2 no significant cleavage was observed

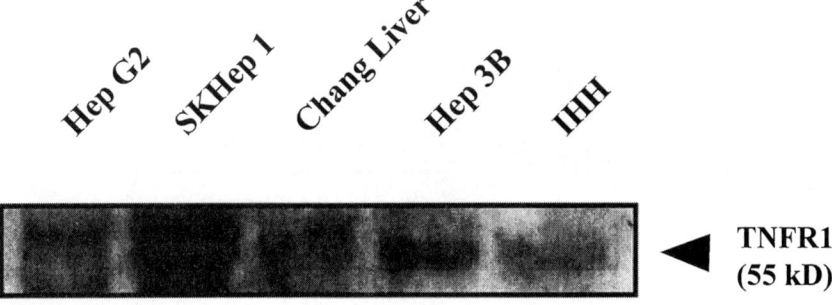

Figure 5 Immunoblotting of TNF-R1 in HepG2, SKHep1, Chang Liver, Hep3B and IHH cell lines. TNF-R1 is present in all five cell lines

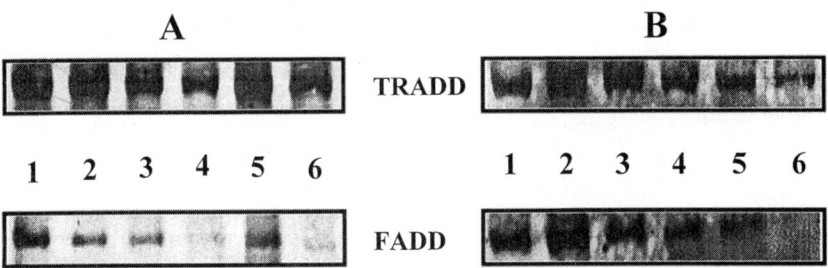

Figure 6 Immunoblotting of transducing proteins TRADD and FADD: (**A**) in HepG2 cells, (**B**) in IHH cells, after 24 h of treatment. Lines 1: control; 2: TNF-α (50 IU/ml); 3: TNF-α (200 IU/ml); 4: actD (0.8 μM); 5: actD (0.8 μM) + TNF-α (50 IU/ml); 6: actD (0.8 μM) + TNF-α (200 IU/ml). The two proteins are present in untreated cell lines; their expression varied according to the treatment (for details see Results)

and FADD were present in HepG2 and IHH, the two cell lines which were resistant to TNF-α and actD-induced apoptosis (Fig. 6). However if, in IHH, TRADD did not decrease after TNF-α alone, whatever the dose, a decrease was observed with actD alone and the decrease was more pronounced when TNF-α was added, especially with a dose of 200 IU/ml. The situation was different for HepG2, where actD alone induced a slight decrease of TRADD, the same decrease being observed when TNF-α was added at 200 IU/ml. Regarding FADD in IHH, no decrease of the protein was observed with TNF-α alone, whatever the dose, while the protein decreased with actD alone and with TNF-α at a dose of 50 IU/ml. For HepG2, TNF-α alone induced a decrease of FADD, particularly at 200 IU/ml. ActD alone strongly decreased FADD expression, but when 50 IU/ml TNF-α was added, the decrease was less pronounced.

Presence of anti-apoptotic proteins Bcl-2 and HSP70

Bcl-2 and HSP70 were studied by immunoblotting in the five cell lines (Fig. 7). While HSP70 was expressed in all five cell lines, Bcl-2 was not present in IHH cells. In addition, we have determined by RPA that HSP70 mRNA levels were

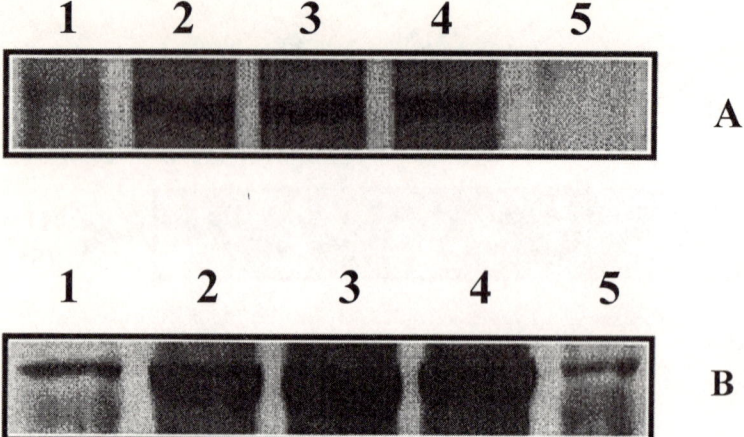

Figure 7 Immunoblotting of anti-apoptotic proteins Bcl-2 (**A**) and HSP70 (**B**) in 1: SKHep1; 2: Chang Liver; 3: Hep3B; 4: HepG2; 5: IHH. HSP70 is present in all five cell lines and Bcl-2 is absent in IHH cells

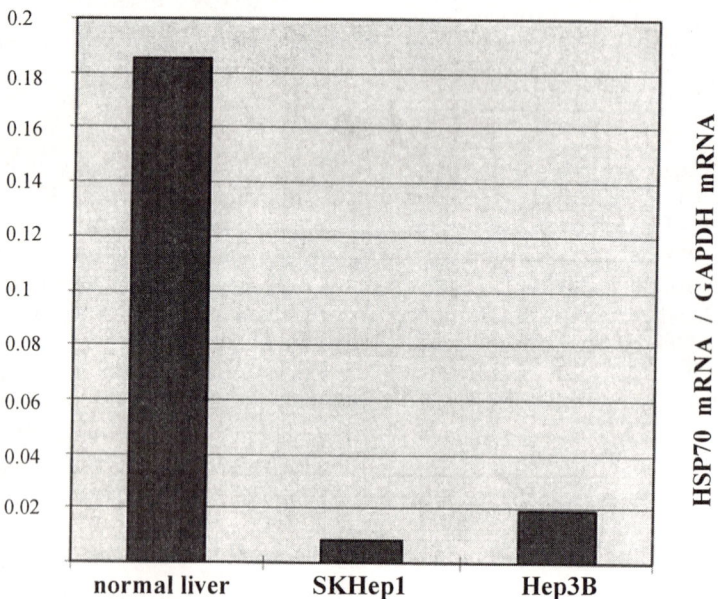

Figure 8 Quantification of HSP70 mRNA in SKHep1, Hep3B and in normal liver. The HSP70 mRNA level is 10 times lower in Hep3B and 20 times lower in SKHep1 cells than in normal liver

10 times lower in Hep3B cells and 20 times lower in SKHep1 cells than in the normal liver (Fig. 8).

DISCUSSION

The aim of this work was to study the effects of TNF-α on five human hepatoma cell lines: Hep3B, HepG2, SKHep1, Chang Liver and IHH. Proliferation was investigated first, and we observed that three cell lines (SKHep1, HepG2 and Chang Liver) were proliferating after TNF-α treatment, a finding which has already been reported in some tumoral cell lines[4] and more recently in hepatocytes[3]. No cytotoxic effect was detected after TNF-α addition in any hepatoma cell line, a finding which has also been described earlier in other tumoral cells[4].

It has been shown that TNF-α was apoptotic in normal hepatocytes only after pretreatment with a transcriptional inhibitor[6]. A similar result was observed with the HepG2 cell line[6]; that is why we decided to sensitize our cell lines to TNF-α by pretreatment with actinomycin D. No cytolysis was observed after 24 or 48 h, even for HepG2 cells. Moreover, no apoptosis was detected for HepG2 cells although the protocol that we used in this work was similar to that used by Leist et al.[6]. However, we did not use the same methods to demonstrate apoptosis: while Leist et al.[6] researched DNA fragmentation, we first investigated apoptosis by a morphological method, DAPI staining, under which regimen apoptotic figures (chromatin condensation and/or nuclear fragmentation) were observed. This method gives satisfactory results, but the typical figures are difficult to analyse when cells are clustered. So apoptosis was also investigated by immunoblotting of PARP, which is a reliable method to detect apoptosis[21], and can be semi-quantified. For the HepG2 cell line these two methods proved negative. While the HepG2 cell line that we used in this work came from ATCC, as did the cell line employed by Leist et al.[6], it is possible that the two cell lines, when cultured, presented some mutations, and so responded differently to TNF-α. In order to explain why HepG2 cells were resistant to TNF-α-induced apoptosis, the presence of transducing proteins TRADD and FADD was demonstrated by immunoblotting. While TRADD was changed slightly after actD pretreatment, a large decrease of FADD was observed after 24 h with TNF-α alone, and was more pronounced when actD was added. This result could explain the resistance of HepG2 cells to TNF-α-induced apoptosis, and it also indicates that FADD has a rapid turnover in HepG2 cells because 24 h of transcriptional inhibition was sufficient to cause a large decrease in its expression. The IHH cell line was also resistant to TNF-α-induced apoptosis and, similarly to HepG2, TRADD and FADD were present when immunoblotting was used. TRADD expression decreased markedly with actD, and when TNF-α was added. A moderate decrease was also observed for FADD with actD and TNF-α. The resistance of HepG2 to TNF-α-induced apoptosis could be explained by the FADD decrease, because of the subsequent inhibition of the caspase cascade. The slight decrease of TRADD and FADD in IHH did not explain the resistance of this cell to apoptosis. Other hypotheses can be suggested to explain IHH resistance: either other proteins of the TNF-α-signalling pathway could be absent or inactive, or actD could stop the synthesis and renewal of other TNF-α-signalling pathway proteins such as caspases. Finally, it is also possible that IHH expresses a high level of anti-apoptotic proteins other than Bcl-2 (see below). In another respect, Hep3B, Chang Liver and SKHep1 were sensitive to TNF-α-induced apoptosis, as shown by DAPI, PARP cleavage and DNA fragmentation.

The presence of two anti-apoptotic proteins Bcl-2 and HSP70 was also investigated by immunoblotting in the five cell lines. While HSP70 was expressed in all five cell lines, Bcl-2 was not expressed in IHH cells. This result is not very surprising because the IHH cell line is very close to the hepatocyte phenotype[20] and it is known that hepatocytes do not express the Bcl-2 protein[23]. A quantification of HSP70 mRNA was realized by RPA in SKHep1 and Hep3B cells in comparison to normal liver. The HSP70 mRNA level was 10 times lower in Hep3B cells, and 20 times lower in SKHep1 cells, than in normal liver. Quantification of Bcl-2 mRNA by RPA in SKHep1 and Hep3B will be possible when some technical problems are overcome. As mentioned in the introduction, it has been shown that inhibition of NF-κB sensitized the cells to TNF-α-induced apoptosis[17,18]. So, after HSP70 and Bcl-2 mRNA quantification, we plan, using an antisense strategy, to inhibit Bcl-2 and HSP70 mRNA in order to sensitize SKHep1 and Hep3B to TNF-α-induced apoptosis. Recent published results suggest that this type of technique could be interesting in the induction of apoptosis in some hepatoma cell lines[24].

References

1. Carswell EA, Old LJ, Kassel RL, Green S, Fiore N, Williamson B. An endotoxin-induced serum factor that causes necrosis of tumors. Proc Natl Acad Sci USA. 1975;72:3666–70.
2. Beutler B, Cerami A. Tumor necrosis, cachexia, shock and inflammation: a common mediator. Annu Rev Biochem. 1988;57:505–18.
3. Yamada Y, Webber EM, Kirillova I, Peschon JJ, Faust N. Analysis of liver regeneration in mice lacking type 1 or type 2 Tumor Necrosis Factor Receptor: requirement for type 1 but not type 2 receptor. Hepatology. 1998;28:959–70.
4. Sugarman BJ, Aggarwal BB, Hass PE, Figari IS, Palladino MA, Shepard HM. Recombinant human tumor necrosis factor-α: effects on proliferation of normal and transformed cells *in vitro*. Science. 1985;230:943–5.
5. Leist M, Gantner F, Naumann H *et al.* Tumor necrosis factor-induced apoptosis during the poisoning of mice with hepatotoxins. Gastroenterology. 1997;112:923–34.
6. Leist M, Gantner F, Bohlinger I, Germann PG, Tiegs G, Wendel A. Murine hepatocyte apoptosis induced *in vitro* and *in vivo* by TNFa requires transcriptional arrest. J Immunol. 1994;153:1778–88.
7. Nagata S, Goldstein P. The Fas death factor. Science. 1995;267:1449–55.
8. Hsu H, Shu H, Pan M, Goeddel DV. TRADD–TRAF2 and TRADD–FADD interactions define two distinct TNF receptor 1 signal transduction pathways. Cell. 1995;81:299–308.
9. Nagata S. Apoptosis by death factor. Cell. 1997;88:355–65.
10. Luo X, Budihardjo I, Zou H, Slaughter C, Wang X. Bid, a Bcl-2 interacting protein, mediates cytochrome c release from mitochondria in response to activation of cell surface death receptors. Cell. 1998;94:481–90.
11. Adams JM, Cory S. The Bcl-2 protein family: arbiters of cell survival. Science. 1998;281:1322–6.
12. Susin SA, Lorenzo HK, Zamzami N *et al.* Molecular characterization of mitochondrial apoptosis-inducing factor. Nature. 1999;397:441–6.
13. Li P, Nijhawan D, Budihardjo I *et al.* Cytochrome c and dATP-dependent formation of Apaf-1/caspase 9 complex initiates an apoptotic cascade. Cell. 1997;91:479–89.
14. Angel P, Karin M. The role of Jun, Fos and AP-1 complex in cell-proliferation and transformation. Biochem Biophys Acta. 1991;1072:129–57.

15. Natoli G, Costanzo A, Guido F, Moretti F, Levrero M. Apoptotic, non-apoptotic and anti-apoptotic pathways of tumor necrosis factor signalling. Biochem Pharmacol. 1998;56:915–20.
16. Van Antwerp DJ, Martin SJ, Tal Kafri, Green DR, Verma IM. Suppression of TNF-α induced apoptosis by NF-κB. Science. 1996;274:787–9.
17. Beg AA, Baltimore D. An essential role for NF-κB in preventing TNF-α-induced cell death. Science. 1996;274:782–4.
18. Bellas RE, Fitzgerald MJ, Fausto N, Sonenshein GE. Inhibition of NF-κB activity induces apoptosis in murine hepatocytes. Am J Pathol. 1997;112:923–34.
19. Mosser DD, Caron AW, Bourget L, Denis-Larose C, Massie B. Role of the human heat shock protein HSP70 against stress induced apoptosis. Mol Cell Biol. 1997;17:5317–27.
20. Schippers IJ, Moshage H, Roelofsen H et al. Immortalized human hepatocytes as a tool for the study of hepatocytic (de-)differentiation. Cell Biol Toxicol. 1997;13:375–86.
21. Cohen GM. Caspases: the executioners of apoptosis. Biochem J. 1997;326:1–16.
22. Kaabache T, Barraud B, Feldmann G, Bernuau D, Lardeux B. Direct solution hybridization of guanidine thiocyanate-solubilized cells for quantitation of mRNAs in hepatocytes. Anal Biochem. 1995;232:225–30.
23. Charlotte F, L'Hermine A, Martin N et al. Immunohistochemical detection of Bcl-2 protein in normal and pathological human liver. Am J Pathol. 1994;144:460–5.
24. Takahashi M, Saito H, Okuyama T et al. Overexpression of Bcl-2 protects human hepatoma cells from Fas-antibody-mediated apoptosis. J Hepatol. 1999;31:315–22.

29
Molecular regulation of liver regeneration

J. H. TREMBLEY, B. T. KREN and C. J. STEER

INTRODUCTION

The liver is unique in its ability to regenerate after injury from chemicals, viruses, other infections, physical trauma or surgical ablation. The restoration of mass, cell population and function constitutes what is commonly referred to as 'regeneration'. The most dramatic form of liver regeneration, and the model that has been most extensively studied, involves organ regrowth after partial hepatectomy. In this model, cell replication occurs in the absence of cell death, fibrosis or inflammatory events. The process is actually a compensatory growth of the remnant liver rather than true 'regeneration' of the resected lobes. A complicated cascade of molecular events occurs in the regenerating liver after partial hepatectomy involving induction of numerous immediate-early, delayed-early and liver-specific genes. A temporal boundary exists between the major growth period of the liver and the time during which elevated levels of liver-specific genes are expressed. In addition, only after significant cell replication does the liver begin an active remodelling phase. Numerous factors have been proposed as potential hepatic growth regulators, including hormones and nutrients, neural stimulation, polypeptide growth factors derived from both serum and liver, and inhibitory factors. No single 'master switch' has been identified which turns regeneration on and off. Instead, the process is controlled by an orchestrated balance of growth controls which maintains liver function during the period of regrowth. The information generated by morphological, physiological and molecular biological approaches has provided enormous insight into the complexities of the process. Ultimately, our knowledge base of this remarkable phenomenon of liver regeneration will help bridge the gap from bench to bedside.

WHAT IS LIVER REGENERATION?

The liver and compensatory hyperplasia

Organ regeneration is a topic which has fascinated scientists for centuries. In the 18th century, scientists observed the ability of lower animals to regrow entire body segments following bisection[1]. The replacement of a limb, complete with the various cell types such as muscle and bone, is an example of classic regeneration. The liver has the remarkable ability to fully replace lost tissue mass and cells after acute injury. The regrowth of the liver following tissue removal or other injury is commonly referred to as regeneration, but is actually compensatory hyperplasia. One key difference lies in the fact that while cell number, cell type and organ mass are faithfully replaced, the original gross morphology is not. This is particularly true of the two-thirds partial hepatectomy model in rodents, where there is regrowth of the remnant liver after removal of the left lateral and median lobes.

The liver is an epithelial organ composed of parenchymal cells, or hepatocytes, and non-parenchymal cell types including Kupffer, Ito, bile duct epithelial (cholangiocytes), and fenestrated endothelial cells. The optimal mass of the liver which is required to perform its many functions is primarily determined by body size, and the liver is remarkably adaptable to changes in demand. Once liver mass falls below the optimal threshold level due to physical, chemical or biological injury, the liver responds by initiating growth until the threshold level is again achieved. Cell replication which is initiated by a mitogenic stimulus without coincident liver cell loss or injury is not a regenerative or compensatory growth response, but rather is termed direct hyperplasia[2].

The regenerative process

Adult hepatocytes are normally quiescent, highly differentiated cells in which mitosis can be detected in only 1 in 10 000 to 20 000 cells in the liver. A variety of injuries can result in liver cell loss, including chemical injuries such as carbon tetrachloride, viral infection and surgical loss. The most studied and well-characterized model for liver regeneration is a 70% partial hepatectomy (PH). After resection of the left lateral and median liver lobes, an ordered sequence of events occurs which is characterized by three major phases. The first phase involves priming the remnant liver cells for growth in which the remaining hepatocytes and non-parenchymal cells synchronously exit their resting G_0 state and enter the G_1 phase of the cell cycle. The second phase includes progression through one or more cell division cycles, and the final phase involves organization of the newly replicated cells and extracellular matrix for normal liver function (Fig. 1). The regenerating liver demands an increased amount of oxygen for mitochondrial oxidative phosphorylation to restore hepatic energy charge. The hepatic venous haemoglobin oxygen saturation index reflects oxygen metabolic status in the remnant liver and could be useful for estimating liver regeneration[3].

The priming events of the first phase include immediate changes in membrane potential, rapid influx of sodium, increased intracellular pH, calcium release from intracellular stores, and an increase in urokinase receptor and urokinase activity within several minutes. Furthermore, signalling through cytokine and/or growth factor pathways occurs within 30 min post-PH and are the catalyst for subsequent events. Almost immediately after PH, latent transcription factors are activated and induce immediate-early gene expression. In phase two there is activation of delayed-early genes followed by DNA synthesis and progression through the cell cycle. Two waves of cell division typically occur after PH. The first major wave is primarily hepatocyte replication while the second wave

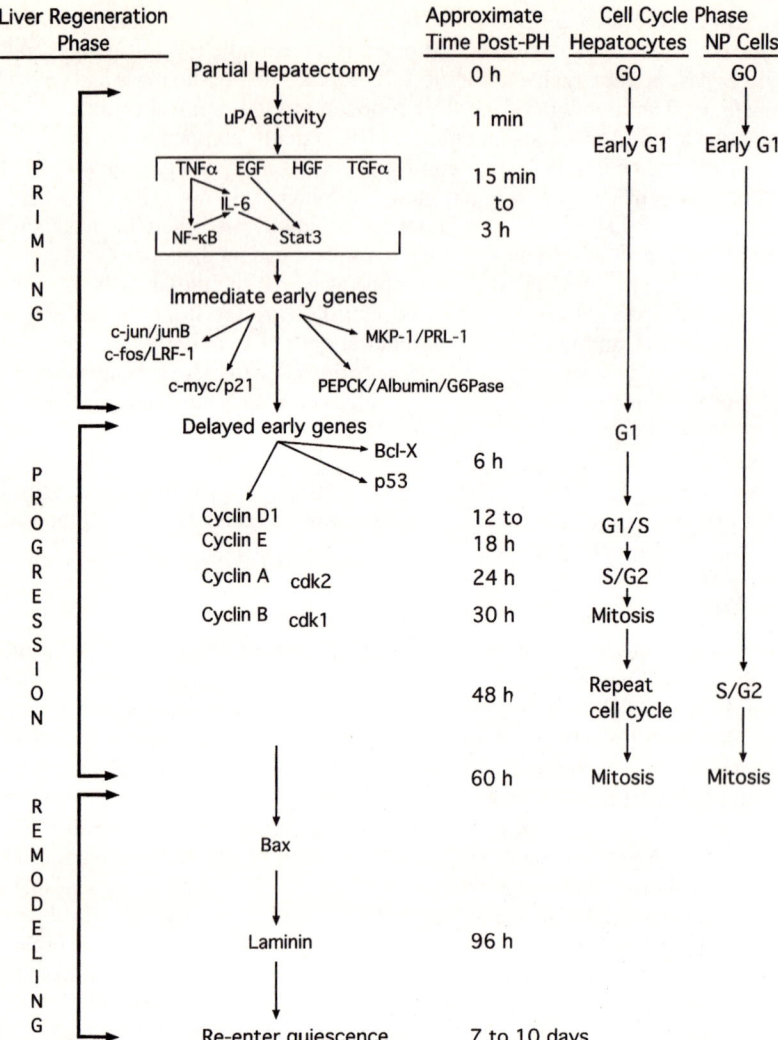

Figure 1 Sequential events after partial hepatectomy in the rat can be characterized into three major phases. The diagram illustrates the types of regulatory events involved, including increased expression of immediate and delayed-early genes, active participation of members of the cyclin family and modulation of certain apoptosis-associated gene products. Cell cycle progression for non-parenchymal (NP) cells is typically delayed approximately 24 h compared to hepatocytes. The complexity of the entire process is as profound as the simplicity of this diagram. Details of the mechanisms are described in the text. PH, partial hepatectomy; uPA, urokinase plasminogen activator; EGF, epidermal growth factor; TGF-α, transforming growth factor alpha; TNF-α, tumour necrosis factor alpha; HGF, hepatocyte growth factor; cdk, cyclin-dependent kinase; IL-6, interleukin-6; LRF, liver regeneration factor; Stat3, signal transducer and activator of transcription-3; NF-κB, nuclear factor-κB; PEPCK, phosphoenolpyruvate carboxykinase; PRL, phosphatase of regenerating liver; G6Pase, glucose-6-phosphatase; MKP, map kinase phosphatase

includes both parenchymal and non-parenchymal cells. DNA syntheses for the rat peak at 18–24 h and 42–48 h post-PH, with the first peak representing a more dramatic and synchronous wave of DNA replication. The time-course of liver regeneration in the mouse is typically delayed by about 12 h compared to the rat. Mitosis typically occurs 6–8 h after DNA synthesis. In young adult rats as many as 95% of the hepatocytes undergo at least a single cycle of replication, and within 4 days the majority of liver cells has been replaced. Finally, in phase three, there is extensive remodelling of the liver microstructure. Within 7–10 days the extracellular matrix microarchitecture and liver mass are restored, and the normal complement of liver-specific gene expression is present. Regulation of gene expression occurs very early, as well as late in the regenerative period, suggesting that certain factors are modulated to function mainly in highly differentiated hepatic cells such as class II phosphoinositide 3-kinase[4].

The hepatocyte as a unipotential stem cell

It is well established that remnant hepatocytes are the source of new hepatocytes in both adult liver regeneration and in postnatal liver development, where the liver mass of rodents increases approximately 10-fold between 1 and 4 weeks of age. Cell replication was monitored in mice transgenic for the human α_1-antitrypsin/β-galactosidase expression construct[5]. Blue transgenic cells which began as singlets or doublets randomly scattered in neonatal livers were later present in large clusters in young adult rats, indicating that the blue-marked cells arise from pre-existing hepatocytes.

Hepatocytes have a remarkable capacity for replication, and are exceedingly long-lived cells. The use of transgenic mice has provided useful information on the clonogenic potential of hepatocytes. Transgenic mice expressing the urokinase plasminogen activator (uPA) gene resulted in elevated plasma uPA and fatal hemorrhaging in newborns[6]. Interestingly, some of the mice survived because of a spontaneous genetic rearrangement which shut down uPA gene expression. Those hepatocytes displayed a marked proliferative advantage and repopulated the livers[7]. The uPA transgenic mice were studied to determine whether adult liver cells rather than neonatal cells could repopulate an impaired liver. Genetically tagged donor hepatocytes were transferred into transgenic uPA mice by splenic injection, and were able to proliferate and replace up to 80% of the recipient parenchyma[8]; furthermore, these livers retained the ability to regenerate following PH. Finally, rat hepatocytes were transplanted into immunosuppressed uPA transgenic mice, which replicated and essentially replaced the recipient mouse liver[9]. It has been reported that rat liver can regenerate at least 12 times, and a single hepatocyte has the clonogenic capacity to undergo at least 34 cell divisions and generate an amazing 50 rat livers[10]. At least a fraction of adult mouse hepatocytes have growth potential similar to that of haematopoietic stem cells exhibiting a minimal number of 69 cell doublings[11]. Interestingly, a zonal regulation of gene expression during liver regeneration was observed in the urokinase transgenic mouse[12]. The diseased microenvironment appears to play an important role in the growth advantage of normal hepatocytes in neighbouring regenerative nodules. These results have exciting potential for gene therapy applications, as discussed in a later section.

One of the striking features of liver regeneration is that these highly differentiated cells simultaneously proliferate and continue to perform most of their normal functions. For example, decreased levels of bile salt uptake systems were associated with a 10-fold increase in plasma bile salt concentration, yet bile flow and bile salt secretion were increased when expressed per gram of liver and unaffected when expressed on the basis of body weight[13]. Remarkably, despite the increased serum bile salt levels, the remnant liver is not cholestatic. Moreover, liver regeneration after 70% PH does not appear to involve stem cell replication. In fact, the oval cell is considered a bipotent stem cell and can differentiate in culture into either hepatocytes or bile ductule cells, and possibly other cell types as well[14]. In contrast, the fully, but not terminally, differentiated adult hepatocyte can replicate only itself in response to regenerative stimuli. Following 60–70% cell loss due to PH, the liver is still able to carry out the necessary functions for organ viability without activation of its stem cells. However, if damage to the liver is so severe that liver function is compromised, and the hepatocytes cannot proliferate, oval cells are required to replicate. For example, exposure of the liver to 2-acetylaminofluorene (AAF) inhibits hepatocyte mitosis after PH, thus provoking replication of oval cells[14]. Interestingly, the c-*kit* receptor tyrosine kinase and its ligand, stem cell factor, both play crucial roles in the development of oval cells[15].

GROWTH FACTORS AND CYTOKINES

The precise role of growth stimulatory and inhibitory factors still remains unclear. A complete mitogen is capable of stimulating DNA synthesis and mitosis of cultured cells in serum-free media, and include transforming growth factor alpha (TGF-α), epidermal growth factor (EGF), and hepatocyte growth factor (HGF), or scatter factor. Hepatic comitogens alone do not induce proliferation, but act to enhance the stimulatory effects of complete mitogens, and include insulin, glucagon, insulin-like growth factors, norepinephrine, various hormones, calcium, vitamin D and certain nutrients. Augmenter of liver regeneration (ALR) is a hepatotrophic protein which appears to be constitutively expressed in hepatocytes in an inactive form, and released from cells in an active form in response to PH[16]. The hepatic ALR levels were independent of mRNA which showed no change. Finally, several hepatic growth inhibitors have been identified such as transforming growth factor beta (TGF-β), inhibin, and interleukin 10 (IL-10).

The role of growth factors in liver cell proliferation has been studied in primary hepatocytes because of the ability to manipulate the cellular environment. However, hepatocytes which are isolated by collagenase perfusion exit G_0 phase and express genes associated with early to mid G_1 including c-*fos*, c-*jun*, c-*myc*, and p53. However, when grown in serum-free media these primary hepatocytes cannot progress through G_1 into DNA synthesis (S phase) without the addition of growth factors. Thus, primary hepatocytes are primed for proliferation and are responsive to growth factors, in contrast to resting or quiescent hepatocytes *in vivo* which are not responsive to growth factors. The mitogen-dependent restriction point in adult rat hepatocytes has been identified in mid to late G_1, or 42–48 h after seeding[17].

Removal of 30% of the liver results in a situation similar to collagenase isolation of primary hepatocytes. The cells in the remnant liver exit G_0 and are primed for DNA synthesis, but require the addition of growth factor(s) to enter S phase. Although quiescent hepatocytes *in vivo* exhibit little response to HGF, EGF, and TGF-α, if the cells are first primed by 30% PH they undergo cell cycle progression[18]. Finally, it has recently been reported that liver regeneration is impaired in inducible nitric oxide synthase (iNOS)-deficient mice[19]. It is proposed that injury-related cytokines induce iNOS and its product NO to protect surviving cells from cytokine-mediated death. NO can prevent TNF-mediated activation of pro-apoptotic protease caspase 3 and protect hepatocytes from cytokine-induced apoptosis.

EGF and TGF-α

Basal levels of EGF RNA are detectable in rat liver using the reverse transcription polymerase chain reaction (RT-PCR)[20]. EGF RNA abundance increases by 10-fold within 15 min post-PH, then diminishes below basal levels around 4 h post-PH. While the EGF transcript is expressed by hepatocytes and Ito cells, the EGF receptor RNA has been detected in hepatocytes, endothelial, Kupffer and Ito cells. Typically, EGF is synthesized as a 140 kDa transmembrane precursor protein that is processed and released from the cell surface as a 6 kDa signalling peptide. However, in regenerating liver, EGF protein accumulates in rat and mouse hepatocytes as a 60 kDa polypeptide[20]. This work established that an autocrine mechanism exists for EGF signalling during liver regeneration.

Both EGF and TGF-α bind to the EGF receptor, resulting in autophosphorylation and exposure of a recognition site for SH2 domain-containing proteins. The phosphorylation of cellular substrates, in turn, modulates transcription. In the rat the number of EGF receptors increases by approximately 2-fold in the first 3 h post-PH, then decreases again until day 4[21]. The majority of EGF in mouse and rat is produced in the salivary glands. Removal of the salivary glands in the mouse 2 weeks prior to PH resulted in a 50% decrease in plasma EGF concentration, abolished the increase in EGF levels post-PH, and greatly delayed peak DNA synthesis[22]. Injection of EGF restored the time-course of the regenerative response. In the rat, sialoadenectomy at the time of PH or 3 h post-PH decreased DNA synthesis and mitosis by 50%, but did not affect the expression of the early response genes c-*jun*, c-*fos* and c-*myc*[23]. If the salivary gland removal was performed 6 h or later post-PH, no reduction in DNA synthesis was observed. Furthermore, administration of EGF from 3 to 9 h post-PH in sialoadenectomized rats was sufficient to restore normal regenerative activity. Diminished EGF levels delayed the regeneration response to PH in the first 24 h, but liver mass in sialoadenectomized rats was similar 7 days post-PH to controls. Thus, the role of EGF in liver regeneration appears to affect early G_1 events which occur after the priming phase from 0 to 3 h post-PH. Jones and colleagues reported a more severe effect of salivary gland removal 24 h pre-PH in rats[24]. They reported that DNA synthesis was inhibited by 90% at 24 h after 33% PH. Thus, it is apparent that EGF signalling during liver regeneration occurs through both autocrine and endocrine mechanisms.

TGF-α mRNA levels increase 4 h following PH and remain elevated for at least 48 h. TGF-α peptide levels increased 2-fold between 24 and 48 h via an autocrine loop mechanism[18]. Hepatocytes produce TGF-α and bind the growth factor through the EGF receptor which is expressed at the plasma membrane. Transgenic mice overexpressing TGF-α demonstrate an increased rate of hepatocyte replication leading to increased liver size. This is compensated for after 3–5 months of life by increased cellular turnover[18]. Furthermore, by 15 months of TGF-α overexpression, 85% of the mice exhibit hepatic tumours. In contrast, TGF-α knockout mice develop normally, except for abnormal hair growth[25].

HGF

HGF is produced by mesenchymal cells in the body, which in the liver is represented by Ito, Kupffer and endothelial cells. Blood levels of HGF increase 20-fold by 1 h post-PH[10]. However, proteolytic processing of the inactive single-chain form of HGF to the active form may occur as early as 1 min post-PH. Active urokinase-type plasminogen activator is responsible for the cleavage and this protein is detected 1 min post-PH[26]. The importance of this growth factor is highlighted from HGF knockout mice which die during embryonic development between days 13 and 16. In these embryos the liver is reduced in size, there is extensive loss of hepatocytes, and placental development is impaired[27,28]. Homozygous deletion of the HGF receptor, c-Met, also results in embryonic lethality[29]. Overexpression of HGF in transgenic mice produced a phenotype in which liver regrowth following PH occurred 2–3 times faster than wild-type. The livers were larger than normal and contained smaller hepatocytes with diploid DNA content[30,31]. Moreover, the proliferative stimulus of prolonged HGF expression resulted in the formation of hepatocellular adenomas and carcinomas in most transgenic mice beyond 1.5 years of age[31]. Finally, overexpression of a truncated c-Met receptor containing the regulatory and catalytic cytoplasmic domains causes a block to apoptosis and permits immortalization of these transgenic hepatocytes[32]. These results indicate that HGF may play an essential role in liver morphogenesis and that deregulated HGF signalling is oncogenic for hepatocytes.

TNF-α and IL-6

The cytokines tumour necrosis factor (TNF)-α, IL-6, and IL-10 are also expressed by non-parenchymal cells of the liver and expression of these factors increases within 3 h post-PH[33]. Signalling through TNF receptor type 1 using a pathway that involves nuclear factor-κB (NF-κB), IL-6 and STAT3 is required for the initiation of liver regeneration[34]. TNF acts as a primer to sensitize hepatocytes to the proliferative effects of growth factors and offers a mechanism to explain the initiation and progression phases of liver regeneration after PH. In addition, TNF may increase mitochondrial oxidant production after PH, which promotes the induction of antioxidant factors such as uncoupling protein-2 in regenerating hepatocytes[35]. IL-6 affects the process of regeneration by recruiting, and possibly synchronizing the entry of hepatocytes into cell cycling, which quickly restores liver mass. However, this robust response generates superfluous hepatocytes, which are eliminated by apoptosis, similar to many other processes involving organ growth[36]. Recent data strongly support a signal pathway(s) in which TNF-α, IL-6 and IL-10 interact in regulating each other. EGF and IL-6 activate the transcription factor signal transducer and activator of transcription-3 (Stat3), and TNF-α induces NF-κB transcription factor activation[37–39]. Mice homozygous for an IL-6 gene deletion are developmentally normal, but exhibit a dramatic decrease in the number of S phase hepatocytes during liver regeneration[40]. In conjunction with a decreased response in DNA synthesis, these mice demonstrate no Stat3 activation and decreased c-*fos*, *jun*B, c-*myc* and cyclin D1 expression. In contrast to the effect of IL-6 depletion on hepatocyte proliferation during liver regeneration, non-parenchymal cells exhibited DNA synthesis and gene expression patterns similar to wild-type mice. One further effect of IL-6 deficiency was the development of necrotic areas in the liver. Liver regeneration does eventually occur in these IL-6-negative mice, and injection of IL-6 prior to PH restores Stat3 activation and nearly normal hepatocyte pro-liferation. The IL-6 knockout mice exhibit increased death rates following PH. Specifically, 40% died post-PH versus 10% mortality in wild-type and 8% death in knockout mice which received an IL-6 injection pre-PH.

Treatment of rats with antibodies to TNF-α prior to surgery inhibited liver regen-eration after PH. The effects of antibody injection included decreased DNA synthe-sis at 24 h post-PH, significantly decreased IL-6 serum concentrations, and diminished induction of activator protein-1 (AP-1) transcription factor activity[41]. Mice deficient in type 1 TNF-α receptor (TNF-R1) also exihibit severely impaired DNA synthesis as well as no detectable activation of Stat3 or NF-κB and decreased AP-1 activity and IL-6 levels[42]. Furthermore, 50% of these animals died between 3 and 5 days post-PH, and the surviving mice demonstrated slower than normal liver regeneration. The loss of TNF-α receptors can be compensated for by injection of IL-6 at 30 min before PH, which restores DNA synthesis and the Stat3 pathway, but not NF-κB DNA binding. Normally, TNF-α levels are down-regulated post-transcriptionally by IL-10 and TGF-β_1. Treatment of rats with gadolineum chloride (GdCl) depletes the liver of active Kupffer cells and results in increased levels of TNF-α and TNF-α-inducible cytokines such as IL-6. After PH in GdCl-treated rats, induction of IL-10 is greatly decreased, TNF-α is transiently overexpressed, and the regenerative response is greater than normal[33]. Since TGF-β_1 expression is not significantly affected by the GdCl treatment prior to PH, TGF-β_1 is thought to affect TNF-α down-regulation in these animals.

The results of TNF-α and IL-6 on liver regeneration suggest a signalling pathway in which PH induces expression of TNF-α, followed by activation of NF-κB which induces IL-6. IL-6 causes activation of Stat3, and the activation of Stat3 and NF-κB together initiates immediate-early gene expression. The expres-sion of both IL-10 and TGF-β_1 acts to prevent TNF-α overexpression. Furthermore, increased stress-activated protein kinase activity following PH might play a positive role in proliferative signalling during regeneration, pos-sibly by stimulating IL-6 production[43]. Ischaemia dramatically impairs the regen-erative capacity of the liver in both mice and rats. IL-6 administration completely restored the normal parameters of regeneration. This cytokine appears to be a key protective molecule in reducing injury and promoting regeneration following combined tissue loss and ischaemia[44].

Growth inhibitors

There is increased expression of the growth-inhibiting cytokines TGF-β_1, TGF-β_2 and TGF-β_3 following PH[45]. TGF-β_2 and TGF-β_3 peak early post-PH, whereas TGF-β_1 expression peaks around 48 h. TGF-β mRNA isoforms are transcribed by both non-parenchymal and parenchymal cells following PH; however, TGF-β polypeptide released by hepatocytes is in the latent form, whereas non-parenchymal cells release active TGF-β. TGF-β_1 is the best characterized of the three TGF-β isoforms, and receptors for this molecule are present on virtually all cells. Transgenic mice in which a mature form of porcine TFG-β_1 under control of the mouse albumin promoter was expressed exhibited increased hepatocyte mitotic and apoptotic activity and hepatic fibrosis[46]. Furthermore, high plasma expression levels of the transgene negatively affected other organs, most notably the kidneys. Finally, inhibin-βC is a recently identified TGF-β family member whose gene expression is down-regulated following PH by at least 8-fold in the mouse[47].

IMMEDIATE-EARLY GENE EXPRESSION

The regenerating liver uses multiple signal transduction pathways and many of those signalling pathways begin with ligand binding to specific receptors. The event transduces signals by a variety of mechanisms including receptor auto-phosphorylation and subsequent binding of protein complexes, kinase activity of the receptor, or coupling of the receptor to other signalling systems such as G proteins. For example, binding of receptor tyrosine kinases by the growth factors EGF, TFG-α and HGF following PH are most probably key events initiating early growth response pathways. The early growth response is dependent upon immediate-early gene expression, and has been extensively investigated in regenerating liver. However, a number of other early events occur during liver regeneration after PH. For example, system A, the sodium-dependent neutral amino acid transport activity, has a 3-fold increase in its initial uptake velocity into hepatocytes following PH[48]. The results suggest that system A transport activity functions primarily to provide amino acids to fuel liver-specific biochemical pathways and to increase cell volume.

The primary growth response by remnant liver after PH consists of the transcriptional activation of immediate-early genes, which is initially accomplished through activation of latent transcription factors. By definition, immediate-early genes do not require protein synthesis for their activation. Pre-existing factors within liver cells function to activate genes normally quiescent in these mature, differentiated cells. It is generally accepted that increased circulation of growth factors like those described above triggers this response. Two key transcriptional activators are Stat3 and partial hepatectomy factor (PHF)/NF-κB, a liver-specific form of NF-κB[49]. Both of these DNA-binding factors are activated by phosphorylation events. Stat3 activation and nuclear translocation occur by phosphorylation of a tyrosine residue, and phosphorylation of the inhibitor protein IκB-α or RL/IF-1 results in release of PHF/NF-κB. PHF/NF-κB DNA-binding activity peaks at 30–60 min post-PH, whereas Stat3 activity is induced by 30 min but peaks 2–3 h post-PH.

Many transcription factors are induced as immediate-early genes, resulting in a transcriptional cascade during the G_1 phase of the initial liver regeneration cell cycle. For example, the expressions and activities of several CCAAT/

enhancer-binding proteins (C/EBP) fluctuate in the regenerating liver[50]. They appear to be actively involved in the regulation of many hepatocyte mitogens and co-mitogens, which in turn regulate C/EBP activity. They also appear to modulate gene expression in both hepatocyte and non-parenchymal cells of the liver. C/EBPβ –/– livers showed reduced expression of immediate-early growth-control genes including *Egr-1* transcription factor, *MKP-1* and *HRS*, the delayed-early gene that encodes an mRNA splicing protein[51]. CREM (cAMP-responsive promoter element modulator) is activated by phosphorylation at a serine residue by certain kinases. CREM expression is powerfully induced during liver regeneration, and its absence results in delayed S-phase entry, thereby impairing the synchronization of proliferation[52]. It is associated with dysregulation of a number of cell cycle-dependent factors including many of the cyclins. Leucine zipper transcription factors which dimerize to form AP-1 type transcriptional complexes are important participants in this induction. High levels of AP-1 DNA-binding complexes containing the proteins c-Jun, JunB, Fos, and the liver-specific partner protein liver regeneration factor-1 (LRF-1) are detected for several hours after the G_0/G_1 transition[49]. Recently, it has been reported that certain splicing factor proteins are also modulated during liver regeneration[53]. HRS/SRp40, an SR protein and delayed early gene in liver regeneration, mediates alternative splicing of fibronectin mRNA. Transcription of the gene is induced about 5-fold during liver regeneration after PH, similar to the observed levels of steady-state mRNA. Heavy metal-responsive transcriptional activator MTF-1 regulates the basal and heavy metal-induced expression of met-allothioneins[54]. Embryos lacking MTF-1 die *in utero* and show impaired development of hepatocytes and liver degeneration.

Two other immediate-early genes involved in proliferative signalling include EGF and c-*myc*. The functions of EGF in liver regeneration are discussed in the previous section. The transcriptional activator protein c-Myc is a proto-oncogene which plays a role in both cell proliferation and cell death. The role of two immediate-early genes, map kinase phosphatase (MKP)-1 and phosphatase of regenerating liver (PRL)-1, which encode protein tyrosine phosphatases, has yet to be delineated[49]. However, it has been shown that Egr-1 (early growth response factor) expression increased in concert with PRL-1 gene transcription and trans-activates the *PRL-1* promoter[55]. The discovery of novel phosphatase gene activation during liver regeneration is intriguing because of the role played by the cdc25 phosphatase family in activating cyclin/cyclin-dependent kinase (cdk) complexes during cell proliferation. The parallel induction of most immediate-early genes in hepatocytes as well as non-parenchymal cells provides evidence that the exit from G_0 is simultaneous for all cells in the remnant liver[56]. Moreover, because DNA synthesis in non-parenchymal cells occurs in the second wave of cell proliferation, these data suggest a prolonged G_1 phase in non-parenchymal cells. Interestingly, activation of NF-κB and AP-1 and expression of TNF-α are specific to the compensatory hyperplastic response since these effects are not observed in direct hyperplasia induced by nafenopin or cyproterone acetate[57].

The orchestrated modulation of gene expression post-PH is involved in maintaining normal liver function. For example, several immediate-early genes encode proteins important for glucose regulation and metabolism, thus compensating for the loss in liver mass. These genes include glucose-6-phosphatase, insulin-like growth factor binding protein-1, and phosphoenolpyruvate carboxykinase[49]. Albumin is also expressed as an immediate-early gene. Thus, the combined up-regulation of immediate-early transcription factor and liver function genes allows for the remnant liver to both proliferate and perform its myriad differentiated functions.

POST-TRANSCRIPTIONAL GENE REGULATION

Following the transcriptionally regulated immediate-early gene response occurring from 0 to 3 post-PH, gene expression patterns and regulation become more complex. Seminal studies demonstrated that genes are induced in three expression patterns following PH[56]. The patterns include growth-regulated expression beginning at surgery through 60–72 h post-PH, cell cycle-related expression, and liver-specific gene expression after the growth phase from 60 h post-PH and beyond. Interestingly, genes induced beyond the immediate-early phase of liver regeneration are predominantly regulated at the post-transcriptional level by several different and potentially additive mechanisms. In addition, a number of studies have reported an uncoupling between protein and transcript expression.

The alteration of steady-state transcript levels in the regenerating liver following PH for a number of genes involves modulation of the rate of decay of their transcript[58]. Even transcript levels of the immediate-early gene c-*myc* are controlled both transcriptionally and post-transcriptionally following PH. The rate of decay of a transcript can be affected by many factors[59]. The association of a mRNA with ribosomes appears to be an integral step in modulating the rate of decay of a transcript. Polysome distribution appears to significantly affect post-transcriptional control of gene expression in the quiescent and regenerating liver.

Polysomes exist in hepatocytes as either free, cytoskeletal- or membrane-bound. The abundance of p53 and c-*myc* mRNA in the three discrete polysome populations has been shown to be quite dynamic in the regenerating liver after PH (unpublished observations). For example, in quiescent liver most of the p53 transcript was associated with free polysomes and not with the cytoskeletal- or membrane-bound populations. Following 70% PH, the distribution among the three polysome populations changed significantly. The free fraction increased by 3 h, fluctuated and returned to baseline by 24 h. The membrane-bound polysome abundance of p53 increased 12-fold by 3 h, showed a moderate return by 6 h and then remained unchanged through 24 h. The loss of the p53 transcript from the free polysomes 6 h post-PH was associated with an 8-fold increase in cytoskeletal-bound p53 mRNA. In contrast to the differential polysome distribution of the p53 transcripts, c-*myc* mRNA was evenly distributed at 0 time. In the regenerating liver, c-*myc* transcript increased 7-fold in the free, 30% in the cytoskeletal- and 4-fold in the membrane-bound polysomes at 3 h. By 24 h the transcript abundance and distribution returned to baseline.

The decay of both the p53 and c-*myc* transcripts in the three polysome fractions *in vitro* at 0 time exhibited a similar pattern to that determined *in vivo* using α-amanitin and Northern blot analysis[58]. In short, the decay rate of c-*myc* was rapid while the loss of p53 transcript occurred more slowly. The c-*myc* mRNA half-life with the membrane-bound polysomes at 0 h was 2-fold longer than that observed in the other two populations. At 6 h post-PH there was a decreased transcript decay rate for p53 in the free polysomes. This was also apparent in the cytoskeletal-bound fraction where the relative increase in half-life was slightly greater than that observed in the free polysomes. Membrane-bound p53 mRNA also showed a significant decrease in decay activity with no detectable loss of transcript. The c-*myc* transcript half-life increased in both the 6 h post-PH free and cytoskeletal-polysome populations. Interestingly, no significant decay of the membrane-bound associated c-*myc* transcript was observed in the 6 h post-PH *in vitro* decay reactions.

Western blot analysis of the membrane-polysome populations used for the decay studies indicated that the abundance of c-*myc* mRNA and steady-state protein levels was coupled. This suggested that translational activity of the membrane-bound c-*myc* transcript potentially increases the transcript half-life. Translational gradient analysis of the c-*myc* mRNA indicated that the membrane-bound polysomes contain a greater percentage of the transcript associated with fractions bound to more ribosomes than the free and cytoskeletal populations. The coupling of increased p53 protein levels and transcript decay rates was also observed in the 6 h post-PH free and cytoskeletal-bound polysome populations. Interestingly, Western blot analyses of the same membrane-bound polysome populations used in the decay assays indicated a 20% decrease in p53 protein in this fraction relative to 0 time. Thus, translational activity is only one of many potential factors determining mRNA turnover rates following PH. The c-*myc* and p53 transcript decay rates and protein levels were also differentially regulated by polysome population association at 3 and 24 h post-PH. The distribution and flux of a transcript through the polysome population in regenerating liver appears to be unique to an individual transcript. Moreover, polysomal trafficking of the mRNA population appears to be one method that the liver uses to modulate gene expression post-transcriptionally.

An interesting example for alternate gene regulation following PH involves the genes for ornithine decarboxylase (ODC) and connexin 32 (Cx32). ODC is an RNA helicase belonging to the DEAD box family and is the rate-limiting enzyme for polyamine biosynthesis which is required for maximal DNA synthetic activity[60]. ODC transcript levels increase by 3 h post-PH and continue to increase steadily until they reach peak expression at 24 h which is 37-fold over non-regenerating levels. ODC transcript expression then steadily declines until baseline levels are again achieved by 96 h[58]. ODC transcription rate did not change post-PH; however, the *in vivo* chemical half-life increased from 2.5 h in non-regenerating liver to greater than 12 h at 24 h post-PH. Furthermore, at times of increased ODC mRNA stability and expression levels, the gene exhibited demethylation at *Hin*P1 I restriction sites and the transcript was located on heavier polysomes, suggesting increased translation[58,59]. Moreover, the rate of poly(A) tail removal for ODC transcripts was greatly increased in non-regenerating liver when the mRNA half-life was the shortest in comparison to a time-point post-PH of increased half-life.

Cx32 transcripts from the β_1 gap junction gene represent an example of complementary regulation to that of ODC. Gap junction proteins form intercellular channels which allow cell-to-cell communication. Cx32 transcripts are abundant in non-regenerating liver, and cycle in their pattern of expression post-PH with very low levels at 12 and 48 h, and abundant expression in the intervening time-points[61]. This pattern is consistent with those for other gap junction proteins during liver regeneration. Fladmark and colleagues proposed that the advantage to down-regulation of gap junctions during liver regeneration-induced cell cycling may be in maintaining separate pools of metabolites and signalling molecules between replicating hepatocytes and those which are maintaining liver-specific functions[62]. The Cx32 gene exhibited no change in transcription rate during liver regeneration, but the mRNA half-life decreased concordant with the decrease in transcript abundance at 12 h post-PH, from 10.9 to 3.8 h[59]. Furthermore, Cx32 transcripts were associated with heavier polysome fractions in non-regenerating liver, suggesting greater mRNA stability. In contrast, the rate of poly(A) tail shortening increased at 12 h post-PH, consistent with decreased mRNA stability. Cx32 protein expression levels paralleled the transcript levels in a slightly delayed manner[61]. These data are summarized in Table 1, and illustrate that many post-transcriptional mechanisms of gene regulation are employed during liver regeneration to affect the dramatic fluctuations observed in gene expression. Thus, the liver has many levels of gene regulation available for manipulation. Interestingly, the paradigm of coordinate and opposite control of ferritin and transferrin receptor by iron regulatory proteins is contradicted in liver regeneration, thereby preserving an essential iron-storage compartment for replicating hepatocytes[63].

THE ROLE OF THE CELL CYCLE

Several laboratories have investigated the cell cycle regulatory family of cyclins and cdks during liver regeneration. Cyclins form complexes with members of another family of genes, the cdks. The cyclin subunit plays a regulatory

Table 1 Inverse modulation of ODC and Cx32 gene expression in the regenerating liver after 70% partial hepatectomy

	Quiescent liver		Regenerating liver	
	ODC	Cx32	ODC	Cx32
Transcript expression	↓	↑	↑	↓
Transcription rate	—	—	No change	No change
mRNA half-life	2.5 h	10.9 h	> 12 h 24 h post-PH	3.8 h 12 h post-PH
Relative translation	↓	↑	↑	↓
Poly(A) tail shortening rate	↑	↓	↓	↑
Genomic methylation	↑	N.D.	↓	N.D.

No change in transcription rate is relative to that in the quiescent liver. In addition to ODC, increases in mRNA half-lives for p53, c-*myc* and H-*ras* were also associated with decreased genomic methylation, suggesting a potential role for DNA methylation in post-transcriptional gene regulation. ODC, ornithine decarboxylase; Cx32, connexin 32; N.D., not determined

activating role, and the serine/threonine protein kinase catalyses the final phosphorylation reaction. It is apparent that most, if not all, of the transitions and checkpoints in the eukaryotic cell cycle involve cyclin/cdk activity. Cyclins and their partner cdks form complexes which are active at specific times during the cell cycle. Targets for cyclin/cdk kinase activity include the retinoblastoma tumour suppressor protein, histone H1, E2F-1 and RNA polymerase II[64]. In quiescent cells many of the cyclins and their associated cyclin-dependent kinases are located primarily in the cytoplasm. During liver regeneration after PH, their activation is associated with a significant translocation from cytosol to nucleus[65]. This is particularly true for cyclin D–cdk4 and cyclin E/A–cdk2 complexes during rat liver regeneration.

At the transcript level, most of the cyclins and cdks exhibit cell cycle-dependent expression which peaks at cell cycle time-points in which they are known to be active[66–68]. However, the cycling pattern of transcript expression exhibited by these genes is not due to changes in transcription rate as detectable by nuclear run-on assays; and changes in mRNA stability only partially account for the transcript fluctuations observed[66,69]. Furthermore, cyclin steady-state protein levels do not consistently correlate with the mRNA expression pattern[67]. For example, in contrast to the transcript expression, cyclin B1 protein is readily detectable in non-regenerating liver and the total liver expression level does not change appreciably during regeneration[68]. However, the steady-state expression pattern for cdk1 does occur in a cell cycle-related manner, and cyclin B/cdk1 kinase activity is detected at the appropriate mitotic phase during the first wave of regeneration[67,68]. Cyclin A is also detected in resting liver, and a unique tyrosine-phosphorylated form was detected during the G_2 phase of the first wave of cell proliferation following PH[70].

p53

The p53 tumour suppressor gene product is a critical component in cellular pathways for DNA damage-induced G_1 and G_2 arrest, as well as for apoptosis. p53 is a transcription factor which binds to and activates various response genes in a signal-specific manner, including the cdk inhibitor *p21* and the apoptosis gene *bax*[71]. Mice in which the p53 gene has been knocked out are viable, but exhibit pronounced tumour formation. Steady-state mRNA and protein levels are loosely coupled for p53 during liver regeneration. The p53 gene is induced in a delayed-early manner, and transcript expression peaks at 6 h post-PH exhibiting a 35-fold increase over non-regenerating liver RNA expression[58]. p53 transcript levels then exhibit two further peaks in expression 24 and 42 h post-PH, which represent 15–20-fold increases over baseline expression. Protein levels for p53 peak 5-fold over baseline 6–12 h post-PH, and 40-fold over baseline 30 h post-PH in the rat[72]. Thus, the maximum p53 protein expression in regenerating liver corresponds to cell cycle phases of G_1 and mitosis in the first wave of cell division.

It is recognized that p53 plays a role in sensitizing hepatocytes to both growth and death signals. Quiescent hepatocytes from p53 null mice are phenotypically normal. However, once these cells are released from G_0 by isolation for culture, a greater proportion of p53 null cells enter DNA synthesis than wild-type hepatocytes[73]. Induction of liver regeneration by carbon tetrachloride in p53 knockout mice also resulted in greater DNA synthetic activity. Furthermore, isolated p53 null cells are less responsive than wild-type cells to the addition of the mitogens EGF, insulin and fetal bovine serum, as well as to mitosuppressive agents such as TGF-β. In contrast, the livers of p53 null mice were more responsive *in vivo* to a non-genotoxic mitogen.

p53 plays an integral role in G_1 and G_2 checkpoint arrest in gamma-irradiated hepatocytes. Gamma irradiation of mice 48 h after carbon tetrachloride-induced liver regeneration (late G_1 phase of the cell cycle) resulted in reduced hepatocyte G_1/S arrest in p53 null versus wild-type mice[73]. This was followed by a striking rise in the mitotic index 24 h after irradiation, indicating no significant G_2 arrest in response to DNA damage. However, many of the mitotic figures were abnormal, suggesting that the mitotic peak resulted from damaged hepatocytes proceeding to and arresting in mitosis. p53 appears to be important in the regulation of proliferating, but not quiescent, hepatocytes.

p21

p21 is a member of the cdk inhibitor (CKI) family of genes. The CKI proteins can inhibit cyclin/cdk kinase activity by binding to either the complex or the cdk alone. As mentioned previously, the *p21* gene contains p53-binding sites and the p21 protein product is hypothesized to be a key downstream mediator of p53 regulatory pathways. In correspondence with this notion, p21 is induced by many of the same cellular signals which induce p53. Alternatively, p21 is also induced during cellular senescence[64]. It was observed that *p21* transcripts were barely detectable in mouse and rat liver pre-PH, but the abundance increased by 1 h post-PH[74]. Transcript levels decreased at the onset of DNA synthesis in both rodents, then increased again. Dietary protein deprivation also resulted in increased *p21* mRNA expression. Moreover, the same pattern of *p21* induction was exhibited in both p53 null and wild-type mice post-PH. However, following protein deprivation, the increase in *p21* transcript expression after PH was p53-dependent. p21 expression was induced in cycloheximide pre-treated mice subjected to PH, defining *p21* as an immediate-early growth response gene. *p21* transcript expression post-PH is predominantly regulated at the post-transcriptional level, which suggests why the *p21* gene response in PH-stimulated regenerating liver is independent of p53[74].

A liver-specific minigene construct was used to create transgenic mice overexpressing p21 in the liver[75]. Endogenous p21 was undetectable in the liver by two methods, whereas the transgenic livers expressed readily detectable p21 in the hepatocytes. Transgenic mice exhibited decreased liver mass by 49–62%, overall stunted growth, and a shorter lifespan. Furthermore, there were fewer hepatocytes and more non-parenchymal cells than normally observed, along with an abundance of oval cells. This is consistent with the notion stated earlier that, if hepatocytes proliferation is impaired, oval cell replication will increase. The majority of cyclin D1 and cdk4 proteins in hepatocytes were found in complex with p21, which indicates that phosphotransfer activity is inhibited for this kinase. No detectable increase in apoptosis was observed. Following PH in the p21 overexpressing mice, DNA synthesis was less than 15% of normal values and occurred mainly in oval cells. Furthermore, no mitoses were observed, indicating a possible G_2 block as well. Thus, p21 overexpression results in a dominant negative effect in the normal regenerative response to PH. Additionally, mice lacking p21 develop normally but exhibit defective G_1 arrest in response to DNA damage or nucleotide pool perturbation[76].

APOPTOSIS!?

Hepatocytes demonstrate well-characterized signal-specific responses to apoptotic stimuli. Several gene products have been identified which have an anti-apoptotic effect, including the retinoblastoma (Rb) tumour suppressor, Bcl-2, and Bcl-X_L. Rb is a key regulatory protein for the progression from G_1 to S phase of the cell cycle, and also plays a role in development[77]. The functions of Rb are controlled through fluctuations in the protein's phosphorylation status where hypophosphorylation inhibits and hyperphosphorylation allows cell cycle progression through S phase. Loss of functional Rb in the cell results in deregulation of transcriptional activity and either tumorigenesis or apoptosis. Mice lacking the Rb gene die during embryogenesis and demonstrate increased cell division and programmed cell death in the haematopoietic and nervous systems, liver, and skeletal muscle precursor cells.

Rb appears to play a protective role against apoptosis in hepatocytes. Rb protein expression peaks at 12, 30, and 72 h post-PH in the rat, and expression at 30 h is greater than 100-fold increase over non-regenerating levels[72]. Rb transcript expression is uncoupled from that of its protein[78]. TGF-β_1 treatment inhibits Rb gene expression and protein phosphorylation in culture, while Rb protein expression is inhibited in regenerating liver[72,79]. TGF-β_1-induced decrease in Rb abundance and phosphorylation was associated with apoptosis in both primary rat hepatocytes and in HuH-7 human hepatoma cells[79]. Furthermore, depletion of Rb protein expression by antisense oligonucleotides also resulted in hepatocyte death by apoptosis. Overexpression of Rb inhibited the apoptosis of hepatic cells induced by TGF-β_1, Rb antisense, and REC2, a DNA recombinase[72,79,80].

The bcl-2 gene family members Bcl-2 and Bcl-X_L also act to protect cells from apoptosis. Overexpression of either of these genes can block apoptosis[81]. Bcl-2 and bcl-X_L gene expression occurs early during regeneration, with maximal expression 6 h following PH[82]. Bcl-2 transcripts are expressed by non-parenchymal cells and exhibit less than 2-fold induction, whereas Bcl-X_L transcripts are expressed by hepatocytes and exhibit greater than 20-fold induction. Bcl-2 and Bcl-X_L protein levels do not fluctuate significantly during regeneration. Bcl -X_L transcript and protein expression are a delayed-early response and coupled following PH in the mouse[83]. The functions performed by Bcl-2 in other cell types may be fulfilled by Bcl-X_L in hepatocytes. Interestingly, BAG-1, an antiapoptotic protein, associates with the c-Met receptor for HGF, thus linking the antiapoptotic effects of HGF with the survival branch of the bcl-2 family[84].

Other members of the bcl-2 family are proapoptotic in function. These gene products include Bax, Bad, and Bak. Bax homodimers promote cell death, while Bax heterodimers formed with Bcl-2 or Bcl-X_L do not. Bad and Bak can also bind to Bcl-2 and Bcl-X$_L$, thus promoting the formation of Bax homodimers and cell death. Bax transcript and protein abundance increase following PH in the rat in a stepwise fashion[82]. The Bax protein is most abundant in regenerating liver after proliferation but during reorganization of the liver in which apoptosis appears to play a key role. Similarly, Bax protein levels increase following withdrawal of the drug clofibrate, an inducer of direct hyperplasia, and are associated with apoptosis of the 'unnecessary' hepatocytes[82].

p53 is a key cellular status sensor which can halt the cell proliferation machinery in order to effect repairs, but can also induce apoptosis. Cultured p53 null hepatocytes are able to survive and proliferate under conditions in which wild-type cells cease to proliferate and undergo apoptosis[73]. Liver cells can also undergo Fas ligand/receptor-mediated cell death. Hep 3B human hepatoma cells, which lack p53, can still undergo apoptosis in response to apoptotic stimuli[79,80]. Interestingly, Fas-signalling events at the level or upstream of caspase-3 activity are suppressed during liver regeneration, resulting in delayed hepatocyte apoptosis[85]. TNF-α acts as one of the protective factors against Fas-mediated hepatocyte apoptosis.

REMODELLING AND THE EXTRACELLULAR MATRIX

The reproduction of liver mass and function also requires regulation of apoptosis and the extracellular matrix (ECM) to effect the remodelling of parenchymal and non-parenchymal cells into functional units. Remodelling occurs during embryo development, tissue repair, and regeneration, and requires coordination of matrix degradation, apoptosis, matrix deposition, and cell proliferation. The hepatocyte is the only epithelial cell in the body not separated from the vascular space by two continuous basement membranes, which may allow for the rapid exchange of components between the plasma and the hepatocytes[86]. Hepatic failure due to cirrhosis results, in great part, from the formation of basement membrane between hepatocytes and the vascular space.

The processes of cell division and subsequent remodelling of the hepatocytes intuitively requires remodelling of the pre-existing ECM. Activation of uro-kinase plasminogen activator (uPA) occurs within 5 min post-PH and this, in turn, is proposed to initiate a proteolytic cascade resulting in hepatic biomatrix degradation and release of active HGF[10]. Four days post-PH, mitotic activity has ceased and the hepatocytes exist as clusters of 10–14 cells which lack sinusoids and extracellular matrix[86]. Furthermore, by this point the cell to ECM ratio has greatly increased. Laminin-positive Ito cells become detectable and appear to extend processes to invade the hepatocyte clusters. Fenestrated endothelial cells then penetrate the clusters and separate the hepatocytes into cell plates, thus restoring normal hepatocyte vascular structure. Once this is accomplished, laminin is no longer produced. Along with the hepatic plates the biliary tree must also regenerate in the hepatectomized liver. Intrahepatic bile duct epithelial cells, or cholangiocytes, line the intrahepatic biliary tree and function to modify bile. In these cells, DNA synthesis increased by 1 day, peaked on day 3 and returned to control values by 28 days post-PH[87]. By 10 days post-PH the normal distribution of ECM and regrowth of the biliary tree are complete.

CONCLUSIONS

There are a number of issues involved in liver regeneration which remain unanswered. For example, what are the critical signals occurring within minutes of surgery which catalyse the entire regenerative process? It is unlikely that a single 'master' signal is the causative agent, and we now know that even a change in membrane potential is not a critical event[88]. Following PH, the blood flow to the remnant liver increases 3-fold relative to before surgery, and is probably responsible for delivery of necessary signalling agents for regeneration. In this regard, studies performed almost half a century ago revealed that, when the circulations of two rats are joined, PH of one of the rats causes proliferation in the intact liver of the other rat. Furthermore, regeneration proceeds periportal to pericentral, in the direction of portal blood flow within the remnant lobes. How do liver cells maintain their differentiated functions and yet exit quiescence to begin proliferating? How does the liver sense when the optimal mass has been achieved and hepatic proliferation ceases? Many genes, such as those for proto-oncogenes and tumour suppressors appear to be involved in multiple cellular processes, including cell proliferation, development and apoptosis. While this seems antithetical, it also reflects an economy of function in the cell. A change in the intricate balance between signals for proliferation and apoptosis can be swiftly acted upon by key proteins capable of functioning in either pathway.

The capacity for regeneration in most vertebrates is limited to a few tissues, such as bone, skeletal muscle and, of course, liver. For bone and muscle, regeneration in some ways recapitulates embryonic differentiation from stem cells. In contrast, it is widely accepted that the liver is able to regenerate without activation of those stealth stem cells. We also know that hepatocytes can undergo partial dedifferentiation, allowing them to re-enter the cell cycle while maintaining critical differentiated functions. It will be important to identify the cellular and molecular differences that distinguish tissue embryogenesis from wound repair from regeneration. Why do tissues scar rather than regenerate? They may even contain cells competent to undergo replication, but lack the stimulatory signals to effect regeneration. On the other hand, they may be receptive to signals that suppress regeneration and promote scarring. It seems that most tissues appear to lack the critical cells required for regeneration. However, is it conceivable that they simply lie dormant with all the machinery necessary for regeneration – waiting for just the right combination of stimuli? Perhaps we should take a closer look at livers and urodeles and learn from them how to induce regeneration in other tissues. In the future we may ultimately develop the technology to regenerate vital organs. The fun and excitement will be in getting there!

References

1. Brockes JP. Amphibian limb regeneration: rebuilding a complex structure. Science. 1997;276: 81–7.
2. Columbano A, Shinozuka H. Liver regeneration versus direct hyperplasia. FASEB J. 1996;10: 1118–28.
3. Yoshioka S, Miyazaki M, Shimizu H *et al*. Hepatic venous hemoglobin oxygen saturation predicts regenerative status of remnant liver after partial hepatectomy in rats. Hepatology. 1998;27:1349–53.

4. Ono F, Nakagawa T, Saito S *et al.* A novel class II phosphoinositide 3-kinase predominantly expressed in the liver and its enhanced expression during liver regeneration. J Biol Chem. 1998;273:7731–6.
5. Kennedy S, Rettinger S, Flye MW, Ponder KP. Experiments in transgenic mice show that hepatocytes are the source for postnatal growth and do not stream. Hepatology. 1995;22:160–8.
6. Heckel JL, Sandgren EP, Degen JL, Palmiter RD, Brinster RL. Neonatal bleeding in transgenic mice expressing urokinase-type plasminogen activator. Cell. 1990;62:447–56.
7. Sandgren EP, Palmiter RD, Heckel JL, Daugherty CC, Brinster RL, Degen JL. Complete hepatic regeneration after somatic deletion of an albumin–plasminogen activator transgene. Cell. 1991;66:245–56.
8. Rhim JA, Sandgren EP, Degen JL, Palmiter RD, Brinster RL. Replacement of diseased mouse liver by hepatic cell transplantation. Science. 1994;263:1149–52.
9. Rhim JA, Sandgren EP, Palmiter RD, Brinster RL. Complete reconstitution of mouse liver with xenogeneic hepatocytes. Proc Natl Acad Sci USA. 1995;92:4942–6.
10. Michalopoulos GK, DeFrances MC. Liver regeneration. Science. 1997;276:60–6.
11. Overturf K, Al-Dhalimy M, Ou C-N, Finegold M, Grompe M. Serial transplantation reveals the stem-cell-like regenerative potential of adult mouse hepatocytes. Am J Pathol. 1997;151:1273–80.
12. Locaputo S, Carrick TL, Bezerra JA. Zonal regulation of gene expression during liver regeneration of urokinase transgenic mice. Hepatology. 1999;29:1106–13.
13. Vos TA, Ros JE, Havinga R *et al.* Regulation of hepatic transport systems involved in bile secretion during liver regeneration in rats. Hepatology. 1999;29:1833–9.
14. Thorgeirsson SS. Hepatic stem cells in liver regeneration. FASEB J. 1996;10:1249–56.
15. Matsusaka S, Tsujimura T, Toyosaka A *et al.* Role of c-*kit* receptor tyrosine kinase in development of oval cells in the rat 2-acetylaminofluorene/partial hepatectomy model. Hepatology. 1999;29:670–6.
16. Gandhi CR, Kuddus R, Subbotin VM *et al.* A fresh look at augmenter of liver regeneration in rats. Hepatology. 1999;29:1435–45.
17. Loyer P, Cariou S, Glaise D, Bilodeau M, Baffet G, Guguen-Guillouzo C. Growth factor dependence of progression through G_1 and S phases of adult rat hepatocytes *in vitro*. Evidence of a mitogen restriction point in mid-late G_1. J Biol Chem. 1996;272:11484–92.
18. Fausto N, Laird AD, Webber EM. Role of growth factors and cytokines in hepatic regeneration. FASEB J. 1995;9:1527–36.
19. Rai RM, Lee FYJ, Rosen A *et al.* Impaired liver regeneration in inducible nitric oxide synthase-deficient mice. Proc Natl Acad Sci USA. 1998;95:13829–34.
20. Mullhaupt B, Feren A, Fodor E, Jones A. Liver expression of epidermal growth factor RNA. Rapid increases in immediate-early phase of liver regeneration. J Biol Chem. 1994;269:19667–70.
21. Fausto N, Webber EM. 1994. Liver regeneration. In: Arias IM, Boyer JL, Fausto N, Jakoby WB, Schachter D, Shafritz DA, editors. The Liver: Biology and Pathobiology. New York: Raven Press; 1994:1059–84.
22. Noguchi S, Ohba Y, Oka T. Influence of epidermal growth factor on liver regeneration after partial hepatectomy in mice. J Endocrinol. 1991;128:425–31.
23. Lambotte L, Saliez A, Triest S *et al.* Effect of sialoadenectomy and epidermal growth factor administration on liver regeneration after partial hepatectomy. Hepatology. 1997;25:607–12.
24. Jones DE Jr, Tran-Patterson R, Cui D-M, Davin D, Estell KP, Miller DM. Epidermal growth factor secreted from the salivary gland is necessary for liver regeneration. Am J Physiol. 1995;268:G872–8.
25. Russell WE, Kaufmann WK, Sitaric S, Luetteke NC, Lee DC. Liver regeneration and hepatocarcinogenesis in transforming growth factor-α-targeted mice. Mol Carcinogen. 1996;15:183–9.
26. Mars WM, Liu M-L, Kitson RP, Goldfarb RH, Gabauer MK, Michalopoulos GK. Immediate early detection of urokinase receptor after partial hepatectomy and its implications for initiation of liver regeneration. Hepatology. 1995;21:1695–701.
27. Schmidt C, Bladt F, Goedecke S *et al.* Scatter factor/hepatocyte growth factor is essential for liver development. Nature. 1995;373:699–702.
28. Uehara Y, Minowa O, Mori C *et al.* Placental defect and embryonic lethality in mice lacking hepatocyte growth factor/scatter factor. Nature. 1995;373:702–5.

29. Bladt F, Riethmacher D, Isenmann S, Aguzzi A, Birchmeier C. Essential role for the c-*met* receptor in the migration of myogenic precursor cells into the limb bud. Nature. 1995;376: 768–71.

30. Shiota G, Wang TC, Nakamuro T, Schmidt EV. Hepatocyte growth factor in transgenic mice: effects on hepatocyte growth, liver regeneration and gene expression. Hepatology. 1994;19: 962–72.

31. Sakata H, Takayama H, Sharp R, Rubin JS, Merlino G, LaRochelle WJ. Hepatocyte growth factor/scatter factor overexpression induces growth, abnormal development, and tumor formation in transgenic mouse livers. Cell Growth Differ. 1996;7:1513–23.

32. Amicone L, Spagnoli FM, Späth G et al. Transgenic expression in the liver of truncated Met blocks apoptosis and permits immortalization of hepatocytes. EMBO J. 1997;16:495–503.

33. Rai RM, Loffreda S, Karp CL, Yang S-Q, Lin H-Z, Diehl AM. Kupffer cell depletion abolishes induction of interleukin-10 and permits sustained overexpression of tumor necrosis factor alpha messenger RNA in the regenerating rat liver. Hepatology. 1997;25:889–95.

34. Webber EM, Bruix J, Pierce RH, Fausto N. Tumor necrosis factor primes hepatocytes for DNA replication in the rat. Hepatology. 1998;28:1226–34.

35. Lee FYJ, Li Y, Zhu H et al. Tumor necrosis factor increases mitochondrial oxidant production and induces expression of uncoupling protein-2 in the regenerating rat liver. Hepatology. 1999;29:677–87.

36. Sakamoto T, Liu Z, Murase N et al. Mitosis and apoptosis in the liver of interleukin-6-deficient mice after partial hepatectomy. Hepatology. 1999;29:403–11.

37. Tewari M, Dobrzanski P, Mohn KL et al. Rapid induction in regenerating liver of RL/IF-1 (an IκB that inhibits NF-κB, RelB-p50, and c-Rel-p50) and PHF, a novel κB site-binding complex. Mol Cell Biol. 1992;12:2898–908.

38. Ruff-Jamison S, Zhong Z, Wen Z, Chen K, Darnell JE Jr, Cohen S. Epidermal growth factor and lipopolysaccharide activate stat3 transcription factor in mouse liver. J Biol Chem. 1994;269:21933–5.

39. FitzGerald MJ, Webber EM, Donovan JR, Fausto N. Rapid DNA binding by nuclear factor κB in hepatocytes at the start of liver regeneration. Cell Growth Differ. 1995;6:417–27.

40. Cressman DE, Greenbaum LE, DeAngelis RA et al. Liver failure and defective hepatocyte regeneration in interleukin-6-deficient mice. Science. 1996;274:1379–83.

41. Akerman P, Cote P, Yang SQ et al. Antibodies to tumor necrosis factor-α inhibit liver regeneration after partial hepatectomy. Am J Physiol. 1992;263:G579–85.

42. Yamada Y, Kirillova I, Peschon JJ, Fausto N. Initiation of liver growth by tumor necrosis factor: deficient liver regeneration in mice lacking type I tumor necrosis factor receptor. Proc Natl Acad Sci USA. 1997;94:1441–6.

43. Spector MS, Auer KL, Jarvis WD et al. Differential regulation of the mitogen-activated protein and stress-activated protein kinase cascades by adrenergic agonists in quiescent and regenerating adult rat hepatocytes. Mol Cell Biol. 1997;17:3556–65.

44. Selzner M, Camargo CA, Clavien P-A. Ischemia impairs liver regeneration after major tissue loss in rodents: protective effects of interleukin-6. Hepatology. 1999;30:469–75.

45. Bissell DM, Wang S-S, Jarnagin WR, Roll FJ. Cell-specific expression of transforming growth factor-β in rat liver. Evidence for autocrine regulation of hepatocyte proliferation. J Clin Invest. 1995;96:447–55.

46. Sanderson N, Factor V, Nagy P et al. Hepatic expression of mature transforming growth factor β1 in transgenic mice results in multiple tissue lesions. Proc Natl Acad Sci USA. 1995;92: 2572–6.

47. Esquela AF, Zimmers TA, Koniaris LG, Sitzmann JV, Lee S-J. Transient down-regulation of inhibin-βC expression following partial hepatectomy. Biochem Biophys Res Commun. 1997;235:553–6.

48. Freeman TL, Ngo HQ, Mailliard ME. Inhibition of system A amino acid transport and hepatocyte proliferation following partial hepatectomy in the rat. Hepatology. 1999;30: 437–44.

49. Taub R. Transcriptional control of liver regeneration. FASEB J. 1996;10:413–27.

50. Diehl AM. Roles of CCAAT/enhancer-binding proteins in regulation of liver regenerative growth. J Biol Chem. 1998;273:30843–6.

51. Greenbaum LE, Li W, Cressman DE et al. CCAAT enhancer-binding protein β is required for normal hepatocyte proliferation in mice after partial hepatectomy. J Clin Invest. 1998;102:996–1007.

52. Servillo G, Della Fazia MA, Sassone-Corsi P. Transcription factor CREM coordinates the timing of hepatocyte proliferation in the regenerating liver. Genes Dev. 1998;12:3639–43.

53. Du K, Leu JI, Peng Y, Taub R. Transcriptional up-regulation of the delayed early gene *HRS/SRp40* during liver regeneration. Interactions among YY1, GA-binding proteins, and mitogenic signals. J Biol Chem. 1998;273:35208–15.

54. Günes Ç, Heuchel R, Georgiev O *et al.* Embryonic lethality and liver degeneration in mice lacking the metal-responsive transcriptional activator MTF-1. EMBO J. 1998;17:2846–54.

55. Peng Y, Du K, Ramirez S, Diamond RH, Taub R. Mitogenic up-regulation of the *PRL-1* protein–tyrosine phosphatase gene by Egr-1. Egr-1 activation is an early event in liver regeneration. J Biol Chem. 1999;274:4513–20.

56. Haber BA, Mohn KL, Diamond RH, Taub R. Induction pattern of 70 genes during nine days after hepatectomy define the temporal course of liver regeneration. J Clin Invest. 1993;91: 1319–26.

57. Menegazzi M, Carcereri-De Prati A, Suzuki H *et al.* Liver cell proliferation induced by nafenopin and cyproterone acetate is not associated with increases in activation of transcription factors NF-κB and AP-1 or with expression of tumor necrosis factor α. Hepatology. 1997;25:585–92.

58. Kren BT, Trembley JH, Steer CJ. Alterations in mRNA stability during rat liver regeneration. Am J Physiol. 1996;270:G763–77.

59. Kren BT, Steer CJ. Posttranscriptional regulation of gene expression in liver regeneration: role of mRNA stability. FASEB J. 1996;10:559–73.

60. Diehl AM, Wells M, Brown ND, Thorgeirsson SS, Steer CJ. Effect of ethanol on polyamine synthesis during liver regeneration in rats. J Clin Invest. 1990;85:385–90.

61. Kren BT, Kumar NM, Wang S-q, Gilula NB, Steer CJ. Differential regulation of multiple gap junction transcripts and proteins during rat liver regeneration. J Cell Biol. 1993;123:707–18.

62. Fladmark KE, Gjertsen BT, Molven A, Mellgren G, Vintermyr OK, Døskeland SO. Gap junctions and growth control in liver regeneration and in isolated rat heptocytes. Hepatology. 1997;25:847–55.

63. Cairo G, Tacchini L, Pietrangelo A. Lack of coordinate control of ferritin and transferrin receptor expression during rat liver regeneration. Hepatology. 1998;28:173–8.

64. MacLachlan TK, Sang N, Giordano A. Cyclins, cyclin-dependent kinases and cdk inhibitors: implications in cell cycle control and cancer. Crit Rev Euk Gene Exp. 1995;5:127–56.

65. Jaumot M, Estanyol J-M, Serratosa J, Agell N, Bachs O. Activation of cdk4 and cdk2 during rat liver regeneration is associated with intranuclear rearrangements of cyclin–cdk complexes. Hepatology. 1999;29:385–95.

66. Albrecht JH, Hoffman JS, Kren BT, Steer CJ. Cyclin and cyclin-dependent kinase 1 mRNA expression in models of regenerating liver and human liver diseases. Am J Physiol. 1993;265: G857–64.

67. Loyer P, Glaise D, Cariou S, Baffet G, Meijer L, Guguen-Guillouzo C. Expression and activation of cdks (1 and 2) and cyclins in the cell cycle progression during liver regeneration. J Biol Chem. 1994;269:2491–500.

68. Trembley JH, Ebbert JO, Kren BT, Steer CJ. Differential regulation of cyclin B1 RNA and protein expression during heptocyte growth *in vivo*. Cell Growth Differ. 1996;7:903–16.

69. Trembley JH, Kren BT, Steer CJ. Posttranscriptional regulation of cyclin B messenger RNA expression in the regenerating rat liver. Cell Growth Differ. 1994;5:99–108.

70. Rinaudo JAS, Thorgeirsson SS. Detection of a tyrosine-phosphorylated form of cyclin A during liver regeneration. Cell Growth Differ. 1997;8:301–9.

71. Levine AJ. p53, the cellular gatekeeper for growth and division. Cell. 1997;88:323–31.

72. Fan G, Xu R, Wessendorf MW, Ma X, Kren BT, Steer CJ. Modulation of retinoblastoma and retinoblastoma-related proteins in regenerating rat liver and primary hepatocytes. Cell Growth Differ. 1995;6:1463–76.

73. Bellamy COC, Clarke AR, Wyllie AH, Harrison DJ. p53 deficiency in liver reduces local control of survival and proliferation, but does not affect apoptosis after DNA damage. FASEB J. 1997;11:591–9.

74. Albrecht JA, Meyer AH, Hu MY. Regulation of cyclin-dependent kinase inhibitor p21[WAF1/Cip1/Sdi1] gene expression in hepatic regeneration. Hepatology. 1997;25:557–63.

75. Wu H, Wade M, Krall L, Grisham J, Xiong Y, Van Dyke T. Targeted in vivo expression of the cyclin-dependent kinase inhibitor p21 halts hepatocyte cell-cycle progression, postnatal liver development, and regeneration. Genes Dev. 1996;10:245–60.

76. Deng C, Zhang P, Harper JW, Elledge SJ, Leder P. Mice lacking p21$^{CIP1/WAF1}$ undergo normal development, but are defective in G1 checkpoint control. Cell. 1995;82:675–84.

77. Herwig S, Strauss M. The retinoblastoma protein: a master regulator of cell cycle, differentiation, and apoptosis. Eur J Biochem. 1997;246:581–601.

78. Kren BT, Teel AL, Steer CJ. Transcriptional rate and steady-state changes of retinoblastoma mRNA in regenerating rat liver. Hepatology. 1994;19:1214–22.

79. Fan G, Ma X, Kren BT, Steer CJ. The retinoblastoma gene product inhibits TGF-β1 induced apoptosis in primary rat hepatocytes and human HuH-7 hepatoma cells. Oncogene. 1996;12: 1909–19.

80. Fan G, Ma X, Kren BT, Rice M, Kmiec EB, Steer CJ. A novel link between REC2, a DNA recombinase, the retinoblastoma protein, and apoptosis. J Biol Chem. 1997;272:19413–17.

81. Yang E, Korsmeyer SJ. Molecular thanatopsis: a discourse on the BCL2 family and cell death. Blood. 1996;88:386–401.

82. Kren BT, Trembley JH, Krajewski S, Behrens TW, Reed JC, Steer CJ. Modulation of apoptosis-associated genes *bcl*-2, *bcl*-x, and *bax* during rat liver regeneration. Cell Growth Differ. 1996;7:1633–42.

83. Tzung S-P, Fausto N, Hockenberry DM. Expression of Bcl-2 family during liver regeneration and identification of Bcl-x as a delayed early response gene. Am J Pathol. 1997;150:1985–95.

84. Bardelli A, Longati P, Albero D *et al.* HGF receptor associates with the anti-apoptotic protein BAG-1 and prevents cell death. EMBO J. 1996;15:6205–12.

85. Takehara T, Hayashi N, Mita E *et al.* Delayed Fas-mediated hepatocyte apoptosis during liver regeneration in mice: hepatoprotective role of TNF-α. Hepatology. 1998;27:1643–51.

86. Martinez-Hernandez A, Amenta PS. The extracellular matrix in hepatic regeneration. FASEB J. 1995;9:1401–10.

87. LeSage G, Glaser SS, Gubba S *et al.* Regrowth of the rat biliary tree after 70% partial hepatectomy is coupled to increased secretin-induced ductal secretion. Gastroenterology. 1996;111: 1633–44.

88. Minuk GY, Kren BT, Xu R *et al.* The effect of changes in hepatocyte membrane potential on immediate-early proto-oncogene expression following partial hepatectomy in rats. Hepatology. 1997;25:1123–7.

30
New aspects of signal transduction in the liver

D. A. BRENNER, E. HATANO, C. A. BRADHAM, T. QIAN, R. SCHWABE, K. BEHRNS and J. J. LEMASTERS

INTRODUCTION

Cell survival is dependent on the complex integration of multiple intracellular signalling pathways that are responsive to extracellular stimuli. Cellular stressors, including radiation, oxidative stress, tumour necrosis factor alpha (TNF-α), and Fas ligand may dramatically alter cell signalling such that apoptotic cell death ensues. Apoptosis is characterized by a highly orchestrated, caspase cascade that proteolytically cleaves substrates that either propagate a caspase cascade or result in cleavage of DNA or the cellular cytoskeleton. The apoptogenic pathway, however, may only be activated with concomitant inhibition of cell survival factors such as nuclear factor kappa B (NF-κB). This review will focus on molecular signalling of TNF-α and Fas-induced hepatocyte apoptosis with emphasis on NF-κB signalling, the caspase cascade, inhibitors of apoptosis, and the role of mitochondria in cell death.

TNF-α-receptor-mediated apoptosis occurs with ligand–receptor interaction and trimerization of the type I TNF-α receptor (TNFRI)/, TNFRI. With receptor activation interacts with TRADD (TNF-associated death domain) which is necessary for TNF-α-mediated apoptosis and NF-κB activation[1]. TNF-α-mediated NF-κB activation is dependent on the association of TRADD with TRAF2 (TNF-associated factor 2), but TNF-α-induced apoptosis is dependent on TRADD– FADD (Fas-associated death domain) association[2], but not TRADD–TRAF2 interaction. Thus, the NF-κB and apoptogenic signals of TNF-α appear to diverge at TRADD (see Fig. 1).

TNF-α induction of TRAF2 leads to activation of the NF-κB pathway that sequentially includes a MEKK1 kinase, probably NIK (NF-κB-inducing kinase[3], IκB kinase complex[4] with phosphorylation of IκB at serines 32 and 36. Phosphorylation of IκB results in ubiquitination and proteasome degradation with release of NF-κB for translocation to the nucleus.

The Fas receptor (Apo-1, CD95) is a type I transmembrane protein and a member of the TNF-receptor superfamily. Ligand binding of CD95 plays a

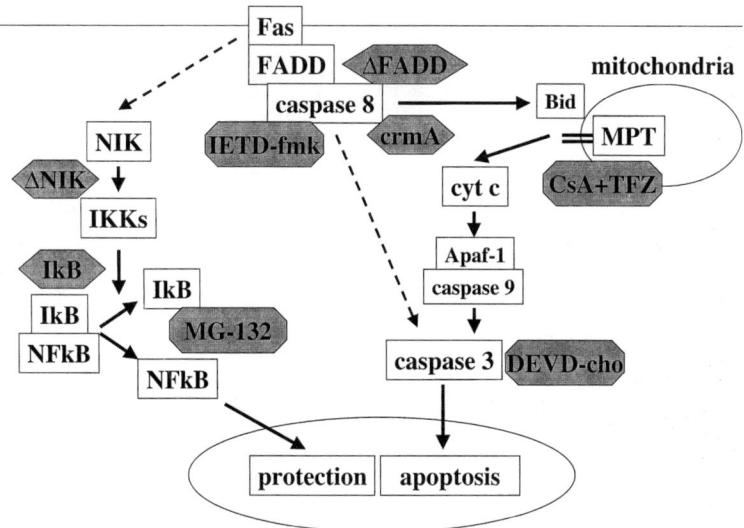

Figure 1   A model of signal transduction by TNF-α binding hepatocytes

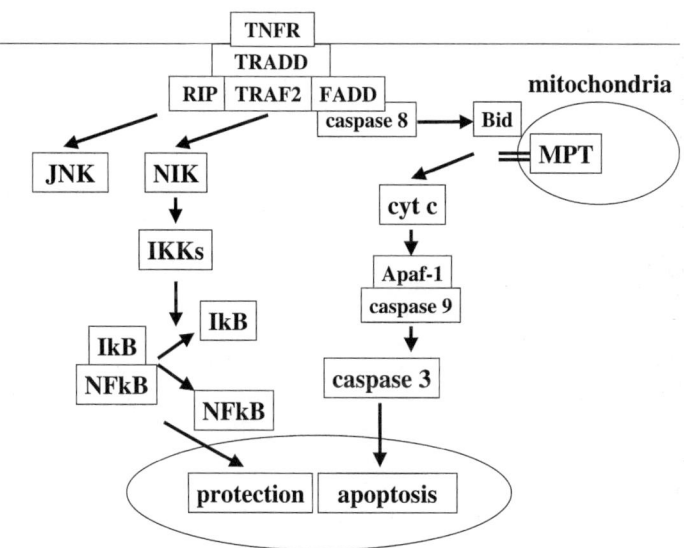

Figure 2   A model of signal transduction of fasL binding to fas in hepatocytes

prominent role in homeostasis of the immune system, but has also been shown to induce hepatocyte apoptosis[5]. The intracellular component of Fas contains a death domain, homologous with the TNFRI death domain, that is critical for the induction of apoptosis and binds FADD[6,7]. The caspase cascade is initiated with interaction between FADD and pro-caspase-8 (FLICE)[8,9] which together form the death-inducing signalling complex (DISC)[10] (see Fig. 2). A potential alternative Fas-induced death pathway involves Daxx, which can enhance Fas-mediated apoptosis by ASK1 activation of the JNK kinase cascade[11]. Confirmatory evidence for apoptosis via this pathway, however, is lacking.

TNF-α and Fas-mediated activation of the caspase cascade occur with the conversion of procaspase-8 to the proteolytically active caspase-8 at the DISC. Caspase-8 cleaves Bid, a member of the pro-apoptotic Bcl-2 family, and the activated form of Bid (p15) traverses the mitochondrial membrane. Bid is responsible for mitochondrial membrane permeability transition (MPT) with creation of a large membrane pore and release of cytochrome-c[12–14]. The importance of Bid in this signalling pathway was addressed in a recent study which demonstrated that Bid-deficient mice do not exhibit hepatocyte apoptosis in response to Fas stimulation[15]. Changes in the MPT and release of cytochrome-c result in the creation of an 'aptostat' complex of cytochrome-c, procaspase-9, and Apaf-1 which collectively activate caspase-9, which in turn cleaves caspase-3 to its active form. Activation of caspase-3 results in proteolysis of ICAD (inhibitor of caspase-activated deoxyribonuclease [CAD]) from CAD, which translocates to the nucleus where it mediates DNA degradation into olignucleosomes[16]. Although this signalling pathway is operative in many cell types (designated type II cells), other cell systems (designated type I cells) do not require mitochondrial and apostat activation, but have abundant, direct caspase-8-induced activation of caspase-3[17].

Although apoptosis is protective for the organism, control of cell death through cell survival signalling provides homeostatic balance against the caspase cascade. Many cell signalling pathways have been implicated as cell survival mechanisms, but NF-κB has received considerable attention as an anti-apoptotic transcription factor. For example, Romanshkova and Makarov[18] have demonstrated that platelet-derived growth factor not only acts as a cell survival factor, but also induces NF-κB as an anti-apoptotic signal through a Ras/PI(3) K/Akt/IKK/NF-κB pathway. Furthermore, other NF-κB anti-apoptotic responsive genes include TRAF1, TRAF2, cIAP1, cIAP2[19], IEX-IL[20], and iNOS[21]. Another family of proteins that is important in the inhibition of apoptosis is the IAP (inhibitors of apoptosis proteins) family. Human family members include NAIP, cIAP1/HIAP-2, cIAP2/HIAP-1, XIAP/hILP, survivin, and BRUCE[22]. These anti-apoptotic factors may act by direct caspase inhibition or by interfering with cell survival signalling such as NF-κB and the JNK pathway[22]. Further investigation of these inhibitors of apoptosis will be important in understanding mechanisms of cellular growth control.

Even though apoptosis is an operative mechanism of hepatocyte death for many stressors, some cellular toxins (viral hepatitis) may induce cell death that share features of apoptosis and necrosis. Recent evidence suggests that these mechanisms of cell death may be viewed as a continuum, and the term 'necrapoptosis' has been introduced to show shared pathways between apoptosis and necrosis[23]. Both forms of cell death can induce the mitochondrial permeability transition (MPT), but with rapid induction of the MPT and cellular depletion of adenosine triphosphate (ATP) necrosis (cellular swelling and lysis) occurs, whereas slow onset of the MPT in the presence of ATP results in apoptosis (cellular resorption)[23].

The aim of this review is to examine the role of NF-κB signalling and the MPT in TNF-α and Fas-mediated hepatocyte apoptosis.

MATERIALS AND METHODS

Primary hepatocyte cultures

Primary rat hepatocytes were isolated by collagenase protein and cultured as described previously[24]. C57B16 male mice were anaesthetized with ketamine/ acepromazine malate administered by intraperitoneal injection. Hepatocytes were then isolated by a retrograde, non-recirculating *in-situ* collagenase perfusion of livers cannulating through the inferior vena cava by a procedure modified from Moldeus *et al.*[25]. A total of 5×10^5 cells were plated on six-well plates coated with mouse collagen type I in Waymouth's medium containing 10% fetal bovine serum, 0.1 μM insulin, and 0.1 μM dexamethasone. After 2 h the culture was washed with PBS and changed to hormonally defined medium (HDM) containing 0.1 μM insulin, 2 mM L-glutamine, 5 μg/ml transferrin, 3 μM selenium, and 10 nM free fatty acids in RPMI basal medium. Cells were infected with recombinant adenoviruses in HDM containing 30 pfu/cell for 2 h at 37°C and then changed to HDM containing recombinant murine TNF-α (R&D Systems, Minneapolis, MN), Jo-2 (Pharmingen, San Diego, CA) or other treatments. All animals received humane care in compliance with the guidelines of University of North Carolina.

Adenoviruses

The adenovirus 5 variants Ad5IκB, Ad5LacZ, Ad5ΔFADD, Ad5ΔNIK, and Ad5crmA expressing HA-IκB-α (S32A, S36A), β-galactosidase, a truncated form of FADD, or truncated form of NIK, and crmA, respectively, have been described elsewhere[26,27].

Measurement of apoptosis

For quantitation of cell viability (presented as mean ± SEM), cells were infected and treated as described above. After 17–20 h of TNF-α or Jo-2 treatment, cell viability was determined by exclusion of trypan blue. Viable cells were counted in three different 200 × power fields and the percentage of treated viable cells to untreated viable cells was determined as a percentage of control viability. For propidium iodide nuclear staining, cells were fixed in 3:1 methanol/acetic acid, stained with 10 μg/ml popidium iodide, and viewed with an Olympus fluorescence microscope using a rhodamine filter set. To assess DNA ladder formation, 2×10^6 cells were digested overnight at 37°C in 0.5 mg/ml proteinase K, 0.5% arcosyl in PBS, treated with 10 μg RNase for 1 h at 37°C, then gently extracted with phenol and chloroform, and analysed on 2% agarose gels.

Confocal microscopy

Cell loading and confocal microscopy were carried out as described previously[28]. Briefly, 1–2 × 10^6 hepatocytes plated on collagen-coated 40 mm diameter glass coverslips were infected with Ad5IκB in HDM supplemented with 50 mM HEPES (pH 7.0) to stabilize pH during the confocal measurements. The cells were loaded with 250 nM tetramethylrhodamine methyl ester (TMRM, Molecular Probes, Eugene, OR) and 1 μM calcein-acetoxymethyl ester (Molecular Probes) in KRH buffer for 15 min at 37°C. The coverslips were mounted on a Nikon microscope (Nikon, Melville, NY) in HDM-HEPES containing 100 nM TMRM, and the temperature was maintained at 37°C. The first image (time-point 0) was then recorded. Subsequently, TNF-α or Jo-2 was added to the medium, and images were collected at given time-points. Calcein and TMRM fluorescence was excited with an argon laser through a double dichroic reflector at 488 nm and 568 nm, respectively. TMRM was imaged through 590-nm long path emission filter using a Bio-Rad MRC-600 confocal system (Bio-Rad Laboratories, Hercules, CA). Calcein fluorescence was collected through a 515–560 nm bandpath emission filter. A numerical aperture 1.4, 60× objective lens was used, and pinholes were set to 4 in both channels. Laser attenuation and power were set at 0.3% and low, respectively.

RESULTS

Apoptosis model

Rat and mouse hepatocytes resist TNF-α-mediated apoptosis unless they are also treated with a protein synthesis inhibitor such as cycloheximide or actinomycin D[29], which may reflect the protective role of proteins whose expression is stimulated by the transcription factor NF-κB[30]. To render normally resistant hepatocytes sensitive to TNF-α-mediated apoptosis, we blocked NF-κB activation by using an IκB-α (S34A, S36A)-expressing adenovirus (Ad5IκB)[27]. This mutant form of IκB-α is not phosphorylated and targeted for degradation and thus prevents NF-κB activation[31]. When primary rat hepatocytes overexpressing the IκB superrepressor were treated with TNF-α, the cells lost viability after 24 h, as shown by morphological changes including rounding, loss of attachment, and increased refractility in phase-contrast images. Cells expressing the IκB superrepressor but not treated with TNF-α did not lose viability (Fig. 3).

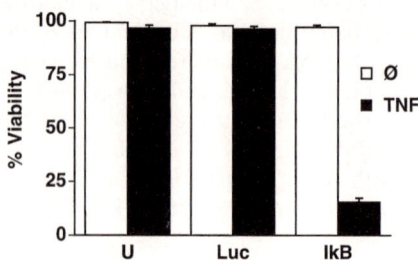

Figure 3   The IκB superrepressor sensitizes hepatocytes to TNF-β-mediated apoptosis. Primary hepatocyte cultures were infected with Ad5IκB or control Ad5Luc and then either not treated or treated with TNF-α (30 mg/ml). Average percentage viability ± SEM

Uninfected cells and cells infected with a control adenovirus (Ad5Luc) were not killed after 24 h of TNF-α treatment, while Ad5IκB-infected hepatocytes treated with TNF-α displayed striking cell death (Fig. 3).

Hepatocytes expressing the IκB superrepressor and treated with TNF-α fulfilled morphological and biochemical criteria of apoptosis. When hepatocytes were fixed and stained with propidium iodide to visualize nuclear morphology, Ad5IκB-infected hepatocytes treated with TNF-α displayed nuclear condensation and fragmentation. Uninfected cells and cells infected with control virus Ad5Luc displayed normal nuclear morphology after exposure to TNF-α, as did untreated Ad5IκB-infected cells. Additionally, we prepared genomic DNA from hepatocytes expressing the IκB superrepressor. DNA ladders were formed in TNF-α-treated but not untreated cells.

TNF-α induces mitochondrial effects during apoptosis. To directly determine the effect of TNF-α on mitochondrial function and membrane permeability, we loaded cells with cationic TMRM, a red-fluorescing, membrane potential-indicating fluorophore, and calcein, a green-fluorescing fluorophore that localizes to the cytosol under the loading conditions used[32] (Fig. 4). After 7 h of treatment with TNF-α the distributions of TMRM (Fig. 4A, top) and calcein (Fig. 5A, bottom) remained normal (for comparison, see ref. 33). Each red TMRM-labelled mitochondrion corresponded to a dark void in the green calcein image, showing that the mitochondria were polarized and impermeable to low-molecular-weight solutes. After 9 h of exposure of TNF-α approximately one-third to one-half of the mitochondria lost TMRM fluorescence, indicating depolarization (Fig. 4b, top). Simultaneously, these mitochondria filled with calcein fluorescence, demonstrating permeabilization of the inner mitochondrial membrane to low-molecular-weight solutes, corresponding to onset of the MPT (Fig. 4B, bottom).

After 11 h of TNF-α treatment more than two-thirds of the mitochondria had undergone these changes (Fig. 5C), and after 12 h virtually all mitochondria were affected (Fig. 4D). Mitochondria in normal hepatocytes (not expressing the IκB superrepressor) treated with TNF-α did not depolarize or undergo MPT,

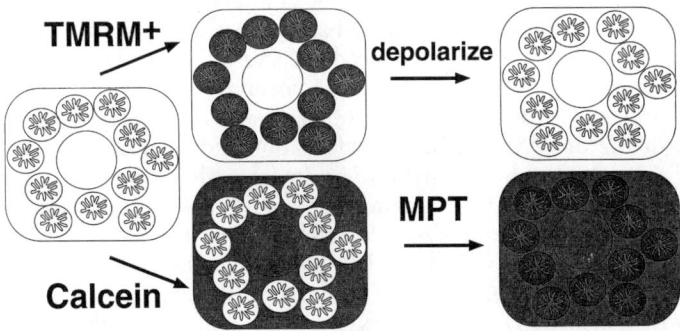

Figure 4 Confocal microscopy of hepatocytes to demonstrate the MPT and mitochondrial depolarization. MPT is demonstrated by calcein entering the mitochondria. Mitochondrial depolarization is demonstrated by loss of TMRM fluorescence in the mitochondria

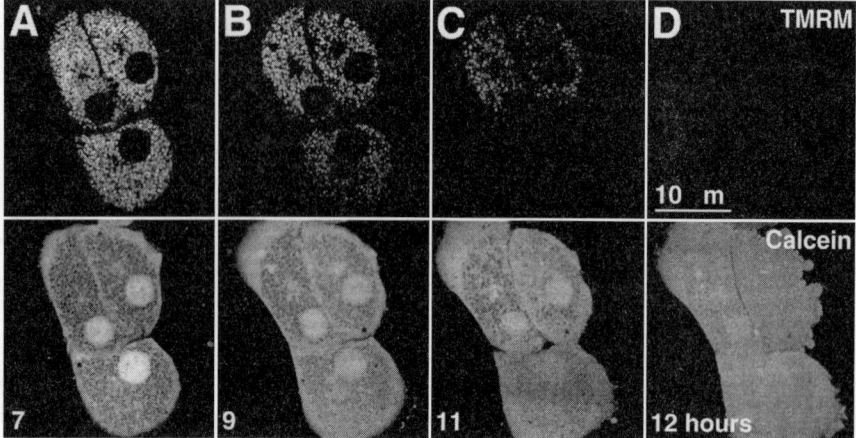

Figure 5 TNF-α induces MPT and mitochondrial depolarization in Ad5IκB-infected hepatocytes. Primary hepatocytes were treated with TNF-α (30 ng/ml) and then loaded with TMRM (top row) and calcein (bottom row). Red and green fluorescence was monitored simultaneously in living cells by confocal microscopy

since TMRM and calcein distributions did not change between 7 h and 13 h of treatment. Overall, these results show that the MPT and mitochondrial depolarization occurred in hepatocytes overexpressing the IκB superrepressor in response to TNF-α. These mitochondrial changes began in a subset of mitochondria between 7 and 9 h after TNF-α treatment and progressed to involve all mitochondria by 13 h of treatment.

NF-κB protects mouse hepatocytes from Fas-mediated apoptosis

To extend these studies into Fas-mediated apoptosis, we switched to primary cultures of adult mouse hepatocytes, since rat hepatocytes only express low levels of Fas. To study the role of NF-κB activation on Fas-mediated apoptosis, we treated mouse hepatocytes with anti-Fas agonist-like antibody Jo2. Ad5IκB plus Jo2 or ActD plus Jo2 rapidly induced massive cell death, whereas Jo2 alone had low cytotoxicity. Furthermore, Jo2 did not induce significant cell death in Ad5LacZ-infected hepatocytes (Fig. 6). The Ad5IκB-infected hepatocytes treated with Jo2 displayed nuclear condensation and fragmentation by propidium iodide staining, characteristic of apoptosis, while uninfected cells displayed normal nuclear morphology after Jo2 treatment. Apoptosis was confirmed by the detection of fragmented chromosome DNA in infected cells after exposure to TNF-α or Jo2. However, no DNA fragmentation was observed in the uninfected cells after Jo2 treatment. Furthermore, we confirmed the role of the IκB/NF-κB system in TNF-α and Fas-mediated apoptosis with a proteasome inhibitor, because proteasome inhibitors block IκB-α degradation and reduce NF-κB activation[34]. MG-132, a potent and specific proteasome inhibitor, promotes TNF-α and Fas-mediated apoptosis.

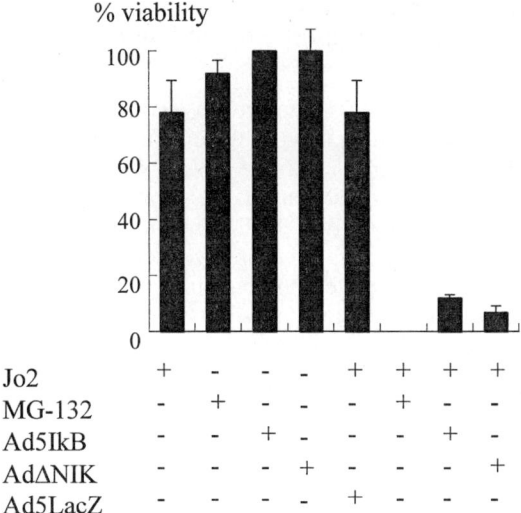

Jo2	+	-	-	-	+	+	+	+
MG-132	-	+	-	-	-	+	-	-
Ad5IkB	-	-	+	-	-	-	+	-
AdΔNIK	-	-	-	+	-	-	-	+
Ad5LacZ	-	-	-	-	+	-	-	-

Figure 6 Inhibition of NF-κB sensitizes hepatocytes to Fas-mediated apoptosis. Primary hepatocyte cultures were infected with Ad5IκB, Ad5ΔNIK, or control Ad5LacZ. Then the cells were not treated or treated with the anti-fas agonist antibody Jo2 or the proteasome inhibitor MG-132

The NF-κB-inducing kinase (NIK) has been identified as a TRAF2-interacting protein that signals for NF-κB activation[35]. Adenovirus (Ad5ΔNIK)-mediated overexpression of the C-terminal NIK fragment (NIKΔ2101) functions as a dominant-negative mutation. Ad5Δ NIK sensitized mouse hepatocytes to TNF-α and Fas-mediated cell death (Fig. 6). These results support a protective role for NF-κB activation in TNF-α and Fas-mediated apoptosis, and indicate that NIK is required for the activation of NF-κB by TNF-α or Fas.

TNF-α and Jo2 induce the MPT and mitochondrial depolarization in Ad5IκB-infected hepatocytes with different time-courses

Primary mouse hepatocytes were treated with TNF-α (30 ng/ml) or Jo2 (0.5 μg/ml) after Ad5IκB infection (30 MOI) and then loaded with calcein to monitor the MPT and TMRM to monitor mitochondrial depolarization. At 3 h after treatment of Jo2, some mitochondria filled with calcein fluorescence, demonstrating permeabilization of the inner mitochondrial membrane, corresponding to onset of the MPT. Simultaneously, these mitochondria lost TMRM fluorescence, indicating depolarization. Finally, after 3.5 h of exposure to Jo2, there was hepatotoxicity with extravasation of calcein. In contrast to Jo2 treatment, TNF-α treatment induced MPT and mitochondrial depolarization at 8–10 h in mouse hepatocytes. These results show that MPT is induced in both TNF-α and Jo2-mediated apoptosis, but at different time-courses.

The combination of cyclosporin A (CsA) and trifenoperazine (TFZ) blocks TNF-α-, but not Fas-mediated cell death in Ad5IκB-infected hepatocytes

To test the ability of CsA plus TFZ to protect against TNF-α and Fas-mediated apoptosis, primary mouse hepatocytes were infected with Ad5IκB and then treated with TNF-α (30 ng/ml) or Jo2 (0.5 μg/ml) with and without CsA (5 μM) and/or TFZ (12.5 μM). The combination of CsA and TFZ significantly protects Ad5IκB-infected hepatocytes from TNF-α-mediated apoptosis, but not from Fas-mediated apoptosis. Although multiple concentrations of CsA (1–10 μM) and TFZ (2.5–25 μM) were tested, the maximal protective effects of CsA plus TFZ on TNF-α and Fas-mediated apoptosis were observed at the above concentrations.

DISCUSSION

Fas and TNF-α are potent mediators of hepatotoxicity *in vivo* and in cultured cells. In our studies we confirmed that treatment of primary cultures of hepatocytes with Fas or TNF-α alone is insufficient to induce cell killing. Both agonists induce NF-κB activation, and this activation must be blocked to reveal an apoptotic pathway. We used four mechanisms for inhibiting NF-κB and each resulted in subsequent apoptosis: the IκB superrepressor, a proteasome inhibitor, a dominant-negative NIK, or the RNA inhibitor actinomycin D. The effectiveness of multiple different blocking agents, the specificity of the adenovirus vectors and the lack of toxicity of control adenoviral vectors provides strong support for the role of NF-κB as an anti-apoptotic pathway for both TNF-α and Fas.

Our studies are consistent with the pathway for TNF-α signal transduction in hepatocytes as outlined in Fig. 1. In this pathway TNF-α interacts with the type I receptor and the associated protein TRADD that in turn activates an upstream kinase in the MEKK family, most likely NIK. Activated NIK in turn activates the IKK signalasome, which in turn phosphorylates IκB-α or S32 and S36. The phosphorylated IκB-α is subsequently ubiquinated and undergoes degradation in proteosomes. The released NF-κB translocates to the nucleus, where it is responsible for the induction of anti-apoptotic genes. Through a separate pathway, TRADD interacts with FADD and activates caspase-8. The caspase-8 signal is transmitted to the mitochondria, through the activation of Bid[15], which produces the mitochondria permeability transition. The MPT is required for TNF-induced apoptosis. Following the MPT there is release of cytochrome-c from the mitochondria with subsequent activation of caspase-3 and then the nuclear changes of apoptosis.

Our studies demonstrate that TNF and Fas recruit similar pathways in hepatocytes, including FADD, the activation of caspase-3 and caspase-8, the induction of MPT, and cytochrome-c release. Thus, it appears that in hepatocytes Fas also induces NF-κB through the activation of NIK, the IKK complex, the phosphorylation and degradation of IκB and the release of NF-κB. Fas also activates FADD to activate caspase-8 which, via Bid[15], induces the MPT with release of cytochrome-c activation of caspase-3 and then again the nuclear apoptotic pathway (Fig. 2).

However, there are major differences between TNF-α and Fas signal transduction. The Fas signalling pathway for apoptosis is more rapid than for TNF-α. The inhibition of the MPT with CsA and TFZ blocks TNF-α-mediated apoptosis, but delays rather than prevents Fas-mediated apoptosis. The MPT markedly decreases cytochrome-c release, but only delays and does not block caspase-3 activation. These observations suggest that parallel pathways contribute to Fas-mediated apoptosis and that the MPT contributes an early and more rapid pathway to apoptotic cell killing, but there is an alternative MPT-independent pathway that also results in apoptosis.

Acknowledgements

This work was supported by Research Fellowships of the Japan Society for the Promotion of Science for Young Scientists (*to* E.H.), and National Institutes of Health Grants GM41804 (*to* D.A.B.), DK34987 (*to* D.A.B. and J.J.L.), AA11605 (*to* D.A.B. and J.J.L.), DK37034 (*to* J.J.L.), and AG07218 (*to* J.J.L.). We thank Dr Robert Currin for technical assistance with the confocal microscopy, and Dr Christian Jobin for supplying the reagents.

References

1. Hsu H, Xiong J, Goeddel DV. The TNF receptor 1-associated protein TRADD signals cell death and NF-kappaB activation. Cell. 1995;81:495–504.
2. Hsu H, Shu HB, Pan MG, Goeddel DV. TRADD–TRAF2 and TRADD–FADD interactions define two distinct TNF receptor 1 signal transduction pathways. Cell. 1996;84:299–308.
3. Ling L, Cao Z, Goeddel DV. NFκB-inducing kinase activates IKK-α by phosphorylation of ser-176. Proc Natl Acad Sci USA. 1998;95:3792–7.
4. Lee F, Peters R, Duang L, Maniatis T. MEKK1 activates both IκB kinase alpha and IκB kinase beta. Proc Natl Acad Sci USA. 1998;95:9319–24.
5. Lacronique V, Mignon A, Fabre M *et al.* Bcl-2 protects from lethal hepatic apoptosis induced by an anti-Fas antibody in mice. Nature Med. 1996;2:80–6.
6. Itoh N, Nagata S. A novel protein domain required for apoptosis. J Biol Chem. 1993;268:10932–7.
7. Tartaglia LA, Ayers T, Wong G, Goeddel DV. A novel domain within the 55 kD TNF receptor signals cell death. Cell. 1993;74:845–53.
8. Boldin MP, Goncharov TM, Goltsev YV, Wallach D. Involvement of MACH, a novel MORT1/FADD-interacting protease, in Fas/APO-1- and TNF receptor-induced cell death. Cell. 1996;85:803–15.
9. Muzio M, Chinnaiyan AM, Kischkel FC *et al.* FLICE, a novel FADD-homologous ICE/CED-3-like protease, is recruited to the CD95 (Fas/Apo-1) death-inducing signal complex. Cell. 1996;85:817–27.
10. Medema J, Scaffidi C, Kischkel FC *et al.* FLICE is activated by association with the CD95 death-inducing signaling complex (DISC). EMBO J. 1997;16:2794–804.
11. Chang H, Nishitoh H, Yang X, Ichijo H, Baltimore D. Activation of apoptosis signal-regulating kinase 1 (ASK1) by the adapter protein Daxx. Science. 1998;281:1860–3.
12. Luo X, Budihardjo I, Zou H *et al.* Bid, a Bcl-2 interacting protein, mediates cytochrome *c* release from mitochondria in response to activation of cell surface death receptors. Cell. 1998;94:481–90.
13. Li H, Zhu H, Xu C, Yuan J. Cleavage of BID by caspase 8 mediates the mitochondrial damage in the Fas pathway of apoptosis. Cell. 1998;94:491–501.
14. Gross A. Caspase-cleaved BID targets mitochondria and is required for cytochrome *c* release, while BCL-XL prevents this release but not tumor necrosis factor-R1/Fas death. J Biol Chem. 1999;274:1156–63.
15. Yin X-M, Wang K, Gross A *et al.* Bid-deficient mice are resistant to Fas-induced hepatocellular apoptosis. Nature. 1999;400:886–91.

16. Enari M, Sakahira H, Yokoyama H *et al*. A caspase-activated DNase that degrades DNA during apoptosis, and its inhibitor ICAD. Nature. 1998;391:143–50.
17. Scaffidi C, Fulda S, Srivastava A *et al*. Two CD95 (Apo-1/Fas) signaling pathways. EMBO J. 1998;17:1675–87.
18. Romashkova J, Makarov S. NF-κB is a target of AKT in anti-apoptotic PDGF signaling. Nature. 1999;401:86–90.
19. Wang C-Y, Mayo MW, Korneluk RG, Goeddel DV, Baldwin Jr AS. NF-κB antiapoptosis: induction of TRAF1 and TRAF2 and c-IAP1 and c-IAP2 to suppress caspase-8 activation. Science. 1998;281:1680–3.
20. Wu M, Ao Z, Prasad K, Wu R, Schlossman SF. IEX-1L, an apoptosis inhibitor involved in NF-κB-mediated cell survival. Science. 1998;281:998–1001.
21. Kim YM, Talanian R, Billiar TR. Nitric oxide inhibits apoptosis by preventing increases in caspase-3-like activity via two distinct mechanisms. J Biol Chem. 1997; 272:31138–48.
22. Deveraux Q, Reed JC. IAP family proteins – suppressors of apoptosis. Genes Dev. 1999;13: 239–52.
23. Lemasters JJ. Mechanisms of hepatic toxicity. V. Necrapoptosis and the mitochondrial permeability transition: shared pathways to necrosis and apoptosis. Am J Physiol. 1999;276:G1–6.
24. Bradham CA, Qian T, Streetz K, Brenner D, Lemasters JJ. The mitochondrial permeability transition is required for TNF-α-mediated apoptosis and cytochrome *c* release. Mol Cell Biol. 1998;18:6353–64.
25. Moldeus P, Hogberg J, Orrenius S. Isolation and use of liver cells. Methods Enzymol. 1978;52:60–71.
26. Bradham CA, Qian T, Streetz K, Trautwein C, Brenner DA, Lemasters JJ. The mitochondrial permeability transition is required for tumor necrosis factor α-mediated apoptosis and cytochrome *c* release. Mol Cell Biol. 1998;18:6353–64.
27. Iimuro Y, Nishiura T, Hellerbrand C *et al*. NFκB prevents apoptosis and liver dysfunction during liver regeneration. J Clin Invest. 1998;101:802–11.
28. Qian T, Nieminen A, Herman B, Lemasters JJ. Mitochondrial permeability transition in pH-dependent reperfusion injury to rat hepatocytes. Am J Physiol. 1997;273:C1783–92.
29. Leist M, Gantner F, Bohlinger I, Germann P, Tiegs G, Wendel A. Murine hepatocyte apoptosis induced *in vitro* and *in vivo* by TNF-α requires transcriptional arrest. J Immunol. 1994;153: 1778–87.
30. Wang CY, Mayo MW, Baldwin Jr AS. TNF- and cancer therapy-induced apoptosis: potentiation by inhibition of NF-kappaB. Science. 1996;274:784–7.
31. Ray CA, Black RA, Kronheim SR *et al*. Viral inhibition of inflammation: cowpox virus encodes an inhibitor of the interleukin-1B converting enzyme. Cell. 1992;69:597–604.
32. Nieminen A, Saylor AK, Tesfai SA, Herman B, Lemasters JJ. Contribution of the mitochondrial permeability transition to lethal injury after exposure of hepatocytes to *t*-butylhydroperoxide. Biochem J. 1995;307:99–106.
33. Lemasters JJ, Nieminen A, Qian T, Trost LC, Herman B. The mitochondrial permeability transition in toxic, hypoxic and reperfusion injury. Mol Cell Biochem. 1997;174:159–65.
34. Jobin C, Hellerbrand C, Licato LL, Brenner DA, Sartor RB. Mediation by NFκB of cytokine induced expression of intercellular adhesion molecule 1 (ICAM-1) in an intestinal epithelial cell line, a process blocked by proteasome inhibitors. Gut. 1998;42:779–87.
35. Malinin NL, Boldin MP, Kovalenko AV, Wallach D. MAP3K-related kinase involved in NFκB induction by TNF, CD95 and IL-1. Nature. 1997;385:540–4.

31
Glutathione homeostasis in liver regeneration

S. C. LU

INTRODUCTION

Glutathione (GSH) is an essential tripeptide and the most abundant intracellular non-protein thiol. It is involved in numerous cellular processes ranging from antioxidant defence to cell growth. This review deals with changes in GSH homeostasis during liver regeneration. A brief discussion on the structure, functions and determinants of hepatic GSH homeostasis is in order prior to describing changes that occur during liver regeneration.

STRUCTURE AND FUNCTIONS OF GSH

Glutathione is a ubiquitous tripeptide, γ-glutamylcysteinyl glycine, found in all mammalian tissues, and is particularly concentrated in the liver. Glutathione exists in the thiol-reduced (GSH) and disulphide-oxidized (GSSG) forms[1]. Eucaryotic cells have three major reservoirs of GSH. Almost 90% of cellular GSH are in the cytosol, 10% is in the mitochondria and a small percentage is in the endoplasmic reticulum[2–4]. In the endoplasmic reticulum, where GSH is implicated in protein disulphide bond formation, the GSH to GSSG ratio[2] is 3:1. In the cytoplasm and mitochondria, ratios[3,4] exceed 10:1. Cytosolic GSH in the rat liver turns over rapidly with a half-life of 1–2 h, whereas mitochondrial GSH turns over with a half-life of 18 min[5].

Two structural aspects of GSH are important for its intracellular stability and function (Fig. 1). The peptide bond linking the N-terminal glutamate and the cysteine residue of GSH is through the γ-carboxyl group of glutamate rather than the conventional α-carboxyl group. This unusual arrangement resists degradation by intracellular peptidases and is subject to hydrolysis by only one known enzyme, namely γ-glutamyltranspeptidase, which is on the external surfaces of certain cell types[1,4]. Furthermore, the C-terminal glycine moiety of GSH protects the molecule against cleavage by intracellular γ-glutamylcyclotransferase[4]. As a consequence, GSH resists intracellular degradation and is only metabolized

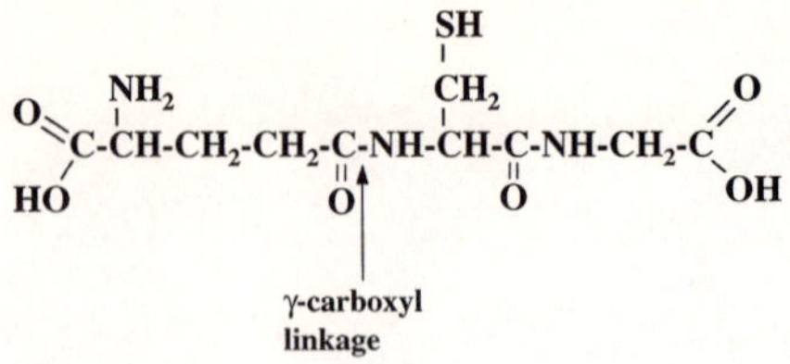

Figure 1 The structure of glutathione, γ-glutamylcysteinyl glycine. The N-terminal glutamate and cysteine are linked by the γ-carboxyl group of glutamate

extracellularly. Extracellular breakdown of GSH liberates cysteine, which is then available for uptake. The sulphydryl group of GSH is intimately involved in the multiple functions of GSH described below.

GSH serves several vital functions including (1) detoxifying electrophiles, (2) maintaining the essential thiol status of proteins by preventing oxidation of –SH groups or by reducing disulphide bonds induced by oxidant stress, (3) scavenging free radicals, (4) providing a reservoir for cysteine, and (5) modulating critical cellular processes such as DNA synthesis, microtubular-related processes, and immune function[1,4,6,7].

BIOSYNTHESIS AND HOMEOSTASIS OF HEPATIC GSH

The liver has one of the highest organ contents of GSH (~6 mM) and is unique in two aspects of GSH biosynthesis. First, the hepatocyte has the unique ability to convert methionine to cysteine through the transsulphuration pathway[1]; and second, the rate of GSH biosynthesis in the hepatocyte is balanced by its rate of export into plasma, bile and mitochondria via distinct GSH transport systems[5,8]. The mitochondrial GSH transporter maintains the GSH pool in the mitochondria, which cannot biosynthesize GSH[8,9]. Pathways that consume GSH, such as formation of GSH conjugates and mixed disulphides, account for very little of the hepatocyte GSH utilization under normal physiological conditions. The importance of hepatic GSH to the inter-organ GSH homeostasis is underscored by the fact that plasma GSH and cysteine levels are largely determined by the sinusoidal efflux of hepatic GSH[5]. Therefore, perturbations of hepatic GSH homeostasis will probably impact on systemic GSH homeostasis. Figure 2 illustrates hepatic GSH homeostasis.

GSH is synthesized from precursor amino acids in the cytosol of virtually all cells[1,4,8]. The synthesis of GSH from its constituent amino acids, L-glutamate, L-cysteine, and L-glycine, involves two ATP-requiring enzymatic steps. In the first and rate-limiting step catalysed by γ-glutamylcysteine synthetase (GCS), glutamate and cysteine are conjugated to form γ-glutamylcysteine. In the second step catalysed by GSH synthetase, GSH is formed from conjugation of γ-glutamylcysteine and glycine. The rate of GSH synthesis is regulated physiologically by two determinants, the activity of the rate-limiting enzyme

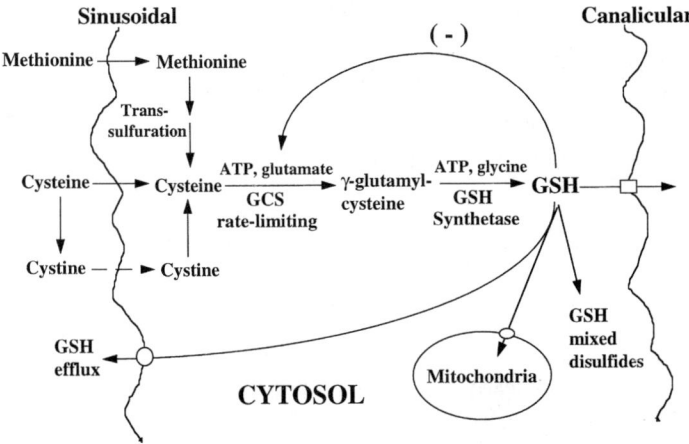

Figure 2 Hepatic GSH homeostasis. Under normal physiological conditions the cellular homeostasis of GSH is maintained by a balance between synthesis and export or utilization such as formation of GSH mixed disulphides. In hepatocytes, cysteine can be derived from uptake of cysteine, cystine or methionine. Normal liver cells do not appear to take up cystine, but this transporter can be induced in culture and under oxidative stress[1]. Methionine is converted to cysteine via the transsulphuration pathway which is limited to a few cell types only[1]. In hepatocytes, efflux of GSH occurs into both the sinusoidal blood and canalicular bile by carrier-mediated mechanisms. There is also a mitochondrial GSH transporter that transports GSH from the cytosol to the mitochondria, where it also plays a major defensive role against oxidative stress

γ-glutamylcysteine synthetase (GCS) and the availability of cysteine[1,4]. The activity of GCS is in turn regulated by the amount of GSH present as GSH exerts a competitive feedback inhibition on GCS[10] with a K_i value[1] of about 2 mM. The apparent K_m values of GCS for glutamate and cysteine are 1.8 and 0.1–0.3 mM, respectively in both rat and human[11,12]. The intracellular glutamate concentration is several-fold higher than the K_m value of GCS for glutamate but the intracellular cysteine concentration approximates the apparent K_m value of GCS for cysteine[1]. Therefore, the availability of intracellular cysteine can influence the rate of GSH synthesis.

Cysteine is derived normally from the diet, protein breakdown and in the liver, from methionine via the transsulphuration pathway[1,13]. Cysteine differs from other amino acids because its sulphydryl form, cysteine, is predominant inside the cell whereas its disulphide form, cystine, is predominant outside the cell. Cysteine readily autoxidizes to cystine in the extracellular fluid and cystine, once it enters the cell, is rapidly reduced to cysteine[13]. Therefore, the key factors that regulate the hepatocellular level of cysteine other than diet include membrane transport of cysteine, cystine and methionine, the activity of the transsulphuration pathway and cysteine breakdown[1,13]. Although glutamate and glycine are also precursors of GSH there is no evidence to suggest their transport influences GSH synthesis, since they are synthesized via several metabolic pathways within hepatocytes[13].

GCS STRUCTURE AND REGULATION

GCS is composed of a heavy (GCS-HS, Mr ~ 73 000) and a light (GCS-LS, Mr ~ 30 000) subunit which are encoded by different genes in both rat and human[14–17]. The enzyme may be dissociated under non-denaturing conditions by treatment with dithiothreitol[18]. The heavy subunit obtained after this treatment exhibits all of the catalytic activity of the isolated enzyme as well as feedback inhibition by GSH[18]. Although the heavy subunit is active catalytically, it has a higher K_m value for glutamate (18.2 vs. 1.4 mM) and a lower K_i value for GSH (1.8 vs. 8.2 mM) as compared to the holoenzyme[19]. Thus, the light subunit plays an important regulatory role for the overall function of the enzyme and allows the holoenzyme to be catalytically more efficient and less subject to inhibition by GSH than the heavy subunit alone.

Recent studies have clearly established the importance of GCS in the overall cellular GSH homeostasis. Changes in GCS activity can result from regulation at multiple levels affecting only the heavy or both the heavy and light subunits. Transcriptional and post-transcriptional regulation of both subunits have been described. This topic has been recently reviewed[1] and will not be discussed further except in the context of liver regeneration.

RELATIONSHIP BETWEEN GSH LEVEL AND CELL PROLIFERATION *IN VITRO*

Many studies involving lymphocytes and fibroblasts showed that an increased GSH level was associated with an early proliferative response and was essential for the cell to enter the S phase[20–26]. However, other studies using CHO cells and various tumour cells did not find a correlation between GSH levels and cell cycle progression[27,28]. To discover whether GSH level correlates with cell cycle in hepatocytes, we first used an *in-vitro* model of liver regeneration, namely plating adult hepatocytes under low cell density, and examined changes in the parameters important for GSH homeostasis[29]. Primary cultures of adult rat hepatocytes shift into the growth phase (G_0 to G_1) when plated at low density (LD)[30–33]. In culture, growth and functions of liver cells are known to be regulated reciprocally by cell density: at high cell density liver-specific functions are expressed and growth is suppressed, whereas the opposite is true at lower cell density[30–33]. We found that, as early as 2 h after plating, there is a striking inverse relationship between cell density and cell GSH[29]. The lower the cell density, the higher the cell GSH (Fig. 3). The increase in cell GSH under LD occurred in the absence of any growth factors or hormones and in either collagen- or matrigel-precoated dishes[29]. The mechanisms involved an increase in the specific activity of GCS and higher cysteine levels at LD, which were blocked by cycloheximide and actinomycin D. By co-culturing cells of different density, thus allowing the medium to mix, the increase in GCS activity under LD was blocked when co-cultured with high-density cells, whereas the increase in cysteine level was unaffected. Thus, the availability of cysteine appears to be regulated by cell–cell contact, whereas the activity of GCS may be modulated by soluble factor(s). In follow-up studies we found the effect of plating under LD on GCS activity was

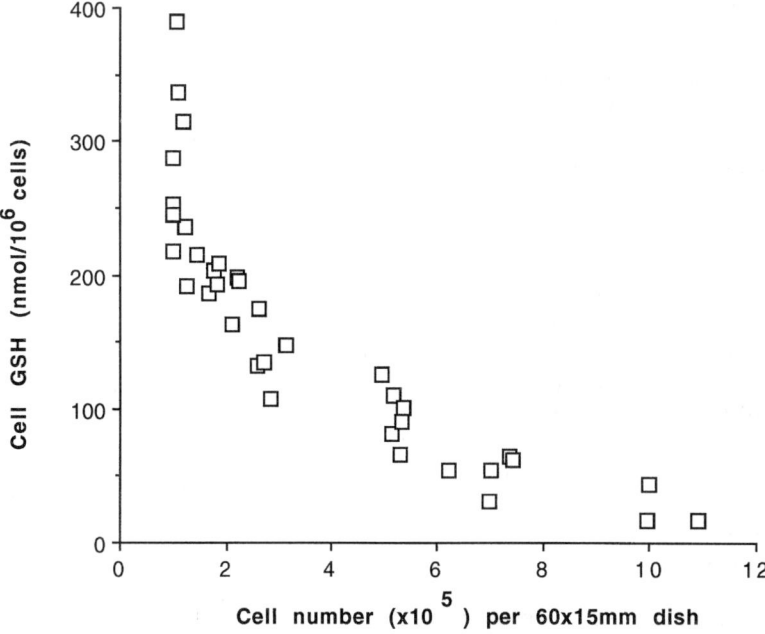

Figure 3 Effects of plating cell density on GSH of cultured rat hepatocytes. Varying numbers of cells in 5 ml DME/F12 + methionine (1 mM) medium were plated on 60 × 15 mm collagen-precoated dishes for 20 h. Data represent combined results of five different experiments

exerted at the gene transcriptional level of GCS-HS[34] without any influence on the gene expression of GCS-LS[35]. This suggests that, in hepatocytes, there may be more light subunit present since alteration in the heavy subunit alone changed the GCS activity and GSH level.

CHANGES IN GSH HOMEOSTASIS DURING LIVER REGENERATION AFTER TWO-THIRDS PARTIAL HEPATECTOMY (PH)

To extrapolate our findings in culture to an appropriate *in-vivo* model, we chose the liver regeneration model after two-thirds PH. Earlier studies showed that transitory elevation in cellular GSH occurred in regenerating rat liver and may have been partially responsible for resistance against several hepatotoxins during liver regeneration following PH[36,37]. More recent studies also showed increased hepatic GSH, although the timing of the increase varied from 24 to 48 h[38,39]. Since DNA synthesis begins around 12 h and peaks around 24 h after hepatectomy[40], whether the increase in GSH precedes or is concurrent with DNA synthesis is unclear. Interestingly, the increase in GSH occurs concurrent with a reduction in enzymes involved in drug and xenobiotic metabolism, including cytochrome P450 and certain glutathione *S*-transferases during the initial phase of liver regeneration[38,41]. Thus, there appears to be a shift from xenobiotic metabolism to increased antioxidant defence.

In our study we examined both biosynthesis of GSH and GSH export[42], two major determinants of GSH homeostasis. Both sinusoidal and canalicular GSH transport are sensitive to membrane potential[8], and a rapid, prolonged depolarization of the membrane potential has been described after hepatectomy[43]. Thus, we were interested to see whether sinusoidal and biliary GSH transport is altered during liver regeneration.

Changes in liver GSH, cysteine levels and DNA synthesis after two-thirds PH

As shown in Fig. 4, both total liver GSH and cysteine levels doubled at 12 h post-PH when compared to sham controls. GSSG levels also increased, but the ratio of GSH to GSSG remained unchanged at ~105–110. At 12 h post-PH, DNA synthesis had not yet begun. Liver GSH level remained doubled at 24 h post-PH, liver cysteine level was still elevated as compared to sham controls but the magnitude of increase was lower than at 12 h (~ 60% increase), and at this time DNA synthesis had increased. By 36 h post-PH, liver GSH level had returned to baseline and liver cysteine level was still slightly elevated[42]. Thus, our study established the temporal relationship of the rise in GSH and cysteine levels to DNA synthesis.

Mechanisms for the increase in liver GSH level after two-thirds PH

GSH export

An increase in the steady-state liver GSH level can result from increased biosynthesis of GSH, decreased GSH utilization intracellularly or decreased GSH export. We measured GSH efflux using the *in-situ* perfused liver model. Perfusions were adjusted for the liver size and the rates of perfusion; O_2 uptakes were not different among the different groups and the values compare closely to those reported previously[42]. Figure 5 summarizes our results regarding changes in GSH efflux, either expressed as per gram liver or per 100 g body weight. When expressed as per gram liver there is no change in sinusoidal efflux at 12 and 24 h after PH. However, expressed as per 100 g body weight, it is clear that the total systemic output of GSH is markedly impaired. Biliary efflux was significantly reduced regardless of how it is expressed. Paracellular permeability is increased after PH[42], which may account for part of the fall in biliary GSH efflux. Hepatic sinusoidal GSH efflux provides a systemic source of GSH and cysteine and is critical to the inter-organ homeostasis of GSH[8]; whereas canalicular GSH efflux is critical in the maintenance of intestinal mucosal GSH homeostasis as diversion of bile in rats leads to a 50% decrease in mucosal GSH level[44]. Thus, the changes in GSH export may impair both systemic and intestinal GSH and cysteine availability.

GSH synthesis capacity

In the cell culture model, increased GSH level was due to increased cysteine availability and GCS activity. The same is also true in the *in-vivo* model. Figure 6 shows that hepatic GCS activity also increased markedly at 12 h post-PH and returned to normal level by 24 h post-PH. To see whether the increase in GCS

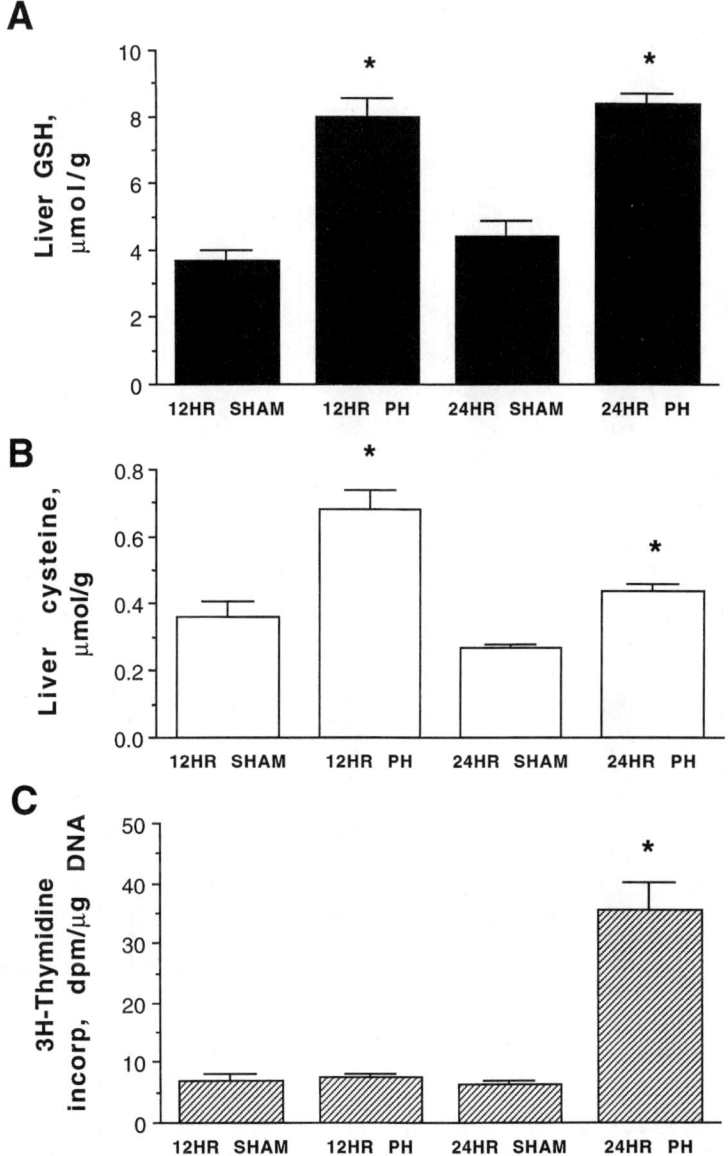

Figure 4 Changes in liver total GSH (**A**), cysteine (**B**) and DNA synthesis (**C**) after two-thirds partial hepatectomy (PH). Male Sprague-Dawley rats underwent two-thirds PH and had liver GSH, cysteine levels measured and DNA synthesis determined at 12 and 24 h afterwards. Control animals had sham operation. Results represent mean ± SE from three to eight animals in each group. *$p < 0.05$ vs. respective sham control groups by ANOVA followed by Fisher's test

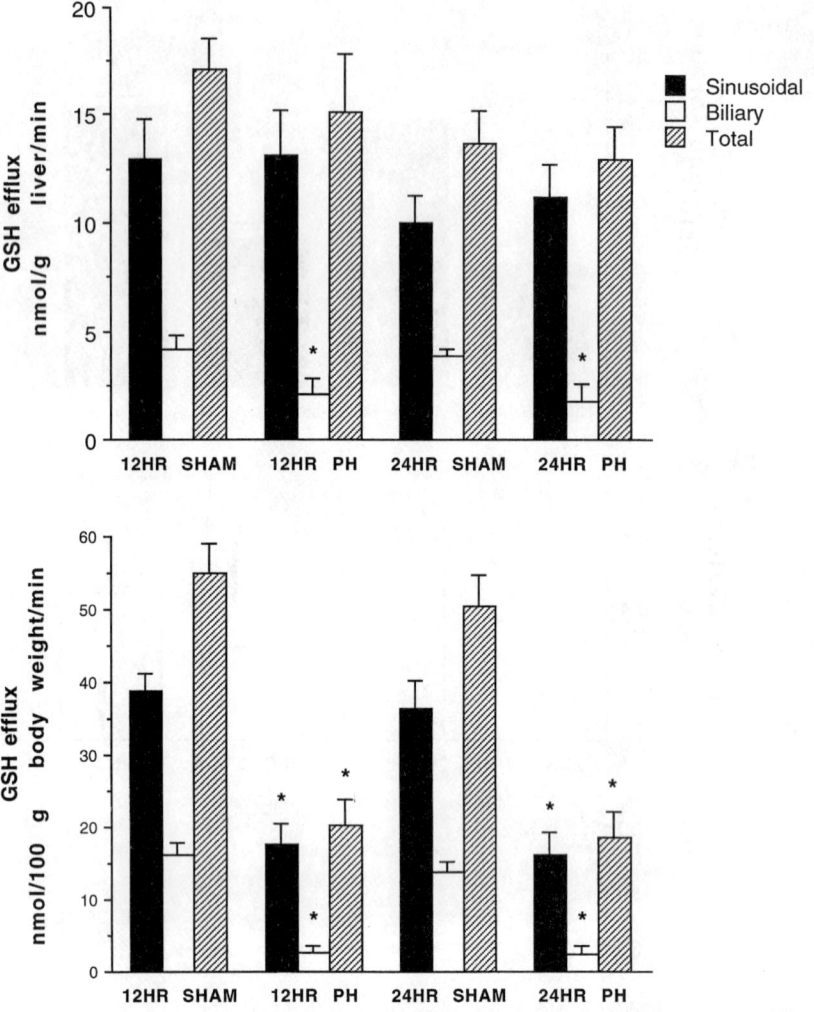

Figure 5 Changes in GSH efflux during liver regeneration. Male Sprague-Dawley rats underwent two-thirds PH or sham operation, and GSH efflux was determined using *in-situ* liver perfusions between 7 and 11 a.m. as described[42]. GSH efflux is expressed as either per gram liver (top panel) or per 100 g body weight (bottom panel). Results represent mean ± SE from three to five animals in each group. *$p < 0.05$ vs. respective sham-operated controls by ANOVA followed by Fisher's test

activity is a result of an increase in the amount of GCS enzyme, we next examined steady-state mRNA levels of the GCS subunits. The mRNA level of the heavy subunit of GCS was increased nearly 3-fold at 12 h post-PH and returned to baseline by 24 h post-PH (Fig. 7) but that of the light subunit was unchanged (Fig. 8). Western blotting analysis confirmed the increase in GCS-HS protein level at 12 h post-PH (Fig. 7).

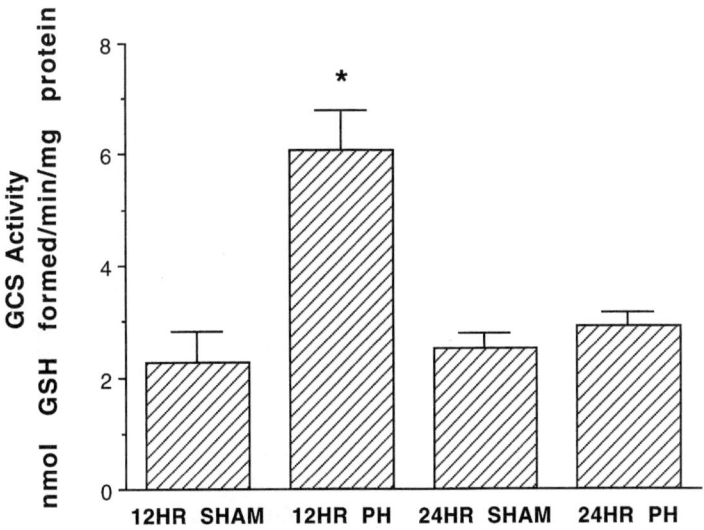

Figure 6 Changes in GCS activity after two-thirds PH. GCS activity was measured in liver cytosol of hepatectomized and sham-operated rats at 12 and 24 h post-surgery. Results represent mean ± SE from three to five animals in each group. *$p < 0.05$ vs. sham control group by ANOVA followed by Fisher's test

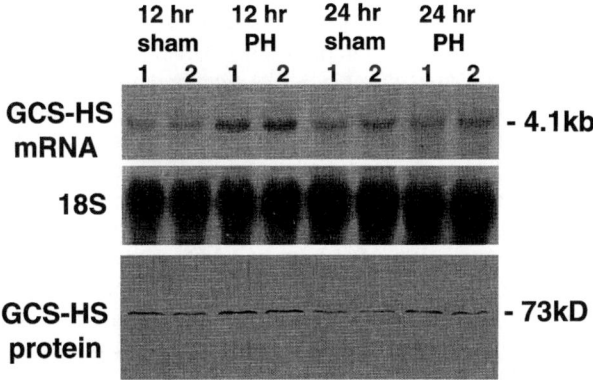

Figure 7 Steady-state GCS-HS mRNA and protein levels in hepatectomized and sham-operated controls 12 and 24 h after surgery. Top panel shows the steady-state GCS-HS mRNA level. Liver RNA (30 μg each lane) samples were analysed by Northern blot hybridization with a ^{32}P-labelled GCS-HS cDNA probe. The same membrane was then rehybridized with a ^{32}P-labelled 18S cDNA probe. The molecular size markers, GCS-HS (~ 4.1 kb) and 18S are as indicated. The bottom panel depicts the steady-state GCS-HS protein level. Liver cytosols (25 μg/lane) were subjected to SDS-PAGE followed by immunoblotting with anti-GCS-HS antibodies. Molecular weight marker (in kDa) is shown on the right. The bands at 73 kDa represent GCS-HS

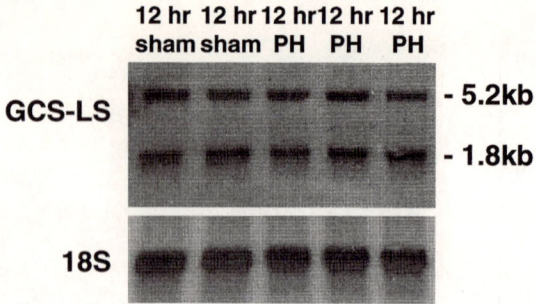

Figure 8 Steady-state GCS-LS mRNA level in hepatectomized and sham-operated controls 12 h after surgery. Poly(A)-RNA (4 μg each lane) were analysed by Northern blot hybridization with GCS-LS and 18S cDNA probes. The molecular size markers, GCS-LS (~ 5.2 and 1.8 kb) and 18S are as indicated

The increase in cysteine level may reflect an increase in cysteine transport via systems ASC and A, as well as an increase in the conversion of methionine to cysteine[39,45]. This, along with an increase in GCS activity, resulted in increased liver GSH at 12 h after PH. The increase in GCS activity is short-lived, however, so that at 24 h after PH it is the increased cysteine availability that appears to be mainly responsible for the increase in GSH.

Significance of the increase in hepatic GSH during liver regeneration

We have recently examined the effect of preventing the increase in liver GSH level on subsequent liver regeneration, as well as the effect of depleting liver GSH on liver regeneration. Many conditions, including chronic alcoholic and non-alcoholic liver diseases[46] and diabetic mellitus[12], have lower hepatic GSH level, so that whether a lower hepatic GSH level hinders liver regeneration becomes an important question. GSH was depleted and synthesis inhibited by the use of buthionine sulphoximine (BSO), an irreversible inhibitor of GCS[4]. Two different regimens were used. First was 900 mg/kg intraperitoneally given 45 min prior to PH and repeated 12 h later, once. This kept the starting GSH level relatively normal and prevented the increase in GSH after PH. The second regimen was 667 mg/kg intraperitoneally given 6 h prior to PH and repeated q. 12 h × 2. This led to a 50% lower starting liver GSH level and prevented the increase in GSH after PH (see Table 1). When sham animals received the same doses of BSO, much more profound depletion in liver GSH occurred 24 h later (data not shown). BSO-treated sham animals did not differ from sham controls in [³H]thymidine incorporation into DNA.

Table 1 summarizes the results of our observations. If the starting liver GSH was kept relatively normal (BSO1) and the increase in GSH prevented, there was a 33% inhibition in DNA synthesis. However, if the starting liver GSH was already 50% depleted and the increase also prevented (BSO2), then DNA synthesis was inhibited by nearly 60%. BSO treatment also blunted or prevented the increase in cysteine (Table 1), which may be due to decreased cysteine uptake as reported by others[47]. Finally, we examined what effect a lower hepatic GSH

Table 1 Effect of BSO on liver GSH, cysteine levels and DNA synthesis after two-thirds PH in the rat

Condition	Liver GSH ($\mu mol/g$)		Liver cysteine ($\mu mol/g$)		[³H]thymidine incorporation
	Time 0	At sacrifice	Time 0	At sacrifice	(dpm/μg DNA)
Sham		4.38 ± 0.49		0.27 ± 0.01	6.35 ± 0.58
Two-thirds PH	6.2 ± 0.23	8.37 ± 0.31*	0.24 ± 0.01	0.44 ± 0.02*	35.5 ± 4.68*
BSO1	4.97 ± 0.26[†]	2.63 ± 0.5[†]	0.25 ± 0.01	0.34 ± 0.04[†]	23.7 ± 4.72[†]
BSO2	2.92 ± 0.53[††]	1.95 ± 0.33[††]	0.21 ± 0.02	0.25 ± 0.02[††]	14.6 ± 2.52[††]

Results represent mean ± SE from five to nine animals for each condition. All animals were fed ad lib and two-thirds PH was performed between 10 and 11 a.m.; animals were sacrificed 24 h later. Methods used for GSH, cysteine and DNA synthesis assays have been previously described[42]. BSO1 = animals received BSO 900 mg/kg intraperitoneally 45 min prior to PH and repeated 12 h later. BSO2 = animals received BSO 667 mg/kg intraperitoneally 6 h prior to PH and repeated every 12 h twice.

*$p < 0.05$ vs. sham-operated control; [†] $p < 0.05$ vs. two-thirds PH controls; [††] $p < 0.05$ vs. two-thirds PH controls and BSO1 group by ANOVA followed by Fisher's test.

Table 2 Effect of initial GSH depletion on the course of liver regeneration

Condition	Percentage liver regeneration	Liver GSH (μmol/g)		Liver cysteine (μmol/g)		Total liver DNA (mg)	
		Time 0	At sacrifice	Time 0	At sacrifice	Time 0	At sacrifice
PH-3D	56 ± 3	5.39 ± 0.1	6.38 ± 0.43	0.24 ± 0.01	0.35 ± 0.02*	20 ± 0.9	16 ± 0.5
PH-7D	106 ± 7	4.82 ± 0.3	5.42 ± 0.1	0.28 ± 0.01	0.25 ± 0.03	19 ± 0.8	25 ± 0.5
BSO-3D	45 ± 2†	1.77 ± 0.21†	5.30 ± 0.5*	0.19 ± 0.01	0.28 ± 0.01	19 ± 1	13 ± 0.5†
BSO-7D	86 ± 2†	2.91 ± 0.6†	4.6 ± 0.23*	0.26 ± 0.04	0.31 ± 0.03	22 ± 0.5	18 ± 1.3†

Results represent mean ± SE from three animals each. All animals were fed ad lib and two-thirds PH was performed between 10 and 11 a.m. All animals were sacrificed between 10 and 11 a.m. either 3 (3D) or 7 days (7D) after PH. BSO-treated animals received BSO 667 mg/kg intraperitoneally 6 h prior to PH and repeated every 12 h twice.

* $p < 0.05$ vs. time 0 by paired t-test; † $p < 0.05$ vs. respective PH control groups (3D or 7D) by ANOVA followed by Fisher's test.

level, and preventing the increase in GSH, had on the course of liver regenera-tion. Rats were treated with BSO2 or vehicle and followed for up to 7 days. As summarized in Table 2, although initial hepatic GSH was much lower in the BSO-treated groups, by the third day after PH the levels were not significantly different from the control group. There was also no toxicity of BSO since both groups of rats lost and gained comparable amounts of weight by 3 and 7 days after PH (data not shown). Liver regeneration was complete by the seventh day in the control group but 20% lower in the BSO-treated group. Similarly, total liver DNA amount was 20–28% lower in the BSO-treated group at 3 and 7 days after PH. Thus, just by the initial lowering of liver GSH and preventing the initial increase in GSH, the long-term course of regeneration was affected.

SPECULATIONS ON THE ROLE OF GSH IN CELL PROLIFERATION

Some speculations can be made about the significance of the increase in hepatic GSH and cysteine levels prior to DNA synthesis. The requirement for increased GSH or thiols prior to DNA synthesis may be related to the fact that prolif-erating cells require increased amounts of pentoses and thiols. DNA synthesis depends absolutely on the formation of pentoses and on their conversion into deoxyribose by ribonucleotide reductase[48]. The activity of this rate-limiting enzyme in DNA synthesis requires reduced glutaredoxin or thioredoxin, which are maintained by GSH with concomitant oxidation to GSSG via glutathione reductase or oxidation of NADPH via thioredoxin reductase, respectively. Alternatively, an increase in the cellular GSH content may change the thiol-redox status of the cell[7], which is proportional to $[GSH]^2/[GSSG]$. A change in the redox state may then affect the expression or activity of factors important for cell cycle progression. Further studies will be required to examine these possibilities.

CONCLUDING REMARKS

Despite the importance of GSH in numerous cellular functions, its role in cell proliferation remains ill-defined. Our studies demonstrate clearly that hepatic GSH level correlates with liver growth, an increase is observed prior to the start of DNA synthesis after two-thirds PH. This increase in hepatic GSH during liver regeneration can be accounted for by both an increase in the availability of cys-teine and the activity of GCS. Changes in GSH export that occur during liver regeneration may impair systemic and intestinal GSH and cysteine availability. Studies with BSO treatments suggest normal and subsequent increase in GSH levels may both be important for normal liver regeneration to occur. Elucidation of the exact molecular mechanisms is important, and may impact on the course of liver regeneration.

Acknowledgements

This work was supported by NIH grant DK-45334 and Professional Staff Association Grant 6-268-0-0, USC School of Medicine. *In-situ* liver perfusions were performed by the Organelle/Perfusion Core of the USC Liver Disease Research Center (NIH DK48522).

References

1. Lu SC. Regulation of hepatic glutathione synthesis: Current concept and controversies. FASEB J. 1999;13:1169–83.
2. Hwang C, Sinsky AJ, Lodish HF. Oxidized redox state of glutathione in the endoplasmic reticulum. Science. 1992;257:1496–502.
3. Meredith MJ, Reed DJ. Status of the mitochondrial pool of glutathione in the isolated hepatocyte. J Biol Chem. 1982;257:3747–53.
4. Meister A. Glutathione. In: Aria IM, Jakoby WB, Popper H, Schachter D, Shafritz DA, editors. The Liver: Biology and Pathobiology, 2nd edn. New York: Raven Press; 1988:401–17.
5. Ookhtens M, Kaplowitz N. Role of the liver in interorgan homeostasis of glutathione and cysteine. Sem Liver Dis. 1998;18:313–29.
6. Suthanthiran M, Anderson ME, Sharma VK, Meister A. Glutathione regulates activation-dependent DNA synthesis in highly purified normal human T lymphocytes stimulated via the CD2 and CD3 antigens. Proc Natl Acad Sci USA. 1990;87:3343–7.
7. Hutter DE, Till BG, Greene JJ. Redox state changes in density-dependent regulation of proliferation. Exp Cell Res. 1997;232:435–8.
8. Fernández-Checa J, Lu SC, Ookhetens M et al. The regulation of hepatic glutathione. In: Tavoloni N, Berk PD, editors. Hepatic Anion Transport and Bile Secretion: Physiology and Pathophysiology. New York: Marcel Dekker;1992:363–95.
9. Feríndez-Checa J, Kaplowitz N, Garcia-Ruiz C et al. GSH transport in mitochondria: defense against TNF-induced oxidative stress and alcohol-induced defect. Am J Physiol. 1997;273: G7–17.
10. Huang CS, Moore WR, Meister A. On the active site thiol of γ-glutamylcysteine synthetase: relationship to catalysis, inhibition, and regulation. Proc Natl Acad Sci USA. 1988;85:2464–8.
11. Misra I, Griffith OW. Expression and purification of human γ-glutamylcysteine synthetase. Protein Exp Purif. 1998;13:268–76.
12. Lu SC, Ge J, Kuhlenkamp J, Kaplowitz N. Insulin and glucocorticoid dependence of hepatic γ-glutamylcysteine synthetase and GSH synthesis in the rat: Studies in cultured hepatocytes and in vivo. J Clin Invest. 1992;90:524–32.
13. Bannai S, Ishii T, Takada A et al. Regulation of glutathione level by amino acid transport. In: Taniguchi N, Higashi T, Sakamoto Y et al., editors. Glutathione Centennial. San Diego: Academic Press; 1989:407–21.
14. Yan N, Meister A. Amino acid sequence of rat kidney γ-glutamylcysteine synthetase. J Biol Chem. 1990;265:1588–93.
15. Huang C, Anderson ME, Meister A. Amino acid sequence and function of the light subunit of rat kidney γ-glutamylcysteine synthetase. J Biol Chem. 1993;268:20578–83.
16. Gipp JJ, Chang C, Mulcahy RT. Cloning and nucleotide sequence of a full-length cDNA for human liver γ-glutamylcysteine synthetase. Biochem Biophys Res Commun. 1992;185:29–35.
17. Gipp JJ, Bailey HH, Mulcahy RT. Cloning and sequence of the cDNA for the light subunit of human liver γ-glutamylcysteine synthetase and relative mRNA levels for heavy and light subunits in human normal tissues. Biochem Biophys Res Commun. 1995;206:584–9.
18. Seelig GF, Simondsen RP, Meister A. Reversible dissociation of γ-glutamylcysteine synthetase into two subunits. J Biol Chem. 1984;259:9345–7.
19. Huang C, Chang L, Anderson ME, Meister A. Catalytic and regulatory properties of the heavy subunit of rat kidney γ-glutamylcysteine synthetase. J Biol Chem. 1993;268:19675–80.
20. Shaw JP, Chou I. Elevation of intracellular glutathione content associated with mitogenic stimulation of quiescent fibroblasts. J Cell Physiol. 1986;129:193–8.
21. Hamilos DL, Zelarney P, Mascali JJ. Lymphocyte proliferation in glutathione-depleted lymphocytes: direct relationship between glutathione availability and the proliferative response. Immunopharmacology. 1989;18:223–35.
22. Messina JP, Lawrence DA. Cell cycle progression of glutathione-depleted human peripheral blood mononuclear cells is inhibited at S phase. J Immunol. 1989;143:1974–81.

23. Atzori L, Dypbukt JM, Sundqvist K *et al.* Growth-associated modification of low-molecular weight thiols and protein sulfhydryls in human bronchial fibroblasts. J Cell Physiol. 1990;143: 165–71.
24. Suthanthiran M, Anderson ME, Sharma VK, Meister A. Glutathione regulates activation-dependent DNA synthesis in highly purified normal human T lymphocytes stimulated via the CD2 and CD3 antigens. Proc Natl Acad Sci USA. 1990;87:3343–7.
25. Iwata S, Hori T, Sato N *et al.* Thiol-mediated redox regulation of lymphocyte proliferation. Possible involvement of adult T cell leukemia-derived factor and glutathione in transferrin receptor expression. J Immunol. 1994;152:5633–42.
26. Poot M, Teubert H, Rabinovitch PS, Kavanagh, TJ. *De novo* synthesis of glutathione is required for both entry into and progression through the cell cycle. J Cell Physiol. 1995;163:555–60.
27. Harris JW, Teng SS. Sulfhydryl groups during the S phase: comparison of cells from G_1, plateau-phase G_1, and G_0. J Cell Physiol. 1972;81:91–6.
28. Lee FYF, Siemann DW, Allalunis-Turner MJ, Keng PC. Glutathione contents in human and rodent tumor cells in various phases of the cell cycle. Cancer Res. 1988;48:3661–5.
29. Lu SC, Ge J. Loss of suppression of GSH synthesis under low cell density in primary cultures of rat hepatocytes. Am J Physiol. 1992;263:C1181–9.
30. Ichihara A. Mechanisms controlling growth of hepatocytes in primary culture. Dig Dis Sci. 1991;36:489–93.
31. Kumatori A, Nakamura T, Ichihara A. Cell-density dependent expression of the c-myc gene in primary cultured rat hepatocytes. Biochem Biophys Res Commun. 1991;178:480–5.
32. Nakamura T, Yoshimoto K, Nakayama Y, Tomita Y, Ichihara A. Reciprocal modulation of growth and differentiated functions of mature rat hepatocytes in primary culture by cell–cell contact and cell membranes. Proc Natl Acad Sci USA. 1983;80:7229–33.
33. Nakamura T, Nakayama Y, Ichihara A. Reciprocal modulation of growth and liver functions of mature rat hepatocytes in primary culture by an extract of hepatic plasma membranes. J Biol Chem. 1984;259:8056–8.
34. Cai J, Sun W, Lu SC. Hormonal and cell density regulation of hepatic γ-glutamylcysteine synthetase gene expression. Mol Pharmacol. 1995;48:212–18.
35. Cai J, Huang Z, Lu SC. Differential regulation of γ-glutamylcysteine synthetase heavy and light subunit gene expression. Biochem J. 1997;326:167–72.
36. Dore M, Atzori L, Congiu L. Glutathione content in regenerating rat liver after surgical and chemical hepatectomy. IRCS Med Sci. 1981;9:576.
37. Roberts E, Ahluwalia MB, Lee G, Chan C, Sarma DSR, Farber E. Resistance to hepatotoxins acquired by hepatocytes during liver regeneration. Cancer Res. 1983;43:28–34.
38. Lee SJ, Boyer TD. The effect of hepatic regeneration on the expression of the glutathione S-transferases. Biochem J. 1993;293:137–42.
39. Teshigawara M, Matsumoto S, Tsuboi S, Ohmori S. Changes in levels of glutathione and related compounds and activities of glutathione-related enzymes during liver regeneration. Res Exp Med. 1995;195:55–60.
40. LaBrecque D. Liver regeneration: a picture emerges from the puzzle. Am J Gastroenterol. 1994;89:S86–96.
41. Srivastava RC, Dwivedi RS, Kaur G, Srivastava R. Haem and drug-metabolizing enzymes in regenerating rat liver. Br J Exp Pathol. 1982;63:1–4.
42. Huang Z, Li H, Cai J, Kuhlenkamp J, Kaplowitz N, Lu SC. Changes in glutathione homeostasis during liver regeneration in the rat. Hepatology. 1998;27:147–53.
43. Zhang XK, Gauthier T, Burczynski FJ, Wang GQ, Gong YW, Minuk GY. Changes in liver membrane potentials after partial hepatectomy in rats. Hepatology. 1996;23:549–51.
44. Aw TY. Biliary glutathione promotes the mucosal metabolism of luminal peroxidized lipids by rat small intestine *in vivo*. J Clin Invest. 1994;94:1218–25.
45. Brand HS, Duetz NEP, Meijer AJ, Jörning GGA, Chamuleau RAFM. *In vivo* amino acid fluxes in regenerating liver after two-thirds hepatectomy in the rat. J Hepatol. 1995;23:333–40.
46. Uhlig S, Wendel A. The physiological consequences of glutathione variations. Life Sci. 1992;51:1083–94.
47. Kang UJ, Enger MD. Buthionine sulfoximine-induced cytostasis does not correlate with glutathione depletion. Am J Physiol. 1992;262:C122–7.
48. Holmgren A. Regulation of ribonucleotide reductase. Curr Top Cell Reg. 1981;19:47–76.

Section III
Pancreas

32
Role of Kupffer cells in acute pancreatitis

B. GLOOR, O. J. HINES, T. A. BLINMAN, D. A. RIGBERG, K. E. TODD, J. S. LANE and H. A. REBER

INTRODUCTION

Acute pancreatitis (AP) can range from a mild disease characterized by limited pancreatic interstitial oedema and rapid recovery to a life-threatening illness distinguished by a systemic inflammatory response syndrome and multi-organ failure. The death rate in patients with severe disease is as high as 20–30%, and it is often associated with pulmonary failure[1,2]. The aetiology of the pulmonary failure remains obscure, although there is increasing evidence that various chemokines and cytokines may cause much of the lung damage. During an episode of AP it is known that cytokines are released from the pancreas[3] into the portal venous system, where they reach the liver. Hepatic Kupffer cells (KC) have been shown to be a major source of cytokines within the liver[4,5], where they can release large amounts of cytokines into the systemic circulation. In a previous study we investigated the effect of KC blockade using a choline-deficient, 0.5% ethionine-supplemented (CDE) diet to induce AP in young female mice. KC blockade with gadolinium chloride lowered the systemic levels of cytokines, and also decreased the mortality rate[6]. In the current study we wished: (1) to confirm the protective effects of Kuppfer cell blockade in a different model of pancreatitis, and (2) to determine the relative pancreatic, hepatic, and pulmonary contributions to the cytokine response.

METHODS

One day before the experiment, female Sprague-Dawley rats (250–275 g) had arterial and venous access established for saline injection in control groups and for gadolinium chloride (GD) (10 mg/kg in saline) in treatment groups. Twenty-four hours after the first saline or GD injection, animals were subject to either sham operation or induction of AP. In anaesthetized animals (sodium pentobarbital, 40 mg/kg), AP was induced by intraductal infusion of 2.5% sodium taurocholate, at constant low pressure and standard volume. The bile duct above the pancreas was temporarily clamped. Sham operation consisted of a laparotomy, a ductal cannulation and a ductal saline infusion under the same conditions. The bile duct clamp was then removed, the cannula withdrawn and the abdomen closed. Two hours later, blood samples from (1) the iliac artery, (2) the portal vein cranial to the entry of the cranial pancreaticoduodenal vein, and (3) hepatic veins were taken. After tissue samples from the pancreas and lung were obtained, animals were sacrificed by an overdose of pentobarbital. Blood was collected in heparinized tubes containing aprotinin, centrifuged at 5000 rpm for 10 min, and the serum separated and stored at $-80C°$ for later assay. Separate tissue samples were either immediately processed, snap-frozen in liquid nitrogen for further assay, or fixed in formaldehyde for subsequent paraffin embedding and staining.

Rats were randomly allocated to five groups (Table 1). Serum TNF-α, IL-1β, and IL-6 were measured by ELISA technique, using commercially available kits specific for rat cytokines. Endotoxin, a potent stimulator of cytokine production, was assessed in the serum by a *Limulus* amoebocyte lysate assay. All assays were run in duplicate.

Neutrophil infiltration in pancreas and lung were determined by a myeloperoxidase (MPO) assay, using a modification of the technique of Andrews and Krinsky as previously described in detail[6]. Lung and pancreatic tissue (5 μm sections) were stained with haematoxylin and eosin. Histological changes were graded in a blinded manner by two observers. For pancreatic tissue we used a scale from 0 to 4 for oedema and inflammatory infiltration and a scale from 0 to 7 for haemorrhage and parenchymal necrosis, consistent with previous reports[7,8]. Lung tissue was graded using a score from 0 to 12 (0 to 4: absent 0; mild 1; moderate 2; severe 3; overwhelming 4) for intra-alveolar oedema, intra-alveolar haemorrhage and neutrophil infiltration.

Pancreas and lung water content were assessed by the tissue wet/dry ratio. Pieces of pancreas or lung were weighed immediately after harvest to obtain the wet weight, and again after desiccation to obtain the dry weight. Desiccation was achieved in an oven at 120°C for 24 h.

Statistical analysis

Serum cytokine levels and lung MPO levels were compared with the ANOVA test. Histological grading and lung wet/dry ratio were analysed with the Mann–Whitney U test. Data are expressed as means ± SEM; p-values < 0.05 were considered significant.

RESULTS

No cytokines were detectable in the control or sham groups (A–C). No endotoxin was detectable in any serum sample in this study. Figure 1 shows the serum cytokine values in animals with AP. IL-1β, IL-6, and TNF-α levels in untreated animals (Fig. 1, group D) were lowest in the portal vein, higher in the hepatic vein and highest in the iliac artery. IL-6 levels were similar in the hepatic vein and iliac artery. Hepatic KC blockade by GD treatment resulted in lower

Table 1 Study design: group specification, injections, surgical procedures, and number of animals

Group name	Group A: Control (n = 6)	Group B: Sham/saline (n = 8)	Group C: Sham/GD treatment (n = 8)	Group D: AP/saline (n = 10)	Group E: AP/GD treatment (n = 10)
Intravenous injection*	Saline	Saline	GD	Saline	GD
Surgical procedure	None	Ductal cannulation	Ductal cannulation	Ductal cannulation	Ductal cannulation
Intraductal infusion	None	Saline	Saline	STC†	STC†
Time of sacrifice	Zero	2 h after sham operation or induction of AP			

* At 24 h before AP induction.
† Sodium taurocholate, 2.5%.
AP = acute pancreatitis; GD = gadolinium chloride.

367

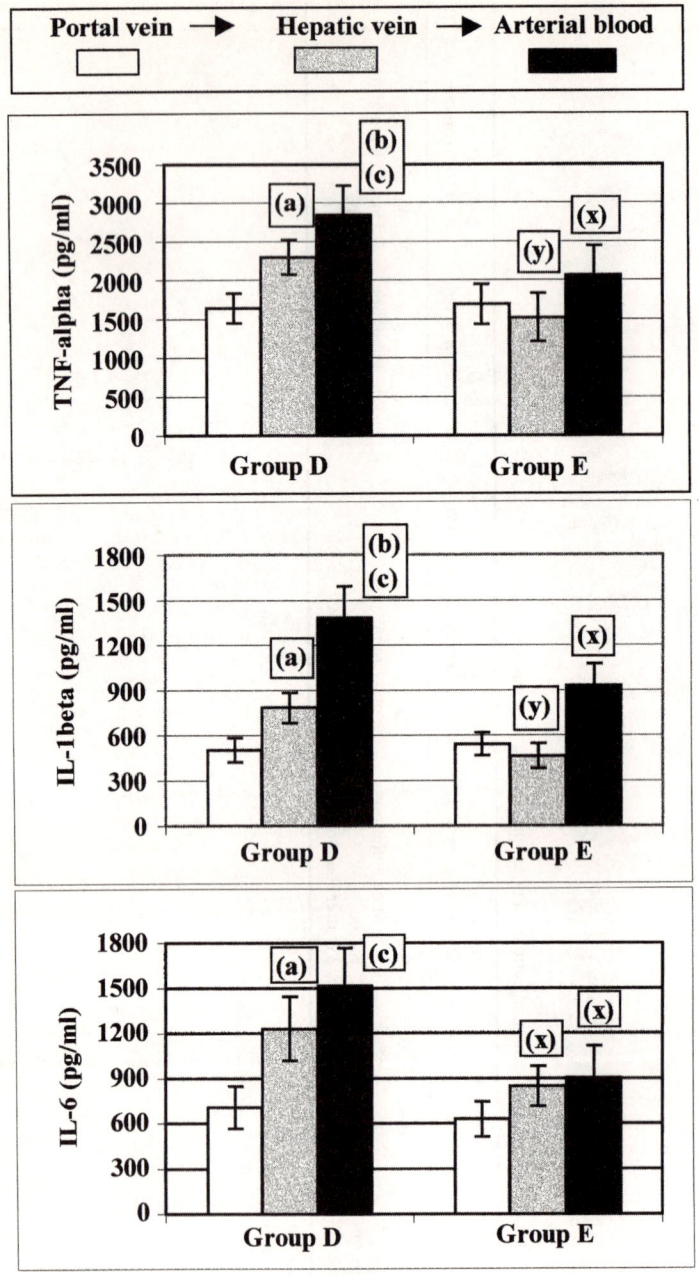

Figure 1 (a), (b) and (c) indicate comparison within group D: (acute pancreatitis and saline, control) (a) $p < 0.05$ vs portal vein, (b) $p < 0.05$ vs hepatic vein, (c) $p < 0.01$ vs portal vein. The differences between the different sites of blood sampling in group E (acute pancreatitis and gadolinium) are not significant. (x) and (y) indicate comparison with the cytokine value from the same site in group D: (x) $p < 0.05$, (y) $p < 0.01$

Table 2 Pancreas and lung histology, neutrophil infiltration, and wet–dry ratio in all five groups

	Group A	Group B	Group C	Group D	Group E
Pancreas					
Histological score	0	0.4 ± 0.1	0.42 ± 0.08	15.1 ± 2.21*	16.3 ± 2.4*
MPO (U/g tissue)	0.2 ± 0.07	0.31 ± 0.09	0.3 ± 0.1	1.1 ± 0.17*	1.0 ± 0.18*
Wet–dry ratio	0.2 ± 0.07	0.31 ± 0.09	0.3 ± 0.1	7.1 ± 0.57*	7.7 ± 0.81*
Lung					
Histological score	0	0.5 ± 0.12	0.6 ± 0.16	8.8 ± 0.9*	6.2 ± 1.1*†
MPO (U/g tissue)	2.1 ± 0.31	2.8 ± 0.53	2.95 ± 0.6	7.3 ± 0.55*	5.3 ± 0.6*†
Wet–dry ratio	3.86 ± 0.12	3.8 ± 0.13	3.95 ± 0.16	4.58 ± 0.1*	4.33 ± 0.11*†

* $p < 0.001$ vs group A, B and C.

† $p < 0.05$ vs group D.

levels for TNF-α, IL-1β, and IL-6 in the systemic circulation and lower levels of TNF-α, IL-1β, and IL-6, in the hepatic vein, compared to untreated animals (Fig. 1, group E).

Pancreas histology, neutrophil infiltration and wet–dry ratio all confirmed a severe AP after sodium taurocholate infusion (group D and E), compared to the control or sham groups, and an equal severity of AP in groups D and E (Table 2).

Lung injury, assessed by histology, neutrophil infiltration and wet–dry ratio, was considerable after AP, but attenuated by KC blockade (Table 2).

DISCUSSION

In this study we blocked KC activity in the liver with gadolinium-chloride. Its mechanism of action and effect on hepatic KCs have been investigated by others[9–13], who found it to be highly specific with few or no effects on peritoneal macrophages or other cells within the portal system[13]. There was also no evidence that the gadolinium treatment itself affected the well-being of the animals in this study. The group C rats, which received gadolinium, appeared well and all the results were comparable to group B rats, which received saline. In untreated animals with AP, serum cytokine levels were higher in the hepatic vein than in the portal vein, and highest in the systemic circulation. This suggested that extrapancreatic cytokine production contributed considerably to the systemic cytokine levels.

Norman and co-workers have examined extrapancreatic cytokine production during experimental acute pancreatitis in mice. They found that mRNA for TNF-α and IL-1β was up-regulated in liver, lung and spleen[14], and postulated that morbidity and mortality from AP was primarily the result of pancreatic parenchymal necrosis and the development of marked pulmonary dysfunction, manifested by an increase of TNF-α and IL-1 in lung tissue. Blocking highly selective TNF-α gene progression resulted in an attenuated increase of IL-1β and TNF-α cytokine concentration in pancreatic and lung tissue[15]. However, their studies did not address the cause of pulmonary cytokine production, while the present study focused primarily on the role of liver KCs in that regard.

In the setting of AP, cytokines are first produced within the pancreas[3]. The mediators not only act locally where they are responsible for pancreatic injury, but they escape from the pancreas and are carried to the liver in the portal vein. We found significant amounts of IL-1β and TNF-α in portal venous blood in the AP animals. Once these cytokines reach the liver they appear to activate KCs in a dose-dependent manner. This has been studied in a more controlled fashion by others. For example, Bautista et al. investigated the effects of a non-lethal dose of TNF-α in an isolated perfused rat liver model. They found that TNF-α-primed liver KCs to release more superoxide anion[16]. Hepatocytes, endothelial cells, as well as either blood or hepatic neutrophils, were not affected by the TNF-α. The hepatic KCs seem also to be responsible for the increased serum levels of TNF-α, IL-1β and IL-6 in the hepatic vein in our untreated animals, since KC blockade prevented an increase of these same cytokines in the venous blood draining the liver[17]. The work of Closa et al. is consistent with our observations that suggest an important role for hepatic cytokines in causing lung injury. They investigated the role of the liver by diverting the portal venous blood to the vena cava in rats with severe experimental AP. Rats with a portacaval shunt suffered minimal pulmonary damage. Those with the portal circulation intact showed significant lung injury as evidenced by both morphological and biochemical studies. The authors suggested that substances derived from the liver might be involved[18].

SUMMARY

We believe that hepatic cytokine release, primarily from KCs, plays a key role in the development of pulmonary damage in the setting of severe AP. The lung is the first organ after the heart exposed to hepatic venous drainage during AP. It seems reasonable to postulate that the pulmonary parenchyma is directly damaged by the high concentration of these noxious substances that perfuse it. A secondary response by resident pulmonary macrophages and neutrophils probably compounds that damage. This would explain why the lung is usually the first extrapancreatic organ injured in the multisystem organ failure associated with the most severe form of AP. It suggests that attempts to attenuate the hepatic cytokine response in severe AP may be a fruitful therapeutic approach in these patients.

References

1. Rau B, Uhl W, Buchler MW, Beger HG. Surgical treatment of infected necrosis. World J Surg. 1997;21:155–61.
2. Bradley ELI. Surgical indications and techniques in necrotizing pancreatitis. In: Bradley ELI, editor. Acute Pancreatitis: Diagnosis and Therapy. New York: Raven; 1994.
3. Norman J, Franz M, Messina J, Gower W, Carey L. Intrinsic production of proinflammatory cytokines by the pancreas during acute pancreatitis. Surg Forum. 1994;XLX:191–4.
4. Saad B, Frei K, Scholl FA, Fontana A, Maier P. Hepatocyte-derived interleukin-6 and tumor-necrosis factor alpha mediate the lipopolysaccharide-induced acute-phase response and nitric oxide release by cultured rat hepatocytes. Eur J Biochem. 1995;229:349–55.
5. Callery MP, Kamei T, Flye MW. Endotoxin stimulates interleukin-6 production by human Kupffer cells. Circ Shock. 1992;37:185–8.

6. Gloor B, Todd KE, Lane JS, Lewis MPN, Reber HA. Hepatic Kupffer cell blockade reduces mortality in acute hemorrhagic pancreatitis in mice. J Gastrointest Surg. 1998;2:430–5.
7. Rongione AJ, Kusske AM, Kwan K, Ashley SW, Reber HA, McFadden DW. Interleukin 10 reduces the severity of acute pancreatitis in rats. Gastroenterology. 1997;112:960–7.
8. Spormann H, Sokolowski A, Letko G. Experimental acute pancreatitis – a quantification of dynamics at enzymic and histomorphologic levels. Pathol Res Pract. 1989;185:358–62.
9. Husztik E, Lazar G, Parducz A. Electron microscopic study of Kupffer cell phagocytosis blockade induced by gadolinium chloride. Br J Exp Pathol. 1980;61:624–30.
10. Koudstaal J, Dijkhuis F, Hardonk M. Selective depletion of Kupffer cells after intravenous injection of gadolinium chloride. In: Wisse E, Knook D, McCuskey, editors. Cells of the Hepatic Sinusoid, vol. 3. Rijswijk; 1991.
11. Lazar G Jr, Lazar G, Kaszaki J, Olah J, Kiss I, Husztik E. Inhibition of anaphylactic shock by gadolinium chloride-induced Kupffer cell blockade. Agents Actions. 1994;41:C97–8.
12. Bouma J, Smit M. Gadolinium chloride selectively blocks endocytosis by Kupffer cells. In: Wisse E, Knook D, Decker K, editors. Cells of the Hepatic Sinusoid, vol. 2. Rijswijk; 1989.
13. Naito M, Nagai H, Kawano S et al. Liposome-encapsulated dichloromethylene diphosphonate induces macrophage apoptosis in vivo and in vitro. J Leukocyte Biol. 1996;60:337–44.
14. Norman JG, Fink GW, Denham W et al. Tissue-specific cytokine production during experimental acute pancreatitis. A probable mechanism for distant organ dysfunction. Dig Dis Sci. 1997;42:1783–8.
15. Denham W, Fink G, Yang J, Ulrich P, Tracey K, Norman J. Small molecule inhibition of tumor necrosis factor gene processing during acute pancreatitis prevents cytokine cascade progression and attenuates pancreatitis severity. Am Surg. 1997;63:1045–9 (discussion 1049–50).
16. Bautista AP, Schuler A, Spolarics Z, Spitzer JJ. Tumor necrosis factor stimulates superoxide anion generation by Kupffer cells. Am J Physiol. 1991;261:G891–5.
17. Gloor B, Todd KE, Lane JS, Rigberg DA, Reber HA. Mechanism of increased lung injury after acute pancreatitis in IL-10 knockout mice. J Surg Res. 1998;80:110–14.
18. Closa D, Bardaji M, Hotter G et al. Hepatic involvement in pancreatitis-induced lung damage. Am J Physiol. 1996;270:G6–13.

33
The role of pro-inflammatory factors in pancreatitis and associated lung injury

M. L. STEER and A. K. SALUJA

INTRODUCTION

Acute pancreatitis is an inflammatory disease of the pancreas which, in Western countries, has been estimated to affect 50–100 patients per million population per year[1]. Recent insights into the pathophysiology of acute pancreatitis have suggested that it is a process which evolves in several phases (Fig. 1). The *triggering phase* involves one of a number of extrapancreatic so-called 'aetiological factors' which, by as-yet-unexplained mechanisms, bring about intrapancreatic derangements within acinar cells. These derangements initiate the *pancreatic phase* of pancreatitis during which digestive enzyme zymogens become activated within acinar cells and, by acting within those cells, these activated enzymes cause cell injury and cell death. This early phase of cell injury/death is associated with an intrapancreatic inflammatory reaction which is characterized

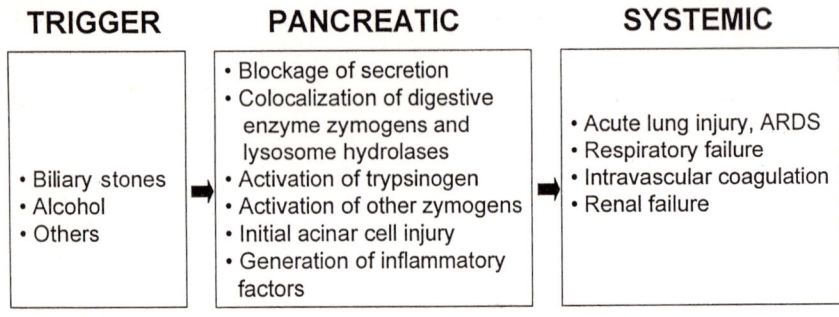

TRIGGER	PANCREATIC	SYSTEMIC
• Biliary stones • Alcohol • Others	• Blockage of secretion • Colocalization of digestive enzyme zymogens and lysosome hydrolases • Activation of trypsinogen • Activation of other zymogens • Initial acinar cell injury • Generation of inflammatory factors	• Acute lung injury, ARDS • Respiratory failure • Intravascular coagulation • Renal failure

Figure 1   Schematic representation of the phases involved in the pathogenesis of acute pancreatitis

by the activation and recruitment of inflammatory cells, generation of various pro-inflammatory factors, and progressive worsening of the extent of acinar cell injury. This local, second phase of acute pancreatitis subsequently evolves into a third or *systemic phase* of pancreatitis during which pro-inflammatory factors generated within the inflamed pancreas act at distant sites to couple acute pancreatic injury to non-pancreatic phenomena including acute lung injury, the adult respiratory distress syndrome, respiratory failure, disseminated intravascular coagulation, and renal failure.

TRIGGERING PHASE

Most patients with acute pancreatitis develop their disease either as a complication of biliary tract stone disease or as a result of prolonged ethanol abuse. Other, less common, causes of pancreatitis include exposure to certain drugs or toxins, pancreatic trauma, hypercalcaemia, hyperlipidaemia, pancreatic duct obstruction and/or hypertension, and pancreatic ischaemia. In some instances no triggering aetiological factor can be identified.

PANCREATIC PHASE

The earliest events in pancreatitis appear to occur within pancreatic acinar cells and to result in the activation of digestive enzyme zymogens[2]. Normally these inactive zymogens, or pro-enzymes (e.g. trypsinogen, chymotrypsinogen, pro-elastase, pro-carboxypeptidase, etc.) are secreted from acinar cells into the ductal space and activation occurs only after they reach the duodenum, where a brush-border enteropeptidase activates trypsinogen, and trypsin catalyses the activation of the other zymogens. In pancreatitis, however, these zymogens are prematurely activated within the acinar cells and the activated digestive enzymes cause the pancreas to undergo digestive necrosis. The mechanisms by which ethanol abuse, biliary tract stones, or other so-called 'aetiological factors' bring about intra-acinar cell activation of digestive zymogens are not entirely known, but there has been considerable recent interest in exploring this issue.

For the most part, studies aimed at identifying those mechanisms have employed one of a number of experimental models of pancreatitis induced in laboratory animals. Studies performed using several otherwise dissimilar models of pancreatitis have all indicated that the earliest acinar cell changes involve the inhibition or blockade of digestive enzyme secretion. This defect in secretion appears to be coupled with a defect in the intracellular trafficking of newly synthesized proteins. As a result the normal segregation process by which lysosomal hydrolases are sequestered from digestive enzyme zymogens during passage through the Golgi stacks is perturbed, and digestive zymogens are co-compartmentalized, along with lysosomal hydrolases, in intracellular membrane-bound spaces or vacuoles. It is believed that this co-localization phenomenon permits the lysosomal hydrolase cathepsin B to activate trypsinogen, trypsin to activate the other zymogens, and activated digestive enzymes to cause cell injury.

MEDIATORS OF INFLAMMATION: AN OVERVIEW

Although the initiation of pancreatitis is believed to involve acinar cell injury mediated by the premature, intracellular activation of digestive enzymes, the subsequent progression of the disease appears to be regulated by factors generated either by the injured acinar cells themselves or by inflammatory cells which become activated as a result of acinar cell injury and which are recruited to the pancreas where they are sequestered. Studies performed by a number of groups[3–8] have indicated that factors such as TNF-α, IL-1, TGF-β, and IL-10 play an important role in regulating the severity of pancreatitis. Our own studies (see below) have focused on a variety of other mediators including adhesion molecules, neutrophils, lymphocytes, chemokines, neurokinins, and complement. In a general sense these various studies have provided insights into the balance of both pro- and anti-inflammatory factors which, when taken together, determine the ultimate severity of the pancreatic injury in pancreatitis and the coupling of that injury to systemic events such as acute lung injury (Fig. 2).

EXPERIMENTAL MODELS

Our current understanding of the role of inflammatory mediators in pancreatitis is the result of studies performed by a number of groups. Many of those studies have provided important insights into this issue, and they should be consulted by the interested reader[3–7,9–13]. The remainder of this review, however, will focus on work performed in the authors' laboratory over the past 5 years.

Our work has employed several models of acute pancreatitis. Most of our studies have employed the secretagogue-induced model of pancreatitis[14,15] in which either mice or rats are given a dose of the CCK analogue caerulein which exceeds the dose required to induce a maximal rate of digestive enzyme secretion from the pancreas. When rats are infused with this supramaximally stimu-

Pro-inflammatory	Anti-inflammatory
IL-1	C5a
IL-6	IL-10
PAF	IL-11
CCR1 ligands	
Substance P	
ICAM-1	
P and E selectins	
Neutrophils	
Lymphocytes	

Figure 2 Inflammatory factors involved in the pathogenesis of acute pancreatitis and associated lung injury

lating dose of caerulein for 3.5 h, a reversible, non-lethal form of interstitial pancreatitis is induced which is characterized by hyperamylasaemia, pancreatic oedema, acinar cell vacuolization, neutrophil sequestration within the pancreas, moderate acinar cell necrosis, and an intrapancreatic inflammatory response[16]. Mice given hourly injections of a supramaximally stimulating caerulein dose (between four and 12 hourly injections) develop a similar but more severe pancreatitis which is characterized by more extensive necrosis and intrapancreatic haemorrhage[15]. Pancreatitis, in the mouse as well as in the rat caerulein model, is associated with lung injury that is characterized by an increase in lung water content, an increase in pulmonary microvascular permeability, and sequestration of neutrophils within the lung[17]. This latter phenomenon can be quantitated by measuring lung myeloperoxidase concentration.

In addition to the secretagogue-induced model of pancreatitis, some of our studies have employed a diet-induced model[18] in which young female mice are fed a choline-deficient ethionine-supplemented diet. This results in the induction of severe, frequently lethal, pancreatitis and that pancreatitis is also associated with significant lung injury[19]. The final model which we have employed involves the induction of biliary/pancreatic duct obstruction in the American opossum[20]. Duct obstruction in that animal results in time-dependent pancreatic acinar cell injury/necrosis, as well as acute lung injury, both of which evolve over several days[21]. From an anatomical standpoint this model appears to most closely mimic the events in clinical gallstone pancreatitis.

THE ROLE OF ICAM-1 AND NEUTROPHILS

The role of ICAM-1 in acute pancreatitis and lung injury was evaluated using genetically altered mice that do not express ICAM-1[22]. Pancreatitis was induced either by supramaximal secretagogue stimulation or by administration of the choline-deficient ethionine-supplemented diet. The role of neutrophils was evaluated by comparing changes in control animals with those obtained after administration of antineutrophil serum (ANS) to deplete neutrophils. We found that ICAM-1 levels are increased in serum, pancreas, and lung during pancreatitis and that the severity of both the pancreatitis and of the associated lung injury is blunted in knockout mice that lack ICAM-1. Neutrophil depletion of ICAM-1-sufficient animals results in similar protection against pancreatitis as well as lung injury. The combination of neutrophil depletion and ICAM-1 deficiency, however, does not reduce the severity of either the pancreatitis or of the lung injury beyond that obtained with either intervention by itself. Furthermore, we found that neither pancreatitis nor its associated lung injury is completely prevented by ICAM-1 deficiency, neutrophil depletion, or combined ICAM-1 deficiency plus neutrophil depletion. These studies led us to conclude that both ICAM-1 and neutrophils play an important role in regulating the severity of pancreatitis and lung injury, and that both may act by similar mechanisms, i.e. that ICAM-1 acts by facilitating neutrophil sequestration in the pancreas and in the lung during pancreatitis. Our studies also indicate that ICAM-1 and neutrophil-independent events play an important role in pancreatitis and associated lung injury.

THE ROLE OF LYMPHOCYTES

Although a role for neutrophils in pancreatitis and lung injury has been generally accepted, surprisingly little attention has been directed at the role of lymphocytes in this process. Mayer *et al.*, in a recently reported study, found that SCID mice, which lack both T and B lymphocytes, are protected against pancreatitis-associated lung injury but not against secretagogue-induced pancreatic injury[23]. Our own studies in this area have employed athymic nude mice which lack only T lymphocytes[24]. We have found that these animals are also protected against pancreatitis-associated lung injury but not against secretagogue-induced pancreatitis itself. Taken together, these two studies indicate that neither T nor B lymphocytes play a critical role in regulating the severity of secretagogue-induced pancreatic injury, but that T lymphocytes (but probably not B lymphocytes) play a critical role in coupling pancreatitis to lung injury. The mechanisms by which T lymphocytes play this role, and the subsets of T lymphocytes involved, remain to be identified.

THE ROLE OF CHEMOKINES

The β-chemokines and their receptors mediate activation and trafficking of a variety of leucocytes, including lymphocytes and macrophages, during the inflammatory process. We have examined the role of the β-chemokine receptor CCR-1, which recognizes the chemokines MIP-1α and RANTES, in pancreatitis and associated lung injury[25]. In our studies we induced pancreatitis and lung injury by supramaximal secretagogue stimulation of mice and compared the results obtained in wild-type mice to those noted when knockout mice lacking CCR-1 were used. We found that genetic deletion of CCR-1 reduces the sequestration of neutrophils in the pancreas during pancreatitis but that it does not otherwise alter the severity of secretagogue-induced pancreatitis. On the other hand, deletion of CCR-1 markedly reduces the severity of pancreatitis-associated lung injury, indicating that this B chemokine receptor, and the ligands acting via it, play an important role in regulating the severity of pancreatitis-associated lung injury.

THE ROLE OF NEUROKININS

The neurokinin substance P, acting via neurokinin-1 receptors (NK-1R) plays an important role in mediating a variety of inflammatory processes[26]. It is believed to be the major mediator of so-called neurogenic inflammation. To evaluate the role of substance P in pancreatitis, we induced pancreatitis by supramaximal secretagogue stimulation in wild-type NK-1 sufficient mice and compared the results obtained with those noted when knockout NK-1R deficient mice were used[27]. We found that substance P as well as NK-1 receptors are markedly increased in the pancreas of wild-type mice during pancreatitis and that deletion of NK-1R reduces the severity of the pancreatitis as well as the associated lung injury. These observations indicate that substance P, acting via NK-1R in the pancreas, and probably in the lung as well, plays an important role in regulating the severity of pancreatitis and of pancreatitis-associated lung injury.

THE ROLE OF COMPLEMENT

During the cascade process of complement activation, the potent anaflatoxin C5a is generated. This peptide, released during processing of complement factor C5, is generally believed to function as a pro-inflammatory factor by promoting the activation as well as the recruitment of inflammatory cells, and by promoting an increase in microvascular permeability in areas of inflammation. To evaluate the role of C5a in pancreatitis we employed mice which lack C5a receptors and mice which do not express C5. Pancreatitis was induced by supramaximal secretagogue stimulation. The severity of pancreatitis and of pancreatitis-associated lung injury in these animals was compared to that noted in wild-type animals. We found that deletion of either C5 or of C5a receptors increases the severity of both the pancreatitis and the pancreatitis-associated lung injury[28]. This surprising observation indicates that, at least in pancreatitis, C5a plays an anti-inflammatory role. The nature of that role, however, has yet to be identified.

THE ROLE OF PLATELET ACTIVATING FACTOR

Platelet activating factor (PAF) is a potent phospholipid pro-inflammatory factor generated by many types of cells including neutrophils, macrophages, platelets, and endothelial cells. It promotes the activation and recruitment of inflammatory cells, generation of chemokines and cytokines, and increases in microvascular permeability. We evaluated the role of PAF in pancreatitis by administering a recombinant form of the enzyme PAF-acetyl hydrolase, which hydrolyses PAF and terminates its action, to opossums 2 days after pancreatitis had been initiated by bile/pancreatic duct obstruction[29]. We found that administration of PAF-AH could delay the progression of pancreatitis and prevent the development of pancreatitis-associated lung injury even if the PAF-AH administration was begun after the onset of pancreatitis. These studies indicate that PAF plays an important role in regulating the severity of pancreatitis and of pancreatitis-associated lung injury. Furthermore, these studies indicate that termination of the action of PAF may have clinical value in the treatment of established pancreatitis.

References

1. Glazer G. Contentious issues in acute pancreatitis. In: Glazer G, Ransen JHC, editors. Acute Pancreatitis. London: Baillière Tindall; 1988;1–36.
2. Steer ML. Frank Brooks Memorial Lecture: The early intraacinar cell events which occur during acute pancreatitis. Pancreas. 1998;17:31–7.
3. Norman J, Franz M, Messina JM et al. Interleukin-1 receptor antagonist decreases severity of experimental acute pancreatitis. Surgery. 1995;177:648–55.
4. Norman JG, Fink GW, Messina J, Carter G, Franz MG. Timing of tumor necrosis factor antagonism is critical in determining outcome in murine lethal acute pancreatitis. Surgery. 1996;120:515–21.
5. Sandoval D, Gukovskaya A, Revey P et al. The role of neutrophils and platelet-activating factor in mediating experimental pancreatitis. Gastroenterology. 1996;111:1081–91.
6. Rongione AJ, Kusske AM, Kwan K, Ashley SW, Reber HA, McFadden DW. Interleukin 10 reduces the severity of acute pancreatitis in rats. Gastroenterology. 1997;112:960–7.
7. Schölmerich J. Interleukins in acute pancreatitis. Scand J Gastroenterol. 1996;31(Suppl. 219):37–42.

8. Gukovskaya AS, Gukovsky I, Zaninovic V *et al.* Pancreatic acinar calls produce, release, and respond to tumor necrosis factor-α. J Clin Invest. 1997;100:1853–62.

9. Grewal HP, Mohey el Din A, Gaber L, Kotb M, Gaber AO. Amelioration of the physiologic and biochemical changes of acute pancreatitis using an anti-TNF-alpha polyclonal antibody. Am J Surg. 1994;167:214–18.

10. Grady T, Liang P, Ernst SA, Logson CD. Chemokine gene expression in rat pancreatic acinar cells is an early event associated with acute pancreatitis. Gastroenterology. 1997;113:1966–75.

11. Kruger B, Lerch MM, Tessenow W. Direct detection of premature protease activation in living pancreatic acinar cells. Lab Invest. 1998;78:763–64.

12. Schnekenburger J, Mayerle J, Simon P, Domschke W, Lerch MM. Protein tyrosine dephosphorylation and the maintenance of cell adhesions in the pancreas. Ann NY Acad Sci. 1999;880:157–65.

13. Steinle AU, Weidenbach H, Wagner M, Adler G, Schmid RM. NF-kappaB/Rel activation in cerulein pancreatitis. Gastroenterology. 1999;116:420–30.

14. Lampel M, Kern J. Acute interstitial pancreatitis in the rat induced by excessive doses of a pancreatic secretagogue. Virchows Arch [A]. 1977;373:97–117.

15. Kaiser A, Saluja A, Sengupta A, Saluja M, Steer ML. Relationship between severity, necrosis and apoptosis in five models of experimental acute pancreatitis. Am J Physiol. 1995;269: C1295–304.

16. Grady T, Saluja A, Kaiser A, Steer M. Pancreatic edema and intrapancreatic activation of trypsinogen during secretagogue-induced pancreatitis precedes glutathion depletion. Am J Physiol. 1996;271:G20–6.

17. Guice KS, Oldham KT, Caty MG, Johnson KJ, Ward PA. Neutrophil-dependent, oxygen-radical mediated lung injury associated with acute pancreatitis. Ann Surg. 1989;210:740–7.

18. Lombardi B, Estes LW, Longnecker DW. Acute hemorrhagic pancreatitis (massive necrosis) with fat necrosis induced in mice by *dl*-ethionine fed with a choline-deficient diet. Am J Pathol. 1975;79:465–80.

19. Bhatia M, Saluja AK, Hofbauer B, Lee HS, Frossard JL, Steer ML. The effects of neutrophil depletion on a completely noninvasive model of acute pancreatitis-associated lung injury. Int J Pancreatol. 1998;24:77–83.

20. Senninger N, Moody FG, Coelho JC, Van Buren DH. The role of biliary obstruction in the pathogenesis of acute pancreatitis in the opossum. Surgery. 1986;99:688–93.

21. Lerch MM, Saluja AK, Runzi M, Dawra R, Saluja M, Steer ML. Pancreatic duct obstruction triggers acute necrotizing pancreatitis in the opossum. Gastroenterology. 1993;104:853–61.

22. Frossard J, Saluja A, Bhagat L *et al.* The role of intercellular adhesion molecule 1 and neutrophils in acute pancreatitis and pancreatitis-associated lung injury. Gastroenterology. 1999;116:694–701.

23. Mayer J, Laine JO, Rao B *et al.* Systemic lymphocyte activation modulates the severity of diet-induced acute pancreatitis in mice. Pancreas. 1999;19:62–8.

24. Bhagat L, Saluja AK, Hietaranta AJ *et al.* T-Lymphocytes are critical to the development of pancreatitis-associated but not endotoxin-induced lung injury. Pancreas. 1999 (abstract; in press).

25. Gerard C, Frossard J, Bhatia M *et al.* Targeted disruption of the β-chemokine receptor CCR1 protects against pancreatitis-associated lung injury. J Clin Invest. 1997;100:2022–7.

26. Change MM, Leeman SE. Isolation of a sialogogic peptide from bovine hypothalamic tissue and its characterization as substance P. J Biol Chem. 1970;245:4784–90.

27. Bhatia M, Saluja A, Hofbauer B *et al.* Role of substance P and the neurokinin 1 receptor in acute pancreatitis and pancreatitis-associated lung injury. Proc Natl Acad Sci USA. 1998;95:4760–5.

28. Bhatia M, Saluja A, Hofbauer H *et al.* Deletion of C5A receptor (C5aR) increases the severity of acute pancreatitis and pancreatitis-associated lung injury. Pancreas. 1997;15:428.

29. Hofbauer B, Saluja A, Bhatia M, Forssard JL, Lee H, Steer ML. Effect of recombinant platelet-activating factor acetylhydrolase on two models of experimental acute pancreatitis. Gastroenterology. 1998;115:1238–47.

34
Effects of hedgehog signalling on pancreas development

M. HEBROK, S. K. KIM and D. A. MELTON

During vertebrate embryogenesis, tissues and signalling pathways interact to regulate cell differentiation and morphogenesis of complex organ structures. Communication between mesoderm and endoderm-derived tissues is required for development of the pancreas, a vital organ involved in food digestion and glucose homeostasis. Cells in the exocrine pancreas secrete enzymes into the gut lumen while endocrine cells produce hormones, including insulin and glucagon, that participate in blood glucose regulation[1]. Pancreas organogenesis can be divided into three main phases: initiation, morphogenesis and maturation. During initiation the endodermal sheet that will give rise to the mature endocrine and exocrine pancreatic cell types is in close contact with the mesodermally derived notochord[2,3], a known source of inducing molecules[4,5]. The first morphogenetic sign of pancreas development is a dorsal evagination of the foregut endoderm posterior to the stomach anlage[1,6]. Shortly afterwards ventral buds form on the opposite site close to the liver diverticulum. When gut and stomach rotate the ventral bud moves around to the dorsal side where it comes in close contact with the dorsal anlage to form the mature organ[1]. By studying pancreas development we seek to understand the general principles of organogenesis to explain and prevent formation of pancreatic diseases, including pancreatic cancer and diabetes mellitus.

Our initial studies have shown that the notochord is required for initiation of pancreas formation in chick embryos[7]. Two notochord factors, activin βB, a member of the transforming growth factor family (TGF-β), and FGF-2, a member of the fibroblast growth factor family, can mimic the notochord effect and induce pancreas marker expression in isolated endoderm[8]. These findings are supported by several other studies, indicating that both signalling pathways can regulate pancreas development in mammals[9-13]. Furthermore, we could demonstrate that endodermal signalling molecules respond to Notochord factors, thereby regulating pancreas formation. It had been previously reported that *Sonic hedgehog (Shh)*, a member of the Hedgehog family of signalling molecules involved in patterning and differentiation of several embryonic structures[14], is expressed in endoderm adjacent to but excluded from pancreatic tissue in

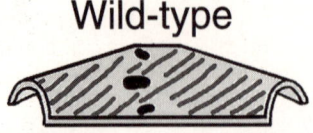

Activin ⊣ *Shh* ⊣ *Ptc* ⊣ *Smo* → target genes

Wild-type

ActR mutant

stomach pancreas duodenum

stomach pancreas duodenum

Figure 1 Interaction of activin and Hedgehog signalling pathways. *Shh* activates transcription of its target genes by blocking the activity of its own receptor *Ptc*. In the absence of ligands Ptc functions by binding and blocking the activity of its co-receptor Smoothened (Smo). Activin interferes with this signalling cascade by down-regulating *Shh* expression in pancreatic tissue (represented by three dark-coloured dots corresponding to *Pdx-1* expression in dorsal and ventral pancreas buds), thereby allowing the formation of a normal pancreas in wild-type embryos. In activin receptor (ActR) mutants, where activin signaling is obliterated, expression of *Shh* and its target genes is increased and pancreas development is attenuated

mice[15–17]. In chick embryos *Shh* can be found in endoderm along the anteroposterior axes, although it is suppressed in the dorsal-most region where endoderm touches the notochord[7], indicating that Shh function might interfere with pancreas development. This is supported by the finding that activin inhibits expression of *Shh* in the chick node region, thereby establishing asymmetric gene expression leading to left–right asymmetry[18]. We were able to demonstrate that in the pancreas anlage, activin βB governs proper pancreas formation by blocking endodermal *Shh* expression[8], while ectopic expression of *Shh* in pancreas interferes with normal development[17] (Fig. 1). These studies provided evidence that early pancreas development is regulated by the interaction of positive, activin and FGF, and negative, hedgehog, signalling pathways.

To understand if these pathways also play a role during maturation and adult pancreas function we decided to investigate mice mutant for specific members of the activin and hedgehog pathways. Activins signal through binding to serin/threonine cell surface receptors. Two receptors, ActRIIA and ActIIB, have a high affinity to activin ligands[19,20], and we have used mice carrying mutations in both genes for our investigations. Consistent with the results obtained from experiments in chicks, we observe a decrease in pancreas size and number of endocrine marker genes, including *Pancreatic and duodenal homeobox gene-1 (Pdx-1)*, insulin and glucagon, in ActR mutants. Furthermore, the severity of the pancreas phenotype depends on the number of intact activin receptor alleles present. While $A^{+/+}/B^{+/-}$ mutants are comparable to wild-type littermates, pancreas size is decreased in $A^{+/+}/B^{-/-}$ mutants and even more compromised in $A^{+/-}/B^{-/-}$ embryos. In addition to these developmental changes we also observed transformations in mature pancreas architecture accompanied by impaired organ function. The average islet area in wild-type littermates is 3-fold and 5-fold larger when compared with islets from $A^{+/+}/B^{-/-}$ and $A^{+/-}/B^{+/-}$ mutants, respectively, and these alterations correlate with impaired pancreas function. Mutants injected with a concentrated glucose solution display a decrease in glucose tolerance when compared with wild-type animals. In compound heterozygous

$A^{+/-}/B^{+/-}$ mice glucose tolerance is more attenuated than in ActRIIB$^{-/-}$ mutants, suggesting that several ligands with binding affinities to both receptor types can regulate pancreas formation and function. However, the basal blood glucose levels after overnight starvation are similar in mutant and wild-type animals, indicating that glucose homeostasis can be maintained under normal conditions. Therefore, these animals might provide a novel polygenic model system for impaired glucose control[21].

Results obtained from chick experiments suggested that activin promotes pancreas organogenesis by blocking expression of *Shh* in pre-pancreatic endoderm[8]. These findings led us to investigate if the changes in pancreas development and function in ActR mutants are due to increased Hedgehog signalling. As anticipated, we do observe an enlarged expression domain of *Shh* extending from the anterior stomach towards the pancreas anlage, although no Hedgehog expression in mutant pancreas has yet been detected. However, it remains to be determined if this ectopic expression alone is sufficient to cause the mutant phenotype, or if other signalling pathways necessary for pancreas development also depend on activin signalling.

In an alternative approach we have looked at mice carrying targeted mutations in factors of the Hedgehog signalling pathway, including *Shh, Indian hedgehog (Ihh)* and *Patched*-1(*Ptc*), a Hedgehog receptor. Hedgehogs transmit their signal through a negative cascade in which binding of the ligands to its receptor releases a co-factor, *Smoothened (Smo)*, thereby activating downstream target genes[22,23] (Fig. 2). Our studies are aimed at understanding if hedgehog signalling interferes with pancreas development and function in mammals and if blocking of negative factors such as *Ptc* can lead to changes in pancreas morphology and performance. As mentioned earlier, two hedgehog molecules, *Shh* and *Ihh*, have been shown to be expressed adjacent to, but are excluded from, pancreatic tissue, and we decided to investigate pancreas organogenesis in mice carrying targeted deletions in both genes. The size and weight of *Shh*$^{-/-}$ embryos is reduced to a third when compared to wild-type embryos (Fig. 2) and development of several organs, including endoderm-derived lungs and oesophagus, is greatly compromised[24,25]. While the organs of the intestinal tract are also affected, and stomach weight is reduced 3-fold, pancreas size and weight is similar in wild-type and mutant embryos throughout development (Fig. 2), indicating that pancreas is relatively increased approximately 3.5-fold when compared to other organs[26]. Dorsal and ventral pancreas are easily distinguishable in *Shh*$^{-/-}$ embryos, although pancreas tissue is more condensed, leading to a large number of clustered islets in the centre of the organ. Islet architecture is conserved, with insulin-producing cells located in the centre and glucagon-positive cells surrounding them[26].

We have analysed if endocrine development is positively affected by the loss of *Shh* and counted insulin- and glucagon-producing cells in islets of E18.5 mouse embryos. Interestingly, the absolute number of endocrine cells is almost identical between wild-type and mutants, although the mutant embryo is 3 times smaller. When adjusted to body weight the relative number of insulin and glucagon-positive cells is increased approximately 4-fold, displaying a significant expansion of endocrine cells in these mutants. Blocking of hedgehog signalling in chick embryos with Cyclopamine, a steroid alkaloid similar to cho-

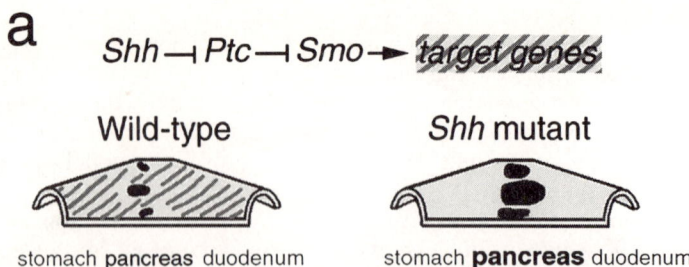

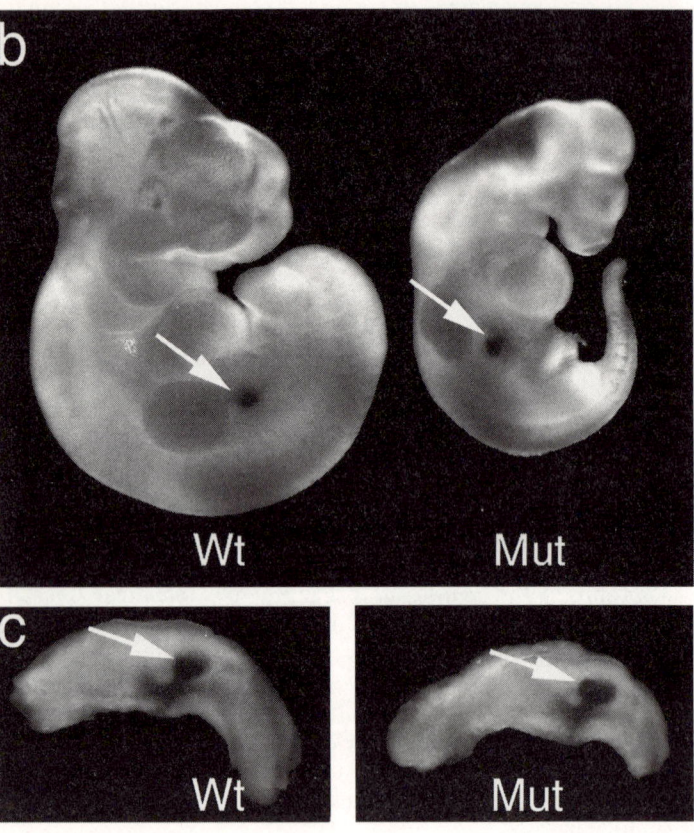

Figure 2 Pancreas is relatively increased in *Shh* mutants. (**a**) Shh interferes with pancreas development. In *Shh* mutants pancreas size is relatively increased when compared to adjacent organs including stomach and duodenum. (**b**) Comparison of E10.5 wild-type and *Shh* mutant embryos. Development of embryonic structures in *Shh* mutants is disturbed and overall size is reduced 3-fold. In contrast, pancreas size, as visualized by β-galactosidase staining of *LacZ* expressed under control of the *Pdx-1* promoter (arrows), is similar in wild-type and mutants. (**c**) Higher magnification of dorsal pancreas buds (arrows) isolated from E10.5 wild-type and mutant embryos. Wt, wild-type; Mut, *Shh*$^{-/-}$

lesterol and presumably a general inhibitor of Hedgehog signalling[27], leads to an increase in endocrine cell numbers and formation of ectopic pancreas in stomach and duodenum[28]. In mice however, even in $Shh^{-/-}/Ihh^{+/-}$ double mutants lacking an additional copy of the *Indian* hedgehog gene, no ectopic pancreas development is detected. An explanation for this discrepancy might be that our studies are limited by the fact that $Shh^{-/-}/Ihh^{-/-}$ double homozygotes die early during development, before pancreas morphogenesis can be investigated, and the homo–heterozygous embryos still contain one intact *Ihh* allele.

To test if other tissues show changes in endocrine development we have investigated glucagon expression in tissues adjacent to pancreas that depend on Hedgehog signaling. While stomach development is severely attenuated in $Shh^{-/-}$ embryos we found twice as many glucagon-positive cells in mutant tissue compared to wild-type littermates. When adjusted to body weight this accounts for a significant 7-fold increase, suggesting that Shh can interfere with endocrine development in non-pancreatic tissues.[26]

Other types of pancreas abnormalities are observed in *Ihh* mutants that display only modest reductions in embryo size. These mice suffer from defects in proliferation and differentiation of chondrocytes, indicating a role of *Ihh* in bone formation[29]. The intestinal tract is proportionally reduced in size and pancreas gross morphology is similar to wild-type littermates. Surprisingly, in 42% of *Ihh* mutants we observed an extension of ventral pancreas tissue around the duodenum, a phenotype similar to a rare human disorder known as annular pancreas[30] (Fig. 3). In humans and *Ihh* mutants most often a band of pancreatic tissue completely encircles the duodenum. However, we have not yet found any pancreas tissue interspersed in duodenal muscularis, a change in gut morphology commonly described in human patients[30]. Furthermore, $Ihh^{-/-}$ embryos die shortly after birth[29]; therefore, we are unable to investigate if annular pancreas can lead to duodenal atresia and stenosis, complications that are frequently found in humans[31].

So far the aetiology of this disorder has remained elusive, although several theories have been proposed to explain its development[30]. These theories include hypertrophy of the ventral and dorsal bud that can result in complete constriction as well as fixation of the tip of the ventral bud to the duodenum prior to rotation. We have used a transgenic mouse line in which the *E. coli LacZ* gene is under control of the *pancreatic and duodenal homeobox gene-1 (Pdx-1)* promoter[32] (Fig. 3). The expression of *Pdx-1* is confined to the caudal stomach, pancreas and duodenum. Heterozygous embryos were used to visualize annular pancreas formation at different stages of embryogenesis. Our results show that only ventral pancreas participates in formation of the disorder. In some cases the already lobulated ventral bud splits to generate an additional anlage that will encircle the duodenum. In other cases the ventral duct leading to the main pancreas duct branches to form another ventral bud, indicating that at least two mechanisms are involved in formation of annular pancreas[26].

An interesting and poorly understood aspect is the association of this disorder with other congenital malformations, including intestinal malrotation, cardiac defects and imperforate anus in humans[34]. Depending on the genetic background these malformations are also found in *Shh* mice mutants together with annular pancreas (M. Ramalho-Santos, A. P. McMahon and D. A. Melton, unpublished

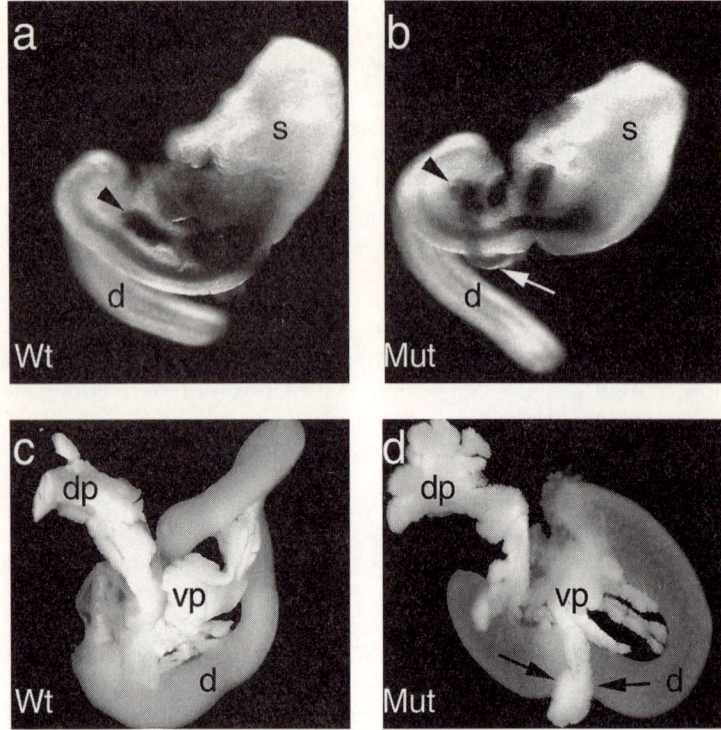

Figure 3 Annular pancreas formation in *Ihh* mutants. (**a, b**) *β*-Galactosidase staining of *Pdx-1-LacZ* reveals formation of a ventral pancreas bud (black arrowhead) extension that encircles the duodenum in *Ihh* mutants (**b**, white arrow) but not wild-type embryos (**a**) at E13.5. **c, d.** Wild-type (**c**) and mutant (**d**) intestinal at E18.5. Only ventral tissue contributes to annular pancreas formation in *Ihh* mutants, completely encircling the duodenum in most cases (black arrows); (**d**), duodenum; dp, dorsal pancreas bud; s, stomach; vp, ventral pancreas bud

results)[35], suggesting a general role for hedgehog signalling during annular pancreas formation. In addition, annular pancreas is one of the most prevalent conditions in patients suffering from Down syndrome[36,37]. Our studies, in combination with reports describing familial annular pancreas, suggest a genetic transmission of this anomaly[30].

Previously, we and others have used *in-situ* hybridization to show that *Shh* and *Ihh* are expressed in stomach and duodenum during embryogenesis, but that both genes are excluded from pancreatic tissue[8,15,17]. Here we have used the more sensitive reverse transcriptase–polymerase chain reaction (RT-PCR) to investigate if low-level hedgehog signalling might be involved in the development of the described phenotypes. As expected, we do not detect *Shh* expression in cDNAs generated from pancreas tissue; however, low levels of *Ihh* and *Ptc* transcripts can be found in pancreas throughout development and in mature tissue, including islets of Langerhans. This finding suggests that Hedgehog signaling not only attenuates pancreas formation but is also required for normal organ development[33]. Future work, involving tissue-specific targeted recombination experiments, will show if the presence of hedgehog ligands in regions adjacent to pancreatic tissue is sufficient for proper morphogenesis, or if low-level pancreatic *Ihh* expression is required to prevent annular pancreas development.

The unexpected finding of *Ptc* expression in pancreatic tissue prompted us to investigate *Ptc* function during organogenesis. We used heterozygous adult mice carrying the *LacZ* gene under the control of the *Ptc* promoter to visualize *Ptc* expression in pancreatic tissue. Interestingly, *Ptc-LacZ* staining is found in distinct regions of the mature organ, including ducts and islets of Langerhans, where its expression overlaps with insulin-producing cells. This specific expression in endocrine pancreas could point to a functional requirement of hedgehog signalling during glucose homeostasis. Injection of adult male *Ptc* heterozygotes with concentrated glucose solution revealed an impaired glucose tolerance, suggesting that *Ptc* haploid insufficiency might be correlated with glucose intolerance in humans. However, blood glucose concentrations after overnight starvation are at the wild-type level, indicating that pancreas functions are impaired only under extreme conditions[26]. Human *Ptc* has been identified and linked to several severe conditions, including basal cell carcinoma, brain tumours, craniofacial defects and spina bifida[23]. Future work will show if changes in glucose tolerance are found in humans carrying mutations in genes of the hedgehog signalling pathway.

The expression of *Ptc* in pancreatic islets and insulin-producing cells presents circumstantial evidence that pancreas dysfunction can lead to the observed changes in glucose tolerance under stress conditions. Alternatively, it is possible that peripheral insulin resistance might cause this change in glucose homeostasis. Therefore, we decided to analyse if other features of pancreas formation are affected in *Ptc* mutants. The development of homozygous embryos is severely compromised, leading to their resorption at approximately 9–9.5 days of development. At this early stage only a few pancreas marker genes are expressed, including *Pdx*-1 and glucagon. Both gene products are easily identified in the pancreas region of wild-type littermates, whereas no expression of these markers can be found in age-matched *Ptc*$^{-/-}$ embryos, indicating that pancreas development and differentiation of endocrine cells is impaired if not abolished[26].

Our results provide evidence that hedgehog signalling governs pancreas development and function. In *Shh*$^{-/-}$ and *Shh*$^{-/-}$/*Ihh*$^{+/-}$ mutants pancreas size and number of endocrine cells is relatively increased and more glucagon-positive cells are found in stomachs of *Shh*$^{-/-}$ embryos. Therefore, as expected from our studies performed in chicks, hedgehog signalling can interfere with pancreas development and might be necessary to restrict pancreas size during development. In *Ihh* mutants we frequently observe the formation of an annular pancreas, suggesting that hedgehog signalling participates in the regulation of pancreas morphogenesis. Furthermore, we find low levels of *Ihh*, but not *Shh*, expression in embryonic and mature pancreatic tissue, similar to *Ptc* expression. Blocking of hedgehog signalling, either through its own receptor or by interaction with activin signals, increases pancreas development and endocrine differentiation. Finally, chick embryos treated with cyclopamine develop ectopic pancreas tissue in stomach and duodenum accompanied by other embryonic malformations, including holoprosencephaly. In humans, holoprosencephaly is observed in patients suffering from Smith–Lemli–Optiz syndrome, a disorder characterized by a defect in cholesterol synthesis. Interestingly, nesidioblastosis and hypoglycaemia are additional problems found in these patients, indicating that misregulation of Hedgehog signalling might impair pancreatic development and function in humans.

Acknowledgements

We thank members of the Melton and Kim laboratory for helpful suggestions and stimulating discussion, and thank Guolin Chen and Olga Martinez for excellent assistance. We thank Andrew McMahon for providing the *Ihh* and *Shh* mutant mice, Chris Wright for sending the *Pdx-LacZ* mice and the *Pdx*-1 antibody, and Matthew Scott for the *Ptc-LacZ* mice. M.H. was supported by a Howard Hughes Medical Institute (HHMI) postdoctoral fellowship and S.K.K. by a Physician Postdoctoral Fellowship, a Pew Biomedical Scholars award and the Donald E. and Delia Baxter Foundation. D.A.M. is an investigator in the HHMI.

References

1. Slack JMW. Development biology of the pancreas. Development. 1995;121:1569–80
2. Wessells NK, Cohen JH. Early pancreas organogenesis: morphogenesis, tissue interactions, and mass effects. Dev Biol. 1967;15:237–70.
3. Pictet RL, Clark WR, Williams RH, Rutter WJ. An ultrastructural analysis of the developing embryonic pancreas. Dev Biol. 1972;29:436–67.
4. Placzek M, Furley A. Neural development: patterning cascades in the neural tube. Curr Biol. 1996;6:526–9.
5. Pourquie O, Coltey M, Teillet MA, Ordahl C, LeDouarin NM. Control of dorso-ventral patterning of somite derivatives by notochord and floorplate. Proc Natl Acad Sci USA. 1993;90: 5242–6.
6. Kim SK, Hebrok M, Melton DM. Early pancreas development in the chick embryo. Cold Spring Harbour Symp Quant Biol. 1997;62 (In press).
7. Kim SK, Hebrok M, Melton DA. Notochord to endoderm signaling is required for pancreas development. Development. 1997;124:4243–52.
8. Hebrok M, Kim SK, Melton DA. Notochord repression of endodermal Sonic hedgehog permits pancreas development. Genes Dev. 1998;12:1705–13.
9. Böttinger EP, Jakubeczak JL, Roberts IS *et al.* Expression of a dominant-negative mutant TGF-beta type II receptor in transgenic mice reveals essential roles for TGF-beta in regulation of growth and differentiation in the exocrine pancreas. EMBO J. 1997;16:2621–33.
10. Celli G, LaRochelle WJ, Mackem S, Sharp R, Merlino G. Soluble dominant-negative receptor uncovers essential roles for fibroblast growth factors in multi-organ induction and patterning. EMBO J. 1998;17:1642–55.
11. Le Bras S, Miralles F, Basmaciogullari A, Czernichow P, Scharfmann R. Fibroblast growth factor 2 promotes pancreatic epithelial cell proliferation via functional fibroblast growth factor receptors during embryonic life. Diabetes. 1998;47:1236–42.
12. Yamaoka T, Idehara C, Yano M *et al.* Hypoplasia of pancreatic islets in transgenic mice expressing activin receptor mutants. J Clin Invest. 1998;102:294–301.
13. Shiozaki S, Tajima T, Zhang YQ *et al.* Impaired differentiation of endocrine and exocrine cells of the pancreas in transgenic mouse expressing the truncated type II activin receptor. Biochim Biophys Acta. 1999;1450:1–11.
14. Hammerschmidt M, Brook A, McMahon AP. The world according to hedgehog. Trends Genet. 1997;13:14–21.
15. Bitgood MJ, McMahon AP. *Hedgehog* and *BMP* genes are coexpressed at many diverse sites of cell–cell interaction in the mouse embryo. Dev Biol. 1995;172:126–38.

16. Ahlgren U, Pfaff SL, Jessell TM, Edlund T, Edlund H. Independent requirement for ISL1 in formation of pancreatic mesenchyme and islet cells. Nature. 1997;385:257–60.
17. Apelqvist A, Ahlgren U, Edlund H. Sonic hedgehog directs specialised mesoderm differentiation in the intestine and pancreas. Curr Biol. 1997;7:801–4.
18. Levin M, Pagan S, Roberts DJ et al. Left/right patterning signals and the independent regulation of different aspects of situs in the chick embryo. Dev Biol. 1997;189:57–67.
19. Mathews LS, Vale WW. Expression cloning of an activin receptor, a predicted transmembrane serine kinase. Cell. 1991;65:973–82.
20. Attisano L, Wrana JL, Cheifetz S, Massagué J. Novel activin receptors: distinct genes and alternative mRNA splicing generate a repertoire of serine/threonine kinase receptors. Cell. 1992;68:97–108.
21. Kim SK, Hebrok M, Li E et al. Activin receptor patterning of foregut organogenesis. Genes Devel. 2000;14:1866–71.
22. Marigo V, Davey RA, Zuo Y, Cunningham JM, Tabin CJ. Biochemical evidence that patched is the Hedgehog receptor. Nature. 1996;384:176–9.
23. Goodrich LV, Milenkovic L, Higgins KM, Scott MP. Altered neural cell fates and medulloblastoma in mouse patched mutants. Science. 1997;277:1109–13.
24. Litingtung Y, Lei L, Westphal H, Chiang C. Sonic hedgehog is essential to foregut development. Nat Genet. 1998;20:58–61.
25. Pepicelli CV, Lewis PM, McMahon AP. Sonic hedgehog regulates branching morphogenesis in the mammalian lung. Curr Biol. 1998;8:1083–6.
26. Hebrok M, Kim SK, St-Jacques B, McMahon AP, Melton DA. Hedgehog signaling is essential for pancreas development. 2000 (Submitted).
27. Cooper MK, Porter JA, Young KE, Beachy PA. Teratogen-mediated inhibition of target tissue response to Shh signaling. Science. 1998;280:1603–7.
28. Kim SK, Melton DA. Pancreas development is promoted by cyclopamine, a hedgehog signaling inhibitor. Proc Natl Acad Sci USA. 1998;95:13036–41.
29. St-Jacques B, Hammerschmidt M, McMahon AP. Indian hedgehog signaling regulates proliferation and differentiation of chondrocytes and is essential for bone formation. Genes Dev. 1999;13:2072–86.
30. Hill D, Lebenthal E. Congenital abnormalities of the exocrine pancreas. In: Go VLW, Dimagno EP, Gardner JD, Lebenthal E, Reber HA, Scheele GA, editors. Pancreas: Biology, Pathobiology, and Disease. New York: Raven Press; 1993:1029–40.
31. Gross RE, Chisholm TC. Annular pancreas producing duodenal obstruction. Ann Surg. 1944;119:759–69.
32. Offield MF, Jetton TL, Labosky PA et al. PDX-1 is required for pancreatic outgrowth and differentiation of the rostral duodenum. Development. 1996;122:983–95.
33. Hebrok M, Kim SK, Melton DM. Screening for novel pancreatic genes expressed during embryogenesis. Diabetes. 1999;48:1550–6.
34. Kiernan PD, ReMine SG, Kiernan PC, ReMine WH. Annular pancreas: Mayo Clinic experience from 1957 to 1976 with review of the literature. Arch Surg. 1980;115:46–50.
35. Chiang C, Litingtung Y, Lee E et al. Cyclopia and defective axial patterning in mice lacking sonic hedgehog function. Nature. 1996;383:407–13.
36. Levy J. The gastrointestinal tract in Down syndrome. Prog Clin Biol Res. 1991;373:245–56.
37. Kallen B, Mastroiacovo P, Robert E. Major congenital malformations in Down syndrome. Am J Med Genet. 1996;65:160–6.

35
Transdifferentiation and transformation of acinar cells in transforming growth factor α transgenic mice – a model for pancreatic cancer development

R. M. SCHMID, M. WAGNER, F. R. GRETEN, S. KOSCHNICK and G. ADLER

DYSPLASIA–CARCINOMA SEQUENCE

While in colon cancer a multistep model of carcinogenesis, based on a definitive progression from hyperplasia and dysplasia through benign tumours to malignant invasive carcinoma, is generally accepted, such a sequence is so far not established for pancreatic cancer[1]. Changes in ductal epithelium, ranging from papillary hyperplasia and atypia to carcinoma *in situ*, are observed in cases of ductal adenocarcinoma, but our current understanding of pancreatic cancer does not allow us to define a clear relationship between the hyperplastic lesions and unequivocal carcinoma[2–4]. The problem is that papillary hyperplasia without atypia can be seen frequently at autopsy in otherwise 'normal' pancreas, or in patients with chronic pancreatitis[3,5]. These lesions were thus suspected to be reactive rather than premalignant changes. However, the characterization of genetic changes revealed the presence of K-ras mutations in ductal lesions in chronic pancreatitis, classifying them as potentially neoplastic[6]. These observations point towards these lesions representing an initial event in the multistep process towards invasive pancreatic carcinoma. In support of this idea it is interesting that the risk of pancreatic cancer is significantly elevated in subjects with chronic pancreatitis[7].

TRANSDIFFERENTIATION OF PANCREATIC ACINAR CELLS TO DUCT-LIKE CELLS

Another matter of debate is the question of whether mature pancreatic acinar cells have the potential to alter their phenotype towards ductal cells. This question has received much attention, especially with regard to pancreatic cancer, whose origin from ducts is defined on the basis of morphological studies[8]. It remains unclear whether ductal adenocarcinomas can develop from acinar cells. It has been demonstrated that a small stem cell population exists which can divide and subsequently differentiate into acinar, duct, or islet cells[9–11]. *In-vitro* data clearly show that mouse acinar cells grow in culture, but they lose their typical cytoplasmic ultrastructure and an antigen specific for mature acinar cells, while acquiring a more duct cell-like phenotype and expressing a duct cell-specific antigen[12]. These changes may reflect a process of retrodifferentiation of the acinar cell to a duct cell-like state. Interestingly, after confluency, the duct cell-specific antigen is lost and the acinar-specific antigen reappears. A similar transdifferentiation of acinar cells to a ductal phenotype has been described in a primary culture of human exocrine pancreas[13,14]. Hall and Lemoine reported that within 4 days all epithelial cells lost amylase immunoreactivity and gained expression of cytokeratin 19, specific for duct cells[13]. In another study an increase in the duct-specific mRNAs for CFTR and carboanhydrase II have been detected in cultured human pancreatic epithelial cells. Using monoclonal antibodies the cytokeratin pattern of the culture suggested a phenotypic switch to cytokeratin 7 and cytokeratin 19 positive cells[14]. These studies clearly indicate that acinar cells, when cultured *in vitro*, gain a duct-like phenotype.

TRANSDIFFERENTIATION OF ACINAR CELLS IN TRANSFORMING GROWTH FACTOR ALPHA (TGF-α) TRANSGENIC MICE

The overexpression of TGF-α in the pancreas causes a progressive fibrosis and the formation of so-called tubular complexes[15–19]. At 4 weeks of age these tubular complexes, which are three-dimensional accumulations of ductular structures, develop interspersed within areas of normal-appearing pancreas. These areas show a dilatation of the acinar lumen, which is lined by a monolayer epithelium mostly composed of flattened acinar cells and cells which display an intermediate phenotype of acinar and duct-like cells. In older animals (6 months old) these transitional forms between acinar cells and duct-like cells disappear in favour of ductal cells, which completely lose ultrastructural criteria typical for mature acinar cells. The secretory granules are missing, the endoplasmic reticulum becomes less abundant and the apical membrane gains microvilli. Interestingly, these cells are strongly positive for carboanhydrase activity, which is specific for duct cells. Furthermore, tubular complexes show immunoreactivity for the Duct-1 antibody. The *de novo* expression of these duct cell markers indicates that the tubular complexes formed in the TGF-α overexpressing mice represent a transdifferentiation process rather than a state of dedifferentiation. Whether these changes are due to a direct effect of TGF-α on the acinar cell, or mediated by an unknown autocrine and/or paracrine mechanism, is unclear.

THE FORMATION OF TUBULAR COMPLEXES

This phenotypic transition is somewhat similar to the changes reported *in vitro*[12–14]. However, *in vitro* this phenomenon may be explained by the lack of cell–cell contacts and/or growth factors controlling acinar cell differentiation and maintenance of the differentiated state. In addition, most probably the matrix upon which these cells grow, and the influence of other differentiating factors, is important[20]. De Listle and Logsdon reported that, after reaching confluency, some degree of differentiation towards acinar morphology occurs in their system[12]. This plasticity of acinar cells has also been observed *in vivo* during acute pancreatitis, several experimental models of pancreatic injury and cystic fibrosis[21–26]. In acute pancreatitis the formation of tubular complexes represents a form of acinar cell degeneration besides necrosis and apoptosis. At the ultrastructural level these tubular complexes were composed of flattened acinar cells surrounding enlarged lumina similar to those observed in human chronic pancreatitis. These duct-like cells revealed a loss of pancreatic enzymes, an increased expression of keratin and actin, as well as weak staining for CEA[27]. Further evidence for the plasticity of the acinar cells *in vivo* come from transgenic mice overexpressing interferon-gamma (IFN-γ) under control of an islet-specific promoter[28]. Inflammatory destruction of islets is followed by local overexpression of epidermal growth factor (EGF), TGF-α and the EGF-receptor in neighbouring acinar cells, and a transdifferentiation to a ductal phenotype and appearance of endocrine cells.

The occurrence of such tubular complexes has initially been interpreted as a result of proliferation or reduplication of intralobular ducts. Careful reconstruction of the relationship between ducts and acini concluded that acini are not tagged to the duct system like grapes to the stem, but rather are arranged in branching and anastomosing tubules with various diameters[29]. This arrangement of the normal pancreas suggests that under pathological conditions a decrease in acinar cell height and an increase in acinar lumen diameter could induce the formation of tubular complexes.

CELLS TRANSFORM WITHIN TUBULAR COMPLEXES IN TGF-α TRANSGENIC MICE

We have recently demonstrated that the overexpression of TGF-α in the pancreas of transgenic mice finally progresses to malignant transformation[18,19]. Pancreatic tumours originate from multiple foci and display a mixed cystic–papillary phenotype. Tumours originate from cells within tubular complexes and are highly positive for carboanhydrase activity and ductal markers indicative of ductal carcinomas. These observations provide strong arguments in favour of tubular complexes being precursors of invasive carcinoma. Duct-like tubular structures have been observed in pancreatic carcinoma and in TGF-α transgenic mice[2,30–32].

Furthermore, cells within tubular complexes, as well as the tumour, express the EGF-receptor. Since overexpression of the EGF-receptor and TGF-α is common in pancreatic cancer as well as in chronic pancreatitis this provided additional evidence that an autocrine loop involving the EGF-receptor/TGF-α pathway may play a key role in hyperplastic and malignant changes of the pancreas[33,34]. This establishes for the first time an acinar–ductal–carcinoma sequence in an animal model. Since tumour formation is a rather late event, and not obligatory, the important problem remains to define events determining the progression to invasive cancer in some, but clearly not the majority of, cases.

WHICH CELL TYPE GIVES RISE TO PANCREATIC CANCER?

These findings raise again the question of the very earliest lesions of pancreatic cancer, and in particular the cellular origin of this neoplasm. There are three different possibilities: pancreatic cancers arise from duct cells, alternatively an undifferentiated stem cell is the origin of cancer, and finally there is the possibility that centroacinar cells or the acinar cells retro/transdifferentiate. The first possibility is based on the fact that pancreatic carcinomas usually display a ductal phenotype and lack characteristics of acinar cells. Consequently, an origin from normal ductal epithelium has been proposed. In addition, several authors have identified 'early lesions' in the ducts of human pancreas[2–5]. These ductal lesions include papillary structures lined with cuboidal, mucin-producing cells displaying various dysplastic changes ranging from hyperplasia to carcinoma *in situ*. These duct lesions have been proposed to be the earlier precursors of pancreatic cancer. The presence of genetic alterations such as activating K-ras mutations in these lesions supports this hypothesis[6].

In addition to the mouse model described here, there is some evidence that the main pancreatic ducts are not the primary site of origin of pancreatic neoplasia. Acinar cell hyperplasia has been described in the human pancreas[35]. Ultrastructural studies suggest that the earliest lesions in the hamster model involve the centro-acinar cells[36] or cells of acinar origin[37]. In the hamster cancer model there is evidence that centro-acinar cells are the origin for tubular complex formations. The hypertrophy and hyperplasia of centro-acinar cells, with formation of initially tiny and long processes that overlie and underlie the adjacent acinar cells, are the early neoplastic lesion[36]. In the hamster a gradual transformation of acinar cells, which lose their apical cytoplasmic portion and zymogen granules, is not observed, indicating that tubular complexes may form differently in TGF-α overexpressing mice. However, both models provide support for the hypothesis that acinar cells may represent the target population for carcinogenic events in the pancreas.

While it is clear that the pancreas originally develops from an undifferentiated duct cell-like progenitor or 'stem' cell, the evidence for a stem cell in the adult pancreas is far from being established. The duct cell compartment appears to be the most likely location of the putative stem cells. Only duct cells have been shown to be able to give rise to endocrine cells[38–40]. Additional evidence supporting the presence of stem cells in the adult pancreas is the capacity of the adult pancreas to regenerate to a modest extent after partial pancreatectomy[41]. This regeneration involves a greater proliferation of endocrine cells than of exocrine cells[42]. Since the evidence for a stem cell in the mature pancreas is only indirect, the hypothesis that pancreatic cancer might originate from such cells has to remain speculative.

GENETIC ALTERATIONS CAUSING PANCREATIC CANCER DEVELOPMENT IN MICE

In the hamster model mutated K-ras at codon 12 and 13 have been demonstrated and suggested to occur early; this may even be the initiating event in this model[43]. It is interesting that TGF-α binding to the EGF-receptor activates a signalling pathway involving the activation of Ras. Therefore similar signalling cascades might be responsible for the formation of tubular complexes in these models. The activation of this pathway might therefore be an initial event in the multistep process of carcinogenesis in the pancreas. In contrast, transgenic animals bearing an elastase c-myc construct develop carcinomas of a mixed acinar ductal phenotype[44]. Interestingly, mice heterozygous for the APC mutation and null alleles for p53 develop adenocarcinoma of the exocrine pancreas[45]. In TGF-α transgenic mice acinar cells show initially dysplastic and malignant changes, and only later in tumour progression do duct-like structures resembling tubular complexes occur[17,18]. Again these cells are positive for ductal markers, suggesting a retrodifferentiation of acinar to ductal cells in this case under malignant circumstances.

According to the multistep model of colorectal cancer the accumulation of a number of critical mutations is important for tumour development. Therefore it is very likely that additional mutations occur in the transgenic models for pancreatic cancer. So far we find a possible alteration in the expression pattern of p53 upon histochemistry, but further investigations to define a somatic mutation are necessary[18]. Furthermore, K-ras mutations at codon 12 are absent in TGF-α transgenic mice. Since transgenic overexpression of TGF-α in skin keratinocytes bypasses the need of an additional H-Ras mutation in skin tumorigenesis[46] other pathways are possibly involved in tumour promotion in this model.

In summary, the overexpression of TGF-α in the pancreas induces a trans-differentiation of acinar cell to duct cells based on lineage-specific markers. The development of ductal carcinoma establishes the possibility of an acinar–ductal–carcinoma sequence. Since tumour formation is a rather late event, and not obligatory, other genetic events are likely to determine the progression to invasive cancer.

Acknowledgements

We are indebted to Sonja Aigner for preparing the manuscript. R.M.S. is supported by grants from Deutsche Forschungsgemeinschaft und Bundesministerium für Bildung und Forschung.

References

1. Vogelstein B, Fearon ER, Hamilton SR et al. Genetic alterations during colorectal-tumor development. N Engl J Med. 1988;319:525–32.
2. Cubilla AL, Fitzgerald PJ. Morphological lesions associated with human primary invasive nonendocrine pancreatic cancer. Cancer Res. 1975;35:2234–48.
3. Klöppel G, Bommer G, Rückert K, Seifert G. Intraductal proliferation in the pancreas and its relationship to human and experimental carcinogenesis. Virchow's Arch Pathol Anat. 1980;387:221–3.
4. Kozuka S, Sassa R, Taki T et al. Relation of pancreatic duct hyperplasia to carcinoma. Cancer. 1979;43:1418–28.
5. Sommers SC, Murphy SA, Warren S. Pancreatic duct hyperplasia and cancer. Gastroenterology. 1954;27:629–40.
6. Yanagisama A, Ohtake K, Ohashi K et al. Frequent c-Ki-ras oncogene activation in mucous cell hyperplasias of pancreas suffering from chronic pancreatitis. Cancer Res. 1993; 53:953–6.
7. Lowenfels AB, Maisonneuve P, Cavallini G et al. The International Pancreatitis Study Group. Pancreatitis and the risk of pancreatic cancer. N Engl J Med. 1993;328:1433–7.

8. Klöppel G. Pathology of nonendocrine pancreatic tumors. In: Go VL, DiMagno EP, Gardner JD, Lebenthal E, Reber HA, Scheele GA, editors. The Pancreas – Biology, Pathology, and Disease, 2nd edn. New York: Raven Press; 1993;46:871–98.

9. Githens S. The pancreatic duct cell: proliferative capabilities, specific characteristic, metaplasia, isolation, and culture. J Pediatr Gastroenterol Nutr. 1988;7:486–506.

10. Githens S, Pictet R, Phelps P, Rutter WJ. 5-Bromodeoxyuridine may alter the differentiative program of the embryonic pancreas. J Cell Biol. 1976;71:341–56.

11. Jamieson JD, Ingber DE, Muresan V et al. Cell surface properties of normal, differentiating, and neoplastic pancreatic acinar cells. Cancer. 1981;47:1516–25.

12. De Listle BC, Logsdon CD. Pancreatic acinar cells in culture: expression of acinar and ductal antigens in a growth-related manner. Eur J Cell Biol. 1990;51:64–75.

13. Hall PA, Lemoine NR. Rapid acinar to ductal transdifferentiation in cultured human exocrine pancreas. J Pathol. 1992;166:97–103.

14. Vila MR, Lloreta J, Real FX. Normal human pancreas cultures display functional ductal characteristics. Lab Invest. 1994;71:423–31.

15. Sandgren EP, Luetteke NC, Palmiter RD, Brinster RL, Lee DC. Overexpression of TGF-α in transgenic mice: induction of epithelial hyperplasia, pancreatic metaplasia, and carcinoma on the breast. Cell. 1990;61:1121–35.

16. Jhappan C, Stahle C, Harkins RN, Fausto N, Smith GH, Merlino GT. TGF-α overexpression in transgenic mice induces liver neoplasia and abnormal development of the mammary gland and pancreas. Cell. 1990;61:1137–46.

17. Bockman DE, Merlino G. Cytological changes in the pancreas of transgenic mice overexpressing transforming growth factor α. Gastroenterology. 1992;103:1883–92.

18. Wagner M, Lührs H, Klöppel G, Adler G, Schmid RM. Malignant transformation of duct-like cells originating from acini in transforming growth factor α transgenic mice. Gastroenterology. 1998;115:1254–62.

19. Schmid RM, Klöppel G, Adler G, Wagner M. Acinar–ductal–carcinoma sequence in transforming growth factor-α transgenic mice. Ann NY Acad Sci. 1999;880:219–30.

20. Arias AE, Bendayan M. Differentiation of pancreatic acinar cells into duct like cells in vitro. Lab Invest. 1993;69:518–30.

21. Churg A, Ward RR. Early changes in the exocrine pancreas of the dog and rat after ligation of the pancreatic duct. Am J Pathol. 1971;63:521–34.

22. Bockman DE, Black O Jr, Mills LR, Webster PD. Origin of tubular complexes during developing induction of pancreatic adenocarcinoma by 7,12-dimethylbenz(a)antracene. Am J Pathol. 1978;90:645–51.

23. Mudlos S, Adler G, Schaar M, Koop I, Arnold R. Exocrine function in oleic acid-induced pancreatic insufficiency in rats. Pancreas. 1986;1:29–36.

24. Elsässer HP, Adler G, Kern HF. Time course and cellular source of pancreatic regeneration following acute pancreatitis in the rat. Pancreas. 1986;1:421–9.

25. Porta EA, Stein AA, Patterson P. Ultrastructural changes of the pancreas and liver in cystic fibrosis. Am J Clin Pathol. 1964;42:451–65.

26. Willemer S, Elsässer HP, Kern HF, Adler G. Tubular complexes in cerulein and oleic acid induced pancreatitis in rats: glycoconjugate pattern, immunocytochemical and ultrastructural findings. Pancreas. 1987;2:669–75.

27. Willemer S, Adler G. Histochemical and ultrastructural characteristics of tubular complexes in human acute pancreatitis. Dig Dis Sci. 1989;34:46–55.

28. Arnush M, Gu D, Baugh C et al. Growth factors in the regenerating pancreas of gamma interferon transgenic mice. Lab Invest. 1996;74:985–90.

29. Bockman DE, Boydston WR, Parsa I. Architecture of human pancreas: implication for early changes in pancreatic disease. Gastroenterology. 1981;85:55–61.

30. Reddy JK, Rao MS. Pancreatic adenocarcinoma in inbred guinea pigs induced by N-methyl-N-nitrosourea. Cancer Res. 1975;35:2269–77.

31. Rao MS, Reddy JK. Histogenesis of pseudoductular changes induced in the pancreas of guinea pigs treated with N-methyl-N-nitrosourea. Carcinogenesis. 1980;1:1027–34.

32. Parsa I, Longnecker DS, Scarpelli DG, Pour P, Reddy JK, Lefkowitz M. Ductal metaplasia of human exocrine pancreas and its association with carcinoma. Cancer Res. 1985;45:1285–90.

33. Barton CM, Hall PA, Hughes CM, Gullick WJ, Lemoine NR. Transforming growth factor alpha and epidermal growth factor in human pancreatic cancer. J Pathol. 1991;163:111–16.

34. Lemoine NR, Hughes CM, Barton CM *et al*. The epidermal growth factor receptor in human pancreatic cancer. J Pathol. 1992;166:7–12.

35. Longnecker DS, Shinozuka H, Dekker A. Focal acinar cell dysplasia in human pancreas. Cancer. 1980;45:534–40.

36. Pour PM. Mechanism of pseudoductular (tubular) formation during pancreatic carcinogenesis in the hamster model. Am J Pathol. 1988;130:335–44.

37. Flaks B. Histogenesis of pancreatic carcinogenesis in the hamster: ultrastructural evidence. Environ Health Perspect. 1984;56:187–203.

38. Dudek RW, Lawrence IEJ, Hill RS, Johnson RC. Induction of islet cytodifferentiation by fetal mesenchyme in adult pancreas ductal epithelium. Diabetes. 1991;40:1041–8.

39. Gu D, Sarvetnick N. Epithelial cell proliferation and islet neogenesis in IFN-γ transgenic mice. Development. 1993;118:33–46.

40. Wang RN, Rehfeld JF, Nielsen FC, Klöppel G. Expression of gastrin and transforming growth factor-alpha during duct to islet cell differentiation in the pancreas of duct-ligated adult rats. Diabetologia. 1997;40:887–93.

41. Lehv M, Fitzgerald PJ. Pancreatic acinar cell regeneration. IV. Regeneration after surgical resection. Am J Pathol. 1968;53:513–35.

42. Brockenbrough JS, Weir GC, Bonner-Weir S. Discordance of exocrine and endocrine growth after 90% pancreatectomy in rats. Diabetes. 1988;37:232–6.

43. Cery WL, Mangold KA, Scarpelli DG. Activation of K-ras in transplantable pancreatic ductal adenocarcinomas of Syrian golden hamsters. Carcinogenesis. 1990;11:2075–9.

44. Sandgren EP, Quaife CJ, Paulovich AG, Palmiter RD, Brinster RL. Pancreatic tumor pathogenesis reflects the causative genetic lesion. Proc Natl Acad Sci. 1991;88:93–7.

45. Clarke AR, Cummings MC, Harrison DJ. Interaction between murine germline mutations in p53 and APC predisposes to pancreatic neoplasia but not to increased intestinal malignancy. Oncogene. 1995;11:1913–20.

46. Vassar R, Hutton ME, Fuchs E. Transgenic overexpression of transforming growth factor alpha bypasses the need for c-Ha-ras mutations in mouse skin tumorigenesis. Mol Cell Biol. 1992;12:4643–53.

36
Peptide growth factors in regeneration after acute pancreatitis

A. MENKE, R. VOGELMANN and G. ADLER

ACUTE PANCREATITIS

The mechanisms leading to complete pancreatic regeneration after acute inflammation are still fascinating but little understood. Recent studies have focused on the importance of peptide growth factors in regulation of these processes. In this chapter we summarize data regarding the influence of different growth factors on regeneration after acute pancreatitis.

The importance of growth factors in the subsequent regenerative process in acute pancreatitis is analysed mainly in experimental models such as caerulein-induced pancreatitis in rats, as well as in *in-vitro* experiments.

Experimentally induced pancreatitis is characterized by destruction of the regular tissue structure and development of focal necrosis. In these areas proliferation of fibroblasts and production of collagen can be observed, resulting in a transient fibrosis. Later, this extracellular matrix (ECM) is degraded and after a few weeks complete functional and structural regeneration of the pancreas can be found[1,2]. The connective tissue which transiently replaces parts of the pancreas is the result of altered biosynthesis, deposition and destruction of ECM proteins, namely collagen type I, type III and fibronectin, and to a lesser extent collagen type IV and laminin. Different experiments on protein levels, such as immunfluorescence studies, hydroxyproline measurements and Western blot analyses, confirmed the synthesis and deposition of ECM as early as 24 h after induction of pancreatitis. The maximal collagen content was found on the third day, decreasing continuously during further regeneration, and 2 weeks after induction of pancreatitis the collagen content returned to normal values[3,4].

In addition to the production of ECM proteins, the collagen content is regulated by altered degradative events. Matrix metalloproteinases (MMPs), as well as their natural inhibitors (TIMPs), are present in this coordinated turnover. During regeneration after acute pancreatitis MMP-2, the 72 kDa collagenase type IV, and MMP-3, stromelysin, were overexpressed accompanied by a parallel rise of TIMP-2, the MMP-2 inhibitor. In correlation with the expression data, MMP-2 and MMP-3 activities were found to be elevated in the regenerative process as measured by zymographies. MMP-2 was significantly activated 2 days after induction of pancreatitis, with maxima between days 3 and 5. MMP-3 and also MMP-9, the 92 kDa collagenase type IV, activities were observed earlier between 2 and 3 days after induction. Thus, MMP-2, MMP-3 and MMP-9 seem to be involved in the removal of ECM during regeneration from caerulein-induced pancreatitis[5].

TGF-β-EXPRESSION AND ITS INFLUENCE ON COLLAGEN CONTENT

Mediators in fibrotic events during regeneration in many tissues, such as liver, kidney and skin, are the transforming growth factors beta (TGF-β)[6–10]. This protein family contains three isoforms in mammalians, and stimulates the transcription and synthesis of ECM proteins. In addition TGF-βs are involved in the regulation of cell proliferation[6,11].

TGF-β_1 and TGF-β_2 transcription and secretion, but not TGF-β_3 expression, increased very early after induction of pancreatitis (12–24 h)[4,12,13]. *In-situ* hybridization revealed that acinar cells were the sources of TGF-β production in pancreatitis[3,14]. The intracellular effects of TGF-β are mediated by activation of transmembrane receptor proteins. At least TGF-β receptors type I and II containing serine/threonine kinase activity seem to be involved in the phosphorylation and activation of different SMAD proteins, which transmit the cellular effects of TGF-β[15–18]. Examination of TGF-β receptor concentrations demonstrated an increase after acute pancreatitis[19]. In agreement with the expression maxima of TGF-β_1 and TGF-β_2, both receptors were slightly overexpressed during regeneration. The neutralization of TGF-β_1 activity decreased the expression of the TGF-β receptors, confirming the hypothesis that TGF-β_1 stimulates the expression of its own receptors[20,21]. These data suggest that TGF-β induces an autocrine stimulation of pancreatic acinar and ductal cells.

To study the functional involvement of TGF-β, its activity was neutralized by injection of an antibody against the growth factor. A reduction of collagen deposition of about 35% in the pancreas was determined by mRNA studies (Fig. 1) and measurement of hydroxyproline contents[4], supporting the functional involvement of TGF-β_1 and TGF-β_2 in expression, production and deposition of ECM during regeneration. Besides collagen reduction, a diminished pancreatic expression of TGF-β_1 and TGF-β_2 mRNAs could be shown. Similar results have been reported by Border and co-workers, who described a reduction of TGF-β_1 RNA and expression of ECM components in experimental glomerulonephritis after treatment with neutralizing TGF-β_1 antibody and the natural inhibitor decorin[10,22]. This phenomenon as described above has been attributed to an autocrine loop in which TGF-β induces its own synthesis in an autoregulatory way[23,24]. In agreement with these data, the pancreas-specific overexpression of TGF-β_1 in transgenic mice revealed a progressive deposition of connective tissue in the pancreas[25–27]. Recurrent episodes of caerulein-induced pancreatitis in TGF-β transgenic mice resulted in a dramatically enhanced fibronectin deposition but only a moderate elevation of collagen type I and type III.

The detailed mechanisms by which TGF-β_1 is involved in the regulation of ECM turnover are little understood. Whether TGF-β exerts its effects by direct or indirect mechanisms is controversial. Recently, the connective tissue growth factor (CTGF) was described as a downstream acting factor of TGF-β responsible for the enhanced production of ECM, even in the pancreas[28].

PANCREATIC STELLATE CELLS

Recently we identified a cell type responsible for ECM production. After activation these pancreatic stellate cells (PSC), named because of their similarity to hepatic stellate cells, are characterized by a prominent endoplasmic reticulum, enhanced expression of smooth muscle actin and increased synthesis of collagen and fibronectin[29]. Pancreatic stellate cells may represent the target cells of elevated TGF-β_1 concentrations in the transgenic mouse model as well as in pancreatitis. TGF-β stimulates these cells to produce large amounts of collagen and fibronectin. Interestingly, not only TGF-β but also FGF-2 and less effective PDGF and TGF-α stimulated fibronectin mRNA and protein concentrations in isolated PSC[29].

To postulate a causal link between PSC and pancreatic fibrosis, further analyses are required to discover how TGF-β_1 and other peptide growth factors influence matrix production in the pancreas.

TGF-β-RELATED GROWTH FACTORS

The data discussed above indicate involvement of other regulators in the ECM turnover during pancreatic regeneration. Members of the TGF-β superfamily are candidates which may be involved in regenerative processes. Bone morphogenetic proteins (BMP) have been implicated in the patterning of the mesoderm during embryogenesis[30]. Examination of mRNA levels demonstrated an overexpression of BMP2 and to a lower extent BMP7, but not BMP4 or BMP6, during regeneration from experimentally-induced acute pancreatitis. Expression of activins (also TGF-β-related growth factors well characterized during embryogenesis[31]), in particular activin βc and activin βe, was elevated during pancreatic regeneration. Besides reports concerning activin involvement in wound repair[32], to date there is no information on the functional relation of these TGF-β-related growth factors to regenerative processes, especially in the pancreas.

GROWTH FACTORS SIGNALLING VIA RECEPTOR TYROSINE KINASE

Growth factors signalling via receptor tyrosine kinases represent another important group of regulators, mainly described in the control of growth and differentiation during development. However, there is growing evidence concerning their involvement in regenerative events[33–35]. Whereas numerous reports have been published on the involvement of peptide growth factors in pancreatic cancer and chronic pancreatitis, little is known regarding their role in acute pancreatitis.

Comparative analysis demonstrated that most analysed growth factors were expressed even at low levels in normal pancreas (FGF-1, FGF-2, HGF, IGF-1, IGF-2, TGF-α, PDGF B). During regeneration PDGF B, IGF-2 and EGF revealed only minor, not significant, alterations in their expression, whereas the transcript levels of FGF-1 and -2, IGF-1, TGF-α and HGF showed significant increases. Expression of FGF-2 demonstrated the most pronounced (about 20-fold) transcriptional elevation; in contrast IGF-1 was the first growth factor overexpressed 12 h after starting caerulein infusion[36].

The different expression maxima (IGF-1 12 h, HGF 72 h, TGF-α 48 h, FGF-1 72 h, FGF-2 36 h after induction of pancreatitis) may implicate the existence of different target cells for these growth factors. It was shown 10 years ago by Elsässer, Adler and Kern that cell proliferation shows a biphasic pattern in regeneration after acute pancreatitis. Fibroblasts proliferate earlier than acinar and centroacinar cells[1]. The correlation of proliferation data and reported time-courses of the growth factor expression patterns may lead to the speculation that early-expressed growth factors such as TGF-α and FGF-2 lead directly or indirectly to proliferation of fibroblasts, whereas HGF may stimulate epithelial cell growth. The involvement of growth factors in other processes such as induction of differentiation could be an additional explanation for the different time-courses of the factors studied, and this should be considered in future studies.

In contrast to elevated expression of their ligands, protein concentrations of most receptors remained unchanged. Only in the case of c-*met*, the HGF receptor, was an overexpression detectable during regeneration[36].

FUNCTIONAL ASPECTS OF FGF AND HGF

In recent experiments with isolated pancreatic cells under cell culture conditions the overexpression of FGF-2 and HGF was associated with functional aspects.

Primary pancreatic fibroblasts were obtained by outgrowing from small pancreatic samples. Incubation of these fibroblasts with FGF-2 revealed a dose-dependent stimulation of DNA synthesis. Using isolated pancreatic acinar cells Hoshi and Logsdon[37] demonstrated FGF-2 and to a lower extent FGF-1 as potent mitogens for epithelial cells. Examination of mRNA contents of fibroblasts and PSC stimulated with 1.0 nM FGF-2 revealed increased collagen and fibronectin expression. In contrast to TGF-α or PDGF AB, FGF-2 stimulated the mRNA concentration of collagen type I and III and fibronectin but had no effect on laminin and collagen IV. Costimulation of these fibroblasts with TGF-β and FGF-2 showed a more pronounced gene expression of collagen and fibronectin compared to stimulation with single growth factors. These results propose a regulatory function of FGF-2 together with TGF-β in production and deposition of ECM in the regenerative process, as well as a proliferative stimulus for mesenchymal and epithelial pancreatic cells under culture conditions.

Hepatic growth factor (HGF), as well as its receptor, seem to promote different epithelial cancers, i.e. pancreatic cancer, as shown by many groups[38–40]. The involvement in acute pancreatitis was demonstrated by Ueda et al.[41]. They

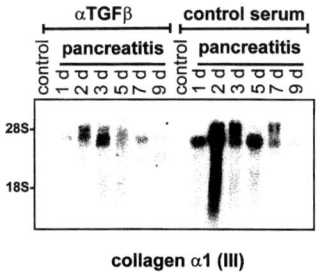

collagen α1 (III)

Figure 1 Messenger RNA concentration of the α1 chain of collagen type III in the regenerative process after caerulein-induced pancreatitis. A representative Northern blot hybridization is shown with a collagen type III-specific probe. During regeneration after pancreatitis a significant increase in collagen III mRNA is visible. This increase is reduced in pancreatic samples from animals treated with anti-TGF-β antibody during and after caerulein infusion compared to animals which received control antibody

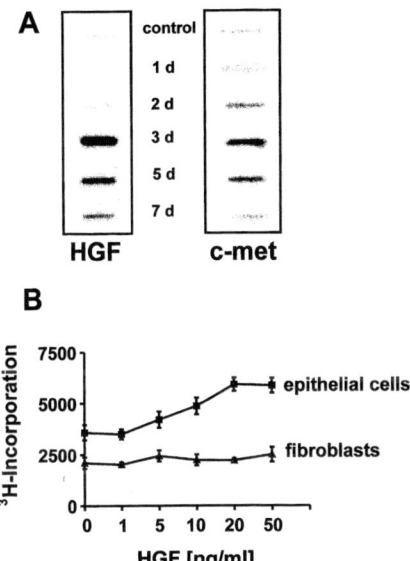

Figure 2 Hepatocyte growth factor (HGF) and its receptor c-*met* are overexpressed in the regenerative process. **A**: Slot–blot analyses revealed a distinct increase of HGF and c-*met* mRNA 3 days after induction of pancreatitis. **B**: HGF stimulated DNA synthesis of cultured pancreatic epithelial cells in a dose-dependent manner

reported elevated HGF levels in the serum of patients with acute pancreatitis. During regeneration from experimentally induced pancreatitis in rats HGF was strongly overexpressed 3 days after caerulein infusion, c-*met* mRNA levels increased after 2 days (Fig. 2A). Under cell culture conditions HGF was able to induce elevated proliferation of cultured primary pancreatic epithelial cells

(Fig. 2B), suggesting the functional relevance of HGF in induction of epithelial cell proliferation during pancreatic regeneration[36].

SUMMARY

The precise role of peptide growth factors in regeneration after acute pancreatitis is still unknown. New data concerning their function in formation and degradation of ECM, regulation of proliferation of mesenchymal and epithelial cells, as well as tissue differentiation, have been presented in recent years. More insights into the effects of different growth factor combinations or expression patterns may provide new ideas concerning the regulatory steps leading to chronic or acute pancreatitis on the one hand, and pancreatic cancer on the other.

References

1. Elsässer HP, Adler G, Kern HF. Time course and cellular source of pancreatic regeneration following acute pancreatitis in the rat. Pancreas. 1986;1:421–9.
2. Elsässer HP, Adler G, Kern HF. Fibroblast structure and function during regeneration from hormone-induced acute pancreatitis in the rat. Pancreas. 1989;4:169–78.
3. Gress TM, Müller-Pillasch F, Elsässer HP et al. Enhancement of transforming growth factor beta 1 expression in the rat pancreas during regeneration from caerulein-induced pancreatitis. Eur J Clin Invest. 1994;24:679–85.
4. Menke A, Yamaguchi H, Gress TM, Adler G. Extracellular matrix is reduced by inhibition of transforming growth factor β1 in pancreatitis in the rat. Gastroenterology. 1997;113:295–303.
5. Müller-Pillasch F, Gress TM, Yamaguchi H, Geng M, Adler G, Menke A. The influence of transforming growth factor β1 on the expression of genes coding for extracellular matrix metalloproteinases and tissue inhibitors of metalloproteinases during regeneration from caerulein-induced pancreatitis. Pancreas. 1997;15:168–75.
6. Roberts AB, Flanders KC, Heine UI et al. Transforming growth factor-beta: multifunctional regulator of differentiation and development. Phil Trans R Soc Lond B Biol Sci. 1990;327:145–54.
7. Gressner AM, Krull N, Bachem MG. Regulation of proteoglycan expression in fibrotic liver and cultured fat-storing cells. Pathol Res Pract. 1994;190:864–82.
8. Bachem MG, Sell KM, Melchior R, Kropf J, Eller T, Gressner AM. Tumor necrosis factor alpha (TNF alpha) and transforming growth factor beta 1 (TGF beta 1) stimulate fibronectin synthesis and the transdifferentiation of fat-storing cells in the rat liver into myofibroblasts. Virchows Arch B Cell Pathol Incl Mol Pathol. 1993;63:123–30.
9. Gressner AM, Bachem MG. Cellular sources of noncollagenous matrix proteins: role of fat-storing cells in fibrogenesis. Semin Liver Dis. 1990;10:30–46.
10. Border WA, Okuda S, Languino LR, Sporn MB, Ruoslahti E. Suppression of experimental glomerulonephritis by antiserum against transforming growth factor beta 1. Nature. 1990;346:371–4.
11. Roberts AB, Heine UI, Flanders KC, Sporn MB. Transforming growth factor-beta. Major role in regulation of extracellular matrix. Ann NY Acad Sci. 1990;580:225–32.
12. Konturek PC, Dembinski A, Warzecha Z et al. Expression of transforming growth factor-beta 1 and epidermal growth factor in caerulein-induced pancreatitis in rat. J Physiol Pharmacol. 1997;48:59–72.
13. Riesle E, Friess H, Zhao L et al. Increased expression of transforming growth factor betas after acute oedematous pancreatitis in rats suggests a role in pancreatic repair. Gut. 1997;40:73–9.
14. Friess H, Lu Z, Riesle E et al. Enhanced expression of TGF-betas and their receptors in human acute pancreatitis. Ann Surg. 1998;227:95–104.
15. ten Dijke P, Miyazono K, Heldin CH. Signaling via hetero-oligomeric complexes of type I and type II serine/threonine kinase receptors. Curr Opin Cell Biol. 1996;8:139–45.
16. Zhang Y, Feng XH, Wu RY, Derynck R, Feng X, We R. Receptor-associated Mad homologues synergize as effectors of the TGF-β response. Nature. 1996;383:168–72.

17. Lagna G, Hata A, Hemmati Brivanlou A, Massagué J. Partnership between DPC4 and SMAD proteins in TGF-beta signalling pathways. Nature. 1996;383:832–6.
18. Macias Silva M, Abdollah S, Hoodless PA, Pirone R, Attisano L, Wrana JL. MADR2 is a substrate of the TGFbeta receptor and its phosphorylation is required for nuclear accumulation and signaling. Cell. 1996;87:1215–24.
19. Menke A, Geerling I, Giehl K, Vogelmann R, Reinshagen M, Adler G. Transforming growth factor-β-induced upregulation of transforming growth factor-β receptor expression in pancreatic regeneration. Biochim Biophys Acta. 1999;1449:178–85.
20. Van Obberghen Schilling E, Roche NS, Flanders KC, Sporn MB, Roberts AB. Transforming growth factor beta 1 positively regulates its own expression in normal and transformed cells. J Biol Chem. 1988;263:7741–6.
21. Norgaard P, Spang Thomsen M, Poulsen HS. Expression and autoregulation of transforming growth factor beta receptor mRNA in small-cell lung cancer cell lines. Br J Cancer. 1996;73: 1037–43.
22. Border WA, Noble NA, Yamamoto T et al. Natural inhibitor of transforming growth factor-beta protects against scarring in experimental kidney disease. Nature. 1992;360:361–4.
23. Berrou E, Quarck R, Fontenay Roupie M, Levy Toledano S, Tobelem G, Bryckaert M. Transforming growth factor-beta 1 increases internalization of basic fibroblast growth factor by smooth muscle cells: implication of cell-surface heparan sulphate proteoglycan endocytosis. Biochem J. 1995;311:393–9.
24. Guvakova MA, Yakubov LA, Vlodavsky I, Tonkinson JL, Stein CA. Phosphorothioate oligodeoxynucleotides bind to basic fibroblast growth factor, inhibit its binding to cell surface receptors, and remove it from low affinity binding sites on extracellular matrix. J Biol Chem. 1995;270:2620–7.
25. Vogelmann R, Ruf D, Wagner M et al. Development of pancreatic fibrosis in a TGFβ transgenic mouse. Gastroenterology. 1999;116:A1174.
26. Lee MS, Gu D, Feng L et al. Accumulation of extracellular matrix and developmental dysregulation in the pancreas by transgenic production of transforming growth factor-beta 1. Am J Pathol. 1995;147:42–52.
27. Sanvito F, Nichols A, Herrera PL et al. TGF-beta 1 overexpression in murine pancreas induces chronic pancreatitis and together with TNF-alpha, triggers insulin-dependent diabetes. Biochem Biophys Res Commun. 1995;217:1279–86.
28. Wenger C, Ellenrieder V, Alber B et al. Expression and differential regulation of connective tissue growth factor in pancreatic cancer cells. Oncogene. 1999;18:1073–80.
29. Bachem MG, Schneider E, Gross H et al. Identification, culture, and characterization of pancreatic stellate cells in rats and humans. Gastroenterology. 1998;115:421–32.
30. Lyons KM, Hogan BL, Robertson EJ. Colocalization of BMP 7 and BMP 2 RNAs suggests that these factors cooperatively mediate tissue interactions during murine development. Mech Dev. 1995;50:71–83.
31. Kaufmann E, Paul H, Friedle H et al. Antagonistic actions of activin A and BMP-2/4 control dorsal lip-specific activation of the early response gene XFD-1′ in *Xenopus laevis*. EMBO J. 1996;15:6739–49.
32. Hübner G, Hu QJ, Smola H, Werner S. Strong induction of activin expression after injury suggests an important role of activin in wound repair. Dev Biol. 1996;173:490–8.
33. Michalopoulos GK, DeFrances MC. Liver regeneration. Science. 1997;276:60–6.
34. Husmann I, Soulet L, Gautron J, Martelly I, Barritault D. Growth factors in skeletal muscle regeneration. Cytokine Growth Factor Rev. 1996;7:249–58.
35. Schott RJ, Morrow LA. Growth factors and angiogenesis. Cardiovasc Res. 1993;27:1155–61.
36. Menke A, Yamaguchi H, Giehl K, Adler G. Hepatocyte growth factor and fibroblast growth factor 2 are overexpressed following cerulein-induced acute pancreatitis. Pancreas. 1999;18: 28–33.
37. Hoshi H, Logsdon CD. Direct trophic effects of fibroblast growth factors on rat pancreatic acinar cells in vitro. Biochem Biophys Res Commun. 1993;196:1202–7.
38. Furukawa T, Duguid WP, Kobari M, Matsuno S, Tsao MS. Hepatocyte growth factor and Met receptor expression in human pancreatic carcinogenesis. Am J Pathol. 1995;147:889–95.
39. Di Renzo MF, Poulsom R, Olivero M, Comoglio PM, Lemoine NR. Expression of the Met/hepatocyte growth factor receptor in human pancreatic cancer. Cancer Res. 1995;55:1129–38.

40. Kiehne K, Herzig KH, Folsch UR. c-Met expression in pancreatic cancer and effects of hepato-cyte growth factor on pancreatic cancer cell growth. Pancreas. 1997;15:35–40.
41. Ueda T, Takeyama Y, Toyokawa A, Kishida S, Yamamoto M, Saitoh Y. Significant elevation of serum human hepatocyte growth factor levels in patients with acute pancreatitis. Pancreas. 1996;12:76–83.

Index